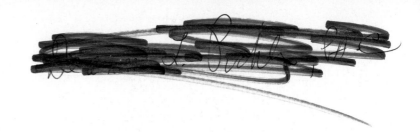

A Comprehensive Review
for the Certification and
Recertification Examinations
for Physician Assistants

A Comprehensive Review for the Certification and Recertification Examinations for Physician Assistants

THIRD EDITION

Published in Collaboration with AAPA and PAEA

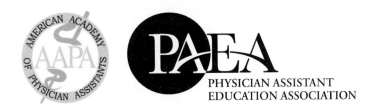

PHYSICIAN ASSISTANT
EDUCATION ASSOCIATION

Volume Editor
Claire Babcock O'Connell, MPH, PA-C

Associate Professor
University of Medicine and Dentistry of New Jersey
Physician Assistant Program
Piscataway, New Jersey

Consulting Editor
Sarah F. Zarbock, PA-C

Medical Writer and Editor
Editor in Chief of JAAPA
Lakeville, Connecticut

Wolters Kluwer | Lippincott Williams & Wilkins
Health

Philadelphia • Baltimore • New York • London
Buenos Aires • Hong Kong • Sydney • Tokyo

Acquisitions Editor: Nancy Anastasi Duffy
Development Editor: Stacey Sebring
Associate Managing Editor: Liz Stalnaker
Marketing Manager: Emilie Moyer
Production Editor: Gina Aiello
Designer: Doug Smock
Compositor: International Typesetting and Composition
Printer: Data Reproduction Corp.

Library of Congress Cataloging-in-Publication Data

A comprehensive review for the certification and recertification
examinations for physician assistants / volume editor, Claire Babcock
O'Connell ; consulting editor, Sarah F. Zarbock. —3rd ed.
    p. ; cm.
  Includes bibliographical references and index.
   ISBN-13: 978-0-7817-6767-5
   ISBN-10: 0-7817-6767-9
   1. Physicians' assistants—Examinations, questions, etc.   I.
O'Connell, Claire Babcock.   II. Zarbock, Sarah F.   III. American Academy
of Physician Assistants.   IV. Association of Physician Assistant
Programs.
   [DNLM: 1. Physician Assistants—Examination Questions.   2.
Certification—Examination Questions.   W 18.2 C7385 2007]
   R697.P45C66 2007
   610'.76—dc22

                                                  2006101492

Dedication

In memory of my father, Thomas G. Babcock, Jr.
Claire Babcock O'Connell

To the Physician Assistant profession: joining it was life-transforming.
Sarah F. Zarbock

Preface

Taking certification and recertification examinations are a fact of life for physician assistants (PAs). The certification examination is taken upon graduation from an accredited physician assistant program, and the recertification examination is taken every 6 years thereafter. The National Commission on the Certification of Physician Assistants (NCCPA), using test data from the National Board of Medical Examiners (NBME) as well as the experience and aptitude of test-item writers, develops the two examinations and refines them on an annual basis to keep current with clinical practice and medical advances.

Traditionally, test-preparation books have consisted of practice questions, answers, and explanations. This format provided the opportunity for both new and experienced PAs to improve their test-taking ability by becoming more accustomed to the test experience, and by reading the answers and explanations provided with each question, the candidate could learn from his or her successes and mistakes.

Although all three editions of this book have similar goals, the second and third editions have moved several important steps toward achieving these goals. First, a pretest has been added, and the posttest continues to be available but on an enclosed CD-ROM in a format that simulates the NCCPA exam. Both tests have been written by experienced, NBME-trained PA educators and compiled using the proportions per subject area and skills areas as delineated in the NCCPA guidelines. Each test question also is written according to the NCCPA structure for multiple-choice format, an especially important feature of the second and third editions. For further information and explanation of the NCCPA subject and skills areas, see http://www.nccpa.net.

In addition to the practice questions and answers, this book provides, in a condensed outline format, all the necessary information not only to take and successfully complete either of the tests but also to refer to, on a day-to-day basis, in clinical practice. The third edition also includes three important new chapters on surgery, pediatrics, and geriatrics, making the third edition even more comprehensive and able to be used as a quick and easy-to-read reference. In other words, this book is a practical, "real-time" educational tool for busy practitioners—a handy resource to be used on the front line of patient care.

The chapters are carefully formatted to give general characteristics of diseases (e.g., incidence, pathophysiology, prognosis), clinical signs and symptoms, diagnostic and laboratory evaluation, and treatment. These chapters, as well as the accompanying questions and their explanations, closely mirror the body of knowledge that is tested on the certification examinations and is needed for the reality of clinical practice. Regardless of their practice setting, PAs can use this book to review and test themselves on the material most likely to be included in either examination. For instance, more extensive information and questions are provided in cardiology, because patients with cardiac problems are more common in clinical practice.

The American Academy of Physician Assistants (AAPA) and the Physician Assistant Education Association (PAEA) have continued their close collaboration in the development of this book. This partnership serves to enhance the value and credibility of the book and to ensure that it meets certification and continuing medical education needs of the PA constituency.

We believe that you will find this book helpful in preparing to take either of the NCCPA examinations. Equally important, however, we hope that you use this book as a quick and valuable reference in clinical practice. We encourage you to make the book a permanent addition to your library not only upon graduation and every 6 years thereafter but also on a daily basis for the most important use of all—providing quality care to your patients.

Contributors

Frank Acevedo, PA-C, M.S.
Associate Director/Academic Coordinator
Assistant Professor
Department Physician Assistant Studies
New York Institute of Technology
Old Westbury, NY

Petar Breitinger, PA-C, MPAS
Clinical Assistant Professor
University of Florida Physician Assistant Program
Gainesville, Florida

Edward D. Huechtker, PhD, MPA, PA-C
Chair, Department of Critical Care
Acting Chair, Department of Diagnostic and
    Therapeutic Sciences
School of Health Professions
University of Alabama at Birmingham
Birmingham, Alabama

Kathy Kemle, MS, PA-C
Assistant Professor
Department of Family Medicine
Division of Geriatrics
Mercer University School of Medicine
Medical Center of Central Georgia
Macon, Georgia

Susan LeLacheur, MPH, PA-C
Assistant Professor
Department of Health Care Science
Physician Assistant Program
The George Washington University
Washington, District of Columbia

William H. Marquardt, MA, PA-C
Associate Professor & Chair
Physician Assistant Department
Nova Southeastern University
Fort Lauderdale, Florida

Bob McNellis, MPH, PA
Director, Clinical Affairs and Education
American Academy of Physician Assistants
Alexandria, Virginia

Matthew A. McQuillan, MS, PA-C
Associate Professor
University of Medicine and Dentistry of
    New Jersey
School of Health Related Professions
Physician Assistant Program
Piscataway, New Jersey

Claire Babcock O'Connell, MPH, PA-C
Associate Professor
University of Medicine and Dentistry of
    New Jersey
School of Health Related Professions
Physician Assistant Program
Piscataway, New Jersey

Nancy E. Orr, PA-C
Retired Academic Coordinator
PA Program
Cuyahoga Community College
Parma, Ohio

Patti Pagels, MPAS, PA-C
Assistant Professor
Division of Physician Assistant Studies
University of North Texas Health Science Center
Ft Worth, Texas

Lori Parlin Palfreyman, MS, PA-C
Assistant Professor
University of Medicine and Dentistry of
    New Jersey
School of Health Related Professions
Physician Assistant Program
Piscataway, New Jersey

Jennifer Roach, MS, PA-C
Instructor, University of Medicine and Dentistry of
 New Jersey
School of Health Related Professions
Physician Assistant Program
Piscataway, New Jersey

Rebecca Lovell Scott, PhD, PA-C
Clinical Coordinator
Northeastern University Physician Assistant Program
Boston, MA

Melanie Trecartin, MS, PA-C
Assistant Professor
University of Medicine and Dentistry of
 New Jersey
Physician Assistant Program
Piscataway, New Jersey

Reviewers

Frank Acevedo, PA-C, M.S.
Associate Director/Academic Coordinator
Assistant Professor
Department of Physician Assistant Studies
New York Institute of Technology
Old Westbury, NY

Phyllis L. Barks, MPH, PA
Assistant Professor & Technology Development Coordinator
Division of Physician Assistant Education
School of Medicine
Oregon Health & Science University
Portland, Oregon

Kenneth W. Betzing, MPAS, PA-C
Assistant Professor, Louisiana State University
    Health Sciences Center
Physician Assistant Program
Shreveport, Louisiana

Meredith Schierer Burke, MS, PA-C
Instructor, University of Medicine and Dentistry of
    New Jersey
School of Health Related Professions
Physician Assistant Program
Piscataway, New Jersey

Sheryl L. Geisler, MS, PA-C
Assistant Professor, University of Medicine and
    Dentistry of New Jersey
School of Health Related Professions
Physician Assistant Program
Piscataway, New Jersey

Dawn LaBarbera, PhD, PA-C
Associate Professor, University of Saint Francis
School of Health Sciences
Physician Assistant Program
Fort Wayne, Indiana

Ellen D. Mandel, MPA, MS, PA-C, RD, CDE
Assistant Professor, Seton Hall University
School of Graduate Medical Education
Physician Assistant Program
South Orange, New Jersey

Matthew A. McQuillan, MS, PA-C
Associate Professor, University of Medicine and
    Dentistry of New Jersey
School of Health Related Professions
Physician Assistant Program
Piscataway, New Jersey

Lori Parlin Palfreyman, MS, PA-C
Assistant Professor
University of Medicine and Dentistry of New Jersey
School of Health Related Professions
Physician Assistant Program
Piscataway, New Jersey

Harry Pomeranz, MS, PA-C
Assistant Professor, City University of New York
York College Physician Assistant Program
Jamaica, New York

Jennifer Roach, MS, PA-C
Instructor, University of Medicine and Dentistry of New Jersey
School of Health Related Professions
Physician Assistant Program
Piscataway, New Jersey

Christina M. Robohm, MS, PA-C
Director of Admissions
Assistant Professor, Department of Pediatrics
University of Colorado at Denver and Health Sciences Center
Child Health Associate/Physician Assistant Program
Aurora, Colorado

Carol J. Sadley, M.Ed., PA-C
Associate Professor
University of Medicine and Dentistry of New Jersey
School of Health Related Professions
Physician Assistant Program
Piscataway, New Jersey

Melanie Trecartin, MS, PA-C
Assistant Professor
University of Medicine and Dentistry of New Jersey
School of Health Related Professions
Physician Assistant Program
Piscataway, New Jersey

Marianne Vail, MS, PA-C
Assistant Professor
Massachusetts College of Pharmacy and Health Sciences
School of Health Sciences
Physician Assistant Studies
Boston, Massachusetts

Eric Vangsnes, MS, PA-C
Assistant Professor
Physician Assistant Program
Western Michigan University
Kalamazoo, Michigan

Erich Vidal, MS, PA-C
Assistant Professor
University of Medicine and Dentistry of
    New Jersey
School of Health Related Professions
Physician Assistant Program
Piscataway, New Jersey

Amy Warren, PA-C
Shreveport, Louisiana
awarr1@cox.net

Acknowledgments

The effort involved in putting together this edition has been tremendous. However, the assistance, support, and encouragement from excellent colleagues has guided those efforts and succeeded in producing a high-quality text and review book. I am in debt to my program directors, Ruth Fixelle and Jill Reichman, and my fellow faculty at the University of Medicine and Dentistry of New Jersey. Their confidence in me has been a constant presence throughout my career as a physician assistant. I am also grateful to the contributing authors; the personnel at Lippincott Williams & Wilkins; and the leadership of the Physician Assistant Education Association and American Academy of Physician Assistants. Sarah Zarbock continues to be an excellent mentor and instrumental in guiding me throughout such a large task—and I thank her for her diligence and inspiration. Finally, I wish to thank my family for their endless patience and constant support and love.

—*Claire Babcock O'Connell*

Developing a third edition is just as exciting, challenging, and rewarding as beginning from scratch for the first edition. In addition to working with many of the first- and second-edition authors, I had the opportunity to meet some wonderful new and dedicated colleagues. Claire O'Connell, my coeditor, continues to be at the top of my list. She helped immeasurably in finding new authors, reviewing manuscripts, providing feedback and encouragement, and authoring one of the chapters. Claire combines a level of patience and hard work that is extraordinary, and she has a unique ability in helping authors stay on track. Needless to say, I feel very fortunate to have teamed up with her again. I am also indebted to all the authors—both those who returned to revise and update their chapters and others who just came on board. All these efforts were accomplished in their "spare" time—that is, when they were not working in their clinical practices, teaching PA students, or participating in professional activities. I am especially grateful to Greg Thomas, Vice President, Clinical and Scientific Affairs, and Ken Brady, Director, Strategic Business Development and Marketing, at the AAPA. They continually provided encouragement and managed the behind-the-scenes aspects that were crucial to developing this third edition. I want to give special thanks to my colleagues at Lippincott Williams & Wilkins. Donna Balado, Senior Acquisitions Editor, enthusiastically supported the need for a third edition and carefully shepherded the proposal until its acceptance. The baton was then passed to Stacey Sebring, Senior Managing Editor, who worked diligently and patiently to guide us through the process, and to Liz Stalnaker, Associate Managing Editor, who took on the project in its last stages, readying it for release to the production team. I would also like to thank my family, friends, and PA colleagues—all of whom helped me take some of the important steps along the way. Finally—and this may seem odd—I'd like to thank myself. I read the book from cover to cover, reviewed all of the practice test questions and explanations, and passed the Recertification Exam in October 2005—25 years after graduating from PA school!

—*Sarah F. Zarbock*

Contents

Pretest

Directions: Each of the numbered items or incomplete statements in this section is followed by a list of answers or completions of the statement. Select the ONE lettered answer or completion that is BEST in each case.

1. In a patient with elevated blood pressure, which of the following physical examination findings most strongly indicates a need for workup for secondary hypertension?
   A. S3 gallop
   B. Flank bruits
   C. CVA tenderness
   D. Retinal exudates

2. A 30-year-old man returns from an extended trip to Mexico and complains of 3 weeks of mild diarrhea, mostly after breakfast. The stool is described as bulky, greasy, frothy, and malodorous; it is free of blood or pus. He has upper abdominal discomfort, cramps, distention, and excessive flatus and has lost several pounds. He is afebrile. What is the treatment of choice?
   A. Albendazole
   B. Metronidazole
   C. Nitazoxanide
   D. Paromomycin

3. An unstable tibial and fibular shaft fracture was initially immobilized in a long leg, non-weight-bearing cast. It is improving after 6 weeks. What type of immobilization should be continued for the next phase of healing?
   A. Posterior splint
   B. Removable walking boot
   C. Short leg, weight-bearing cast
   D. Long leg, non-weight-bearing splint

4. A 25-year-old woman undergoes echocardiography for nonspecific chest pain and palpitations. Results indicate a floppy mitral valve. What finding was most likely present on the physical exam?
   A. Fixed split S_1
   B. Midsystolic click
   C. Late diastolic rumble
   D. Early systolic ejection sound

5. A 30-year-old white woman presents with fatigue and generalized weakness for several weeks. Physical examination reveals mucosal pallor and an atrophic appearance to the tongue. Laboratory data show a microcytic, hypochromic appearance to the RBCs. What is the treatment of choice?
   A. Vitamin B_{12} supplements
   B. Ferrous sulfate
   C. Folic acid
   D. Prednisone

6. A 36-year-old man presents 2 weeks after a prolonged upper respiratory infection complaining of chest pain, which he describes as sharp and worsening with deep breaths or lying flat. Examination reveals a low-grade fever and a friction rub. Which of the following drug classes should be prescribed?
   A. Antibiotics
   B. Nonsteroidal anti-inflammatory drugs
   C. Diuretics
   D. Antiarrhythmics

7. In an adult with ventricular fibrillation, which of the following is the recommended initial defibrillator setting?
   A. 200 Joules
   B. 300 Joules
   C. 360 Joules
   D. 400 Joules

8. A 27-year-old woman gives a history of unilateral throbbing headaches that occur perimenstrually. Which of the following is LEAST appropriate as part of her management?
   A. Restrict foods rich in tyramine
   B. Reduce stress
   C. Standardize sleep and wake cycles
   D. Increase caffeine intake

9. A 44-year-old man complains of fatigue, low-grade fever, and headaches for several months. Examination reveals splenomegaly. Laboratory tests identify a persistent leukocytosis and thrombocytosis with circulating immature granulocytes. Bone marrow aspiration and biopsy reveal the Philadelphia chromosome in dividing marrow cells. What is the most likely diagnosis?

A. Acute lymphocytic leukemia
B. Acute myeloblastic leukemia
C. Chronic lymphocytic leukemia
D. Chronic myelogenous leukemia

10. Which of the following statements should be a component of patient education for a patient diagnosed with irritable bowel syndrome?
A. It can be cured with proper diet and medication.
B. The condition will progress to a more serious disease.
C. Psychological counseling is necessary for improvement.
D. It is a chronic disorder of exacerbation and quiescence.

11. An elderly farmer complains of an enlarging skin lesion on the dorsum of his hand that occasionally bleeds. Physical examination reveals a single, 2-cm, red, hard nodule with central ulceration. Which of the following management options would be most effective?
A. Radiation therapy
B. Topical tretinoin
C. Surgical excision
D. Cryosurgery

12. A 35-year-old woman complains of galactorrhea for 2 months. She denies trauma to the breast, is taking no medications, and is not pregnant. Physical examination demonstrates galactorrhea bilaterally. Which of the following visual field defects would best support a pituitary tumor as the cause of the galactorrhea?
A. Homonymous quadratic defect
B. Bitemporal hemianopia
C. Homonymous hemianopia
D. Horizontal defect

13. Physical examination of a 34-year-old woman reveals visual fields defects. A follow-up skull radiograph is reported to show sellar enlargement. Elevation of which of the following substances is most likely?
A. ACTH
B. TSH
C. Prolactin
D. Growth hormone

14. Which of the following laboratory tests is the primary screening method for neural tube defects during pregnancy?
A. Pelvic ultrasonography
B. Maternal serum α-fetoprotein
C. Chorionic villus sampling
D. Amniocentesis

15. A 34-year-old man has noted a painless "bump" on his wrist that has become progressively larger over the past few months. He denies any known injuries. Physical examination reveals a 2.5-cm mass on the dorsal aspect of the wrist joint that limits flexion of his wrist because of pain. Transillumination of the mass results in a homogenous, red glow throughout the mass. Which of the following is most appropriate at this time?
A. Radiography
B. Ultrasound
C. Bone scan
D. No further studies

16. Which of the following medications is the best initial treatment for deep venous thrombosis confirmed by ultrasound?
A. Aspirin
B. Heparin
C. Warfarin
D. Ibuprofen

17. A patient began treatment 4 months ago for pulmonary tuberculosis. The patient now complains of difficulty seeing and of distorted areas in his central visual fields. Which of the following is the most likely cause of this complaint?
A. Ethambutol
B. Rifampin
C. Isoniazid
D. Pyrazinamide

18. On postoperative day 2 after an exploratory laparotomy under general anesthesia, a patient has a low-grade fever with decreased bibasilar breath sounds. The patient is not coughing and denies any shortness of breath. Which of the following diagnoses is the most likely cause?
A. Atelectasis
B. Pneumonia
C. Pulmonary embolus
D. Congestive heart failure

19. Which of the following is consistently abnormal in acute delirium?
A. CT scan of head
B. EEG
C. Lumbar puncture
D. MRI of the head

20. Patients with lower extremity rheumatoid arthritis should be counseled and encouraged in sports and exercises designed to preserve joint motion and muscular strength. Which of the following exercises would best meet this goal?
A. Jogging
B. Swimming
C. Cycling
D. Walking

21. A steelworker presents to the clinic immediately after getting foreign material in his eyes. He is complaining of pain and photophobia in his left eye. Fluoroscein stain reveals an area that stains a deeper green than the surrounding cornea. Which of the following is the most likely diagnosis?

A. Corneal erosion
B. Corneal abrasion
C. Corneal ulcer
D. Keratitis

22. A 64-year-old man presents to an ambulatory clinic with worsening pain in his right calf that occurs after walking short distances and resolves with rest. Diminished distal pulses in the right lower extremity are noted. Which of the following diagnostic studies is most appropriate to perform initially?
    A. Ankle-brachial index
    B. Arteriography
    C. Lymphangiography
    D. Ultrasonography

23. A 61-year-old woman stopped menstruating approximately 8 years ago and declined postmenopausal hormone replacement. She comes into the office for evaluation of a recent onset of vaginal bleeding. Physical examination reveals mild atrophy of the vaginal walls and a smooth, pale cervix with a small amount of blood at the os. What is the most beneficial diagnostic test to perform at this time?
    A. Pap smear
    B. Endometrial biopsy
    C. FSH and estradiol level
    D. Colposcopy-directed biopsy

24. A 35-year-old man presents with palpitations and weakness. Additional symptoms include dyspnea on exertion and near-syncope. He has been drinking alcohol daily because of the recent loss of his job, and his pulse is irregularly irregular. Which of the following is the most likely diagnosis?
    A. Atrial fibrillation
    B. Paroxysmal supraventricular tachycardia
    C. Ventricular bigeminy
    D. Premature atrial complexes

25. A female athlete presents with a history of worsening, burning, right heel pain for the last 2 weeks. She states the pain is worse when she gets out of bed or after prolonged sitting, and she denies any foot numbness. The pain is reproduced with palpation of the area and passive dorsiflection of the toes. Which of the following is the most likely diagnosis?
    A. Plantar fasciitis
    B. Heel contusion
    C. Calcaneal fracture
    D. Tarsal tunnel syndrome

26. A 60-year-old man of Mediterranean descent has a history of benign prostatic hyperplasia. He develops increased frequency and dysuria. Urine microscopy shows 50–100 WBCs per high-power field and Gram-negative rods. A 3-day course of antibiotic is given; 4 days later, the patient returns with acute fatigue.

Laboratory tests reveal hgb 8.5 g/dL, hct 25.5%, and haptoglobin 20 mg/dL; peripheral smear shows Heinz bodies. This presentation is likely a result of administering which of the following drugs?
    A. Acetaminophen
    B. Azithromycin
    C. Prazocin
    D. Trimethroprim/sulfamethoxazole

27. A 15-month-old child presents with inspiratory stridor audible without a stethoscope and a respiratory rate of 40 bpm. There are moderate intercostal retractions, and there is no cyanosis. After aerosolized racemic epinephrine administration, which of the following is the next best management plan?
    A. Cool mist room humidification
    B. Dexamethasone IM, one dose
    C. Aerosolized ribavirin
    D. Chest physical therapy

28. A 61-year-old data entry manager gives a history of chronic pain in his hands for many years. The pain grows worse as the day progresses and is relieved by naproxen. He denies edema or stiffness. Which of the following physical examination findings is most likely in this patient?
    A. Thenar atrophy
    B. Heberden's nodes
    C. Boutonniere deformity
    D. Dupuytren's contracture

29. A patient describes unpredictable, acute episodes of intense fear and a sense of impending doom. Episodes are associated with palpitations, dyspnea, and diaphoresis. The events begin abruptly and last for about 20 minutes. Which of the following is the best choice for long-term therapy?
    A. Alprazolam (Xanax)
    B. Imipramine (Tofranil)
    C. Paroxetine (Paxil)
    D. Phenelzine (Nardil)

30. Which of the following is the most common early manifestation of left ventricular failure?
    A. Ascites
    B. Anorexia
    C. Leg edema
    D. Exertional dyspnea

31. A 73-year-old woman complains of progressive urinary incontinence, which she describes as an intense feeling of urgency that cannot be delayed, accompanied by urinary leakage. Which of the following is the recommended treatment?
    A. α-Blocking agent
    B. Topical estrogen cream
    C. Detrusor relaxant medication
    D. Surgical intervention

32. Occlusion of which of the following arteries is most likely to result in an anterior wall infarction?
   A. Left anterior descending
   B. Right coronary
   C. Left circumflex
   D. Left marginal

33. A 63-year-old man who smokes complains of an insidious onset of vague, epigastric pain over the past several months. Which of the following additional descriptions of the pain would most strongly support a diagnosis of carcinoma of the pancreas?
   A. Cramping quality after eating
   B. Relief with sitting and leaning forward
   C. Absence of pain radiation
   D. Referral to the right lower quadrant

34. A 3-week old infant is evaluated for persistent projectile vomiting. She is hungry and nurses avidly; her vomit consists of breast milk without bile or blood. The abdomen is distended before vomiting, and a small mass is palpable after vomiting. Upper GI series reveals a narrowed distal stomach with double tract of barium. What is the treatment of choice?
   A. Barium enema
   B. Duodenal dilation under fluoroscopy
   C. Erythromycin therapy
   D. Pyloromyotomy

35. Which of the following is the typical presentation of nonbullous impetigo?
   A. Edematous, red, indurated spreading lesion
   B. Inflammatory hot lesion with diffuse erythema
   C. Vesiculopustular lesion that follows a dermatome
   D. Vesicular, honey-colored, crusted superficial lesions

36. A 60-year-old presents with acute unilateral loss of vision. Funduscopic examination reveals vein dilation, intraretinal hemorrhages, and cotton-wool spots. Which of the following is the most likely diagnosis?
   A. Retinal vein occlusion
   B. Macular degeneration
   C. Retinal detachment
   D. Hypertensive retinopathy

37. A 43-year-old female presents with RUQ pain. She is febrile and today cardiac; there is a + Murphy's sign on exam. Which of the following likely presented this condition?
   A. Large, fatty meals
   B. High-fiber meal
   C. Spicy foods
   D. Alcohol

38. A 23-year-old patient with diabetes type-1 who has been taking her insulin reliably for years comes in for advice because her early morning sugars have been high. She has been gradually increasing her evening insulin to prevent this, but her morning sugars have continued to increase significantly. She is concerned that her insulin levels are getting "too high." What is the most likely assessment of this patient?
   A. Somogyi effect
   B. Waning phenomenon
   C. Munchausen syndrome
   D. Dawn phenomenon

39. A routine ECG performed on a healthy, asymptomatic, 65-year-old reveals from three to five unifocal nonconsecutive premature ventricular complexes per minute. These decrease in frequency with exercise. Which of the following is the most appropriate intervention?
   A. Start propranolol
   B. Start procainamide
   C. Administer lidocaine
   D. Reassure patient that treatment is unnecessary

40. A patient presents for renewal of topical medications for chronic atopic dermatitis. Where on the physical examination are lesions most likely to be found?
   A. Palms and soles
   B. Knees
   C. Gluteal cleft
   D. Antecubital fossae

41. Endometrial hyperplasia has been associated with prolonged exposure to unopposed estrogen and is associated with an increased risk of endometrial cancer. Which of the following patients would be at high risk for endometrial hyperplasia?
   A. A 45-year-old woman who has been on oral contraceptives for 7 years
   B. A 39-year-old patient with anorexia nervosa who has had amenorrhea for the past 2 years
   C. A 16-year-old girl with 2 weeks of heavy bleeding after 3 months of amenorrhea
   D. A 45-year-old woman who is obese, hypertensive, and diabetic and has a 4-month history of heavy bleeding

42. A 17-year-old female presents with fever, generalized pelvic pain, and malodorous vaginal discharge for 2 hours. Examination reveals marked suprapubic tenderness with rebound and cervical motion tenderness. Vaginal discharge is dark, thick, and foul-smelling. Vitals include T 104°F, P 110, BP 80/50 mm Hg. She is cool and clammy. Which of the following is the most likely diagnosis?
   A. Septic abortion
   B. Ectopic pregnancy
   C. Pelvic inflammatory disease
   D. Ruptured tubo-ovarian abscess

43. A mother brings her 1-year-old infant to the clinic with complaints of "large testicles." Physical examination reveals bilateral inguinal hernias. A positive finding during which of the following examination procedures indicates the need for immediate surgical intervention?

A. Palpation of the abdomen
B. Auscultation of the scrotum
C. Percussion of the urinary bladder
D. Valsalva maneuver while the infant is standing

44. Which of the following foods should be avoided by patients with celiac disease?
    A. Barley
    B. Egg
    C. Grapefruit
    D. Rice

45. A 63-year-old woman presents with painful vesicles on her right cheek, forehead, and the tip of her nose. The eye on the affected side is red and tearing; vision is blurred. Which of the following is the most appropriate initial intervention?
    A. Prescribe acetaminophen with codeine and compresses with Burow's solution.
    B. Refer immediately to an ophthalmologist.
    C. Recommend topical capsaicin cream to control the pain.
    D. Prescribe a 3-week tapering course of prednisone.

46. A 70-year-old woman is brought to the emergency department with altered mental state. Her son reports that she has been in good mental and physical health all her life. At the suggestion of her local health food store salesperson, she began taking pills to improve her bone strength. The results of blood work show renal impairment and marked elevation in both serum calcium and phosphates. Chest radiography shows areas of calcification. Which of the following is the most likely etiology?
    A. Riboflavin toxicity
    B. Vitamin A toxicity
    C. Vitamin B_6 toxicity
    D. Vitamin D toxicity

47. A 24-year-old woman at 32 weeks gestation presents with new onset of seizures, blood pressure of 155/95 mm Hg, lower and upper extremity edema, and 3+ proteinuria. Which of the following is the most likely diagnosis?
    A. Eclampsia
    B. Preeclampsia
    C. Primary seizure disorder
    D. Pregnancy-induced hypertension

48. Which of the following is the most appropriate initial treatment for a corneal abrasion?
    A. Pilocarpine hydrochloride, 0.25% solution
    B. Tobramycin/dexamethasone, 0.1% suspension
    C. Polymyxin-B sulfate ophthalmic ointment
    D. Tropicamide, 1% solution

49. Initial evaluation of a 3-year-old reveals a female child with short stature, round face, obesity, short fourth metacarpals, and mental retardation. She is sitting happily on her mother's lap. Her teeth are in good repair with normal eruptive pattern. She has never been on any long-term medication. She has a good appetite and eats well. Laboratory evaluation, including a comprehensive metabolic panel, calcium, and TSH, is normal. What is the recommended intervention?
    A. 24-hour urine collection for calcium
    B. Further evaluation for pituitary disorders
    C. Genotyping analysis
    D. No further diagnostic or lab tests

50. A 30-year-old African American complains of bloating, abdominal cramps, and flatulence that occur 1 to 2 hours after meals containing any milk or cheese products. The hydrogen breath test is positive. Which of the following is the most likely diagnosis?
    A. Bacterial overgrowth
    B. Celiac sprue
    C. Lactose intolerance
    D. Pancreatic insufficiency

51. Four days ago, a mother brought her 4-year-old boy to the clinic for impetigo. She returns with the child today because the penicillin-V "just isn't working." She has been soaking and removing the crusts and following hand-washing instructions. The child still has extensive honey-colored, crusted lesions on his hands, arms, and face. Which of the following is the most appropriate course of action?
    A. Substitute oral clindamycin for the penicillin-V.
    B. Substitute mupirocin ointment for the penicillin-V.
    C. Substitute oral ciprofloxacin for penicillin-V.
    D. Tell the mother to continue the penicillin-V for another 4 days.

52. Which of the following is the initial treatment for terminating symptomatic PSVT in a hemodynamically stable patient?
    A. Digoxin
    B. Catheter ablation
    C. Carotid sinus massage
    D. Direct current cardioversion

53. A 12-year-old boy complains of pain and fullness in the periorbital area. He has had cold symptoms with low-grade fever, dry cough, and congestion for 3 days. Today, he has a temperature of 102°F and thick, purulent nasal discharge. Which of the following is the most appropriate first-line antibiotic?
    A. Amoxicillin
    B. Erythromycin
    C. Ampicillin
    D. Tetracycline

54. A 60-year-old woman presents with bilateral shoulder and hip pain. The pain started in the left shoulder about 6 weeks ago and has since spread to both shoulders and hips. Morning stiffness lasts about 2 hours, and the pain grows worse with rest and improves with activity. She also has a low-grade fever and fatigue. Physical

examination elicits tenderness over the affected muscles with painful, limited range of motion of the hip and shoulder. Laboratory tests reveal ESR 60 mm/hr, normochromic anemia, and a negative rheumatoid factor. Which of the following is the most likely diagnosis?

A. Multiple myeloma
B. Osteomalacia
C. Polymyalgia rheumatica
D. Sarcoidosis

55. Which of the following statements is true concerning type 2 diabetes mellitus?
A. Islet cell antibodies are common in type 2 diabetes mellitus.
B. Type 2 diabetes mellitus is linked to HLA markers on the sixth chromosome.
C. Endogenous insulin in patients with type 2 diabetes is adequate to prevent ketoacidosis.
D. Fewer than 40% of people with type 2 diabetes mellitus are obese.

56. Which of the following mechanisms is most commonly associated with a whiplash injury to the neck?
A. Hyperextension of the neck
B. Contusion to the neck
C. Extreme rotation of the cervical spine
D. Strangulation

57. Which of the following is considered to be the best method of screening for diabetic nephropathy?
A. Serum creatinine
B. Urine protein electrophoresis
C. Overnight urine for microalbumin
D. Renal biopsy

58. A hospital worker developed tuberculosis and was started on drug therapy. Which of the following should be included in the continued management of this patient?
A. The patient should have a chest radiograph every 3 months to monitor treatment response.
B. The patient should rest and remain isolated at home for the full duration of drug therapy.
C. A bacillus-Calmette-Guerin vaccine should be given to prevent reactivation of the disease in the future.
D. Evaluation for drug side effects should be obtained monthly for the first few months.

59. A type I, second-degree artrioventricular block is best characterized by which of the following electrocardiographic findings?
A. Accordion-appearing QRS morphology
B. Progressive lengthening of the PR interval
C. Ventricular rate of less than 50 bpm
D. Widened QRS complexes

60. Which of the following serum markers is most likely to be elevated within 6 hours of an acute myocardial infarction?

A. Creatine kinase
B. Alanine transaminase
C. Aspartate transaminase
D. Lactic dehydrogenase

61. A 23-year-old man with a 2-year history of mild depression has recently lost his job because of erratic behavior, including irrational paranoia, nonsensical conversations, and inability to focus or complete tasks. He admits to auditory hallucinations and delusions of persecution. Which of the following is the most appropriate first-line treatment?
A. Carbamazepine (Tegretol)
B. Haloperidol (Haldol)
C. Lithium
D. Risperidone (Risperdal)

62. A 58-year-old, postmenopausal woman comes into the office with a rash on her left breast. On examination, a diffuse area of swelling in the upper quadrant of the left breast is noted, but no mass is found. The skin over this swelling is erythematous, edematous, and warm. Which of the following is the recommended management?
A. Refer the patient for mammography.
B. Initiate antibiotics for an infection.
C. Refer the patient for a biopsy to rule out an inflammatory carcinoma.
D. Use warm compresses three times per day, and return within 2 weeks.

63. The varicella-zoster virus belongs to which of the following families?
A. Papovaviruses
B. Picornaviruses
C. Poxviruses
D. Herpes viruses

64. During the evaluation of an unconscious patient who has a head injury, which of the following is the most important diagnostic test?
A. Skull radiography
B. CT of head
C. Cervical spine radiography
D. Lumbar puncture

65. A 28-year-old female with normal CBC, platelet count, and international normalized ratio (INR) before surgery is noted to have excessive bloody drainage in a Hemovac drain following abdominal surgery. Repeat CBC, platelet counts, and INR continue to be normal, but bleeding time is prolonged. What is the recommended treatment?
A. Desmopressin
B. Factor VIII
C. Factor IX
D. Vitamin K

66. A 36-year-old flight attendant returns to the United States from Southeast Asia. Within 2 days, the patient develops severe diarrhea, which is becoming

progressively worse. The patient describes the diarrhea as watery with flecks of mucous, but he denies any blood. He also denies fever but has had four episodes of emesis. Examination reveals signs of dehydration with active bowel sounds. Laboratory results reveal an increased hematocrit, creatinine, and BUN. Electrolyte panel reveals an exceptionally low bicarbonate. Which of the following is the most likely diagnosis?
A. *Escherichia coli*
B. *Entamoeba histolytica*
C. *Salmonella typhi*
D. *Vibrio cholerae*

67. A 79-year-old man with a history of hypertension controlled using hydrochlorthiazide and mild COPD presents with dyspnea. He states it began 2 days ago on exertion and has progressed over the last 12 hours to dyspnea at rest. Physical examination reveals 2.1-cm JVD and 2+ pitting edema to the ankles. Which of the following is most likely to be found on cardiac exam?
A. An ejection click
B. The presence of a thrill
C. A third heart sound (S_3)
D. A fourth heart sound (S_4)

68. A 26-year-old woman presents with a painful swelling of her right eyelid. There is a tender erythematous swelling around the eyelashes that involves the lid margin. Which of the following is the most likely diagnosis?
A. Chalazion
B. Hordeolum
C. Pinguecula
D. Xanthelasma

69. A healthy 22-year-old presents with mild jaundice. Which of the following additional historical factors best supports the diagnosis of Gilbert's disease?
A. Family history of recurrent mild jaundice
B. Family history of sickle-cell trait
C. History of fatty food intolerance
D. Recent fever, malaise, and myalgias

70. A patient with Addison's disease is awaiting surgical repair of a fractured acetabulum sustained in a motor-vehicle crash. Which of the following adjustments in this patient's medication regimen is necessary to avoid life-threatening complications?
A. Parenteral dose of hydrocortisone
B. Double oral dose of hydrocortisone
C. Parenteral dose of fludrocortisone
D. Double oral dose of fludrocortisone

71. The constellation of tingling of the lips and hands, muscle and abdominal cramps, carpopedal spasms, and psychological changes, as well as the existence of tetany, would most likely occur in association with which of the following situations?

A. Chronic states of hypocapnia
B. Following thyroidectomy
C. Irradiation of the neck
D. Malignancy-associated hypercalcemia

72. A healthy 40-year-old primipara presents at 8 weeks of gestation for her first prenatal appointment. Her physical examination is consistent with an 8-week pregnancy. Which of the following would be the most appropriate next step in this patient's care?
A. Give a follow-up appointment in 2 weeks.
B. Schedule an ultrasound to confirm dating.
C. Refer the patient for genetic counseling.
D. Obtain a serum α-fetoprotein.

73. In a patient with newly diagnosed rheumatoid arthritis that has failed NSAID therapy, which of the following is the best second-line medication?
A. Methotrexate
B. Hydroxychloroquine
C. Corticosteroids
D. Gold salts

74. A 17-year-old student presents with frequent episodes of interdigital tinea pedis. He relates frequent episodes of maceration and irritation and desires information to prevent its irritating occurrence. He is a competitive diver on the high school team and practices almost daily. What advice should be offered?
A. Daily application of steroid ointment
B. Regular cleansing with isopropyl alcohol
C. Regulation diving shoes to minimize exposure to chlorine
D. Shower shoes when showering at home or the gym

75. A patient comes to the emergency department after exposure to ammonia in the left eye. First responders have been irrigating the eye for 40 minutes. What diagnostic study should be performed initially on arrival at the emergency department?
A. Tonometry
B. pH measurement
C. Fluorescein staining
D. Funduscopic examination

76. A 30-year-old woman presents with a 15-year history of unilateral throbbing headaches that occur once or twice monthly and last from 1 to 3 days. These headaches often are preceded by a sensation of flashing lights. She is asymptomatic at this time. Which of the following is the most likely diagnosis?
A. Sinus headache
B. Cluster headache
C. Migraine headache
D. Muscle tension headache

77. A 63-year-old former smoker complains of pain in the lower calves that occurs with exertion. Ankle-brachial

index is 0.63. Which of the following would be harmful in the management of the patient?

A. Lipid-lowering medication
B. Elastic support hose
C. Regular exercise
D. Aspirin therapy

78. A generally healthy 20-year-old man presents with a nonpruritic rash on his upper thighs. Examination reveals small, yellow, grouped pustules surrounded by erythema; each lesion is pierced by a hair. He recently spent time in a hot tub while on vacation. Which of the following is the recommended treatment?

A. Oral dicloxacillin
B. Topical isotretinoin
C. Oral indomethacin
D. No treatment needed

79. A 77-year-old man is seen in the hospital and complains of increasing pain in his right great toe. The toe appears erythematous and warm and is extremely tender. Which of the following medications is the most appropriate initial treatment for this patient?

A. Allopurinol
B. Naproxen
C. Prednisolone
D. Probenecid

80. Which of the following patients meets the criteria requiring an exercise stress test before initiating an exercise program?

A. A 30-year-old woman at ideal body weight with a distant history of asthma
B. A 40-year-old man at 25% above ideal body weight with controlled hypertension
C. A 42-year-old man at 10% above ideal body weight with osteoarthritis in both knees
D. A 50-year-old woman at 15% above ideal body weight with irritable bowel syndrome

81. A patient with diabetes is complaining of throbbing rectal pain for the last several days. Digital rectal examination reveals a tender area of swelling of uncertain dimension anteriorly. Which of the following is the best intervention at this time?

A. Antibiotic therapy that covers anaerobes
B. Office incision and drainage
C. Surgical intervention
D. Warm sitz baths and analgesics

82. A patient presents with left upper quadrant pain described as boring and radiating to the back. Which of the following organs is most likely to be involved?

A. Gallbladder
B. Pancreas
C. Small bowel
D. Duodenum

83. A 19-year-old woman presents with a complaint of painful sores on the vulva. On physical exam, she has multiple, exquisitely painful, shallow, erythematous ulcers on the vulva and perineal area. A Tzanck smear demonstrates multinucleated giant cells. Which of the following is most appropriate for treatment?

A. Azithromycin (Zithromax)
B. Doxycycline (Vibramycin)
C. Acyclovir (Zovirax)
D. Benzathine penicillin G (Bicillin LA)

84. A 27-year-old woman presents for her annual Pap and pelvic exam. She is currently on Ortho-Cyclen without any problems. Her husband is concerned because she has been on the pill for more than 5 years, and he was told women should occasionally take a "pill holiday" to prevent long-term complications. She does not wish to become pregnant for another 5 years. Which of the following advice is most appropriate?

A. She should discontinue the pill for 3 months to give her body a rest. She should use barrier methods in the meantime.
B. She should discontinue the pill as soon as possible, because she has already been on them too long and may not be able to get pregnant as a result.
C. She does not need to discontinue the pill. Pill holidays are recommended after 20 years of continuous use.
D. Studies have shown it is safe for a healthy young woman to take a low-dose pill for 10–20 years without a problem; use of the pill will not effect her ability to get pregnant in 5 years.

85. Cardiac auscultation of a 3-year-old child reveals a III/VI systolic murmur that is short, vibratory, and high pitched and is best heard midway between the apex and the left lower sternal border while the patient is supine. The murmur disappears when the child stands erect. This murmur most likely represents which of the following?

A. Aortic stenosis
B. Atrioventricular septal defect
C. Mitral valve prolapse
D. Functional murmur (Still's)

86. Which of the following agents is responsible for most cases of endocarditis in IV drug users?

A. HACEK organisms
B. Nonalbicans candida
C. *Serratia marcescens*
D. *Staphylococcus aureus*

87. Which of the following physical manifestations is most suggestive of thyroid carcinoma?

A. Painful, diffuse swelling in the thyroid region
B. Rapidly enlarging thyroid mass
C. Symmetrical thyroid gland enlargement
D. Multiple soft thyroid nodules

88. What is the most common cause of acute upper GI bleeding in the United States?

A. Erosive gastritis
B. Gastric neoplasm

C. Esophageal varices

D. Peptic ulcer disease

89. An 8-year-old boy presents with fever, malaise, and severe pain in the knee joint. Examination reveals a tender, warm, and swollen joint. Synovial fluid analysis shows a leukocyte count of 45,000 cells/µL with a predominance of neutrophils. Which of the following organisms is most likely to be responsible?

A. Group A streptococci

B. *Enterococcus* spp.

C. *Staphylococcus aureus*

D. *Streptococcus pneumoniae*

90. A 31-year-old woman, G4 P3003, presents to the clinic at 34 weeks of gestation. She has not felt the baby move all day. What is the initial step in evaluating fetal well-being?

A. Biophysical profile

B. Fetal kick counts

C. Nonstress test

D. Oxytocin challenge test

91. A 16-year-old boy with a 1-week history of sore throat now presents with pain in his leg, fever, and general malaise. Examination reveals redness and swelling over the left tibia with limited range of motion of the knee because of pain. The WBC, CRP, and ESR are elevated; MRI demonstrates separation of the periosteum and bone. What is the best treatment of this patient?

A. Oral macrolide

B. Parenteral nafcillin plus third-generation cephalosporin

C. Open surgical drainage

D. Combination of a cephalosporin and semisynthetic penicillin orally

92. A 35-year-old patient presents with a 3-month history of numbness and tingling in the first three digits of the right hand. On physical examination, there is a positive Tinel's sign and Phalen's sign. Which of the following is the most appropriate test to recommend for confirmation of the suspected diagnosis?

A. Magnetic resonance imaging

B. Electromyography

C. Radiography

D. Arthrocentesis

93. What is the normal respiratory rate in the newborn?

A. 20–30 breaths/min

B. 30–60 breaths/min

C. 60–80 breaths/min

D. 80–100 breaths/min

94. A 43-year-old man complains of a 2-month history of nocturia (twice nightly), a sense of incomplete bladder emptying, weak stream, and a need to strain to begin urination. Which of the following is considered to be optional in the initial evaluation of this patient?

A. Digital rectal examination

B. Prostate-specific antigen

C. Serum creatinine

D. Urinalysis

95. A 25-year-old woman presents with paroxysmal episodes of palpitations and rapid heart rate that occur in no particular pattern. She has no current symptoms, and her ECG shows a sinus rhythm with a rate of 72 bpm. There are no pathologic Q waves or ST-segment elevation or depression; PR interval is 0.11 second and there is a delta wave at the onset of a slurred QRS complex. Which of the following is the most likely diagnosis?

A. First-degree AV block

B. Paroxysmal atrial tachycardia

C. Lown-Ganong-Levine syndrome

D. Wolff-Parkinson-White syndrome

96. Which of the following presents the greatest risk for dissection of the aorta?

A. Hypertension

B. Aortic stenosis

C. Hyperlipidemia

D. Diabetes mellitus

97. After a day of skiing, a 29-year-old man presents with a complaint of left knee pain. He states he fell during the last run of the day, felt a pop, and experienced sudden pain on the inside of his knee. He is unable to bear weight on the left leg. Which of the following techniques will best evaluate this injury?

A. Lachman's test

B. Valgus stress test

C. Thumb sign

D. McMurray test

98. An American college student spends 2 weeks in a rural area of India recently devastated by an earthquake. Two weeks after returning home, she notes fatigue, nausea, anorexia, and vague right upper quadrant pain. Her fatigue and nausea continue to worsen, her urine becomes dark, and friends comment that she "appears yellow." Physical examination reveals jaundice and hepatic tenderness. She denies injection drug use, sexual activity, or blood transfusions. Which of the following is the most likely diagnosis?

A. Hepatitis A

B. Hepatitis B

C. Hepatitis C

D. Hepatitis D

99. In an adolescent patient with comedonal acne, which of the following statements should be included as part of patient education?

A. Discontinue use of oil-based cosmetics.

B. Avoid chocolate, coffee, and greasy foods.

C. Use alcohol and other dehydrating agents to reduce acne.

D. Use abrasive cleaners to promote exfoliation and reduce comedones.

100. The vast majority of cases of acute infective endocarditis in patients with native valves is caused by which of the following?
A. *Streptococcus viridans*
B. *Staphylococcus aureus*
C. Enterococci
D. *Pseudomonas aeruginosa*

101. A 63-year-old presents with acute fever and productive cough. Lung exam reveals diffuse rales with rhonchi in the right middle lung. Which of the following is most consistent with the suspected diagnosis?
A. Consolidation
B. Kerley B lines
C. Blunting of the costophrenic angle
D. Visceral pleural line

102. A 16-year-old, despondent girl is brought in by her mother with weight loss greater than 30% of body weight over the past 3 months. Her mother has repeatedly caught her vomiting during the past 3 weeks. The patient's resting pulse is 38 bpm. Which of the following is the next step in this patient's management?
A. Start her on an antidepressant.
B. Admit her to the hospital for further testing.
C. Order a complete metabolic profile, and see her in 1 week.
D. Order an outpatient psychiatric consult within 2 weeks.

103. A 45-year-old woman presents to the emergency department 1 week after abruptly discontinuing chronic prednisone therapy. She complains of persistent nausea, vague abdominal pain, increasing weakness, and a 5-pound weight loss. Which of the following blood pressure findings will most likely be observed in this patient?
A. 20 mm Hg pressure difference between the right and left arms
B. 40 mm Hg increase in diastolic pressure compared to past pressures
C. 40 mm Hg fall in systolic pressure when the patient stands from a seated position
D. 80 mm Hg difference between systolic and diastolic pressures

104. A 70-year-old woman with coronary artery disease has a total cholesterol of 196 mg/dL, an HDL of 33 mg/dL, and an LDL of 135 mg/dL. She has followed a low-fat, low-cholesterol diet for 6 months. Which of the following is most appropriate at this time?
A. Continue current diet.
B. Prescribe gemfibrozil (Lopid).
C. Add oat bran.
D. Prescribe atorvastatin (Lipitor).

105. A 4-month-old infant presents with an acute onset of tachypnea, cough, rhinorrhea, and expiratory wheezing. Which of the following is the most likely cause?
A. Influenza
B. Adenovirus
C. *Streptococcus pneumoniae*
D. Respiratory syncytial virus

106. During a routine physical examination, a currently asymptomatic patient states that she had rheumatic fever as a child. This patient is at risk for developing which of the following conditions?
A. Dilated cardiomyopathy
B. Viral myocarditis
C. Mitral stenosis
D. Pulmonary embolism

107. A 56-year-old woman complains of vaginal irritation and dyspareunia for the past week. Physical examination reveals vaginal mucosal erythema, a cystocele, and a scant, pink-tinged discharge in the vaginal vault. Urinalysis is significant only for microscopic hematuria. Which of the following is the most likely diagnosis?
A. Atrophic vaginitis
B. Bacterial vaginosis
C. Vaginal candidiasis
D. Trichomonas vaginalis

108. An 18-year-old patient has a history of asthma. Nasal polyps are discovered. What other condition should be suspected in this patient?
A. Adenocarcinoma
B. Aspirin hypersensitivity
C. Cystic fibrosis
D. Rhinitis medicamentosa

109. A 58-year-old patient presents with insidious dyspnea and dry cough for 1 year. The patient gives a 10-year history of smoking, quitting more than 25 years ago. Physical examination reveals a thin patient with mild tachypnea, digital clubbing, and late inspiratory crackles. Which of the following is the most likely diagnosis?
A. Chronic obstructive pulmonary disease
B. Idiopathic pulmonary fibrosis
C. Sarcoidosis
D. Tuberculosis

110. Which of the following behavior descriptions is most characteristic of schizotypal personality disorder?
A. Hypersensitivity, excessive self-importance, and rigidity
B. Submissiveness, unable to make decisions, pessimism, and self-doubt
C. Withdrawal, oversensitivity, shyness, and detachment
D. Emotional instability, overreactivity, and self-dramatization

111. A 3-year-old child with a history of recurrent febrile seizures presents today with a temperature of 103°F. After treating the underlying cause of the fever, which of the following treatments is most appropriate?
    A. Diazepam
    B. Phenytoin
    C. Carbamazepine
    D. Ethosuximide

112. A 1-month-old infant has adherent white plaques on the buccal mucosa. She is feeding well, gaining weight, and otherwise healthy. Removal of the plaques reveals underlying erythematous mucosa. Which of the following is the most appropriate initial intervention?
    A. Amoxicillin
    B. Nystatin
    C. Ketoconazole
    D. Amphotericin B

113. A 19-year-old G1P0 at 32 weeks gestation returns to the clinic for routine prenatal care. Her last visit was two weeks ago. She has gained 10 pounds since then. Her weight gain is most likely a result of which of the following?
    A. A genetically large baby
    B. Eating too much
    C. Edema
    D. Rapid fetal growth

114. An otherwise healthy 56-year-old man presents to the clinic with chest pain. Myocardial infarction is not evident on ECG or enzymes. He is found to have left main coronary artery stenosis of 65%. Which of the following is the best long-term treatment for this patient?
    A. Prescribe daily aspirin to prevent myocardial infarction.
    B. Initiate nitrate therapy for angina.
    C. Begin aggressive risk factor reduction.
    D. Refer for coronary artery revascularization.

115. Which of the following exercises is most beneficial in preventing osteoporosis?
    A. Swimming
    B. Stair climbing
    C. Riding a bicycle
    D. Weight lifting

116. A 57-year-old woman complains of headaches and scalp tenderness. Examination reveals a fever with a normal WBC and an elevated ESR. Which of the following is the most likely diagnosis?
    A. Polymyalgia rheumatica
    B. Temporal arteritis
    C. Wegener's granulomatosis
    D. Sjögren's syndrome

117. A patient is diagnosed with hepatitis A. Which of the following medications should be administered to close contacts of this patient?

A. Chloramphenicol
B. Immune globulin
C. Corticosteroids
D. Interferon-α

118. Which of the following is indicated initially to establish the diagnosis in patients with orthostatic hypotension unaccompanied by syncope?
    A. Basal metabolic temperature
    B. Electrophysiologic testing
    C. Exercise stress testing
    D. Tilt-table testing

119. A 25-year-old woman complains of persistent abdominal and flank pain. She has been treated for numerous urinary tract infections in the past 3 years. Examination reveals palpable kidneys bilaterally. Urinalysis reveals microscopic hematuria. Which of the following diagnostic tests would be most helpful in confirming the suspected diagnosis?
    A. Abdominal plain-film radiography
    B. IV pyelography
    C. Retrograde urethrography
    D. Renal ultrasonography

120. A patient in her first pregnancy is admitted to labor and delivery with contractions every 4 minutes lasting 45 seconds. On admission, she was 4 cm dilated; 1 hour later, she is 5 cm dilated. Which of the following best describes her labor pattern?
    A. Labor is progressing too rapidly.
    B. She has reached the second stage of labor.
    C. There is adequate progress for the latent phase of labor.
    D. There is good progress for a first delivery.

121. Pituitary adenomas requiring surgical resection typically are removed via which approach?
    A. Subfrontal approach
    B. Subsphenoidal approach
    C. Transfrontal approach
    D. Transphenoidal approach

122. A 44-year-old man presents with frontal bossing, mandibular enlargement with prognathism, and increasing ring and shoe sizes. What is the best initial evaluation?
    A. CT of the abdomen
    B. Cerebral angiography
    C. MRI of the sella turcica
    D. Ultrasound of the neck

123. A patient presents for evaluation after right knee trauma. The anterior drawer sign results in a moderate degree of forward motion of the right knee compared to the left. What other physical examination finding is likely to be present in this patient?
    A. Lachman's sign
    B. McMurray's test

C. Abduction stress test
D. Medial/lateral stress test

124. A 63-year-old man with a history of atrial fibrillation describes a brief episode of confusion, hemiparesis, and unilateral visual loss. He is asymptomatic at this time. Which of the following studies would be most beneficial in the evaluation of this patient?
A. CT of the head
B. Cerebral angiography
C. Cardiac catheterization
D. Transesophageal echocardiogram

125. A 72-year-old woman presents with fatigue, dyspnea, and angina. Physical examination reveals pale conjunctivae, a grade II/VI pulmonary flow murmur, glossitis, and decreased vibratory sensation in the lower extremities. The CBC shows macrocytic indices and pancytopenia with macro-ovalocytes and hypersegmented neutrophils. Reticulocyte count is less than 2%. A deficiency of which of the following substances is most likely?
A. Vitamin B_{12}
B. Folic acid
C. G6PD
D. Iron

126. Which of the following best describes the pathology of Alzheimer's disease?
A. Gliosis and neuronal loss in the basal ganglia
B. Demyelinization and plaque formation
C. Plaques and neurofibrillary tangles
D. Degeneration of the dopaminergic nigrostriatal system

127. A 17-year-old woman presents to the clinic complaining of painful vulvar "sores," dysuria, and difficulty walking secondary to the pain. Her symptoms started this morning and were preceded by some mild tingling and itching last night. Pelvic examination reveals multiple vesicular lesions on an erythematous base on both labia minora. Which of the following is appropriate therapy?
A. Tetracycline
B. Metronidazole
C. Fluconazole (Diflucan)
D. Valacyclovir (Valtrex)

128. An 8-year-old child has a 3-day history of ear pain, which began after swimming in a neighbor's pool. There is severe tenderness upon movement of the pinna. Which of the following is the most appropriate initial treatment?
A. Auralgan otic solution
B. Carbamide peroxide (Debrox) otic solution
C. Oral cephalosporin
D. Ofloxacin otic solution

129. Which of the following is an example of proliferative diabetic retinopathy?
A. Microaneurysms and exudates
B. New vessels arising from the retina

C. White appearance to the retinal vessels
D. Retinal hemorrhage and edema

130. Women who are obese and older than 40 years are at higher risk for which of the following conditions?
A. Nephrolithiasis
B. Peptic ulcer disease
C. Pancreatitis
D. Cholelithiasis

131. Which of the following symptoms suggests diarrhea of an inflammatory etiology?
A. Large volume (>1 L/day)
B. Bloody diarrhea
C. Nausea and vomiting
D. Steatorrhea

132. A 72-year-old with adenocarcinoma of the lung located in the superior mediastinal area presents with headache, dizziness, visual loss, stupor, and near-syncope. Which of the following is most likely to be found on physical exam?
A. Bradycardia
B. Rhinophyma
C. Scattered rhonchi and wheeze
D. Swelling of the face and neck

133. Which of the following is the primary treatment of choice for a neonate with hyaline membrane disease?
A. RBC replacement with packed cells
B. 24 hours under biliary lamp
C. Surfactant replacement therapy
D. Provision of adequate supplemental oxygen

134. A patient with sarcoidosis presents with central nervous system symptoms and hypercalcemia. Which of the following is the treatment of choice?
A. Broad-spectrum antibiotics
B. Corticosteroids
C. Anticoagulants
D. Antivirals

135. Which of the following diseases is characterized by the presence of free light chains in the urine (Bence-Jones proteins) and abnormal serum proteins?
A. Acute lymphocytic leukemia
B. Hodgkin's lymphoma
C. Multiple myeloma
D. Non-Hodgkin's lymphoma

136. A 4-year-old child presents with acute onset of fever to 101°F. Physical examination reveals an erythematous tympanic membrane. Which of the following is the best additional physical examination technique to establish the diagnosis of otitis media?
A. Weber test
B. Auditory acuity
C. Pneumatic otoscopy
D. Retraction of the auricle

137. A 12-year-old male presents with a history of waking suddenly this morning with severe scrotal pain and edema of the scrotal sac, which has continued for 2 hours. He has had similar pain before, but it usually subsided without intervention. Physical examination reveals a tender, swollen, retracted testis. A routine urine examination is normal. Which of the following is the most appropriate next step?
A. Scrotal support and ice packs
B. Immediate surgical intervention
C. Initiation of antibiotic therapy
D. Technetium-99m pertechnetate scan

138. A 42-year-old woman who plays racquetball regularly presents with elbow pain. She complains of pain with wrist extension and lifting from the elbow. Examination reveals tenderness over the left lateral epicondyle. What is the most appropriate treatment?
A. Surgery
B. NSAIDs
C. Antibiotics
D. Injectable steroids

139. A 13-year-old girl presents with three slightly elevated papules on her face that are flat-topped, skin-colored, and 2 to 3 mm in diameter. Which of the following treatments is the best choice?
A. Bleomycin intradermal injection
B. Electrocautery
C. 40% salicylic acid plaster
D. Topical tretinoin cream

140. Which major neurotransmitter is most implicated in tobacco addiction?
A. Dopamine
B. Acetylcholine
C. Norepinephrine
D. Nicotinic acid

141. A 33-year-old patient presents with a hard, nontender swelling at the border of the upper eyelid. Which of the following test results would most clearly indicate that this lesion is a chalazion?
A. Biopsy showing granulomatous tissue consistent with chronic infection
B. Gram's stain of lesion contents showing Gram-positive cocci in clusters
C. Conjunctival scrapings with cytologic evidence of trachoma
D. Culture specimen of lesion positive for *Pseudomonas aeruginosa*

142. A 43-year-old patient who is overweight complains of dull achiness of the lower legs whenever standing for prolonged periods of time. Which of the following is most likely to be found on physical examination?
A. Decreased posterior tibia and dorsalis pedis pulses
B. Dilated tortuous veins in the posterior thigh and leg

C. Loss of pigment over the thighs and shins
D. Pitting edema in bilateral ankles

143. A 26-year-old, sexually active woman has been successfully treated for her third uncomplicated UTI in the past year. Physical examination is normal. Which of the following interventions would best prevent recurrence?
A. Urethral dilation
B. Condom usage with nonoxynol-9
C. Diaphragm usage with nonoxynol-9
D. Voiding immediately following intercourse

144. Which of the following medications increases both lower esophageal sphincter pressure and gastric emptying in the treatment of reflux esophagitis?
A. Antacids
B. H_2-receptor blockers
C. Metoclopramide (Reglan)
D. Proton-pump inhibitors

145. Which of the following prenatal screening tests is best obtained specifically between 24 and 28 weeks of gestation?
A. Urinalysis
B. Ultrasonography
C. α-Fetoprotein
D. Glucose tolerance screening

146. A patient presents in cardiogenic shock secondary to a large myocardial infarction. Which of the following is the expected finding on the echocardiogram?
A. Hyperkinesis of the infarcted segment
B. Hypertrophy of the right atrium
C. Severe regional wall-motion abnormalities
D. Transient increase in left ventricular function

147. A 57-year-old woman presents to the clinic complaining of a slight bloody vaginal discharge that has occurred intermittently for the past 3 months. This is the first bleeding she has experienced since going through menopause at age 51. Pelvic examination reveals an ulcerated lesion on the posterior wall of the lower third of the vagina. What is the most appropriate diagnostic study?
A. Viral culture
B. Endometrial biopsy
C. Lesion biopsy
D. Dark-field microscopy

148. Which of the following conditions will NOT respond to electroconvulsive therapy?
A. Severe depression
B. Psychoses during pregnancy
C. Chronic schizophrenic disorders
D. Catatonic states

149. In a patient with chronic heart failure, where is the apical pulse most likely to be located?

A. Along the left axillary border
B. High in the epigastric region
C. In the right second interspace
D. Under the left nipple

150. A 26-year-old man presents complaining of a stiff right knee that is extremely painful to move. He denies trauma or injury. He is sexually active with inconsistent use of barrier contraception. Examination reveals warmth and swelling in the right knee compared to the left. Aspiration reveals thick, purulent material. What is the next best step in management?
A. Admit to the hospital for IV antibiotics.
B. Administer ceftriaxone 125 mg IM now.
C. Refer to an orthopedic surgeon for evaluation.
D. Refer to a rheumatologist for evaluation.

151. Which of the following risk factors for suicidal behavior places a patient at the highest risk?
A. Alcohol dependence
B. Female gender
C. Previous attempt
D. Age younger than 40 years

152. A 64-year-old woman complains of wrist pain after falling on an outstretched hand. Plain radiographs indicate distal radial fracture with a fragment tilted upward and dorsally but without intra-articular involvement. What is the best management for this type of fracture?
A. A sugar tong splint for 2–3 weeks, followed by a short arm cast for 2-3 weeks
B. Internal surgical reduction and fixation
C. A gutter splint for 2–3 weeks, followed by physical therapy for 2–3 weeks
D. Percutaneous pinning of the fractured bone

153. Which of the following is a predisposing risk factor to thrombophlebitis that can give rise to the development of pulmonary embolism?
A. Von Willebrand's disease
B. Venous dilatation
C. Venous endothelial injury
D. Peripheral IV catheter

154. A 24-year-old woman presents for the first time with complaints of abdominal pain, bloating, and various food intolerance. Early in the conversation, she states she has seen six different health care providers over the past 2 years for her problems. Numerous tests have been run with no positive findings. Review of symptoms is positive for a number of abdominal complaints, periodic joint and back pain, paralysis occurring at various times, pain during intercourse, and menstrual irregularities. Which of the following is the most likely diagnosis?
A. Hypothyroidism
B. Major depression

C. Hypochondriasis
D. Somatization disorder

155. Which of the following test results represents the strongest evidence for the diagnosis of sarcoidosis?
A. Induced sputum cytology demonstrating mononuclear cells
B. Biopsy showing noncaseating granulomas
C. Elevated serum angiotensin-converting enzyme
D. High CD4:CD8 cell ratio by bronchoalveolar lavage

156. Classic pernicious anemia results from a deficiency of what substance?
A. Cobalamin
B. Folic acid
C. Intrinsic factor
D. Vitamin B_{12}

157. A 14-year-old boy presents with bilateral leg pain that has been worsening over the last 2 months. He denies trauma. Pain is exacerbated by running and jumping during basketball practice and typically is worse in the right leg. Examination reveals prominent tibial tubercles with tenderness bilaterally. What is the most likely diagnosis?
A. Patellofemoral dysfunction
B. Osgood-Schlatter disease
C. Osteochondritis dissecans
D. Sever's disease

158. A 43-year-old patient is brought to the emergency department with a steering-wheel injury to the chest following a motor-vehicle accident. Examination reveals that the patient's blood pressure is 130/90 mm Hg at the end of expiration and 114/92 mm Hg at the end of inspiration. Which of the following is the most likely diagnosis?
A. Cardiac tamponade
B. Pulmonary contusion
C. Diaphragmatic rupture
D. Pneumothorax

159. A 38-year-old man presents to the emergency department with his first episode of kidney stones. The pain resolves with ketorolac tromethamine (Toradol), and he is ready for discharge. Which of the following should be included in the discharge instructions?
A. Limiting zinc intake
B. Increasing fluid intake
C. Increasing vitamin D intake
D. Limiting carbohydrate intake

160. Which of the following studies is most useful for determining whether a thyroid nodule is malignant?
A. Thyroid ultrasound
B. Radioisotope scan of the thyroid
C. CT of the thyroid
D. Fine-needle aspiration cytology

161. A 43-year-old man with psoriasis developed severe pain in his lower back. Radiographs of his sacroiliac joints showed soft-tissue swelling, demineralization, erosions, and subchondral cysts. Which of the following medications would be most appropriate for chronic management of this pain?
A. Cyclosporine
B. Methotrexate
C. Intra-articular corticosteroid
D. Sulfasalazine

162. A 5-month-old child is brought to the emergency room for apparent abdominal pain. The child exhibits paroxysms of screaming and drawing up of the knees, followed by vomiting and diarrhea containing blood and mucus. The abdomen is distended, and a small mass is palpable in the upper midabdominal area. What is the recommended treatment?
A. Surgical intervention
B. Enema
C. Reduction via upper endoscopy
D. Fluid resuscitation and observation

163. Delayed primary closure of a laceration is best performed within a certain time interval after the initial wound event. Which of the following is the best time to close a wound using this technique?
A. 1–2 days
B. 2–4 days
C. 4–5 days
D. 7 days

164. A sexually active, monogamous woman has had three annual Pap smears that show no abnormalities. According to the American College of Obstetricians and Gynecologists, the recommended interval for a Pap smear in this woman is how many months?
A. 12 months
B. 18 months
C. 24 months
D. 36 months

165. A newborn has just received his first pertussis vaccination. Which of the following events would be a contraindication to additional doses?
A. Seizures within 5 days of administration
B. Encephalopathy within 7 days of administration
C. Fever of 102°F within 1 day of administration
D. An episode of inconsolable crying for several hours

166. In the evaluation of a patient with hematuria, the presence of RBC casts on microscopic examination of the urine suggests which of the following?
A. Glomerulonephritis
B. Cystitis
C. Pyelonephritis
D. Acute tubular necrosis

167. A stable, ambulatory patient is scheduled to undergo an exercise stress test. In which of the following conditions would the test be contraindicated?
A. Aortic stenosis
B. Essential hypertension
C. Recurrent precordial pain at rest
D. Stable angina

168. High-dose oxygen administration in patients with COPD may precipitate respiratory failure. This is because COPD patients have which of the following?
A. Reduced lung volume
B. Chronic hypercapnia
C. Right heart failure
D. Loss of lung elastic recoil

169. Which of the following is the treatment of choice when weight loss and alcohol restriction have failed to correct obstructive sleep apnea?
A. Uvulopalatopharyngoplasty
B. A tricyclic antidepressant
C. A bronchodilator
D. Nasal continuous positive air pressure

170. A 40-year-old man presents with dysphagia to both solids and liquids with frequent regurgitation of food after meals. He also complains of a nocturnal cough when supine and intermittent chest discomfort without dyspnea or diaphoresis. Barium swallow reveals a dilated esophagus, delayed esophageal emptying, and bird's beak deformity at the lower esophageal sphincter. Which of the following is the most likely diagnosis?
A. Achalasia
B. Esophageal carcinoma
C. GERD
D. Unstable angina

171. Which of the following descriptions is most consistent with uterine fibroids?
A. Normal-size uterus that is slightly softened and tender
B. Diffusely enlarged uterus that is firm and globular in shape
C. Slightly softened, tender, diffusely globular uterine enlargement
D. Firm, irregularly shaped, nontender, enlarged uterus

172. A 66-year-old man presents with a swollen, tender right leg. He denies trauma. Which of the following imaging studies would be the most appropriate initial step in diagnosing this patient?
A. Doppler ultrasound
B. Contrast venography
C. ^{125}I-fibrinogen scan
D. Impedance plethysmography

173. A 47-year-old presents with complaints of nervousness, frequent bowel movements, increased sweating, palpitations, and chest pain. Which of the following is the most likely diagnosis?
    A. Crohn's disease
    B. Adrenocorticoid insufficiency
    C. Irritable bowel syndrome
    D. Hyperthyroidism

174. A 10-month-old infant is brought to the office for evaluation of a day of noisy breathing and a barking cough that gets worse at night. This infant has a 1-week history of rhinorrhea, low-grade fever, and cough. The cough has progressively worsened over the last 3 days. On physical examination, the respiratory rate is 50 breaths/min, temperature is 100.6°F, and there is inspiratory stridor and a barking cough. The remainder of the examination is unremarkable. What is the most likely diagnosis?
    A. Croup
    B. Epiglottitis
    C. Foreign body in trachea
    D. Pneumonia

175. A 66-year-old man presents with a 1-week history of low-grade fever, nausea, vomiting, left lower quadrant abdominal pain, and constipation. Which of the following is the most likely diagnosis?
    A. Diverticulitis
    B. Pancreatitis
    C. Inguinal hernia
    D. Colon cancer

176. A 40-year-old man presents with hematuria and flank pain. Plain-film radiography shows a 2-cm calculus at the renal pelvis. BUN is elevated. Which of the following is the most appropriate intervention?
    A. Pyelolithotomy
    B. Fluids and analgesia
    C. Lithotripsy
    D. Allopurinol

177. A 65-year-old patient presents with progressive, bilateral central visual loss. Amsler grid testing is positive. What is expected on funduscopic exam?
    A. Cupping of the optic disc
    B. Clouded lens
    C. Retinal drusen
    D. Vitreous hemorrhage

178. An 18-year-old patient with a family history of psoriatic arthropathy presents 3 weeks after a minor fall caused an abrasion to her right knee. Although the abrasion was healing well, she now has a pink plaque surrounded by a thin border of fine, silvery scale where the injury had been. What feature does this represent?
    A. Auspitz sign
    B. Koebner's sign

C. Nikolsky's sign
D. Wickham's striae

179. A 68-year-old man with insulin-dependent diabetes mellitus and previously normal blood pressure has had readings of 200/110 mm Hg on two separate visits over the past 2 weeks. Diminished distal lower extremity pulses are noted. Which of the following diagnostic tests would be most helpful at this point?
    A. Serum uric acid
    B. Fasting lipid profile
    C. Renal arteriography
    D. IV pyelography

180. A 35-year-old man complains of gross painless hematuria immediately following a 10-mile run 2 days ago. He denies ever having seen blood in his urine before this occurrence. Which of the following is the most appropriate next step in diagnosing this patient?
    A. Urinalysis and urine culture
    B. PSA level
    C. Abdominal CT
    D. CBC with differential

181. A 25-year-old man presents with vague symptoms, including exertional dyspnea, headache, and leg fatigue gradually progressing in severity over the past 2 months. Physical examination reveals the following blood pressure measurements: RA, 180/100 mm Hg; LA, 148/92 mm Hg; RL, 124/76 mm Hg; and LL, 122/78 mm Hg. What is the most likely diagnosis?
    A. Coarctation of the aorta
    B. Constrictive pericarditis
    C. Dissecting thoracic aorta
    D. Transposition of the great vessels

182. The father of a healthy 6-year-old girl brings her to the clinic because of a "rash" that has been on her face for about 2 weeks. On examination, there are several discrete, oval to dome-shaped, flesh-colored papules on the face and neck, ranging in size from 1 to 5 mm. A plug of cheesy material can be expressed from some lesions. What is the most likely diagnosis?
    A. Milia
    B. Chickenpox
    C. Verruca vulgaris
    D. Molluscum contagiosum

183. Patient education for people with benign thyroid nodules should include which of the following pieces of information?
    A. Expect a thyroidectomy in the future.
    B. Most nodules continue to increase in size.
    C. Benign nodules carry a significant risk of malignant conversion.
    D. Management of benign nodules consists of periodic palpation and rebiopsy, if indicated.

184. Two days ago, a 40-year-old woman injured herself with a garden stake, inducing a laceration of the skin in the right popliteal space. At present, the wound and surrounding tissue appear to be infected. She states that she has never been immunized against tetanus. After cleansing, debridement and dressing of the wound, which of the following is the best treatment?
    A. Admit for IV antibiotics and tetanus immune globulin (TIG).
    B. Administer Td and TIG at separate sites, and discharge with broad-spectrum antibiotics.
    C. Administer TIG now, discharge with oral antibiotics, and return for Td in 6 weeks.
    D. Admit for IV antibiotics and local whirlpool treatments, and monitor for signs of systemic tetanus.

185. Adjunctive heparin therapy is indicated with which of the following thrombolytic agents in the treatment of acute myocardial infarction?
    A. Urokinase
    B. Streptokinase
    C. Anistreplase
    D. Tissue plasminogen activator

186. Chemotherapy is now used as adjunctive treatment of patients with curable breast cancer and positive axillary nodes. What is the objective of this chemotherapeutic treatment?
    A. Cure the breast cancer itself
    B. Prevent metastases from occurring
    C. Eliminate any existing occult metastases
    D. Treat the positive axillary nodes

187. An 18-month-old child is brought to the emergency department several hours after the onset of acute dyspnea, cough, and stridor. Physical examination reveals inspiratory stridor and wheezing over the right upper lobe. Which of the following is most likely to relieve the symptoms?
    A. Bronchoscopy
    B. Oral steroid therapy
    C. Chest postural drainage
    D. Albuterol nebulizer treatment

188. Which of the following symptoms is the most typical manifestation of acoustic neuroma?
    A. Unilateral hearing loss
    B. Rotational vertigo
    C. Tinnitus
    D. Facial numbness

189. A patient with cellulitis of the dorsum of the left hand is noted to have nontender red streaks extending proximally from the site of infection. This is caused by which of the following?
    A. Erysipelas
    B. Lymphangitis

C. Necrotizing fasciitis
D. Thrombophlebitis

190. Which of the following osteoporosis medications may increase bone mineral density in postmenopausal women?
    A. Estrogen
    B. Raloxifene (Evista)
    C. Alendronate (Fosamax)
    D. Calcitonin

191. Clinical or subclinical rubella is associated with a number of congenital and developmental defects. During what time period is contracting this disease most likely to cause defects?
    A. Anytime during pregnancy
    B. During the immediate neonatal period
    C. During the first trimester of pregnancy
    D. During the second trimester of pregnancy

192. Which of the following is the most common causative organism of meningitis in children from 2 to 4 years of age?
    A. *Streptococcus pneumoniae*
    B. Group B β-hemolytic streptococcus
    C. *Haemophilus influenzae*
    D. *Listeria monocytogenes*

193. A 62-year-old woman has diverticula demonstrated on barium enema. What advice or recommendation should be given to this patient to avoid possible future problems?
    A. Follow a high-fiber diet.
    B. Take laxatives regularly.
    C. Follow a low-residue diet.
    D. Limit fluid intake at mealtime.

194. Most sudden cardiac deaths are caused by which of the following arrhythmias?
    A. Atrial tachycardia
    B. Bradycardia
    C. Multifocal atrial tachycardia
    D. Ventricular fibrillation

195. Which of the following is the most specific indication for dialysis in a patient with chronic renal failure?
    A. Anasarca
    B. Severe metabolic acidosis
    C. Hypoalbuminemia
    D. Oliguria

196. A sexually active, 25-year-old man presents with severe dysuria and a thick penile discharge. He reports that he had unprotected sex 1 week ago. A Gram's stain reveals intracellular Gram-negative diplococci. What is the best treatment option?
    A. Benzathine penicillin
    B. Azithromycin (Zithromax)
    C. Doxycycline
    D. Ceftriaxone (Rocephin)

197. Which of the following is indicated for treatment of *Chlamydia trachomatis* cervicitis in a pregnant female?
  A. Oral tetracycline
  B. Oral metronidazole
  C. Vaginal metronidazole
  D. Oral erythromycin

198. A 6-year-old girl presents in early spring with fever and a "slapped-check" appearance and a rash along the extremities, sparing the palms and soles. The caregiver explains that the rash started with small, raised red bumps on the cheeks. About 10 days ago, she had a mild upper respiratory infection. Which of the following treatments is indicated?
  A. Erythromycin
  B. Hospitalization
  C. Supportive care measures
  D. Topical, low-potency steroid cream

199. What is the recommended guideline for the frequency of a clinical foot examination as part of ongoing medical care for patients with diabetes?
  A. Monthly
  B. Quarterly
  C. Yearly
  D. Every other year

200. A 9-year-old child develops hives and shortness of breath after a bee sting. What is the most appropriate first step in management?
  A. Immediate tracheotomy
  B. IV antihistamines
  C. Oxygen under positive pressure
  D. Prompt administration of epinephrine

201. A patient has been treated for 4 weeks with antiulcer medications. The pain and reflux symptoms have not abated. He also complains of diarrhea and weight loss. Which of the following is the diagnostic test of choice for the suspected diagnosis?
  A. Serum gastrin
  B. Serum amylase
  C. Cholecystokinin
  D. Hemoglobin A_{1c}

202. A patient presents to the emergency department complaining of vomiting blood-streaked material. For 2 days, she has been ill and retching. What finding is expected on upper endoscopy?
  A. Linear mucosal tear proximal to the gastric mucosa
  B. Protrusion of pharyngeal mucosa at the pharyngoesophageal junction
  C. Several discrete shallow and deep ulcers
  D. Thin, diaphragm-like membrane in the mid or upper esophagus

203. A 36-year-old schoolteacher presents with an acute onset of fever, chills, malaise, headache, and congestion. She is coughing and sneezing. Conjunctivae are injected; pharyngeal mucosa is edematous and injected. What is expected on examination of the lungs?
  A. Clear lung fields with good air exchange
  B. Diffuse expiratory wheezes
  C. Dullness and rhonchi at the bases
  D. Scattered crackles and inspiratory wheeze

204. Which of the following is a positive sign of pregnancy?
  A. Amenorrhea
  B. Nausea and vomiting
  C. Cyanosis of the vulva and vaginal walls
  D. Palpable fetal movement

205. Which of the following is the best initial intervention for a large tension pneumothorax with cyanosis?
  A. Intubation
  B. Supplemental oxygen via nasal cannula
  C. Needle aspiration
  D. Insertion of a thoracotomy tube

206. A child living with a person newly diagnosed as having active tuberculosis has a negative initial skin test. Which of the following is the most appropriate next step in the management of this child?
  A. Repeat the skin test in 6 months.
  B. Start the child on isoniazid therapy.
  C. Obtain chest radiography.
  D. Obtain sputum cultures.

207. A middle-aged woman's blood work reveals megaloblastic anemia. She has followed a strict vegan diet for the past 10 years and denies having taken any vitamin or mineral supplements. What is the best treatment for her anemia?
  A. Cobalamin
  B. Iron
  C. Folate
  D. Vitamin D

208. A 17-year-old football player presents after an ankle injury. The mechanism of injury was external rotation of the foot. Physical examination reveals localized tenderness over the anterior tibiofibular ligament, swelling, and bruising of the area extending over the dorsum of the foot. Talar tilt and anterior drawer tests indicate no loss of stability, and the patient is able to bear weight. What is the most appropriate treatment for this patient?
  A. Local injection of steroids
  B. Surgical reconstruction
  C. RICE therapy and ROM exercises
  D. Short leg cast for 6–8 weeks

209. A 7-week-old male child develops acute heart failure. Physical examination is significant for weak and delayed femoral pulses, and a late systolic ejection murmur best heard at the base and posteriorly. Which of the following is the most likely diagnosis?

A. Coarctation of the aorta
B. Pulmonary stenosis
C. Tetralogy of Fallot
D. Ventricular septal defect

210. What is the best single screening test for thyroid disease?
A. Free T_4
B. T_3 resin uptake
C. Free T_4 index
D. Thyroid-stimulating hormone

211. In an examination of visual fields by confrontation, a bitemporal hemianopia is noted. A lesion is most likely to be at which of the following locations?
A. Optic nerve
B. Optic chiasm
C. Optic tract
D. Optic radiation

212. An 18-year-old woman presents to the emergency department with vomiting and diarrhea. She states that it started abruptly about 6 hours after attending a family picnic. The patient ate grilled chicken with potato salad and chocolate cream pie. She is afebrile and has active bowel sounds. Which of the following is the most likely diagnosis?
A. *Escherichia coli* O157:H7
B. Rotavirus
C. *Salmonella typhi*
D. *Staphylococcus aureus*

213. A 24-year-old woman complains of pain at the base of her right thumb, which is prohibiting her from picking up her 2-year-old son. Examination reveals tenderness just distal to the radial styloid process without crepitation. Additionally, with the patient clenching her fist over a flexed thumb, forceful ulnar deviation of the hand elicits pain at the radial styloid process. Radiograhic findings are normal. Which of the following is the most likely diagnosis?
A. De Quervain's disease
B. Degenerative joint disease
C. Gonococcal tenosynovitis
D. Carpometacarpal joint fracture

214. A 60-year-old man with a 30 pack-year history of smoking presents with progressive dysphagia for solids over the past 6 months. He states that he has often had to regurgitate his food because of a feeling of a blockage. He has lost 10% of his body weight unintentionally. Which of the following is the initial diagnostic test of choice?
A. Barium esophagography
B. PA chest radiography
C. Ultrasonography
D. Esophageal motility studies

215. A 26-year-old woman required six units of whole blood and 12 units of packed RBCs during a trauma resuscitation and surgical repair of liver and splenic lacerations. The patient is now 6 hours postoperative and has blood oozing from the suture line and IV sites. There is bloody urine in the Foley bag. Laboratory evaluation demonstrates a platelet count of 10,000 cells/µL, prolonged prothrombin level, and the presence of fibrin split products. Which of the following is the most likely diagnosis?
A. Acute ABO incompatibility reaction
B. Disseminated intravascular coagulation
C. Exacerbation of idiopathic thrombocytopenia
D. Inadequate repair of the liver lacerations

216. A mother contacts the outpatient clinic stating that her 8-year-old son is having an asthma attack. She has given him two treatments of 2.5 mg of albuterol by nebulizer 30 minutes apart without relief. He continues to sit very still, leaning forward slightly, and only uses one word answers to her questions. Which of the following would be the most appropriate next step?
A. Instruct the mother to give two additional nebulizer treatments and then call back.
B. Prescribe prednisone, and follow up the next morning.
C. Prescribe salmeterol (Serevent) and a long-acting β_2-agonist.
D. Send him to the emergency department for further evaluation.

217. A 65-year-old patient with resected adenocarcinoma of the colon presents for follow-up. Which of the following tumor markers should be ordered to monitor for the recurrence of colon cancer?
A. α-Fetoprotein
B. Carcinoembryonic antigen
C. Cancer antigen 19-9
D. Cancer antigen 125

218. What is the best advice for prevention of knee osteoarthritis in female athletes?
A. Maintain ideal body weight.
B. Use nonsteroidals early and as often as necessary.
C. Continue in contact sports to stay in shape.
D. Take daily multivitamins containing vitamin A.

219. What bone is most commonly affected by osteosarcoma?
A. Proximal tibia
B. Proximal humerus
C. Scapula
D. Distal femur

220. A 22-year-old, newly married woman with no significant past medical history presents with increasing urinary urgency, frequency, and dysuria. She denies fever, vaginal discharge, flank pain, or a history of similar symptoms. Which of the following is the most likely causative organism?

A. *Escherichia coli*
B. *Klebsiella pneumoniae*
C. *Chlamydia trachomatis*
D. *Pseudomonas aeruginosa*

221. A 52-year-old man complains of fatigue, headache, and dizziness for several weeks. Examination reveals flushed face, retinal vein engorgement, and splenomegaly. The CBC shows the following: WBC 13,000 cells/mcL; Hgb 18 g/dL; Hct 58%; and thrombocytes 750,000 cells/mcL. Smear is normal. Which of the following is the recommended management in this case?
   A. Allopurinol
   B. Diphenhydramine
   C. Phlebotomy
   D. Prednisone

222. On a routine preoperative chest radiograph in a 60-year-old asymptomatic male, a solitary lung nodule is detected. Which of the following is the most likely diagnosis?
   A. AV malformation
   B. Primary lung cancer
   C. Granuloma
   D. Bronchogenic cysts

223. Which of the following arterial blood gases is consistent with a 25-year-old patient suffering from an acute asthma attack at its initial stage?
   A. pH 7.50; PaCO$_2$, 45 mm Hg; PaO$_2$, 55 mm Hg
   B. pH 7.30; PaCO$_2$, 55 mm Hg; PaO$_2$, 75 mm Hg
   C. pH 7.40; PaCO$_2$, 65 mm Hg; PaO$_2$, 77 mm Hg
   D. pH 7.46; PaCO$_2$, 30 mm Hg; PaO$_2$, 99 mm Hg

224. A 21-year-old woman is admitted for inpatient treatment of an eating disorder. She is 24% below the expected weight for her height. Vital signs include T 95.4°F, P 58, R 22, and BP 84/50. Mucous membranes are dry and cracked; eyes are sunken. What is the first consideration in management?
   A. Begin an SSRI.
   B. Restore nutritional status.
   C. Treat the underlying depression.
   D. Begin behavioral therapy.

225. A patient presents to the office at the insistence of his employer. The patient voices marked persecutory delusions and also reveals he hears a voice that tells him who are friends and who are enemies. He is guarded, tense, and reserved. What subtype of schizophrenia is this patient exhibiting?
   A. Catatonic schizophrenia
   B. Paranoid schizophrenia
   C. Disorganized schizophrenia
   D. Undifferentiated schizophrenia

226. Which of the following best describes a precordial thrill?
   A. It almost always represents a normal finding.
   B. It often is an indication of congestive heart failure.

C. It is related to a murmur of at least grade IV/VI.
D. It is best felt with the examiner's finger pads.

227. Which of the following diagnostic tests is best to diagnose trichomonas vaginitis?
   A. Colposcopy
   B. KOH preparation
   C. Wet-mount smear
   D. Dark-field microscopy

228. A patient complains of heartburn relieved with antacids. Which of the following should the patient be told to avoid?
   A. Milk
   B. Smoking
   C. Exercise
   D. High-protein foods

229. Which of the following indicates a need for surgical referral in a patient with varicose veins?
   A. Pain with prolonged standing
   B. Multiple varicosities in both legs
   C. Development of superficial phlebitis
   D. Varicosities in a patient younger than 30 years

230. An elderly woman complains of a scratchy feeling in her eye. Examination reveals an inward turning of the lower lid margin. Which of the following interventions is the most helpful?
   A. Artificial tears
   B. Botulinum toxin injections
   C. Pilocarpine
   D. Topical antibiotics

231. A 30-year-old man has recent-onset diabetes mellitus. He is 5 ft 7 in. tall and weighs 200 lbs. He has polydipsia/polyuria. Urine shows 3+ glucose and no ketones. Fasting blood sugar is 180 gm/dL. Which of the following is the initial treatment of choice?
   A. An oral hypoglycemic agent
   B. Diet and exercise
   C. Long-acting insulin each morning
   D. Short-acting insulin before meals

232. What is the most appropriate initial management for an acute peritonsillar abscess?
   A. Oral antibiotics
   B. Incision and drainage
   C. MRI to assess extent
   D. Supportive care

233. A 22-year-old woman presents for evaluation of urinary frequency and burning following an ocean cruise with her new husband. This morning, she noted gross hematuria. Physical examination is unremarkable. Which of the following is the most likely diagnosis?
   A. Acute cystitis
   B. Nephrolithiasis

C. Bladder carcinoma

D. Acute pyelonephritis

234. A previously healthy, 30-year-old man reports that while having intercourse, he suddenly developed a severe headache. Over the next several minutes, he became increasingly lethargic. He is anxious and confused. Which of the following is the most likely diagnosis?

A. Migraine

B. Meningitis

C. A seizure disorder

D. A subarachnoid hemorrhage

235. A patient is brought to the clinic with a burn on the left upper extremity. The skin of the affected limb appears pearly white and waxy without blistering. On examination, the patient is unable to feel any sensations over the affected area. Which of the following is the correct classification of this patient's burn?

A. First degree

B. Second degree

C. Third degree

D. Minor burn

236. Which of the following is the recommended route of administration for desmopressin in the treatment of central diabetes insipidus?

A. Oral

B. Intravenous

C. Subcutaneous

D. Intranasal

237. A 6-year-old child presents for follow-up care 12 days after discharge following new onset of idiopathic grand mal seizures. The family history is significant for seizure disorder. The child was started on a standard dose of phenobarbital and, other than mild sedation, is seizure-free and symptom-free. Which of the following is now the best choice for ongoing treatment?

A. Discontinue phenobarbital, and begin carbamazepine.

B. Obtain blood today to check for a therapeutic drug level.

C. Add phenytoin to the regimen.

D. Obtain baseline CBC and liver function tests.

238. A 32-year-old presents with monoarticular arthritis of the metatarsal–phalangeal joint of the right first digit. It is warm and tender on examination. Which of the following synovial fluid findings would be diagnostic?

A. WBC count of 50,000 cells/μL

B. Glucose of 23 mg/dL

C. Uric acid crystals

D. 22% PMN count

239. The administration of short-acting anticholinesterase not only will treat this illness but also can be used as a diagnostic tool.

A. Myasthenia gravis

B. Multiple sclerosis

C. Hypokalemic periodic paralysis syndrome

D. Myasthenic syndrome

240. A 22-year-old patient presents with a 2-day history of nasal congestion, headache, clear and watery nasal discharge, and sneezing without fever. Physical examination reveals edematous nasal mucosa with clear watery discharge. Which of the following is the most likely diagnosis?

A. Acute sinusitis

B. Vasomotor rhinitis

C. Viral rhinitis

D. Nasal vestibulitis

241. A synovial fluid analysis performed on a patient with a knee effusion reveals the following results:

Volume	5.0 mL
Clarity	opaque
White blood cells	4,000 cells/μL
Culture	negative

Which of the following is the most likely cause of this patient's condition?

A. Trauma

B. Osteoarthritis

C. Septic arthritis

D. Rheumatoid arthritis

242. A 66-year-old patient complains of fatigue and depression. The TSH is elevated. Which of the following is most likely to also be found in this patient's presentation?

A. Moist skin

B. Hair loss

C. Restlessness

D. Constipation

243. A 66-year-old man with type 1 diabetes mellitus presents with worsening angina pectoris. After 3 days of therapy with propranolol (Inderal), he is symptom-free. On the fourth hospital day, he is difficult to arouse. On examination, his skin is warm and dry, pulse is 52 bpm, and blood pressure is 128/62 mm Hg. He is lethargic, disoriented, and without focal neurologic findings. What is the most important first step in management of this patient?

A. Administer 50% glucose IV.

B. Discontinue administration of propranolol.

C. Perform a lumbar puncture and spinal fluid analysis.

D. Reduce the dosage of propranolol, and administer dopamine.

244. A 40-year-old man presents with a painless, fleshy conjunctival substance that is encroaching on the nasal side of his left cornea. He is a groundskeeper who rarely uses protective goggles while working outside. Which of the following is the most likely diagnosis?

A. Chalazion
B. Conjunctivitis
C. Dacryocystitis
D. Pterygium

245. Which of the following cell forms is responsible for bone resorption?
A. Osteocytes
B. Osteoclasts
C. Osteoblasts
D. Osteophytes

246. A 58-year-old man with an 80-pack-year history of smoking presents with increasing shortness of breath. He has had a productive morning cough for the past 2 years. Physical examination reveals a man who is obese with plethoric facies and wheezes and rhonchi on auscultation. Which of the following is the most likely diagnosis?
A. Bronchial asthma
B. Chronic bronchitis
C. Emphysema
D. Lung cancer

247. A 1-year-old child in day care is found to have an elevated temperature. Physical examination reveals an erythematous tympanic membrane with decreased mobility. This is the infant's first episode of these symptoms. Which of the following is the best recommendation?
A. No treatment necessary
B. Oral ciprofloxacin
C. Cortisporin otic suspension
D. Oral amoxicillin

248. A 2-year-old child presents with diffuse, 2- to 5-mm, nonpruritic maculopapular lesions that started on the trunk and subsequently spread to neck, face, and proximal extremities. During the preceding 3 days, the child had fevers of 101 to 102°F but is afebrile now. Which of the following is the most likely diagnosis?
A. Roseola
B. Measles
C. Rubella
D. Chickenpox

249. A 26-year-old patient presents complaining of itchy, watery eyes and sneezing. Further history shows a pattern of similar symptoms each spring. Which of the following is the best initial treatment?
A. Oral antihistamines
B. Intranasal corticosteroids
C. Oral decongestants
D. Intranasal cromolyn

250. What is the most typical presentation of Hodgkin's disease?
A. Virchow's node
B. Painful inguinal adenopathy
C. Painless progressive dyspnea
D. A painless swelling in the neck

251. A 26-year-old female presents to the emergency department at 10 weeks gestation with complaints of severe cramps and heavy vaginal bleeding. She states she passed some tissue earlier. Examination reveals blood in the vaginal vault and a patent cervical os. Which of the following is the most likely diagnosis?
A. A threatened abortion
B. An inevitable abortion
C. An incomplete abortion
D. A complete abortion

252. A 27-year-old woman presents for evaluation of a rash. Her trunk is covered with multiple red- to copper-colored papulosquamous lesions, and she has discrete, coppery, keratotic papules on the palms of her hands and her tongue. Pelvic examination reveals soft, flat, moist, pinkish nodules on the perineum. Which of the following tests will give the most information about the etiology of these lesions?
A. VDRL or RPR
B. KOH prep
C. HIV test
D. Pap smear with HPV

253. A patient presents with a sudden onset of knee pain after a twisting injury while playing soccer. Physical examination reveals a positive Lachman's test and a bulge sign. Which of the following ligaments is the most likely to be injured?
A. Medial collateral
B. Anterior cruciate
C. Lateral collateral
D. Posterior cruciate

254. Patients with gout may prevent deposition of urate crystal by avoiding which of the following foods?
A. Lettuce and tomatoes
B. Milk products
C. Red meat
D. Refined cereals

255. In a patient with coronary artery disease, which of the following most significantly reduces the risk of heart failure?
A. Daily exercise
B. Control of hypertension
C. Reduced sodium diet
D. Lipid-lowering therapy

256. Which of the following preoperative management options best decreases the risk of postoperative abdominal wound complications?
A. Low-salt, low-cholesterol diet
B. Smoking cessation
C. An aspirin a day
D. Prophylactic antibiotics

257. An elderly man who recently emigrated from a war-torn area of Africa is brought to the clinic by his daughter. She explains that her father's diet was very limited in calories and protein and that he mostly ate corn and very little fresh foods. He has chronic diarrhea. Physical examination reveals pigmented regions on sun-exposed areas and mild dementia. The tongue is smooth and shiny. This patient most likely has a deficiency of which vitamin?
   A. Folate
   B. Niacin
   C. Thiamine
   D. Vitamin K

258. A mother brings in her 4-year-old son for routine care. The boy has red hair and blue eyes. What is the most important advice regarding the boy's long-term skin health?
   A. Use only mild, nonirritating soap.
   B. Avoid sun exposure as much as possible.
   C. Use plenty of moisturizer or other lotions.
   D. Avoid chocolate as the boy approaches adolescence.

259. A patient has a palpable thyroid nodule. What is the best way to determine if the nodule is cystic or solid?
   A. CT of the neck/thyroid
   B. Fine-needle aspiration
   C. Radioactive iodine uptake
   D. Ultrasonography

260. Prinzmetal's (variant) angina is best characterized by which of the following ECG changes?
   A. Transient ST-segment elevations
   B. Transient ST-segment depressions
   C. ST-segment depression without Q waves
   D. ST-segment elevation with Q waves

261. A mother brings in her 5-year-old daughter to the office because of bilateral cheek redness for 2 days. Two days prior, the patient experienced mild fever, headache, and malaise. What can you tell the mother about the most likely course of this illness?
   A. A reticulated or lacy rash may appear on the trunk and extremities.
   B. The cheek erythema will progress to vesicles before crusting over and healing.
   C. She will likely develop red macules on the buccal mucosa and tongue.
   D. A symmetric polyarthritis will likely develop, lasting 2–3 weeks.

262. Which of the following is the most common ECG finding in adults with coarctation of the aorta?
   A. Atrial fibrillation
   B. Tachycardia
   C. Left ventricular hypertrophy
   D. Right-axis deviation

263. A patient is initially charming, likeable, and lively but later becomes seductive, emotionally unstable, and manipulative. This patient most likely has which of the following personality disorders?
   A. Borderline
   B. Histrionic
   C. Narcissistic
   D. Schizoid

264. A 30-year-old man complains of three severe headaches in the past 5 days. He describes the pain as unilateral, knife-like, periorbital pain with tearing and nasal congestion. The pain lasts for 1–2 hours and then abruptly stops. Which of the following is the most likely diagnosis?
   A. Cluster headaches
   B. Paroxysmal hemicrania
   C. Sinus neoplasia
   D. Trigeminal neuralgia

265. A patient presents with nasal congestion with purulent discharge, facial pain, fever, and pain in the upper teeth. What is the most likely diagnosis?
   A. Otitis media
   B. Dental abscess
   C. Acute sinusitis
   D. Allergic rhinitis

266. A nursing home patient has a well-demarcated, shallow ulcer in the sacral area. Necrotic tissue overlies the ulcer and extends through the dermis to the subcutaneous fat. What stage decubitus does this represent?
   A. I
   B. II
   C. III
   D. IV

267. A patient presents with a complaint of painless, bright red blood from the rectum, with small amounts of blood noticed on toilet paper after a bowel movement. What is the most likely diagnosis?
   A. An anorectal fissure
   B. A fistula
   C. A perianal abscess
   D. Internal hemorrhoids

268. A patient has an intense fear of dirt and germs. Her fear has become so great that it affects her ability to maintain relationships or to keep a job. What is the cornerstone of therapy?
   A. Antianxiety medication
   B. Antidepressants
   C. Hypnosis
   D. Desensitization therapy

269. Seventy-two hours after total knee replacement, an otherwise healthy, 57-year-old man develops tachycardia, hand tremor, and nausea. He becomes very anxious, agitated, and tells the nursing staff "millions of

ants are crawling over my skin and sheets." Two hours later, he has a new-onset tonic clonic seizure. Which of the following is the acute treatment of choice?
A. Carbamazepine (Tegretol)
B. Clonidine (Catapres)
C. Diazepam (Valium)
D. Phenytoin (Dilantin)

270. Which of the following is most closely associated with cervical dysplasia?
A. Herpes simplex virus
B. *Trichomonas vaginalis*
C. *Chlamydia trachomatis*
D. Human papilloma virus

271. Which of the following examination findings is most consistent with acute appendicitis?
A. Decreased pain when the patient flexes the hip against resistance
B. Rebound tenderness in the left upper quadrant
C. Increased pain when palpating the right lower quadrant
D. Decreased pain with Valsalva maneuvers

272. A patient presents to the emergency department with epistaxis. Examination reveals bleeding from the anterior nares. External digital pressure for 10 minutes fails to stop the bleeding. Which of the following is the next best step in management?
A. Internal digital compression of Kiesselbach's plexus
B. Packing with petroleum-impregnated gauze
C. Topical nasal application of cocaine and silver nitrate cauterization
D. Topical nasal application of thrombin and packing with gelatin sponge

273. A patient with type 1 diabetes arrives in the emergency department after a rapid onset of frequent urination, excessive thirst, headache, nausea, and vomiting. He gives a history of abdominal pain that has progressively worsened over the last 2 days. Initial laboratory results show that the patient is hyperglycemic, acidotic, and ketotic. Which of the following should be the next intervention?
A. Administer IV replacement fluids and monitor glucose.
B. Administer bicarbonate with an IV bolus, and monitor potassium levels.
C. Start 5% dextrose IV fluids and subcutaneous insulin injections.
D. Start normal saline IV fluids and an insulin IV drip.

274. Lithium therapy requires periodic clinical monitoring. Which of the following is most important to obtain at baseline and then periodically during follow-up in patients receiving lithium?
A. Hemoglobin and hematocrit
B. BUN and creatinine

C. AST/ALT
D. Echocardiogram

275. A 15-year-old patient presents with a 2-day history of low-grade fever, malaise, and cough. The cough was initially dry but has become productive of white sputum with streaks of blood. Physical examination reveals diffuse rhonchi but no wheezing or dullness to percussion. Which of the following is the most likely diagnosis?
A. Bronchiolitis
B. Pneumonia
C. Acute bronchitis
D. Tuberculosis

276. Which of the following findings is most useful in differentiating central from peripheral vertigo?
A. Vertical nystagmus
B. Sensory hearing loss
C. Horizontal nystagmus
D. Conductive hearing loss

277. A 70-year-old male with hypertension complains of urinary hesitancy, decreased force and caliber of stream, frequency, urgency, and nocturia. Which of the following medications would be most beneficial for this patient?
A. ACE inhibitors
B. Calcium channel blockers
C. α-Blockers
D. Direct vasodilators

278. A woman presents for prenatal care. Her LMP was 7 weeks ago. She has had five previous pregnancies with the following outcomes: one elective abortion at 9 weeks; one spontaneous abortion at 12 weeks; one ectopic pregnancy; delivery of a singleton at 40 weeks; and delivery of a singleton at 37.5 weeks. She has two living children. Which of the following correctly designates her obstetric history?
A. G5 P2112
B. G5 P2012
C. G6 P2132
D. G6 P2032

279. Which of the following is most likely to cause an increase in the plasma ratio of BUN to creatinine?
A. Urinary obstruction
B. Congestive heart failure
C. Cefoxitin therapy
D. Trimethoprim/sulfamethoxazole therapy

280. A 50-year-old man presents with persistent and progressive hoarseness over a 2-month period. The history also includes 40 pack-years of smoking. Physical examination reveals a 2-cm, firm, nontender, anterior-cervical chain lymph node. Which of the following is the most likely diagnosis?
A. Laryngitis
B. Thyroid cancer

C. Laryngeal cancer

D. Vocal cord nodules

281. A 42-year-old male complains of epigastric pain described as gnawing. The pain is relieved with food, although his appetite is depressed. Urea breath test is positive. Which of the following is a recommended treatment regimen.

A. Monotherapy with a proton-pump inhibitor for 12 weeks, repeated twice after a 2-week period of no therapy

B. Proton-pump inhibitor and clarithromycin and amoxicillin (metronidazole if penicillin allergic) twice daily for 10–14 days

C. Proton-pump inhibitor plus H_2-receptor agonists for 3 months with amoxicillin (or metronidazole) added after the first month

D. Proton-pump inhibitor plus H_2-receptor agonist and a bland diet for 10–14 days

282. A 3-year-old child has been diagnosed with a third episode of otitis media in 9 months. The parents request advice on nonmedical preventive techniques. Which of the following should be suggested?

A. Place tympanostomy tubes.

B. Humidify the air in the child's bedroom.

C. Administer decongestants.

D. Avoid smoking in the home and near the child.

283. An 85-year-old is admitted to the hospital for confusion of new onset. Physical examination reveals an area in the right upper anterior chest that has dullness to percussion, bronchial breath sounds, and increased tactile fremitus. The rest of the lung fields are clear. He is afebrile. Which of the following is the most likely diagnosis?

A. Pneumonia

B. Pulmonary edema

C. Pulmonary embolism

D. Pulmonary hypertension

284. Which of the following quadrants is the most common site of retinal detachment?

A. Superior temporal

B. Superior medial

C. Inferior temporal

D. Inferior medial

285. A mother brings her 3-year-old daughter to the clinic. The child has lesions in her mouth that have caused pain when eating for the last 2 days. The mother states the child has decreased intake of foods/liquids and a low-grade fever. Examination reveals small, white ulcers on the oral mucosa, red gingivae, and regional lymphadenopathy. Which of the following is the most likely diagnosis?

A. Acute lye ingestion

B. Drug eruption

C. Herpetic gingivostomatitis

D. Herpangina

286. A 34-year-old man has recently been diagnosed with exercise-induced asthma. Which of the following is the best management?

A. Cromolyn inhaler 20 minutes before exercise

B. A β_2-agonist at the onset of symptoms

C. Theophylline daily as prophylaxis

D. Increase conditioning to relieve symptoms

287. A 40-year-old male with no significant medical history is diagnosed with a benign hepatic tumor that has no malignant potential. The tumor was found incidentally during ultrasonography. What is the most likely type of hepatic tumor?

A. Adenoma

B. Hepatoblastoma

C. Mixed hematoma

D. Hemangioma

288. An HIV-positive patient seeks medical care for multiple round, waxy, dome-shaped papules on the face, hands, inner thighs, and genitals. These lesions have a central umbilication. Which of the following is the best choice for managing this skin disorder?

A. No treatment needed

B. Application of liquid nitrogen

C. 40% salicylic acid after paring

D. Paring after warm-water soaks

289. A neonate was born to an Rh-negative mother. Rh immune globulin (Rho-Gam) is most effective if given to the mother within what time frame after delivery?

A. 72 hours

B. 96 hours

C. 5 days

D. 7 days

290. A 28-year-old woman presents with mild left lower quadrant fullness for the past week. Her last menstrual period was 3 weeks ago and was normal. She is not sexually active, has no associated gastrointestinal or genitourinary symptoms, and takes no medications. A pregnancy test is negative. Bimanual examination reveals a nontender, 4-cm ovarian mass. Ultrasound demonstrates a unilocular simple ovarian cyst. What is the recommended management in this case?

A. Observe the patient until after her next menses.

B. Attempt to decompress the cyst manually.

C. Perform an immediate exploratory laparotomy/laparoscopy.

D. Aspirate the cyst fluid with a transvaginal fine needle.

291. A 40-year-old man has one episode of painless gross hematuria. What is the initial management in this case?

A. Tell him to return if the bleeding recurs.

B. Send a urine sample for urinalysis and culture.

C. Schedule him for IVP and cystoscopy.

D. Prescribe antibiotics for probable UTI.

292. A 32-year-old female with SLE presents with low-grade fever and fatigue. Physical examination reveals scleral icterus, generalized lymphadenopathy, and splenomegaly. Laboratory tests reveal a severely depressed hemoglobin and hematocrit, normal platelet count, spherocytes on peripheral smear, and a reticulocyte count of 16%. Which of the following is the most likely diagnosis?
A. Autoimmune hemolytic anemia
B. Congenital spherocytosis
C. G6PD deficiency
D. Hemolytic-uremia syndrome

293. A 33-year-old patient with a history of injection drug use is admitted with fever and a new murmur. Which of the following is most likely to be found on the physical exam?
A. Hairy leukoplakia
B. Papular rash on trunk
C. Pharyngeal pseudomembrane
D. Splinter hemorrhages

294. A 56-year-old male with chronic lymphocytic leukemia (CLL) presents with fatigue, dyspnea, and chest discomfort; physical exam reveals elevated jugular venous pressure, diffuse rates, peripheral edema, scleral icterus, and splenomegaly. Preliminary labs reveal elevated BUN and creatinine, severely hematocrit, normal platelets, and an elevated reticulocyte count. Which of the following lab tests will best support the underlying diagnosis?
A. Direct Coombs' test
B. Direct bilirubin
C. Hemoglobin electrophoresis
D. Osmotic fragility test

295. Which of the following is the recommended initial diagnostic test for acute hepatitis C?
A. Anti-HCV ELISA
B. HCsAg titers
C. HCV RNA by PCR
D. Anti-HCV by Immunoblot

296. A tall, thin man with no significant past medical history presents with mild chest pain and dyspnea upon arising this morning. He denies trauma. He is tachycardic and tachypneic; otherwise, the examination is unremarkable. The ECG is normal. Chest radiography is likely to reveal which of the following?
A. Consolidation
B. Kerley B lines
C. Air bronchograms
D. Visceral pleural line

297. A patient presents complaining of vertigo. Which of the following historical descriptions of vertigo is most consistent with Meniere's disease?

A. Chronic episodes related to head movement lasting for 10–30 seconds
B. Recurrent episodes lasting for several hours with hearing loss
C. Acute onset of severe vertigo lasting for days or weeks
D. Chronic vertigo with progressive, unilateral hearing loss

298. Which segment of the population is at highest risk for anorexia nervosa or bulimia nervosa?
A. Middle-aged, divorced or widowed men
B. Young, white, middle- to upper-class women
C. Low- to middle-class, female adolescents
D. Young men from goal-oriented families

299. A 40-year-old man presents 5 days after an episode of acute epigastric pain he describes as boring straight through to his back. Which of the following serum levels will best support a diagnosis of pancreatitis?
A. Amylase
B. Glucose
C. Lipase
D. Triglycerides

300. A patient with long-standing type 2 diabetes presents with a potassium of 8.5. The ECG reveals tall T waves. Which of the following is contraindicated?
A. IV calcium
B. Sodium polystyrene sulfonate (Kayexalate)
C. Sodium bicarbonate
D. Amiloride (Midamor)

301. A 22-year-old woman was seen 2 days ago and diagnosed with pelvic inflammatory disease. She was given an injection of Rocephin (ceftriaxone), 250 mg IM, and started on doxycycline, 100 mg b.i.d., and metronidazole, 500 mg b.i.d. Today, she states that she does not really feel any better and that she has been unable to keep down the last three doses of her antibiotics because of severe nausea and vomiting. Her temperature today is 39.5°C (103°F). Abdominal and pelvic examinations are unchanged from 2 days ago. Which of the following is the most appropriate management of this patient?
A. Have her continue on the current therapy for 2 more days.
B. Change to different antibiotics.
C. Give her a prescription for an antiemetic, and continue the current therapy.
D. Admit her to the hospital for IV antibiotics.

302. Which of the following is suggestive of early renal failure?
A. Anorexia, fatigue, and weakness
B. Oliguria, shortness of breath, and chest pain
C. Polyuria, polydipsia, and back pain
D. Nausea, pruritus, and abdominal pain

Pretest Explanations

1. The answer is **B** [Cardiovascular].
   A. An S_3 gallop is caused by left ventricular systolic dysfunction and suggests heart failure. It may be caused by uncontrolled essential hypertension.
   B. A flank bruit frequently is caused by atherosclerosis of the renal vasculature. This is the most common cause of secondary hypertension.
   C. Renal vascular disease does not cause CVA tenderness, which indicates inflammation of the kidneys.
   D. Retinal exudates are manifestations of long-term uncontrolled hypertension.

2. The answer is **B** [Gastrointestinal/Nutritional].
   A. Albendazole has shown variable cure rates and, therefore, is not a first-line therapy against *Giardia* sp.
   B. Treatment with metronidazole is effective in more than 90% of patients infected with *Giardia* sp. A single dose of tinidazole provides a shorter, better-tolerated therapy but is very expensive.
   C. Nitazoxanide has been approved for the treatment of Giardia in children.
   D. Cure rates with paromomycin have been mixed. The drug is not absorbed, so it may be a good choice for pregnant females.

3. The answer is **C** [Orthopedics/Rheumatology].
   A. A posterior splint or removable walking boot would not provide sufficient immobilization for this type of injury.
   B. See A for explanation.
   C. At 6 weeks, some shaft fractures are stable enough to be put in short leg, weight-bearing casts (usually a patellar tendon–bearing cast or brace).
   D. Unless the injury shows signs of nonunion, this type of immobilization would be unnecessary.

4. The answer is **B** [Cardiovascular].
   A. See **B** for explanation.
   B. A midsystolic click is the hallmark for prolapse of the mitral valve. The click may be followed by a mid to late systolic murmur, indicating mitral valve regurgitation.
   C. See **B** for explanation.
   D. See **B** for explanation.

5. The answer is **B** [Hematology].
   A. Vitamin B_{12} deficiency causes megaloblastic anemia and neurologic symptoms.
   B. This patient likely has iron deficiency anemia. Ferrous sulfate, 325 mg PO t.i.d., is the treatment of choice. Further studies may be warranted to specify cause.
   C. Folic acid deficiency causes a megaloblastic anemia without neurologic findings.
   D. Prednisone is the treatment for autoimmune hemolytic anemia.

6. The answer is B [Cardiovascular].
   A. Antibiotics play no role in the treatment of pericarditis.
   B. Most patients will respond to NSAIDs administered for 7 days to 3 weeks.
   C. Diuretics play no role in the treatment of pericarditis.
   D. Antiarrhythmics are not warranted unless the underlying etiology is identified.

7. The answer is A [Cardiovascular].
   A. Initial defibrillation in ventricular fibrillation is at 200 Joules. If this fails to resolve the problem, defibrillate at 200 to 300 Joules, then at 360 Joules.
   B. See **A** for explanation.
   C. See **A** for explanation.
   D. See **A** for explanation.

8. The answer is D [Neurology].
   A. Red wine, chocolate, and aged cheeses are precipitating factors in many people subject to migraines.
   B. Stress and emotional upsets often are followed by a migrainous episode.
   C. Vacations and weekends often trigger migraines, because people tend to sleep more or go to bed later.

D. Ingestion of excessive caffeine may trigger migraines. Limiting caffeine to one beverage (minimum caffeine intake) in the morning may reduce the frequency of migraines.

9. The answer is **D** [Hematology].
   A. Acute lymphocytic leukemia is associated with primitive lymphoid cells.
   B. Acute myeloblastic leukemia is associated with Auer bodies.
   C. Chronic lymphocytic leukemia is associated with an absolute lymphocytosis.
   D. Chronic myelogenous leukemia is associated with a left-shift myelopoiesis. The Philadelphia chromosome is present in most cases.

10. The answer is **D** [Gastrointestinal/Nutritional].
    A. It is not a curable disease, but symptoms and exacerbations can be lessened.
    B. It does not develop into more serious diseases.
    C. Psychological counseling may help patients come to terms with having a chronic illness, but it will not affect the pathology.
    D. It is a disorder of varied symptoms that occur and resolve.

11. The answer is **C** [Dermatology].
    A. Radiation therapy is an option only if surgery is not feasible.
    B. Topical tretinoin is appropriate for the management of actinic keratosis, a precursor of squamous cell carcinoma.
    C. Initial surgical excision to include clear margins is the optimal management for squamous cell carcinoma.
    D. Cryosurgery is effective in some cases, but surgical excision has the highest cure rate.

12. The answer is **B** [Neurology].
    A. A homonymous quadratic defect occurs with lesions posterior to the optic chiasm that affect only part of the width of the optic nerve radiation.
    B. A pituitary tumor, the probable diagnosis in this case, would cause galactorrhea and bitemporal hemianopia because of impingement of the optic chiasm.
    C. A homonymous hemianopia would result from a defect posterior to the optic chiasm.
    D. A horizontal defect is seen with occlusions of the superior branch of the retinal artery.

13. The answer is **C** [Neurology].
    A. ACTH is elevated in adrenal dysfunction.
    B. TSH is elevated in hypothyroidism.
    C. Prolactinoma is the most common neoplasia of the pituitary. It is more common in young to middle-aged women and manifests with bilateral hemianopia, oligomenorrhea or amenorrhea, and galactorrhea.

D. Elevations of growth hormone result in acromegaly (adults) and gigantism (children).

14. The answer is **B** [Obstetrics/Gynecology].
    A. Ultrasonography and amniocentesis are helpful in the diagnosis of neural tube defects but are indicated only if the maternal serum α-fetoprotein is elevated to 2.5 or more standard deviations above the mean.
    B. To screen for neural tube defects in the fetus, maternal serum α-fetoprotein levels are measured between 16 and 18 weeks of gestation.
    C. Chorionic villus sampling is used earlier than amniocentesis to evaluate for genetic defects, not for neural tube defects. The risk of complications, such as spontaneous or septic abortion, is greater than that with amniocentesis.
    D. Amniocentesis is a second-line study for neural tube defects if the α-fetoprotein is elevated.

15. The answer is **D** [Orthopedics/Rheumatology].
    A. A radiograph of the wrist is indicated if one suspects inflammatory or degenerative joint disease or a fracture. This patient's history and physical examination findings are more consistent with a ganglion of the wrist and not a fracture.
    B. That the mass transilluminates further supports a cystic mass, which is consistent with a ganglion instead of a neoplasm. An ultrasound would provide further clarification but is not necessary at this point.
    C. Occult fractures not seen by radiography would be visualized with a bone scan, but again, this is not necessary at this point.
    D. No further imaging is necessary in this patient at this point. Reassure and educate the patient that the size of the ganglion changes proportionately to his activity level and, occasionally, that the ganglion may spontaneously resolve.

16. The answer is **B** [Cardiovascular].
    A. Aspirin does not provide enough anticoagulative properties to stop propagation of a thrombus.
    B. Heparin acts rapidly and must be considered as the anticoagulant of choice for short-term therapy.
    C. Warfarin should be used only after the patient is fully anticoagulated with heparin.
    D. NSAIDs interfere with platelet function and prolong bleeding time, but they play no effective role in anticoagulation.

17. The answer is **A** [Pulmonology].
    A. Optic neuritis is the most common toxicity of ethambutol. The likelihood of occurrence is increased with higher doses and length of administration.
    B. Rifampin toxicity primarily is associated with liver dysfunction, rash, and a flu-like syndrome.

C. Isoniazid most commonly produces hepatitis and peripheral neuropathy. Optic neuritis is rare.

D. Hyperuricemia and hepatitis are the most common side effects of pyrazinamide.

18. The answer is **A** [Pulmonology].

A. Atelectasis occurs in up to 70% of patients after thoracotomy and laparotomy. The effects of mechanical ventilation and postoperative analgesia cause depression of the respiratory reflexes, such as coughing, yawning, and periodic deep breathing, that would otherwise expand collapsed alveoli (atelectasis).

B. Although pneumonia may occur secondary to atelectasis or contamination of the bronchial tree, it is less common than atelectasis and would more likely be accompanied by fever.

C. Pulmonary embolus, while a complication of major surgery, is less common than atelectasis. Shortness of breath is a common manifestation. Pulmonary embolus generally does not present with consolidation.

D. This is not a typical presentation of congestive heart failure, which is not a common complication of abdominal surgery. See **A** for explanation.

19. The answer is **B** [Psychiatry/Behavioral Medicine].

A. A CT scan would be positive only if the delirium resulted from a mass lesion or bleed.

B. Invariably, the EEG is diffusely slow in acute delirium and may be very useful in differentiating delirium from depression or psychosis.

C. Lumbar puncture would be positive only in delirium resulting from infection or bleed.

D. An MRI would be positive only in delirium resulting from mass lesions or chronic bleed.

20. The answer is **B** [Orthopedics/Rheumatology].

A. Patients should be advised not to engage in any exercise, such as jogging or cycling, that produces increased joint pain that exacerbates after the exercise has ended.

B. The buoyancy of water permits maximum isotonic and isometric exercise with no more stress on joints than active range-of-motion exercises.

C. See **A** for explanation.

D. Walking may be an acceptable method of exercise, depending on the degree of disease.

21. The answer is **B** [Eyes/Ears/Nose/Throat].

A. Corneal erosions may follow a corneal abrasion that is not adequately treated.

B. A corneal abrasion causes severe pain and photophobia. The abrasion stains deeper green than the surrounding cornea.

C. Corneal ulcers usually result from infections that are inadequately treated.

D. Keratitis usually results from an infection, such as with herpes simplex virus, of the cornea. Fluorescein stain typically reveals multiple diffuse punctate lesions.

22. The answer is **A** [Cardiovascular].

A. An ankle-brachial index is useful in gauging the degree of arterial insufficiency and is performed before any additional imaging studies.

B. This man exhibits signs and symptoms of arterial insufficiency. Arteriography is invasive and, therefore, is not considered to be the initial diagnostic study of choice. Instead, it is used to precisely localize the disease process and, if surgery is warranted, to assist in determining the best invasive surgical procedure for treatment.

C. Lymphatic obstruction typically is associated with prominent, minimally pitting edema, which is not a finding in this case.

D. Duplex ultrasonography provides precise anatomic and flow data of arterial supply. Although it is time-consuming and requires an experienced technician, it may provide a first-line, noninvasive assessment for peripheral arterial disease if an ankle-brachial index is not available.

23. The answer is **B** [Obstetrics/Gynecology].

A. A Papanicolaou smear is used in the diagnosis of cervical pathology. A Pap smear may be performed, but an endometrial biopsy is essential.

B. Any woman with unexplained postmenopausal bleeding must undergo an endometrial biopsy to rule out endometrial cancer.

C. FSH and estradiol levels are used to confirm menopausal status. They are unnecessary in a woman who ceased menstruating 8 years previously.

D. A colposcopy-directed biopsy is appropriate for evaluation of an abnormal Pap smear but not to determine the cause of postmenopausal bleeding.

24. The answer is **A** [Cardiovascular].

A. Acute alcohol excess and alcohol withdrawal in predisposed individuals may precipitate atrial fibrillation. This syndrome is often termed the "holiday heart."

B. Paroxysmal supraventricular tachycardia may result in palpitations, but it typically produces a regular pulse.

C. In ventricular bigeminy, every other cardiac depolarization arises from a ventricular ectopic focus. This produces a regular irregularity in the pulse and does not result in the systemic symptoms.

D. Premature atrial complexes may cause palpitations and an irregularly irregular pulse, but they do not produce systemic symptoms.

25. The answer is **A** [Orthopedics/Rheumatology].

A. Plantar fasciitis occurs most commonly in athletes, military personnel, and the obese as a result of excess stress on the Achilles tendon, which is attached to the plantar fascia. It classically presents with an insidious onset of burning heel pain, described as being worse when bearing weight after a prolonged period of rest (i.e., sleeping).

B. A heel contusion is a soft-tissue injury that results from trauma. Weight bearing, although painful, is tolerable. There is no history of trauma in the case described, and the pain is more severe than would be expected with a contusion.

C. A calcaneal fracture usually occurs after a fall or injury in which axial loading of the calcaneus is evident.

D. Tarsal tunnel syndrome results from entrapment of the posterior tibial nerve, and it presents with medial malleolus pain that may radiate as well as with paresthesias and numbness along the plantar aspect of the foot. Pain is described as worsening during sleep, walking, or dorsiflexion, and paresthesia usually is present.

26. The answer is **D** [Hematology].
A. See **D** for explanation.
B. See **D** for explanation.
C. See **D** for explanation.
D. Sulfonamides, nitrofurantoin, and antimalarials (primaquine and quinine) will cause hemolytic anemia in patients with G6PD deficiency.

27. The answer is **B** [Pulmonology].
A. Cool mist humidification was traditionally recommended, but clinical data supporting its use are lacking.
B. A single dose of dexamethasone (0.15 mg/kg) has been shown to improve symptoms, to permit earlier discharge from the emergency department, and to decrease the length of hospital stay in admitted patients.
C. Aerosolized ribavirin is useful in the treatment of respiratory syncytial virus bronchiolitis, but it is not useful in croup.
D. Chest physical therapy is helpful in patients with asthma or cystic fibrosis to loosen secretions, but it is not useful in the treatment of croup.

28. The answer is **A** [Orthopedics/Rheumatology].
A. Thenar atrophy is associated with median nerve compression.
B. Heberden's nodes are firm and nontender nodes on the dorsal distal interphalangeal joints of the hand and are a characteristic finding in osteoarthritis.
C. Boutonniere deformity is associated with rheumatoid arthritis.
D. Dupuytren's contraction is a thickened plaque overlying the tendon of the ring finger and the little finger.

29. The answer is **C** [Psychiatry/Behavioral Medicine].
A. Alprazolam is effective for short-term use to alleviate the intense anxiety, but it should not be used for chronic management of panic attacks.

B. Tricyclic antidepressants and monoamine oxidase inhibitors are effective in panic attacks, but they have many more side effects than SSRIs.
C. SSRIs are the medication of choice for long-term management of panic attacks. Paroxetine is approved by the FDA for this use.
D. See **B** for explanation.

30. The answer is **D** [Cardiovascular].
A. See **D** for explanation.
B. See **D** for explanation.
C. See **D** for explanation.
D. Exertional dyspnea progressing to orthopnea is the most common early complaint in left ventricular failure. Ascites, anorexia, and leg edema occur with right ventricular failure.

31. The answer is **C** [Urology/Renal].
A. α-Blocking agents may be effective in men with obstructive incontinence resulting from prostatic hyperplasia.
B. Estrogen creams are helpful in patients with stress incontinence resulting from hypoestrogenism of the vagina or urethra. Patients with stress incontinence complain of incontinence with activities that increase intra-abdominal pressure, such as coughing, sneezing, lifting, and exercising.
C. Detrusor relaxant medication, such as oxybutynin, is used to assist in control of urge incontinence. These drugs should be augmented with efforts at behavioral modification.
D. Surgical intervention plays no part in the management of urge incontinence.

32. The answer is **A** [Cardiovascular].
A. The left anterior descending artery supplies the anterior free wall of the left ventricle and the anterior two-thirds of the interventricular septum.
B. The right coronary artery supplies the posterior portion of the heart and the AV node.
C. The left circumflex artery supplies the posterolateral surface of the heart.
D. The left marginal artery supplies the left lateral wall of the heart.

33. The answer is **B** [Gastrointestinal/Nutritional].
A. Postprandial pain more likely indicates pathology of the gallbladder.
B. Sitting up and leaning forward may afford some relief, and this usually indicates that the lesion has spread beyond the pancreas and is inoperable.
C. Pancreatic carcinoma often radiates into the back.
D. Pain that refers or moves to the right lower quadrant most likely indicates appendicitis.

34. The answer is **D** [Gastrointestinal/Nutritional].
A. Barium enema is the treatment for intussusception. Pyloric stenosis is a condition of the upper GI tract.

B. The duodenum is not involved in pyloric stenosis.

C. Erythromycin may contribute to the development of pyloric stenosis in infants younger than 30 days.

D. Pyloromyotomy is the treatment of choice for pyloric stenosis and can be performed laparoscopically.

35. The answer is **D** [Infectious Disease].

A. An edematous, red, indurated, spreading lesion is characteristic of erysipelas.

B. An inflammatory hot lesion with diffuse erythema is characteristic of cellulitis.

C. Vesicopustular lesions that follow a dermatome are characteristic of herpes zoster.

D. Nonbullous impetigo is characterized by vesicular, honey-colored, crusted superficial lesions.

36. The answer is **A** [Eyes/Ears/Nose/Throat].

A. Venous dilation, hemorrhages, and cotton-wool spots with acute loss of vision are the findings in retinal vein occlusion.

B. Macular degeneration gives a mottled appearance to the macula, and loss of vision generally is not acute.

C. Retinal detachment typically will cause unilateral visual loss, as if a blind has closed. Funduscopic examination will show the retina floating in the vitreous.

D. Hypertensive retinopathy, although it may have intraretinal hemorrhages and cotton-wool spots, does not commonly present with acute loss of vision.

37. The answer is **A** [Gastrointestinal/Nutritional].

A. The acute attack of cholecystitis often is precipitated by a large or fatty meal. The pain may gradually subside over a period of 12–18 hours.

B. Fiber is not associated with cholecystitis.

C. Spicy foods may aggravate gastritis, gastroesophageal reflux disease, or peptic ulcer disease.

D. Alcohol more commonly precipitates pancreatitis.

38. The answer is **A** [Endocrinology].

A. The Somogyi effect occurs when patients on relatively high levels of insulin develop nocturnal hypoglycemia. This often produces a surge of counter- regulatory hormones that, in turn, leads to morning hyperglycemia. This may occur simultaneously with the waning and dawn phenomena, causing the patient to become severely hypoglycemic.

B. The waning phenomenon actually is the most common cause of prebreakfast hyperglycemia, but it results from the waning of endogenous circulating insulin levels overnight.

C. Munchausen syndrome involves self-induced symptoms or false physical and/or laboratory findings. Missing the correct diagnosis could lead to poor diabetic control and later complications.

D. The dawn phenomenon presents in about 75% of people with type 1 diabetes, in most people with type 2 diabetes, and in a great many "normal" persons. It refers to reduced tissue sensitivity to insulin between 5 and 8 AM and produces mild hyperglycemia.

39. The answer is **D** [Cardiovascular].

A. See **D** for explanation.

B. See **D** for explanation.

C. See **D** for explanation.

D. In an asymptomatic patient, infrequent premature complexes are not pathological. They typically disappear during exercise. Medical treatment is indicated for frequent PVCs only in the patient with a clinical presentation that is suggestive of cardiac disease, electrolyte abnormality, or other underlying pathology.

40. The answer is **D** [Dermatology].

A. Adult atopic dermatitis occurs on the dorsum of the hands and feet.

B. Adult atopic dermatitis occurs more often in the popliteal fossae. Psoriatic plaques typically occur on the knees.

C. Gluteal cleft lesions are not associated with adult atopic dermatitis. Gluteal cleft lesions are typical in psoriasis.

D. Adult atopic dermatitis has a predilection for the flexures, including the antecubital fossae.

41. The answer is **D** [Obstetrics/Gynecology].

A. Combined oral contraceptives have a protective effect against endometrial hyperplasia and endometrial cancer.

B. This patient has amenorrhea because of too little estrogen as a result of low body fat, not because of unopposed estrogen.

C. A teenager with anovular menstruation is at low risk for endometrial hyperplasia.

D. This woman has four risk factors for endometrial hyperplasia and endometrial cancer: age, obesity, hypertension, and diabetes. The prolonged bleeding is likely related to unopposed estrogen.

42. The answer is **A** [Obstetrics/Gynecology].

A. Septic abortion presents with shock and a foul discharge. Additional investigation of the cervix and upper vagina is warranted to rule out trauma as a result of attempts to induce abortion.

B. Fever is unusual in ectopic pregnancy, occurring in less than 2% of patients. Abnormal uterine bleeding is present in 75% of patients. Discharge is rare; only about 7% of patients will pass a uterine cast.

C. The discharge caused by pelvic inflammatory disease usually is purulent or mucopurulent. Onset of symptoms is somewhat more insidious over 1–3 days, with a less shock-like presentation than in this patient.

D. In a tubo-ovarian abscess, symptoms of pelvic pain or discomfort, fever, and nausea persist for more than a week. With rupture, the patient may present with an acute abdomen and sepsis, but vaginal discharge is unusual.

43. The answer is **B** [Urology/Renal].
A. Palpation does not yield specific information about incarceration of an inguinal hernia.
B. The major complication of inguinal hernias is incarceration of a loop of bowel. Auscultation of the scrotum for bowel sounds can reveal the presence of a loop of bowel descending into the scrotum from the peritoneum.
C. Percussion of the bladder, whether normal or abnormal, is not helpful in diagnosing incarcerated inguinal hernias.
D. A 1-year-old infant cannot follow the instructions to perform a Valsalva maneuver.

44. The answer is **A** [Gastrointestinal/Nutritional].
A. Removal of all gluten from the diet is essential to therapy; all wheat, rye, and barley must be eliminated.
B. Eggs and grapefruit are not implicated in celiac disease, because they do not contain gluten.
C. See **B** for explanation.
D. Rice is not implicated, because it contains no gluten. It is a safe starch alternative in patients with celiac disease.

45. The answer is **B** [Dermatology].
A. See **B** for explanation. Pain control is indicated in herpes zoster with trigeminal involvement, but both ophthalmologic evaluation and administration of a systemic antiherpetic are more pressing interventions.
B. A lesion typical of herpes zoster on the tip of the nose strongly suggests the possibility of ophthalmic involvement, and the injected conjunctiva makes this more likely. Prompt evaluation by an ophthalmologist is essential.
C. Capsaicin cream is only used after skin lesions have healed. It is indicated for amelioration of the pain of postherpetic neuralgia. Application to broken skin would be extremely painful.
D. Although prednisone is used for the treatment of herpes zoster in the immunocompetent patient to decrease pain, it would be more important to prescribe antivirals and send for an evaluation by an ophthalmologist.

46. The answer is **D** [Gastrointestinal/Nutritional].
A. Riboflavin toxicity has not been reported in humans.
B. Vitamin A toxicity is not associated with changes in serum calcium or phosphate.
C. Vitamin B$_6$ toxicity is associated with peripheral neuropathy and photosensitivity.

D. Excess amounts of vitamin D result in abnormally high concentrations of calcium and phosphate, metastatic calcifications, renal damage, and altered mentation.

47. The answer is **A** [Obstetrics/Gynecology].
A. Eclampsia is defined as preeclampsia with the addition of grand mal seizures.
B. Preeclampsia is diagnosed by the presence of hypertension, edema, and proteinuria.
C. Primary seizure disorder is not diagnosed by an isolated occurrence of seizure.
D. Pregnancy-induced hypertension is the finding of hypertension without significant proteinuria.

48. The answer is **C** [Eyes/Ears/Nose/Throat].
A. Pilocarpine is used for reduction of intraocular pressure in the treatment of acute or chronic closed-angle glaucoma.
B. Corticosteroids are used for treatment of inflammatory conditions.
C. Polymyxin-B is used to prevent infections secondary to trauma involving the lids, conjunctivae, or cornea.
D. Tropicamide is used to facilitate initial examination, not to treat ocular problems.

49. The answer is **D** [Endocrinology].
A. A 24-hour urine is not needed. See **B** for explanation.
B. Further evaluation for pituitary disorders is unnecessary. If the patient had hypocalcemia or hyperphosphatemia, further diagnostic evaluation would be in order for pseudohypoparathyroidism. Growth hormone deficiency is characterized by short stature, increased fat, high-pitched voice, and tendency toward hypoglycemia. Cretinism is characterized by mental and growth retardation of iodine-deficient children. One may see delayed tooth eruption, receding chin, and protruding tongue in cretinism and hypopituitarism.
C. Pseudopseudohypoparathyroidism (PPHP) is known to have a genetic defect in the *GNAS-1* gene, located on chromosome 20q13. Genetic analysis could be appropriate but costly and not necessary.
D. This patient meets the diagnostic criteria for PPHP by the physical examination findings and normal laboratory findings. No further diagnostic studies or laboratory tests are needed. The patient may benefit from special services.

50. The answer is **C** [Gastrointestinal/Nutritional].
A. Bacterial overgrowth results in abdominal distention, weight loss, steatorrhea, watery diarrhea, and anemia. The C-xylose breath test is diagnostic.
B. Celiac sprue results in flatulence, diarrhea, weight loss, and weakness. The diagnosis is established by

examining a stool specimen with Sudan stain to detect fat or through serology. Breath tests are not helpful.

C. Lactose intolerance, resulting from a deficiency of lactase, is more prevalent in the African-, Asian-, and Native-American populations. It manifests with abdominal complaints after the ingestion of milk or milk products. Isolated lactase deficiency is not associated with other signs of malabsorption or weight loss, but if the deficiency is very severe, an osmotic diarrhea may occur.

D. Pancreatic insufficiency causes malabsorption and diarrhea with weight loss, flatulence, and large, bulky stools (steatorrhea). It is associated mainly with the malabsorption of triglycerides rather than proteins or carbohydrates.

51. The answer is **A** [Dermatology].

A. Resistant impetigo should be treated with an antimicrobial agent that is effective against *Staphylococcus aureus* (β-lactamase–resistant penicillins or cephalosporins, clindamycin, or amoxicillin/clavulanate) for 7–10 days.

B. Topical treatment is recommended only for localized lesions.

C. Although ciprofloxacin is effective against penicillin-resistant impetigo, it is not approved for use in children.

D. A small percentage of impetigo cases do not respond to penicillin. Improvement should be evident after 4 days of penicillin-V.

52. The answer is **C** [Cardiovascular].

A. Digoxin can be used as chronic therapy for patients with recurrent episodes of PSVT.

B. Radiofrequency catheter ablation is an invasive procedure that is used to treat recurrent PSVT.

C. Carotid sinus massage is a safe and often effective maneuver for termination of tachycardia.

D. Direct current cardioversion is seldom required, except when associated with hemodynamic collapse.

53. The answer is **A** [Eyes/Ears/Nose/Throat].

A. Amoxicillin covers the organisms commonly associated with sinusitis (*Streptococcus* sp., *Haemophilus influenzae*, and *Moraxella catarrhalis*), and it achieves good sinus penetration.

B. Erythromycin does not cover the typical organisms associated with sinusitis.

C. Ampicillin does not achieve good sinus penetration.

D. Tetracycline does not cover the typical organisms associated with sinusitis.

54. The answer is **C** [Orthopedics/Rheumatology].

A. Multiple myeloma presents with bone pain in the lower back or as a pathologic fracture of the femoral neck or vertebrae. Anemia is a common presentation with these patients as well.

B. Osteomalacia is commonly asymptomatic early in the disease; later, patients complain of bone pain and muscle weakness that is continuous throughout the day.

C. Polymyalgia rheumatica presents with proximal, symmetric morning stiffness. The onset may be abrupt or insidious, and it usually involves the shoulders, neck, and pelvic girdle. Malaise, fatigue, and fevers may be present for months before a diagnosis is established. Polymyalgia also can occur with temporal arteritis. Treatment with corticosteroids produces a dramatic response.

D. Sarcoidosis is a systemic disease of unknown cause characterized by granulomatous inflammation of the lung.

55. The answer is **C** [Endocrinology].

A. No immune component is present in type 2 diabetes.

B. No HLA markers have been identified for type 2 diabetes.

C. Circulating endogenous insulin is adequate to prevent ketoacidosis in type 2 diabetes but is inadequate to meet the body's increased need as tissue sensitivity to insulin decreases.

D. Between 60% and 70% of North Americans, Europeans and Africans with type 2 diabetes are obese. Less than 30% of Chinese and Japanese with type 2 diabetes are obese. Nearly 100% of Pima Indians and Pacific Islanders with type 2 diabetes are obese.

56. The answer is **A** [Orthopedics/Rheumatology].

A. A whiplash injury often occurs as a result of motor-vehicle accidents. This consists of rapid flexion followed by hyperextension to the neck.

B. Contusion is likely to cause hematoma and resulting obstruction to nearby structures.

C. Extreme rotation will likely cause sprains and tears.

D. Strangulation causes massive ecchymoses and airway obstruction.

57. The answer is **C** [Endocrinology].

A. Serum creatinine is affected by many processes and is not a reliable means to specifically identify diabetic nephropathy.

B. Urine protein electrophoresis is used in identifying immunoglobulinopathies (i.e., multiple myeloma).

C. Overnight urine collection for quantification of microalbumin correlates directly with diabetic renal disease.

D. Renal biopsy is diagnostic of renal parenchymal and glomerular diseases, but it is not considered to be a routine screening method.

58. The answer is **D** [Pulmonology].

A. Repeated chest radiographs to monitor the response to treatment for tuberculosis are not recommended.

B. The patient is potentially infectious, but isolation is only recommended for active tuberculosis.

C. Bacillus Calmette-Guerin does not reduce the risk of reactivation.

D. Patients should be followed monthly while taking antituberculosis drugs to monitor for the clinical manifestations of drug-induced hepatitis.

59. The answer is **B** [Cardiovascular].
A. Accordion-appearing QRS morphology is seen in torsades de pointes.
B. A type I, second-degree AV block is characterized by progressive lengthening of the PR interval and shortening of the RR interval before a blocked beat.
C. Ventricular rates of less than 50 bpm and wide QRS complexes often are seen in third-degree (complete) heart block.
D. Widened QRS complexes are seen in ventricular arrhythmias and in third-degree (complete) heart block.

60. The answer is **A** [Cardiovascular].
A. Onset of increased creatine kinase activity in the circulation starts 4–8 hours after infarction and peaks as early as 8 hours after the onset of pain.
B. Elevations in alanine transaminase indicate injury to hepatocytes. It may be mildly increased in an acute myocardial infarction without shock or heart failure.
C. Aspartate transaminase activity has an onset of 8–12 hours and peaks at 18–36 hours.
D. Lactic dehydrogenase activity has a late onset of 24–48 hours and peaks at 4–5 days.

61. The answer is **D** [Psychiatry/Behavioral Medicine].
A. Carbamazepine may be helpful in refractory cases if there is no response to first-line medications.
B. Haloperidol is a dopamine-receptor antagonist. It is effective in more than 50% of patients but has a high incidence of adverse side effects.
C. Lithium is an antimanic medication and is not used in schizophrenia.
D. Risperidone is a serotonin/dopamine antagonist. It is highly effective in schizophrenia. It is not associated with extrapyramidal symptoms, causes less sedation, and has fewer anticholinergic side effects than dopamine-receptor antagonists.

62. The answer is **C** [Obstetrics/Gynecology].
A. Although a mammogram may be a part of the evaluation, early biopsy and diagnosis are important.
B. Antibiotics could be started, but if the area does not respond within 1–2 weeks, the patient should be referred for a biopsy.
C. Because of the patient's age, inflammatory carcinoma is much more likely than mastitis or some other infectious process. Referring the patient for a biopsy is necessary to rule out inflammatory carcinoma.

D. Inflammatory carcinoma is the most malignant form of breast cancer. Metastases tend to occur early and widely, so any delay in diagnosis should be avoided.

63. The answer is **D** [Infectious Disease].
A. The papovaviruses include the human papilloma viruses, which cause flat warts, common warts, plantar warts, and condyloma acuminata (genital warts).
B. The picornaviruses include rhinovirus, enterovirus, poliovirus, echovirus, and coxsackieviruses.
C. Poxviruses include smallpox, cowpox, and molluscum contagiosum viruses.
D. The varicella-zoster virus is a member of the herpesvirus family, along with herpes simplex virus I and II, cytomegalovirus, Epstein-Barr virus (herpesvirus 4), and human herpesvirus 6 (rosacea).

64. The answer is **B** [Neurology].
A. Plain-film skull radiography will not identify intracranial bleeding.
B. CT will best identify potentially life-threatening intracranial bleeding as well as mass effect caused by cerebral edema.
C. All patients with head injuries must have cervical spine fractures ruled out, but neck radiographs may be deferred by stabilizing the neck while more urgent conditions are addressed.
D. Lumbar puncture in the presence of increased intracranial pressure may result in transtentorial herniation and, thus, should be avoided.

65. The answer is **A** [Hematology].
A. Desmopressin is the first line treatment for mild von Willebrand's disease.
B. Factor VIII is the treatment for hemophilia A; it is a second line treatment in patients with von Willebrand's disease who do not respond to desmopressin.
C. Factor IX is the treatment for hemophilia B.
D. Patients with a vitamin K deficiency will have a prolonged international normalized ratio. The prothrombin time usually is more prolonged relative to the partial thromboplastin time.

66. The answer is **D** [Infectious Disease].
A. Enterohemorrhaghic *E.coli* produces a severe bloody diarrhea.
B. Diarrhea caused by *Entamoeba* sp. typically does not manifest for 2–6 weeks after ingestion of the cysts.
C. *Salmonella typhi* typically causes a fever before any diarrhea. Most adults have constipation before the diarrhea.
D. The sudden onset of watery diarrhea after a 24- to 48-hour incubation period is characteristic of *Vibrio cholerae*. This is a result of the toxin released by the *Vibrio* sp. Dehydration and electrolyte loss are common.

67. The answer is **C** [Cardiovascular].
   A. An ejection click is indicative of mitral valve prolapse or aortic stenosis.
   B. Thrills often accompany loud, harsh, or rumbling murmurs, such as those of aortic stenosis, patent ductus arteriosus, ventricular septal defect, and mitral stenosis.
   C. An S_3 is highly suggestive of heart failure in adults and results from increased resistance to ventricular filling during passive atrial emptying.
   D. An S_4 occurs when there is increased resistance to ventricular filling during atrial contraction. The causes of an S_4 include hypertensive heart disease, coronary artery disease, aortic stenosis, and cardiomyopathy.

68. The answer is **B** [Eyes/Ears/Nose/Throat].
   A. Chalazion is a chronic inflammation of the meibomian gland and is located inside the eyelid rather than the lid margin.
   B. Hordeolum, or sty, is a tender infection that occurs around the hair follicles of the eyelashes.
   C. Pinguecula is a yellowish nodule in the bulbar conjunctiva. It is painless and harmless.
   D. Xanthelasma may accompany lipid disorders and appears as slightly raised, yellowish plaques in the skin of the upper and lower eyelids.

69. The answer is **A** [Gastrointestinal/Nutritional].
   A. A family history of jaundice or a history of recurrent mild jaundice that resolves spontaneously is most consistent with a familial disorder of bilirubin metabolism, such as Gilbert's, Rotor's, Crigler-Najjar, or Dubin-Johnson syndrome.
   B. Most patients with sickle-cell disease, not sickle-cell trait, develop chronic jaundice from ongoing hemolysis.
   C. History of fatty food intolerance with jaundice is suggestive of acute cholangitis.
   D. The sudden appearance of jaundice in a previously healthy young person, especially if preceded by a brief prodrome of fever, malaise, and myalgias, is likely to be caused by a viral hepatitis.

70. The answer is **A** [Endocrinology].
   A. Whenever a patient with Addison's disease (autoimmune adrenal insufficiency) is under stress, adjustment of the glucocorticoid dosing is necessary to avoid the potential episode of acute adrenal insufficiency. Patients with a major stress (e.g., major trauma or surgery requiring generalized anesthesia) will require at least 10-fold the regular dose of hydrocortisone, administered parenterally in three divided doses. When a major illness is present, the hydrocortisone dose should be doubled for as short a period as possible.
   B. See **A** for explanation.

   C. Fludrocortisone is a synthetic mineralocorticoid and is not adjusted for acute episodes of adrenal insufficiency.
   D. See **C** for explanation.

71. The answer is **B** [Endocrinology].
   A. In chronic cases of hypocapnia, symptomatic findings are those of the primary disease process.
   B. These constellations are indicative of hypocalcemia, and hypocalcemia associated with hypoparathyroidism most commonly occurs following thyroidectomy or surgery for primary hyperparathyroidism.
   C. Hypoparathyroidism rarely follows irradiation of the neck.
   D. Hypercalcemia may be associated with malignancy, but the stated findings are those associated with hypocalcemia, not hypercalcemia.

72. The answer is **C** [Obstetrics/Gynecology].
   A. During the first trimester of pregnancy, follow-up appointments occur every 4 weeks.
   B. Unless there is significant discordance between menstrual dating and uterine size, early ultrasonography for dating is not necessary.
   C. At this maternal age or older, the risk of giving birth to infants with congenital abnormalities increases, which is a major indication for genetic counseling.
   D. A serum α-fetoprotein test is best obtained between 16 and 18 weeks of gestation.

73. The answer is **A** [Orthopedics/Rheumatology].
   A. Many now believe that methotrexate is the treatment of choice for patients with rheumatoid arthritis who fail to respond to NSAIDs. Methotrexate generally is well tolerated and often produces a beneficial effect in 2–6 weeks.
   B. Antimalarials are used to treat rheumatoid arthritis; however, they are reserved for patients with mild, stable disease.
   C. Although corticosteroids usually produce an immediate and dramatic anti-inflammatory effect in rheumatoid arthritis, they do not alter the natural progression of the disease. Furthermore, clinical manifestations of active disease commonly reappear when the drug is discontinued.
   D. Gold salts are reserved for patients who fail to improve on, or who cannot tolerate, methotrexate.

74. The answer is **D** [Dermatology].
   A. Daily steroid cream should not be recommended. Use of Burow's wet dressings or Castellani's paint is effective for prevention.
   B. Washing the feet with benzoyl peroxide directly after showering is effective for prevention. Isopropyl alcohol is not recommended, because it can be damaging to the skin.

C. Chlorine is not associated with recurrence of tinea pedis.

D. Wearing shower shoes while showering is recommended. Arthrospores can survive for 12 months.

75. The answer is **B** [Eyes/Ears/Nose/Throat].
   A. Tonometry is primarily used if increased intraocular pressure is suspected.
   B. Management of a chemical burn to the eye includes initially assessing the pH and repeating the measurement frequently during treatment until it returns to normal (7.4–7.6).
   C. Fluorescein staining is used to detect the presence of a foreign body or corneal abrasion.
   D. Funduscopic examination is not appropriate as an initial study because of the emergency nature of a chemical burn.

76. The answer is **C** [Neurology].
   A. Sinus headaches are rarely associated with visual disturbances.
   B. Cluster headache attacks usually peak in less than 5 minutes, then taper off in less than 1 hour. They are more common in men.
   C. Migraine headaches typically are unilateral, begin in adolescence, and may include visual disturbances. They are more common in women.
   D. Tension headaches often are similar to migraines, but they usually are not associated with visual disturbances.

77. The answer is **B** [Cardiovascular].
   A. Lipid-lowering medication has been shown to decrease new or worsening claudication.
   B. Use of elastic support hose reduces blood flow to the skin and should be avoided in peripheral arterial insufficiency. Elastic support hose are recommended for peripheral venous insufficiency.
   C. Exercise programs often decrease symptoms of claudication by increasing muscle efficiency and stimulating the development of collateral vessels.
   D. Platelet inhibitors, such as aspirin, have been shown to decrease the progression of arterial insufficiency.

78. The answer is **D** [Dermatology].
   A. Dicloxacillin is effective against staphylococcal folliculitis.
   B. Topical isotretinoin may be useful against eosinophilic folliculitis.
   C. Oral indomethacin is helpful in the treatment of eosinophilic folliculitis.
   D. Hot tub *Pseudomonas* folliculitis virtually always resolves without treatment; resistant cases also may be treated with oral antibiotics, such as ciprofloxacin, 500 mg PO b.i.d. for 5 days.

79. The answer is **B** [Orthopedics/Rheumatology].
   A. Allopurinol (xanthine oxidase inhibitor) is a medication used in the prevention of gout.

B. The mainstay for treatment of acute gout is NSAIDs, such as naproxen or indomethacin. Colchicine is also effective, but has a higher side-effect profile.
   C. The alternative for treatment of acute gout or refractory gout is prednisone, a steroid.
   D. Probenecid is a medication used in the prevention of gout.

80. The answer is **B** [Cardiovascular].
   A. At 30 years of age, a resting ECG is not routinely recommended. The history of asthma does not mandate exercise stress test (EST) unless the screening reveals recurrence of the disease. Additionally, EST is not routinely recommended for asymptomatic 30-year-old patients.
   B. Medical screening for initiating an exercise program should include a complete H&P, CBC, urinalysis, blood sugar, creatinine, and cholesterol level. At 50 years of age, a resting ECG is helpful to screen for ischemia, left ventricular hypertrophy, or rhythm disturbances. An EST is a mandatory part of preparing a patient for an exercise program if any of the screening procedures discloses evidence of overt cardiovascular or pulmonary disease. Obesity is a risk factor that should prompt consideration of stress testing; obesity is defined as between 20% to 40% above the ideal body weight (IBW). This patient has two factors that place him in a high-risk category for cardiovascular disease: He is mildly obese, and he has hypertension. He needs to undergo EST before initiating an exercise program.
   C. This patient does not meet any criteria for EST. In fact, the osteoarthritis (OA) in his knees may preclude the use of EST. Depending on the severity of the OA, he will likely require a careful choice of exercise type so as not to further worsen his OA or cause other injuries secondary to decreased functional capacity. At 10% above IBW, he will benefit from exercise but does not meet the obesity definition mandating EST.
   D. At 15% above IBW, this patient is not considered to be obese. As such, this patient does not meet any obvious criteria for EST.

81. The answer is **C** [Gastrointestinal/Nutritional].
   A. Antibiotics alone are ineffective at treating perianal or perirectal infection.
   B. Outpatient incision and drainage of an anorectal abscess would be acceptable if the patient were not diabetic and there was a clear understanding about the extent of infection.
   C. Anorectal abscesses should be treated by surgical drainage as soon as the diagnosis is established. Delayed or inadequate treatment may lead to suppuration with massive tissue necrosis and septicemia. Patients with diabetes are at high risk for disseminated infection.

D. Sitz baths and analgesics are not definitive treatment and only help to relieve discomfort.

82. The answer is **B** [Gastrointestinal/Nutritional].
    A. Right upper quadrant pain is a common symptom in patients with gallbladder pathology.
    B. The major symptom of acute pancreatitis is midepigastric or left upper quadrant pain. It is described most commonly as a constant, boring pain that often radiates to the back as well as to the flanks, chest, or lower abdomen.
    C. Pain of mechanical small bowel obstruction typically is periumbilical or more diffuse.
    D. Burning epigastric pain is the most classic symptom of peptic ulcer disease, which most commonly occurs in the duodenum.

83. The answer is **C** [Dermatology].
    A. Azithromycin is appropriate for the treatment of chancroid.
    B. Doxycycline is appropriate for the treatment of lymphogranuloma venereum.
    C. Acyclovir, valacyclovir, and famciclovir are appropriate for the treatment of genital herpes.
    D. Penicillin G benzathine is appropriate for the treatment of syphilis.

84. The answer is **D** [Obstetrics/Gynecology].
    A. Taking a pill holiday has only put women at higher risk for an unplanned or undesired pregnancy. Pregnancy has a greater morbidity/mortality risk than low-dose pills.
    B. The pill has not been associated with decreased fertility. However, if a woman was started on the pill to regulate her menses, then she may return to her previous irregular menstrual pattern, which may have an underlying cause that is associated with decreased fertility.
    C. See A for explanation.
    D. This is correct.

85. The answer is **D** [Cardiovascular].
    A. Aortic stenosis usually is a grade III/VI, rough, medium-pitched ejection murmur heard loudest at the second intercostal space that transmits to the neck.
    B. Atrioventricular septal defect murmurs are heard best at the left lower sternal border. There also may be an accentuated pulmonary component and a split second sound.
    C. Mitral valve prolapse has a murmur best heard at the apex. There usually is a midsystolic click. The murmur accentuates with squatting.
    D. The Still's murmur often appears around age 2 and persists into adolescence. Although often loud, it is considered to be an innocent or functional murmur.

86. The answer is **D** [Cardiovascular].
    A. HACEK organisms (*Haemophilus, Actinobacillus, Cardiobacterium, Eikenella,* and *Kingella*) are more likely to cause endocarditis in native valves.
    B. Yeasts and fungi tend to cause a subacute endocarditis in native valves.
    C. *Serratia marcescens* is a rare cause of endocarditis.
    D. In injection drug users, *Staphylococcus aureus* accounts for more than 60% of all endocarditis cases.

87. The answer is **B** [Endocrinology].
    A. Swelling or nodules usually are painless in the setting of carcinoma.
    B. Recent and rapid growth of a thyroid mass is suggestive of carcinoma.
    C. Symmetrical enlargement may suggest either hypofunctioning or hyperfunctioning states, but not carcinoma.
    D. A solitary, firm nodule suggests cancer.

88. The answer is **D** [Gastrointestinal/Nutritional].
    A. Erosive gastritis accounts for 1% of upper GI bleeds.
    B. Gastric neoplasm accounts for 1% of upper GI bleeds.
    C. Bleeding esophageal varices account for 10–20% of upper GI bleeds.
    D. Peptic ulcer disease accounts for over 50% of upper GI bleeds.

89. The answer is **C** [Orthopedics/Rheumatology].
    A. Streptococci are responsible for 15–30% of acute nongonococcal bacterial arthritis in all ages.
    B. *Enterococcus* spp. are responsible for less than 1% of acute nongonococcal bacterial arthritis in all ages.
    C. *Staphylococcus aureus* is responsible for 50–70% of acute nongonococcal bacterial arthritis in all ages.
    D. *Streptococcus pneumonia* is responsible for 10–35% of acute nongonococcal bacterial arthritis in all ages.

90. The answer is **C** [Obstetrics/Gynecology].
    A. A biophysical profile may be warranted after the nonstress test. It is an assessment of fetal heart rates and ultrasound monitoring of fetal breathing, fine motor movements, gross motor tone, and amniotic fluid volume.
    B. Expected mothers are encouraged to perform fetal kick counts to assess fetal movement. This woman is already indicating that no fetal movement is occurring.
    C. A nonstress test is the initial investigation into fetal compromise. It also is indicated in preeclampsia, intrauterine growth retardation, multiple gestation, and postterm pregnancy. It assesses fetal heart rate without stimulation and evaluates patterns that may indicate compromise.

D. An oxytocin challenge test is an ancillary test of fetal well-being, but it is not as reliable as the non-stress test.

91. The answer is **B** [Orthopedics/Rheumatology].
    A. See **D** for explanation.
    B. A parenteral, penicillinase-resistant, synthetic penicillin combined with a third-generation cephalosporin is the recommended approach against probable *Staphylococcus aureus* osteomyelitis while awaiting culture results.
    C. Open surgical drainage is indicated in acute osteomyelitis if there is inadequate response to antibiotic therapy or signs of abscess.
    D. IV antibiotics are recommended initially for osteomyelitis.

92. The answer is **B** [Orthopedics/Rheumatology].
    A. An MRI does not demonstrate median nerve compression.
    B. The most common finding on an electromyogram in carpal tunnel syndrome is abnormality in the median nerve distribution.
    C. Radiographs would be indicated in the presence of bony abnormalities.
    D. Aspiration of synovial fluid is not indicated for a diagnosis of carpal tunnel syndrome.

93. The answer is **B** [Pulmonology].
    A. See **B** for explanation.
    B. The normal respiratory rate in the newborn is 30–60 breaths/min.
    C. See **B** for explanation.
    D. See **B** for explanation.

94. The answer is **B** [Urology/Renal].
    A. A digital rectal examination is indicated to evaluate the prostate.
    B. According to recently established practice guidelines, prostate-specific antigen (PSA) would be an optional adjuvant test. There is significant overlap in PSA values between patients with benign prostatic hyperplasia and prostate cancer. The same practice guidelines call for an initial evaluation to include patient history, physical examination, digital rectal examination, urinalysis, creatinine, and optional PSA.
    C. Symptoms are suggestive of obstruction; therefore, renal compromise must be ruled out. See **B** for explanation.
    D. Nocturia is an irritative symptom, and urinalysis would be most valuable in ruling out infection.

95. The answer is **D** [Cardiovascular].
    A. The PR interval in first-degree AV block is greater than 0.20 second.
    B. Paroxysmal atrial tachycardia presents with paroxysmal palpitations and dyspnea. The ECG reveals a P wave different from that of sinus rhythm but no other abnormalities.
    C. Although Lown-Ganong-Levine syndrome can cause supraventricular tachycardia, it is less common and has a short PR interval but no delta wave.
    D. The hallmark of Wolff-Parkinson-White syndrome is a short PR interval with a delta wave. It frequently can cause paroxysmal supraventricular tachycardia.

96. The answer is **A** [Cardiovascular].
    A. Long-standing high blood pressure produces medial degeneration of the aortic wall. These changes are most directly linked to risk of dissection.
    B. Aortic stenosis, by itself, does not increase the risk of aortic dissection.
    C. An increased LDL may contribute to the risk of atherosclerotic disease, but hypertension and its related changes of the arterial wall are linked most directly to the risk of aortic dissection.
    D. Diabetes mellitus contributes to small vessel disease and dyslipidemias.

97. The answer is **B** [Orthopedics/Rheumatology].
    A. Lachman's test evaluates the anterior cruciate ligament.
    B. A valgus stress test is appropriate to assess the medial collateral ligament. A varus stress test assesses the lateral collateral ligament.
    C. Laxity with the thumb sign is indicative of a posterior cruciate ligament tear.
    D. McMurray's test evaluates the meniscus.

98. The answer is **A** [Gastrointestinal/Nutritional].
    A. Hepatitis A is highly contagious and is spread largely by the fecal–oral route, especially in times of poor sanitary conditions. Hepatitis A has become the most common cause of acute hepatitis in the United States; most cases result from direct person-to-person exposure and, to lesser extent, from direct fecal contamination of food or water. High-risk groups include travelers to developing areas of the world.
    B. Although endemic in many areas of the world, such as Southeast Asia, China, and sub-Saharan Africa, hepatitis B is spread predominantly by the parenteral route or by intimate personal contact.
    C. Hepatitis C is spread predominantly by the parenteral route. Injection drug users and persons with multiple parenteral exposures are at highest risk. Sexual transmission occurs but is not common.
    D. Hepatitis D is linked to hepatitis B. Hepatitis D can be spread by the parenteral route and sexually. Persons at greatest risk are chronic carriers of hepatitis B and those with repeated parenteral exposures.

99. The answer is **A** [Dermatology].
  A. Acne vulgaris often is aggravated by externally applied products that may further block sebaceous follicles.
  B. No kind of food has been shown to cause or exacerbate acne.
  C. Skin-cleaning agents are not recommended, because most irritate the skin. Comedolytic agents, such as topical retinoic acid and benzoyl peroxide, are more effective in treating comedonal acne.
  D. See **C** for explanation.

100. The answer is **A** [Cardiovascular].
  A. *Streptococcus viridans*, enterococci, and a number of other Gram-positive and Gram-negative bacilli, as well as yeasts and fungi, tend to cause a subacute endocarditis.
  B. *Staphylococcus aureus* tends to cause a rapidly progressive picture of endocarditis. It commonly results in a destructive infection in which patients present with acute febrile illnesses, acute valvular insufficiency, early embolization, and myocardial abscess formation. It is more common in patients with prosthetic valves or injection drug use.
  C. See **A** for explanation.
  D. See **A** for explanation.

101. The answer is **A** [Pulmonology].
  A. Consolidation is classically associated with bacterial pneumonia.
  B. Kerley B lines are associated with congestive heart failure.
  C. Blunting of the costophrenic angle suggests pleural effusion.
  D. Visceral pleural lines, especially on expiration, are diagnostic of pneumothorax.

102. The answer is **B** [Psychiatric/Behavioral Medicine].
  A. Serotonergic antidepressants and psychiatric counseling are part of the treatment of eating disorders once the patient is stabilized.
  B. Emergency hospitalization is the treatment required for patients who are 15–20% (or more) below expected weight for height and have severe depression, suicide risk, and/or metabolic disturbances (suggested by her resting pulse of 38 bpm).
  C. Metabolic testing is part of the workup for eating disorders to assess the extent of metabolic disturbances. Based on the presentation, however, this patient does not qualify for outpatient management.
  D. See **B** and **C** for explanation.

103. The answer is **C** [Endocrinology].
  A. Pressure differences between arms are seen when arterial compression or obstruction on the side with lower pressure occurs. In this case, it is not likely.
  B. This change in pressure would represent a blood pressure elevation for this patient, enough to be termed hypertensive if repeatedly seen over more

than one visit. Patients with nausea and vomiting typically become hypovolemic, in which case they may become hypotensive, not hypertensive.
  C. This patient has the signs and symptoms associated with acute adrenal insufficiency, especially in light of the recent cessation of a corticosteroid. As such, she will exhibit postural hypotension.
  D. This type of pressure difference is known as a widened pulse pressure and is seen with aortic regurgitation. Although it is possible that she may have this, it is unlikely given the other signs and symptoms.

104. The answer is **D** [Cardiovascular].
  A. This patient has not achieved her dietary goal.
  B. Gemfibrozil is prescribed for isolated hypertriglyceridemia.
  C. The addition of oat bran to an already low-fat, low-cholesterol diet will have little or no effect.
  D. HMG-CoA reductase inhibitors, such as atorvastatin, have been shown to significantly reduce the circulating LDL cholesterol and have an excellent long-term safety profile.

105. The answer is **D** [Pulmonology].
  A. Influenza is less common in younger children, and in neonates, it may present with nonspecific signs and sudden fever.
  B. Adenovirus presents with fever, pharyngitis, conjunctivitis, rhinitis, and cervical adenopathy.
  C. *Streptococcus pneumoniae* is a common cause of bacterial pneumonia in neonates. It presents with cough, high fever, dyspnea, and auscultatory findings of lung consolidation.
  D. These are the classic findings associated with bronchiolitis in the young child. Respiratory syncytial virus is the most common cause of bronchiolitis in a child younger than 2 years.

106. The answer is **C** [Cardiovascular].
  A. Often, no cause can be identified, but chronic alcoholism and myocarditis are common etiologies of dilated cardiomyopathy.
  B. Coxsackieviruses are the most common cause of infectious myocarditis.
  C. Nearly all patients with mitral stenosis have underlying rheumatic heart disease.
  D. Risk factors for the development of pulmonary emboli include venous stasis, injury to the vessel wall, and hypercoagulability.

107. The answer is **A** [Obstetrics/Gynecology].
  A. Atrophic vaginitis resulting from estrogen deficiency may cause inflammation of the vagina, vulva, and urethra as well as a blood-tinged vaginal discharge. Urinalysis should not be abnormal except for hematuria secondary to contamination from the inflamed vulva and vagina.

B. Bacterial vaginosis is characterized by grayish-white, "fishy"-smelling vaginal discharge, which is less likely to be scant in quantity. Wet prep, if prepared, would reveal "clue cells." Urinalysis may show hematuria resulting from contamination.

C. Vaginal candidiasis is characterized by vaginal irritation and a thick, white, curd-like discharge. Wet prep findings of pseudohyphae and spores confirm the diagnosis. Microscopic hematuria may be present.

D. *Trichomonas vaginalis* produces symptoms of vaginal pruritus and a thin, greenish-white, frothy, foul-smelling discharge. Wet prep will confirm the motile protozoa and may reveal red RBCs. Urinalysis may include WBCs and RBCs.

108. The answer is **B** [Pulmonology].

A. Adenocarcinoma of the lung presents as peripheral nodules or masses; these are not associated with asthma or nasal polyps.

B. Aspirin may precipitate bronchospasm in patients with polyps and asthma.

C. Cystic fibrosis typically results in recurrent lung infections; nasal polyps and asthma are not common.

D. Rhinitis medicamentosa occurs with overuse of nasal decongestants (Afrin and others).

109. The answer is **B** [Pulmonology].

A. There generally are fewer physical examination findings in early COPD, which is much more closely linked to recent cigarette smoking.

B. Idiopathic pulmonary fibrosis (i.e., idiopathic fibrosing interstitial pneumonia) has a very insidious process but then is rapidly fatal. Digital clubbing is seen in up to 50% of patients at presentation. Histology is necessary to identify specific type.

C. Sarcoidosis typically presents with fever, malaise, and dyspnea or symptoms referable to the skin, eyes, peripheral nerves, liver, kidney, or heart.

D. Tuberculosis is more likely to manifest with malaise, weight loss, and fever/sweats.

110. The answer is **B** [Psychiatry/Behavioral Medicine].

A. Hypersensitivity, excessive self-importance, and rigidity are characteristic of narcissistic personality disorder.

B. Patients with schizotypal personality disorder are submissive and pessimistic. They have strong self-doubt, are unable to make decisions, and dislike being left alone.

C. Withdrawal from others, oversensitivity, shyness, and detachment are characteristic of avoidant personality disorder.

D. Emotional instability, overreactivity, and self-dramatization are characteristic of borderline personality disorder.

111. The answer is **A** [Neurology].

A. Febrile seizures can be prevented with oral diazepam (0.5 mg/kg in divided doses) for the duration of the febrile illness. Phenobarbital is given prophylactically after febrile seizures if the child exhibits neurologic deficits or prolonged seizures or has a family history of epilepsy.

B. Phenytoin and carbamazepine have not shown effectiveness in the treatment of febrile seizures.

C. See **B** for explanation.

D. Ethosuximide is used to treat absence seizures.

112. The answer is **B** [Infectious Disease].

A. Amoxicillin has the potential to exacerbate an overgrowth of *Candida* sp. by decreasing normal flora.

B. Nystatin is fungistatic and poorly absorbed by the GI tract. It is the first-line treatment for oral candidiasis in an infant.

C. Oral ketoconazole can cause liver abnormalities. It is reserved for resistant chronic candidiasis.

D. Amphotericin B has a high incidence of side effects. It should be used only in immunosuppressed patients with disseminated candidiasis.

113. The answer is **C** [Obstetrics/Gynecology].

A. See **C** for explanation.

B. See **C** for explanation.

C. Rapid weight gain in pregnancy most commonly is the result of fluid; this patient needs to be evaluated for preeclampsia.

D. See **C** for explanation.

114. The answer is **D** [Cardiovascular].

A. Daily aspirin plays a prominent role in decreasing the risk of infarction, but it is not the preferred treatment for this patient because of the significant level of stenosis.

B. Nitrate therapy is an effective therapy for angina, but it is not the best long-term treatment for this patient.

C. Aggressive risk factor reduction is important to initiate in this patient, but it is not the most timely or best choice.

D. Although medical therapy is important, this patient meets one of the generally accepted criteria for revascularization: stenosis of greater than 50% involving the left main coronary artery.

115. The answer is **B** [Orthopedics/Rheumatology].

A. Swimming maintains muscle tone but is a non-weight-bearing exercise; therefore, it does not help prevent osteoporosis.

B. An important measure to prevent osteoporosis is regular, modest weight-bearing exercise. Stair climbing has been shown to increase bone density in women.

C. Bicycling is a non-weight-bearing exercise.

D. Weight lifting does not necessarily load the bones/joints that are most affected by osteoporosis (i.e., spine and hips).

116. The answer is **B** [Cardiovascular].
    A. Polymyalgia rheumatica is based on pain and stiffness of the shoulder and pelvic girdle areas, frequently associated with fever. Almost 50% of these patients also have giant cell arteritis.
    B. Classic symptoms of giant cell arteritis (temporal arteritis) include headache, scalp tenderness, visual symptoms, jaw claudication, and throat pain. Fever is always present, with a normal WBC count and an elevated ESR.
    C. Wegener's granulomatosis presents with upper or lower respiratory tract symptoms (or both) along with glomerulonephritis.
    D. Sjögren's syndrome is characterized by dryness of the eyes, mouth, and other areas covered by mucous membranes and frequently is associated with a rheumatic disease, most often rheumatoid arthritis.

117. The answer is **B** [Gastrointestinal/Nutritional].
    A. Antibiotics, such as chloramphenicol, play no beneficial role in viral conditions.
    B. Immune globulin should be given routinely to all close personal contacts of a patient with hepatitis A. A recommended dose of 0.02 mL/kg IM has been found to be protective if given during incubation.
    C. Corticosteroids have no benefit in patients with viral hepatitis, including those with fulminant disease.
    D. Interferon-α is effective in the treatment of acute hepatitis C.

118. The answer is **D** [Cardiovascular].
    A. Basal metabolic temperature is useful in assessing gynecologic fertility issues, not syncope.
    B. Electrophysiologic testing may be needed, but it is invasive, expensive, and should be reserved for a later date.
    C. Stress testing is useful to determine cardiac dysfunction, especially in a patient with ischemia.
    D. The tilt-table test and event recorder placement are useful in diagnosing patients (especially those of middle age and older) with orthostatic hypotension. They should be done prior to any invasive procedures.

119. The answer is **D** [Urology/Renal].
    A. Abdominal films may reveal enlarged kidneys but do not give further information.
    B. See **D** for explanation.
    C. See **D** for explanation.
    D. The clinical picture indicates polycystic kidney disease. Ultrasonography easily and accurately can help to identify the presence, nature, and location of parenchymal cysts; if still unclear, CT is recommended.

120. The answer is **D** [Obstetrics/Gynecology].
    A. Dilation of 1 cm/hr is considered to be adequate progression.
    B. The second stage of labor does not begin until 10 cm.
    C. She is in the active stage of labor.
    D. This represents good progress of labor.

121. The answer is **D** [Endocrinology].
    A. See **D** for explanation.
    B. See **D** for explanation.
    C. See **D** for explanation.
    D. A transsphenoidal approach avoids invasion of the cranium and manipulation of the brain.

122. The answer is **C** [Endocrinology].
    A. See **C** for explanation.
    B. See **C** for explanation.
    C. The assessment suggests acromegaly caused by an increased release of growth hormone. The MRI evaluation of sella turcica will search for a pituitary adenoma, a common cause of acromegaly.
    D. See **C** for explanation.

123. The answer is **A** [Orthopedics/Rheumatology].
    A. Lachman's sign typically is positive in the presence of an anterior cruciate tear.
    B. McMurray's test typically is positive in the presence of a medial meniscus injury.
    C. An abduction stress test is likely to be positive with medial collateral ligament injury.
    D. Medial and lateral stress tests typically are positive in the presence of a collateral ligament tear.

124. The answer is **D** [Neurology].
    A. CT is useful if differentiation between ischemia and an active bleed is essential.
    B. Cerebral angiography is useful in diagnosing stenotic areas, particularly of the carotid artery.
    C. Cardiac catheterization is used to reveal ischemic potential of the cardiac muscles because of coronary occlusion. Systemic emboli originate from within the cardiac chambers.
    D. Transesophageal echocardiography is most beneficial in diagnosing cardiogenic emboli. This patient is at risk of cardiogenic emboli because of the atrial fibrillation.

125. The answer is **A** [Hematology].
    A. This patient is exhibiting manifestations of megaloblastic anemia caused by vitamin B_{12} deficiency.
    B. Folic acid deficiency also causes a megaloblastic anemia but without neurologic symptoms.
    C. G6PD deficiency causes a hemolytic anemia when certain drugs or foods are introduced.
    C. Iron deficiency anemia is characterized as microcytic and hypochromic.

126. The answer is **C** [Neurology].
- **A.** Gliosis and neuronal loss in the basal ganglia are associated with cortical basal degeneration.
- **B.** Multiple sclerosis is characterized by demyelinization and plaque formation found in the white matter of the brain and spinal cord.
- **C.** Senile plaques and neurofibrillary tangles are found at autopsy in patients with Alzheimer's disease.
- **D.** Degeneration of the dopaminergic nigrostriatal system in the central nervous system is associated with Parkinson's disease.

127. The answer is **D** [Infectious Disease].
- **A.** Tetracycline is the treatment of choice for *Chlamydia* sp.
- **B.** Metronidazole (Flagyl) is the treatment of choice for *Trichomonas* sp.
- **C.** Diflucan is an antifungal.
- **D.** This is a classic presentation of an initial outbreak of herpes genitalis. It is treated with an antiviral, such as Valtrex, not with antibiotics.

128. The answer is **D** [Eyes/Ears/Nose/Throat].
- **A.** Auralgan otic solution will decrease pain and inflammation in otitis media. It does not have antimicrobial properties.
- **B.** Debrox is a ceruminolytic for softening cerumen. It will not treat otitis externa.
- **C.** An oral cephalosporin has demonstrated efficacy in acute otitis media but not otitis externa.
- **D.** A variety of aural antibiotic drops are effective pharmaceutical therapy for otitis externa.

129. The answer is **B** [Eyes/Ears/Nose/Throat].
- **A.** Background (nonproliferative) retinopathy includes dot hemorrhages (microaneurysms), hard or soft exudates, retinal hemorrhages, edema, and dilated veins.
- **B.** Proliferative retinopathy is characterized by neovascularization, or new-forming blood vessels that grow out from the retina toward the vitreous humor, leading to retinal detachment.
- **C.** Lipemia retinalis is the white appearance of the vessels on the fundus when the serum triglyceride level exceeds 2,000 mg/dL.
- **D.** See A for explanation.

130. The answer is **D** [Gastrointestinal/Nutritional].
- **A.** Male gender, age 30–40 years, and reduced fluid intake are important risk factors for the development of kidney stones.
- **B.** Peptic ulcer disease is more common in men, smokers, and chronic NSAID users.
- **C.** Heavy alcohol intake, metabolic causes, drugs, and abdominal trauma are common risk factors for the development of pancreatitis.
- **D.** Obesity, female gender, and age older than 40 years represent the most common risk factors for the development of gallstones.

131. The answer is **B** [Gastrointestinal/Nutritional].
- **A.** Inflammatory diarrhea is small in volume (<1 L/day) and associated with left lower quadrant cramps, urgency, and tenesmus.
- **B.** The presence of bloody diarrhea (dysentery) indicates colonic tissue damage caused by invasion (*Shigella, Salmonella, Campylobacter* or *Yersinia* infection or amebiasis) or a toxin (*Clostridium difficile, Escherichia coli* O157:H7).
- **C.** Prominent vomiting suggests viral enteritis or *Staphylococcus aureus* food poisoning, both noninflammatory in nature.
- **D.** Steatorrhea is caused by undigested fats in the stool, which most commonly results from malabsorption secondary to pancreatic or liver disease.

132. The answer is **D** [Pulmonology].
- **A.** Patients with superior vena cava syndrome typically are tachycardic.
- **B.** Rhinophyma, or soft tissue and sebaceous hyperplasia of the nose, is common in acne rosacea.
- **C.** Adenocarcinoma causes localized rhonchi and, rarely, wheeze.
- **D.** This patient has developed superior vena cava syndrome secondary to obstruction from the mediastinal mass. Swelling of the face and neck are characteristic, as are headache, dizziness, visual loss, stupor, and syncope.

133. The answer is **C** [Pulmonology].
- **A.** RBC replacement and a biliary lamp are not treatments for hyaline membrane disease.
- **B.** See A for explanation.
- **C.** Surfactant replacement therapy has been shown to decrease mortality.
- **D.** Supplemental oxygen is a required primary intervention and an adjunct to other interventions.

134. The answer is **B** [Pulmonology].
- **A.** No evidence shows beneficial outcomes with antibiotics in sarcoidosis.
- **B.** Corticosteroids are indicated in sarcoidosis when a patient presents with constitutional symptoms, hypercalcemia, iritis, arthritis, central nervous system involvement, granulomatous hepatitis, or cutaneous lesions.
- **C.** No evidence supports beneficial outcomes with anticoagulants in sarcoidosis.
- **D.** Antivirals have no beneficial indications in sarcoidosis.

135. The answer is **C** [Hematology].
- **A.** Acute lymphocytic leukemia is the most common leukemia of childhood and presents with a lymphocytosis.
- **B.** Hodgkin's lymphoma produces Reed-Sternberg cells, which are found on bone marrow biopsy.

C. Multiple myeloma is associated with a monoclonal spike on serum protein electrophoresis.

D. Non-Hodgkin's lymphoma is associated with a paratrabecular lymphoid aggregate in the bone marrow.

136. The answer is **C** [Eyes/Ears/Nose/Throat].

A. The Weber test may be abnormal because of fluid behind the tympanic membrane, but it is nonspecific for otitis media.

B. Auditory acuity may be diminished, but this is not diagnostic of acute otitis media.

C. Fever, crying, and cleaning wax from the ear canal can all cause injected vessels and the appearance of an infected ear. In all of these cases, the eardrum will be normally mobile, unlike the markedly decreased or immobile tympanic membrane characteristic of acute otitis media.

D. Pain with movement of the auricle occurs with otitis externa.

137. The answer is **B** [Urology/Renal].

A. Ice packs cause further vasoconstriction, thereby increasing the risk of infarction.

B. Testicular torsion is most common in adolescent boys and is a surgical emergency. If torsion is complete, a testis can be infarcted in 4–6 hours.

C. Antibiotic therapy has no place in the treatment of torsion.

D. Delaying surgical intervention beyond 4–6 hours can lead to testicular infarction and subsequent infertility. Technetium-99m pertechnetate scans will confirm the presence of torsion; however, Doppler studies are quicker, less invasive, and just as effective to confirm the diagnosis.

138. The answer is **B** [Orthopedics/Rheumatology].

A. Surgery is not indicated initially.

B. Because lateral epicondylitis is an inflammatory disorder resulting from overuse, initial therapy would include NSAIDs and joint rest.

C. Lateral epicondylitis is an inflammatory, not an infectious, process, so antibiotics are not indicated.

D. Injectable steroids may be helpful in refractory cases, but rest and NSAIDs should be used first.

139. The answer is **D** [Dermatology].

A. Bleomycin intradermal injection is reserved for refractory warts, usually on the hands and plantar areas. Additionally, it is expensive and causes severe pain.

B. There is a greater chance of scarring with electrocautery, which is a concern when treating lesions on the face.

C. A 40% salicylic acid plaster is an acceptable treatment for plantar warts. A 6% salicylic acid gel would be acceptable for treating flat warts, as in this scenario.

D. Tretinoin (cream or gel) or topical imiquimod (Aldara) is the best treatment option listed for flat warts on the face.

140. The answer is **A** [Psychiatry/Behavioral Medicine].

A. The dopaminergic system is activated by nicotine (the same system that is affected by cocaine and amphetamine).

B. Although acetylcholine, norepinephrine, and nicotinic acid are involved, they are not the major neurotransmitter implicated in tobacco addiction.

C. See **B** for explanation.

D. See **B** for explanation.

141. The answer is **A** [Eyes/Ears/Nose/Throat].

A. A chalazion is a chronic granulomatous inflammation of a meibomian gland that may follow a hordeolum. It is characterized by a hard, nontender swelling on the lid margin.

B. Hordeolum is caused by acute infection of a meibomian gland, usually with *Staphylococcus aureus* and occasionally with other organisms, such as *Pseudomonas aeruginosa*. *Chlamydia trachoma* conjunctivitis does not present with lid lesions.

C. See **B** for explanation.

D. See **B** for explanation.

142. The answer is **B** [Cardiovascular].

A. Decreased pulses are seen in arterial disease.

B. Varicose veins are either asymptomatic or produce dull pains with exertion.

C. Long-standing varicose veins/venous insufficiency leads to hyperpigmentation and thinning of the overlying skin.

D. Pitting edema denotes pathology of the deeper veins.

143. The answer is **D** [Urology/Renal].

A. Urethral dilation would enhance the mechanical entry of bacteria into the bladder.

B. Condom usage is certainly indicated in a sexually active female but would not prevent the mechanical introduction of bacteria into the bladder.

C. Diaphragm usage has actually been shown to increase the risk of cystitis.

D. Cystitis results from bacterial entry into the bladder. Voiding immediately following intercourse helps to "wash-out" any bacteria that might be present in the urethra.

144. The answer is **C** [Gastrointestinal/Nutritional].

A. Antacids buffer hydrochloric acid and increase lower esophageal sphincter pressure.

B. H_2-receptor antagonists only decrease acid secretion.

C. Prokinetics, such as metoclopramide, increase both lower esophageal sphincter pressure and gastric emptying.

D. Proton-pump inhibitors decrease secretion and volume of acid.

145. The answer is **D** [Obstetrics/Gynecology].
  A. Urinalysis for glucosuria, ketonuria, and protein-uria should be obtained at each prenatal visit. Additionally, testing for bacteria and WBCs may be of some benefit.
  B. Ultrasonography, if performed routinely, is more informative between 18 and 20 weeks.
  C. α-Fetoprotein is best obtained between 16 and 18 weeks.
  D. Glucose screening for gestational diabetes is best obtained between 24 and 28 weeks.

146. The answer is **C** [Cardiovascular].
  A. Myocardial infarction causes hypokinesis in the infarcted area.
  B. No immediate effect in muscle size is noted after a myocardial infarction.
  C. Large areas of infarction cause severe wall-motion abnormalities, which most commonly are seen as hypokinesis.
  D. There usually is a decrease in left ventricular function secondary to myocardial infarction.

147. The answer is **C** [Obstetrics/Gynecology].
  A. The history is inconsistent with a viral infection.
  B. A cervical or endometrial biopsy may be a part of the complete evaluation of this patient but will not establish the diagnosis of cancer of the vagina.
  C. A biopsy of the lesion itself is necessary to establish the initial diagnosis. A complete evaluation may be necessary to establish a primary cancer and to rule out metastasis from another source.
  D. The history is inconsistent with a treponemal infection.

148. The answer is **C** [Psychiatry/Behavioral Medicine].
  A. Major depression, manic episodes, and acute schizophrenia are the three best indications for electroconvulsive therapy.
  B. Electroconvulsive therapy can be used in pregnancy when drugs may be contraindicated.
  C. Electroconvulsive therapy is effective for acute episodes of psychosis in patients with schizophrenia but not for chronic stable disease.
  D. Electroconvulsive therapy also is effective in catatonia, episodic or atypical psychoses, obsessive–compulsive disorder, and delirium.

149. The answer is **A** [Pulmonology].
  A. Chronic heart failure leads to cardiomegaly, which displaces the apical impulse laterally.
  B. Because of the hyperinflated lungs in emphysema, the apical impulse may be displaced to the upper epigastric region.
  C. The right second interspace overlies the aorta, which usually is not affected in chronic heart failure.

D. Under the left nipple is too vague an area, because depending on breast size, the nipple may vary in its location.

150. The answer is **A** [Infectious Disease].
  A. This patient has a septic joint and needs IV antibiotics. Failure to treat in this manner could result in permanent impairment of the knee joint.
  B. A single IM dose of ceftriaxone is the treatment for gonorrhea confined to the genitalia.
  C. An orthopedic surgery consult is not needed at this time. Antibiotics administered in a timely manner will preserve the knee joint.
  D. This patient does not have a rheumatologic condition.

151. The answer is **C** [Psychiatry/Behavioral Medicine].
  A. Additional strong predictive factors associated with increased suicide risk include age (>45 years for men, >55 years for women), male gender, and alcohol dependence.
  B. See **A** for explanation.
  C. A previous suicide attempt is the strongest indicator that a person is at increased risk.
  D. See **A** for explanation.

152. The answer is **A** [Orthopedics/Rheumatology].
  A. This is a classic Colles fracture. Without intra-articular involvement in older patients, this may be sufficiently treated with a sugar tong splint for 2–3 weeks, followed by a short arm cast for 2–3 weeks.
  B. Surgical intervention may be performed with intra-articular manifestation or increased angulation.
  C. See **A** for explanation.
  D. See **B** for explanation.

153. The answer is **C** [Pulmonology].
  A. Von Willebrand's disease is a hypocoagulable state. Hypercoaguable states are at risk for thrombophlebitis.
  B. Venous stasis, not dilatation, is a risk factor for the development of thrombosis.
  C. More than 90% of pulmonary emboli originate as clots in the deep veins of the lower extremities. Physiologic risk factors for venous thrombosis include venous stasis, venous endothelial injury, and hypercoagulability.
  D. A thrombosis of the superficial veins or tributaries does not result in pulmonary embolism.

154. The answer is **D** [Psychiatric/Behavioral Medicine].
  A. Thyroid dysfunction is unlikely given her history and the fact that she has seen numerous providers and had a battery of tests.
  B. Major depression is defined as depressed mood, anhedonia, significant weight change, sleep disturbances, fatigue, and trouble concentrating.
  C. Persons suffering from hypochondria fear they have a serious disease even though no physical evidence

supports their diagnosis. Their fear is consistent and persists despite reassurance and lack of specific findings.

D. Somatization disorder begins before the age of 30. Patients believe themselves to be sick and often see numerous practitioners with no organic pathology found. The complaints usually center around GI symptoms, back and joint pain, cardiopulmonary distress, sexual problems, and menstrual irregularity.

155. The answer is **B** [Pulmonology].

A. Sarcoidosis is a granulomatous disease; therefore, it does not cause any change in pulmonary fluids that can be obtained by sputum induction.

B. Tissue for histopathologic study is the definitive method to diagnose sarcoidosis. Biopsy evidence of a mononuclear cell granulomatous inflammatory process is confirmatory.

C. An elevated angiotensin-converting enzyme level is seen in 40–80% of patients with sarcoidosis. This finding is neither sensitive nor specific enough for diagnosis.

D. Sarcoidosis typically causes a high CD4:CD8 cell ratio, but this also can be seen in other interstitial lung diseases.

156. The answer is **C** [Hematology].

A. Cobalamin is vitamin B_{12}.

B. Folic acid deficiency is another cause of megaloblastic anemia.

C. The underlying pathology in pernicious anemia is the lack of intrinsic factor; this deficiency leads to an inability to absorb vitamin B_{12}.

D. See **C** for explanation.

157. The answer is **B** [Orthopedics/Rheumatology].

A. Patellofemoral dysfunction results from subtle maltracking of the patella with extension and flexion. History typically reveals pain aggravated by climbing, jumping, or prolonged sitting. Examination may reveal a positive patella apprehension sign.

B. Osgood-Schlatter disease results from repetitive injury and small avulsion injuries at the insertion of the patella tendon at the tibial tuberosity. Onset typically is during early adolescence. The patient complains of pain exacerbated by running, jumping, kneeling, and sitting with knees flexed.

C. Osteochondritis dissecans results from repetitive stress causing subchondral stress fractures, typically at the medial femoral condyle. A typical history is pain and stiffness after activity.

D. Sever's disease is caused by repetitive stress and microtrauma to the calcaneal apophysis. It presents with pain in the posterior heal that occurs after activity.

158. The answer is **A** [Cardiovascular].

A. Cardiac tamponade often is manifested by the presence of pulsus paradoxus, an exaggerated response from the normal physiologic drop in systolic blood pressure that occurs with inspiration (>10 mm Hg drop).

B. Pulmonary contusions, diaphragmatic ruptures, and pneumothorax are not associated with pulsus paradoxus.

C. See **B** for explanation.

D. See **B** for explanation.

159. The answer is **B** [Urology/Renal].

A. Intake of carbohydrates and zinc has not been associated with the development of kidney stones.

B. Increased fluid intake will decrease solute concentration and so reduce the likelihood of precipitation and stone formation.

C. Increased vitamin D intake will cause elevated calcium levels, which may cause increased stone formation.

D. See **A** for explanation.

160. The answer is **D** [Endocrinology].

A. An ultrasound of the thyroid can help to determine whether the nodule is solid or cystic, but not whether it is benign or malignant.

B. Nodules that are "hot" on radioisotopic scanning are unlikely to be malignant, and only 20% of cold nodules are found to be malignant.

C. A CT scan can show only the size and consistency of the nodule.

D. Fine-needle cytology from a thyroid nodule has a false-negative rate of only 4–6%, with an overall accuracy rate of 95%.

161. The answer is **D** [Orthopedics/Rheumatology].

A. Cyclosporine has been shown to have some clinical efficacy in spondyloarthropathy, but long-term studies need to be performed.

B. Although there have been clinical reports of improvement, few clinical trials have shown efficacy, and little evidence exists that methotrexate changes the course of axial disease.

C. IM corticosteroids may be used for short-term symptomatic treatment only.

D. This patient has psoriatic spondylitis. Although it is appropriate to administer either aspirin or NSAIDs for short-term treatment, in the presence of more severe disease with radiographic findings of erosive arthritis, a disease-modifying agent should be used. Randomized, controlled trials have produced evidence supporting the use of sulfasalazine, particularly in psoriatic arthritis.

162. The answer is **B** [Gastrointestinal/Nutritional].

A. About 25% of patients with intussusception require surgery after unsuccessful hydrostatic or pneumatic reduction.

B. Barium and air enemas are both diagnostic and therapeutic. Reduction by barium enema should not be attempted if signs of strangulated bowel, perforation, or severe toxicity are present.

C. Upper endoscopy is not an acceptable approach. Intussusception is a condition of the lower intestine.

D. Observation is not appropriate, because intervention should begin as soon as possible to prevent complete obstruction.

163. The answer is **C** [Dermatology].

A. See **C** for explanation.

B. See **C** for explanation.

C. Delayed primary closure is performed after a wound is left open for 4–5 days and then closed.

D. See **C** for explanation.

164. The answer is **C** [Obstetrics/Gynecology].

A. See **C** for explanation.

B. See **C** for explanation.

C. The American College of Obstetricians and Gynecologists currently recommends that all women who are sexually active have annual physical examinations, including Pap smears. After three consecutive normal annual Pap smears, screening may occur every 2 years in monogamous women with no other risk factors.

D. See **C** for explanation.

165. The answer is **B** [Neurology].

A. A seizure occurring within 3 days after vaccination is a precaution for further vaccination, not a contraindication. A seizure occurring 5 days after vaccination is very unlikely to be related to vaccination.

B. The causal relationship between neurologic illness and pertussis vaccine is unclear, but a child who exhibited a clearly neurologic disorder following administration should not receive additional doses.

C. A temperature of 102°F is a common reaction to vaccination and alone is not an indication to prohibit additional doses.

D. Episodes of inconsolable crying are not uncommon after vaccination, but they do not necessarily indicate a neurologic problem. They also do not contraindicate future vaccination unless accompanied by significant neurologic symptoms.

166. The answer is **A** [Urology/Renal].

A. Casts with entrapped red cells are suggestive of glomerulonephritis or vasculitis.

B. Casts are not expected in infections in the lower urinary tract.

C. Leukocyte casts may be seen in pyelonephritis.

D. Granular casts and large numbers of epithelial casts are found in intrinsic renal disease, such as acute tubular necrosis.

167. The answer is **A** [Cardiovascular].

A. Because of the common symptom of effort syncope associated with aortic stenosis, any type of exercise stress test is contraindicated.

B. Hypertension is a common comorbidity in cardiac/angina patients and is not a contraindication.

C. Exercise stress testing commonly is indicated to help diagnose the cause of unknown recurrent chest pain whether related to exertion or not.

D. Stable angina is the most common reason for a patient to undergo an exercise stress test.

168. The answer is **B** [Pulmonology].

A. Patients do not have reduced lung volume with COPD. Total lung capacity is normal, or increased, while the forced expiratory volume in 1 second is decreased.

B. COPD leads to chronic hypercapnia. Changes in bicarbonate levels are then needed to normalize brain pH. These changes decrease the central chemoreceptor sensitivity to changes in arterial $PaCO_2$. Minute ventilation then depends on stimuli from the carotid bodies that function as sensors of arterial oxygenation. High concentrations of inspired oxygen reduce carotid body output, leading to a fall in minute ventilation and, possibly, a rapid rise in $PaCO_2$ and coma.

C. Right heart failure is a complication of COPD in patients with a PaO_2 of less than 50 mm Hg at rest.

D. Loss of lung elastic recoil is part of the pathology of COPD but is not the cause of respiratory failure.

169. The answer is **D** [Pulmonology].

A. Uvulopalatopharyngoplasty is a second-generation surgical procedure and is not considered to be first line. Approximately one-third of patients with sleep apnea benefit.

B. Tricyclic antidepressants are not an appropriate choice for sleep apnea. Sedating tricyclic antidepressants may be effective in patients who have depression and experience insomnia.

C. A bronchodilator is a treatment for asthma but not for obstructive sleep apnea.

D. The most common and successful treatment for sleep apnea is continuous positive airway pressure (CPAP). This therapy uses continuously administered air via nasal mask to splint the airway pneumatically. Maintaining positive air pressure prevents the airway from collapsing during inhalation, when intrathoracic pressure becomes negative.

170. The answer is **A** [Gastrointestinal/Nutritional].

A. A bird's beak deformity at the lower esophageal sphincter is pathognomonic for achalasia.

B. Barium swallow in esophageal carcinoma typically reveals a bulky, eroded, partially obstructing esophageal mass.

C. Recurrent heartburn is the hallmark of gastroesophageal reflux disease; barium swallow would not show a bird's beak deformity.

D. Angina is not associated with deformity on barium swallow.

171. The answer is **D** [Obstetrics/Gynecology].
 A. A normal-size uterus that is slightly softened and tender describes no particular uterine disorder.
 B. A diffusely enlarged uterus that is firm and globular in shape describes no particular uterine disorder.
 C. A slightly softened, tender, diffusely globular uterine enlargement is the classic description of adenomyosis.
 D. A firm, irregularly shaped, nontender, enlarged uterus is the classic description of leiomyoma or fibroids.

172. The answer is **A** [Cardiovascular].
 A. Doppler ultrasound is noninvasive, highly sensitive, and specific for popliteal and femoral thrombi.
 B. Although venography is more sensitive and specific, disadvantages include being an invasive procedure, technical difficulty, and a small risk of morbidity.
 C. ^{125}I-fibrinogen scan only detects active clot formation, and it takes several hours to obtain results.
 D. Although impedance plethysmography may be as accurate as ultrasound, it is less sensitive in detecting thrombi in small vessels, such as calf vein thrombi.

173. The answer is **D** [Endocrinology].
 A. Crohn's disease typically presents insidiously, with intermittent episodes of fever, diarrhea, and lower abdominal pain. Sweating, palpitations, and chest pain do not occur.
 B. Clinical findings of adrenocorticoid insufficiency are weakness, abdominal pain, fever, confusion, nausea, vomiting, and diarrhea.
 C. Clinical findings of irritable bowel syndrome (IBS) are abdominal pain, altered bowel habits, and bloating. IBS is a diagnosis of exclusion and is unlikely to present for the first time in a person older than 40 years.
 D. Clinical findings of hyperthyroidism can include hyperactivity, irritability, heat intolerance, increased appetite, weight loss, weakness, and atrial fibrillation.

174. The answer is **A** [Pulmonology].
 A. This is the classic presentation of laryngotracheitis or croup.
 B. With epiglottiditis, patients will have more acute onset, high fevers, and moderate to severe respiratory distress. It is more typical in an older patient population.
 C. Foreign body aspiration would not have the prodromal upper respiratory infection symptoms, and the barking cough is not suggestive of foreign body.
 D. An infant with pneumonia would likely present with more systemic symptoms, such as a higher fever, malaise, GI symptoms, chills, as well as nasal

flaring, or grunting respirations. Physical examination findings more likely would reveal some consolidation on lung examination.

175. The answer is **A** [Gastrointestinal/Nutritional].
 A. Fever, constipation, nausea, and vomiting with left lower quadrant pain in an elderly patient suggests diverticulitis.
 B. Pancreatitis usually presents with tenderness in the upper abdomen, often with radiation to the back.
 C. Symptoms of inguinal hernia include a gradual onset of cramp-like pain with a palpable mass. Fever usually is not present.
 D. Fever, nausea, and vomiting are unlikely in colon cancer.

176. The answer is **C** [Urology/Renal].
 A. Initial management of renal calculi up to 6 mm in diameter involves at least 6 weeks of conservative management. Invasive procedures such as pyelolithotomy are reserved until spontaneous stone passage has failed.
 B. Increasing fluid intake and analgesia are important in the management of a stone that is passing down the ureter but are not adequate for a stone that is in the pelvis with a rising BUN.
 C. Lithotripsy is the procedure of choice for a renal calculus that is obstructing renal output as evidenced by a rising BUN.
 D. Allopurinol is used only when the presence of uric acid stones is confirmed and if hyperuricemia is present.

177. The answer is **C** [Eyes/Ears/Nose/Throat].
 A. Open-angle glaucoma causes slight cupping of the optic disc or changes in the retinal nerve fiber layer.
 B. Clouding of the lens indicates cataracts, which typically causes diffuse blurring of vision.
 C. The precursor to age-related macular degeneration is age-related maculopathy, of which the hallmark is the development of retinal drusen. The visual loss is central. Amsler grid testing shows metamorphopsia.
 D. Vitreous hemorrhage is suspected with a sudden loss of vision, floaters, or bleeding within the eye.

178. The answer is **B** [Dermatology].
 A. Auspitz's sign refers to the appearance of tiny blood droplets when the scales of psoriasis are removed.
 B. Koebner's phenomenon is the development of new lesions on otherwise normal skin following minor trauma.
 C. Nikolsky's sign is present when the epidermis is dislodged from the dermis by lateral shearing pressure, resulting in erosion. It is associated with blistering disorders, such as toxic epidermal necrolysis.
 D. Wickham's striae are linear markings found on the lesions associated with lichen planus.

179. The answer is **C** [Cardiovascular].
  A. A change in serum uric acid is not commonly associated with secondary hypertension.
  B. A fasting lipid profile is useful in assessing the risk of atherosclerotic disease, but it is nonspecific in evaluating possible secondary hypertension.
  C. Renal arteriography is the definitive test for renal artery stenosis. In a patient with diabetes who has signs of peripheral vascular disease and blood pressure that has become difficult to control, renal artery stenosis is the likely cause.
  D. In a patient with renal insufficiency, intravenous pyelography (IVP) may cause renal failure because of the contrast dye. Creatinine clearance needs to be determined before IVP to rule out renal insufficiency in an at-risk patient.

180. The answer is **A** [Urology/Renal].
  A. A urinalysis and urine culture is the most logical and cost-effective step in the workup of painless hematuria. This patient may have benign hematuria because of exercise. Urinalysis can determine a glomerular or nonglomerular origin, directing the next most logical step in the workup.
  B. A PSA determination has utility, especially when combined with a digital rectal examination, for detecting prostate cancer. Acute onset of hematuria in an otherwise asymptomatic man, however, would not indicate prostate cancer.
  C. CT of the abdomen is expensive and time-consuming. It may be indicated, but generally only after urinalysis and urine culture narrow the differential diagnosis.
  D. A CBC may be indicated to check for anemia resulting from chronic blood loss. Given no prior history, it would not be the next step in diagnosing this patient.

181. The answer is **A** [Cardiovascular].
  A. These symptoms and blood pressure findings are suggestive of coarctation. The diagnosis is more common in males and can be associated with significant complications. If not diagnosed in infancy, patients remain asymptomatic until the hypertension causes heart failure or cerebrovascular events.
  B. Constrictive pericarditis may have similar, nonspecific symptoms, but blood pressure readings usually are not elevated and are the same in the upper and lower extremities.
  C. A dissecting thoracic aorta would present with acute onset of severe chest pain.
  D. Transposition of the great vessels usually is diagnosed at birth (secondary to cyanosis). Other major abnormalities are present and would be apparent by this time.

182. The answer is **D** [Dermatology].
  A. Milia are superficial epidermal inclusion cysts typically found in newborns. They consist of firm, 1- to 2-mm vesicles.

  B. The lesions of varicella typically appear as a "dew-drop on a rose petal," with a fine vesicle sitting on an erythematous base. The vesicle often is excoriated before examination, because the lesions tend to be pruritic. Such lesions are not likely to last 2 weeks.
  C. Common warts typically are well-circumscribed papules with a roughened, irregular, keratinized surface.
  D. Molluscum contagiosum is caused by a DNA pox virus that is transmitted via skin to skin contact and by autoinoculation. They are classically oval or dome-like, opalescent, and flesh-colored or white, they have a central umbilication, and may contain a cheesy exudate.

183. The answer is **D** [Endocrinology].
  A. Thyroidectomy is not indicated in most cases.
  B. About 1% of thyroid nodules increase in size; a few involute.
  C. Conversion to malignancy is rare.
  D. Benign nodules are followed by periodic palpation. If further growth occurs, another biopsy is indicated.

184. The answer is **B** [Infectious Disease].
  A. IV antibiotics are not necessary for this wound, because there are no signs of systemic bacteremia.
  B. Cuts that are prone to tetanus are those more than 6 hours old, contaminated with dirt or debris, with ischemic or necrotic edges, or infected. This patient needs immune globulin to neutralize circulating toxin. She also needs Td now, in 4–6 weeks, and in 6–12 months to complete active immunization. Broad-spectrum antibiotics are warranted for the current cutaneous infection.
  C. See **A** and **B** for explanation.
  D. See **A** and **B** for explanation.

185. The answer is **D** [Cardiovascular].
  A. Urokinase has not been specifically approved for use in treating acute myocardial infarction.
  B. There is no evidence that adjunctive heparin therapy following streptokinase improves the outcome in treatment of myocardial infarction.
  C. Anistreplase is a conjugate of streptokinase; adjunctive heparin therapy does not improve the outcome.
  D. Reocclusion rates are higher with tissue plasminogen activator because of the shorter half-life; therefore, IV heparin is recommended for at least 24 hours.

186. The answer is **C** [Obstetrics/Gynecology].
  A. See **C** for explanation.
  B. See **C** for explanation.
  C. The idea is to eliminate the occult metastases responsible for late recurrences while they are microscopic and, theoretically, most vulnerable to anticancer agents.
  D. See **C** for explanation.

187. The answer is **A** [Eyes/Ears/Nose/Throat].

A. Inspiratory stridor and unilateral wheezing are classic manifestations of obstruction with a foreign body; therefore, rigid bronchoscopy is recommended to locate and remove the foreign body.

B. Asthma is an unlikely diagnosis because of the unilateral findings. Oral steroids require several hours to days to become fully effective. Because this case typifies the presentation of a lower airway obstruction, a delay in its recognition may be fatal.

C. Postural drainage is not recommended, because it may cause the foreign body to become dislodged and obstruct a central airway.

D. Albuterol is not recognized as an effective treatment in relieving a lower airway foreign body obstruction. Delaying bronchoscopy may lead to greater morbidity or mortality in this patient.

188. The answer is **A** [Neurology].

A. Acoustic neuroma presents as unilateral nerve deafness with deterioration of speech. Any middle-aged patient complaining of unilateral hearing loss should undergo MRI.

B. Vertigo and tinnitus do not occur in acoustic neuroma.

C. See **B** for explanation.

D. Facial numbness is present in about one-fourth of patients at the time of diagnosis.

189. The answer is **B** [Dermatology].

A. Erysipelas is a superficial cutaneous cellulitis with marked dermal lymphatic vessel involvement. It presents as a painful, bright red, raised, edematous plaque with advancing borders. The area is sharply demarcated from the surrounding normal skin. The most common sites are the face and lower legs.

B. Lymphangitis is inflammation of the lymphatic vessel. It is characterized by bright red streaks ascending proximally.

C. Necrotizing fasciitis is a deep-seated infection of the subcutaneous tissue. It is manifested by swelling, heat, and redness progressing into blisters and gangrene.

D. Thrombophlebitis is an inflammatory thrombosis of a superficial vein characterized by redness, tenderness, and heat.

190. The answer is **C** [Orthopedics/Rheumatology].

A. Estrogen acts to inhibit osteoclastic bone resorption and prevents bone loss in early and late postmenopausal women.

B. Raloxifene (Evista) is a selective estrogen-receptor modulator that prevents bone loss and may reduce the risk of vertebral fracture.

C. Bisphosphonates (alendronate, etidronate) have demonstrated utility in bone loss prevention and have been reported to increase bone mineral density in postmenopausal women, even at low doses.

D. Studies of calcitonin have shown it to be less potent and less effective than other antiresorptive medications. It should be reserved for those who cannot tolerate the other medications.

191. The answer is **C** [Infectious Disease].

A. See **C** for explanation.

B. See **C** for explanation.

C. Congenital malformations are more likely and more severe when the infection is contracted during the first trimester.

D. See **C** for explanation.

192. The answer is **A** [Neurology].

A. *Streptococcus pneumoniae* is the most common cause of meningitis in children up to age 4. From age 3–18, *Neisseria meningitidis* accounts for a similar number of cases.

B. Group B β-hemolytic streptococcus is the most common causative agent in a newborn.

C. The incidence of *Haemophilus influenzae* meningitis has dropped markedly because of routine immunization in early childhood.

D. *Listeria monocytogenes* is a concern only in immunocompromised children.

193. The answer is **A** [Gastrointestinal/Nutritional].

A. Asymptomatic patients in whom diverticulosis is discovered should be encouraged to increase fluids and follow a high-fiber diet or take fiber supplements (bran powder, psyllium or methylcellulose). Ingestion of 10–12 g of fiber per day often is all that is needed to avoid diverticulitis.

B. Prevention of constipation is preferred over treatment of constipation. Laxatives are a treatment for constipation.

C. Low-residue diets minimize high-fiber foods.

D. At least one to two glasses of fluids should be taken with meals.

194. The answer is **D** [Cardiovascular].

A. See **D** for explanation.

B. See **D** for explanation.

C. See **D** for explanation.

D. The causative arrhythmia in the majority of cases of sudden death is ventricular fibrillation, which usually is preceded by ventricular tachycardia.

195. The answer is **B** [Urology/Renal].

A. Anasarca is a result of protein loss and/or congestive heart failure and is not a specific indication for dialysis.

B. In a patient with chronic renal failure, pH less than 7.20 is an indication for dialysis. Other indications include pericarditis, seizures, and volume overload unresponsive to diuretic treatment.

C. Hypoalbuminemia may be a result of renal protein loss but is not a specific indication for dialysis.

D. Oliguria may occur in both acute and chronic failure. It is not an indication for dialysis unless accompanied by volume overload, severe metabolic acidosis, pericarditis, seizures, or hyperkalemia.

196. The answer is **D** [Urology/Renal].
   A. Because of the high incidence of penicillin-resistant gonorrhea, penicillin is not the drug of choice.
   B. Chlamydia is effectively treated with tetracyclines, erythromycin, or azithromycin (Zithromax). Azithromycin has the benefit of single dosing, improving patient compliance.
   C. See **B** for explanation.
   D. Rocephin is the drug of choice in gonorrhea.

197. The answer is **D** [Obstetrics/Gynecology].
   A. A tetracycline is an appropriate drug for the treatment of chlamydial cervicitis. Its use is contraindicated during pregnancy, however, because it is known to cause tooth discoloration in the child.
   B. Oral metronidazole is used for the treatment of bacterial vaginosis and trichomonal vaginitis, not chlamydial cervicitis. Its use is contraindicated during pregnancy because of the risk of toxicity to the fetus.
   C. Metronidazole, by any route of administration, is ineffective for the treatment of chlamydial cervicitis. Furthermore, concern exists regarding potential teratogenicity.
   D. Erythromycin is an appropriate alternative drug for the treatment of chlamydial cervicitis in patients who are pregnant or allergic to tetracycline.

198. The answer is **C** [Infectious Disease].
   A. The use of antibiotics is not indicated for this viral illness, which spreads via respiratory droplets.
   B. Hospitalization is not indicated in erythema infectiosum.
   C. No treatment is indicated for this condition; use supportive care only.
   D. Steroids are not effective in this condition and should be avoided.

199. The answer is **C** [Endocrinology].
   A. Monthly examinations are likely too often and may cause undue anxiety and a tax on the health care system.
   B. Quarterly examinations may be necessary in a patient with peripheral neuropathy who is at higher risk of ulcer formation or gangrenous changes.
   C. Current guidelines call for routine foot examination one or two times per year by a clinician. Daily examinations by the patient or a family member should be encouraged.
   D. Every other year is not frequent enough and may cause an early lesion to be missed.

200. The answer is **D** [Pulmonology].
   A. Tracheotomy is indicated for severe upper airway obstruction, not anaphylaxis.

B. IV antihistamines may be helpful, but onset of action does not occur for 15–30 minutes.
   C. High-flow oxygen should be administered by face mask.
   D. Immediate subcutaneous administration of epinephrine, 0.3–0.5 mg in a 1:1,000 solution, is indicated if there is no significant circulatory compromise; if signs of shock are present, 0.3–0.5 mg in a 1:10,000 solution, should be administered IV.

201. The answer is **A** [Gastrointestinal/Nutritional].
   A. Fasting serum gastrin concentrations of greater than 150 pg/mL (median, 500–600 pg/mL) are diagnostic for Zollinger-Ellison syndrome. Levels should be obtained when patients are not taking H_2-receptor antagonists for 24 hours or proton-pump inhibitors for 6 days.
   B. Serum amylase is helpful for evaluating acute pancreatitis.
   C. Cholecystokinin administration is useful in diagnosing acalculous cholecystitis.
   D. Hemoglobin A_{1c} is helpful for monitoring glucose control in diabetes.

202. The answer is **A** [Gastrointestinal/Nutritional].
   A. A Mallory-Weiss tear is a result of retching; a linear mucosal tear confirms the diagnosis.
   B. A protrusion of pharyngeal mucosa at the pharyngoesophageal junction is consistent with an esophageal web.
   C. Esophagitis results in several discrete ulcers.
   D. A thin, diaphragm-like membrane is consistent with Zenker's diverticulum.

203. The answer is **A** [Pulmonology].
   A. The lung exam in influenza generally is normal.
   B. Diffuse expiratory wheezes are indicative of bronchospasm (asthma).
   C. Dullness and rhonchi indicate bacterial pneumonia.
   D. Scattered crackles and inspiratory wheeze indicate interstitial disease.

204. The answer is **D** [Obstetrics/Gynecology].
   A. Amenorrhea is a presumptive symptom of pregnancy.
   B. Nausea and vomiting are presumptive symptoms of pregnancy.
   C. Vulvar and vaginal cyanosis are known as Chadwick's sign, which is considered to be presumptive for pregnancy.
   D. Fetal movements are a positive sign of pregnancy.

205. The answer is **C** [Pulmonology].
   A. Intubation is not indicated, because positive pressure ventilation may make the tension pneumothorax worse.

B. Oxygen may increase the rate of resorption in small pneumothoraces but is not the best intervention for a large tension pneumothorax.

C. Aspiration with a large needle can quickly relieve the tension pneumothorax.

D. A thoracotomy tube is the ultimate treatment of a large tension pneumothorax, but insertion may be delayed because of practitioner skills or equipment setup.

206. The answer is **B** [Pulmonology].

A. Failure to begin prophylactic therapy increases the risk that this child will become infected with tuberculosis.

B. Although a child initially has a negative skin test, it is best to begin prophylaxis with isoniazid for 3 months. At that time, repeat the skin test; if it is positive, the preventive therapy should be continued for at least 9 months.

C. Chest radiographs are indicated following a positive skin test.

D. Sputum cultures are reserved for symptomatic disease.

207. The answer is **A** [Gastrointestinal/Nutritional].

A. This patient exhibits a vitamin B_{12} deficiency from lack of animal products related to her vegan diet. Oral cobalamin (vitamin B_{12}), 1-2 mg/day, is the treatment of choice for most patients. This dose is as effective and, possibly, superior to a parenteral regimen in all causes of cobalamin deficiency.

B. Iron deficiency is associated with microcytic anemia.

C. Although folate can cause megaloblastic anemia, it is distributed widely in plants as well as in products of animal origin. Green vegetables are particularly rich sources of folate.

D. Vitamin D is not associated with megaloblastic anemia.

208. The answer is **C** [Orthopedics/Rheumatology].

A. Steroid injection is indicated if there is soft-tissue impingement.

B. Surgical reconstruction may be indicated in severe chronic instability following an ankle injury.

C. Most ankle sprains heal without residual problems. The treatment of a class I sprain, as this is, may include rest, ice, compression, and elevation. Within a few days, the patient should begin simple range-of-motion exercises. The patient may return to normal activities in 6–8 weeks.

D. See **C** for explanation.

209. The answer is **A** [Cardiovascular].

A. Coarctation of the aorta results in strong arterial pulsations in the arms and weaker, delayed pulsations in the legs. Late systolic ejection murmurs may be heard over the area of the cardiac base and posteriorly, especially over the spinous processes.

B. Pulmonary stenosis is associated with a parasternal lift and a loud, harsh systolic murmur and thrill in the left second and third intercostal spaces.

C. Tetralogy of Fallot causes cyanosis and hypoxic spells. The rough ejection murmur is best heard along the left sternal border.

D. Ventricular septal defects cause loud, harsh, holosystolic murmurs in the left third and fourth intercostal spaces.

210. The answer is **D** [Endocrinology].

A. Free T_4 is used mainly to monitor thyroid activity during treatment for hyperthyroidism.

B. T_3 resin uptake is a measurement of thyroid-binding protein and is used to correct a total serum T_4 measurement, creating a free T_4 index ($T_4 \times T_3$ uptake).

C. Free T_4 index ($T_4 \times T_3$ uptake) helps correct for abnormalities of T_4 binding.

D. Thyroid-stimulating hormone is the best single screening test for thyroid disease. It will be increased in hypothyroidism and suppressed in hyperthyroidism, regardless of the underlying cause.

211. The answer is **B** [Eyes/Ears/Nose/Throat].

A. A lesion in the optic nerve would cause total blindness in the affected eye (e.g., right nerve = total blindness in the right eye).

B. A lesion at the optic chiasm would cause bitemporal hemianopia.

C. A lesion in the optic tract would cause either left or right homonymous hemianopia (e.g., right tract = left homonymous hemianopia).

D. A lesion in the optic radiation would cause a partial left or right homonymous hemianopia (e.g., right tract = left homonymous hemianopia).

212. The answer is **D** [Infectious Disease].

A. *Escherichia coli* O157:H7 typically causes hemorrhagic colitis as well as hemolytic-uremic syndrome.

B. Rotavirus typically affects young children and causes the temperature to exceed 101°F.

C. *Salmonella typhi* does not cause symptoms so abruptly. Manifestations occur in a step-like fashion with increased temperature.

D. Staphylococcal food poisoning typically starts 4–6 hours after ingestion of contaminated food. Custard-filled desserts are common food vectors, as are foods left at room temperature for prolonged periods of time.

213. The answer is **A** [Orthopedics/Rheumatology].

A. The patient's history of repetitive pain after use of the short extensor and long abductor tendon of the thumb along with the physical findings and positive Finkelstein test (pain with abduction and ulnar deviation of the thumb) strongly support de Quervain's disease.

B. Osteoarthritis of the carpometacarpal joint in this patient would have been evidenced by radiography and a positive "grind test." Axial compression or extension of the thumb with rotation results in crepitus.

C. The patient did not have complaints of a sore throat, fever, or vaginal discharge. Although gonococcal tenosynovitis may mimic de Quervain's disease, no further physical findings supported this diagnosis (e.g., hemorrhagic papules found on the hand).

D. The radiographic findings negate a carpometacarpal joint (Bennett's) fracture at this point.

214. The answer is **A** [Gastrointestinal/Nutritional].

A. The history of progressive dysphagia for solids with a need to regurgitate suggests an obstruction, most likely carcinoma, and esophagography is mandated. Any irregularity or narrowing indicates obstruction and a need for a biopsy.

B. Because of the abundance of organ shadows, the esophagus is not well visualized on plain-film radiographs.

C. An ultrasound is a good tool for studying the gallbladder, pancreas, and liver, but it is less desirable for studying any air-filled areas, such as the esophagus, stomach, or intestines.

D. Esophageal motility studies are indicated with dysphagia of liquids or where solids can be forced with Valsalva or change in position.

215. The answer is **B** [Hematology].

A. ABO incompatibility results in immediate hemolysis and shock.

B. Disseminated intravascular coagulation is characterized by bleeding from many sites as all coagulation factors are consumed and then broken down. Laboratory findings include decreased fibrinogen level and platelet count, prolonged prothrombin time and partial thromboplastin time, and presence of fibrin split products.

C. Idiopathic thrombocytopenia is characterized by decreased platelet count, but coagulation factors are normal.

D. Bleeding would be localized only and, if lacerations of the liver were not repaired properly, would result in shock.

216. The answer is **D** [Pulmonology].

A. With no response to the first two treatments, other additional medications are indicated.

B. Although steroids will help in the treatment, this option without a comprehensive examination could be dangerous.

C. Salmeterol is good for the prevention of asthma exacerbations.

D. Although moderate asthma may be managed at home with telephone assistance, his speaking only in single words, not moving, and the lack of response to two albuterol treatments indicate a severe and, possibly, progressive state.

217. The answer is **B** [Gastrointestinal/Nutritional].

A. α-Fetoprotein is used to monitor recurrence of hepatocellular carcinoma; mild elevations may be seen in chronic hepatitis.

B. Carcinoembryonic antigen is used to monitor recurrence of colon carcinoma. A preoperative level of greater than 5 ng/mL is a poor prognostic indicator. Elevated levels after resection suggest persistent disease and warrant further investigation.

C. Cancer antigen 19-9 had been used to monitor recurrence of pancreatic carcinoma but has not proved to be sensitive enough. Increased values also are found in acute and chronic pancreatitis and cholangitis.

D. Cancer antigen 125 is used to monitor recurrence of ovarian carcinoma. It also may be elevated in premenopausal women with benign diseases, such as endometriosis.

218. The answer is **A** [Orthopedics/Rheumatology].

A. In women, maintenance of ideal body weight has been shown to reduce the risk of symptomatic knee osteoarthritis.

B. Nonsteroidals are used as treatment after patients fail acetaminophen therapy. Therapy is associated with toxicity; it is not used for prevention.

C. Contact sports increase the risk of osteoarthritis.

D. Multivitamins generally will not affect the risk of osteoarthritis. Maintaining a diet high in vitamin D, however, can reduce the progression of established osteoarthritis.

219. The answer is **D** [Orthopedics/Rheumatology].

A. The proximal tibia is the second most frequently affected bone.

B. The proximal humerus is the third most frequently affected bone.

C. The scapula is rarely affected.

D. The distal femur is the site most commonly affected by osteosarcoma.

220. The answer is **A** [Urology/Renal].

A. The most common and ubiquitous urinary tract pathogen is *Escherichia coli*. This enterobacterial species colonizes the vaginal introitus and is easily misplaced into the urinary bladder during intercourse.

B. *Klebsiella pneumoniae* is a cause of acute pyelonephritis, pneumonia, and other respiratory tract infections in an immunocompromised host.

C. *Chlamydia trachomatis* in women usually involves the cervix and can develop into pelvic inflammatory disease.

D. *Pseudomonas aeruginosa* causes infection in an immunocompromised host, especially in patients with burns, cystic fibrosis, or other respiratory diseases.

221. The answer is **C** [Hematology].
  A. Allopurinol is given to patients with polycythemia who develop secondary hyperuricemia.
  B. Diphenhydramine will help relieve the pruritus but will not affect the disease.
  C. Phlebotomy is the treatment of choice in polycythemia vera. One unit per week is removed until the hematocrit reaches 45%.
  D. Prednisone has no role in the treatment of polycythemia.

222. The answer is **C** [Pulmonology].
  A. See **D** for explanation.
  B. Only 30% of solitary nodules discovered by routine chest radiography in asymptomatic patients are pulmonary malignancies. Of these, 75% are primary, and the remainder are metastatic lesions.
  C. Of the 70% of solitary nodules that prove to be benign, 85–90% are granulomas. Of these, most are tuberculous, but histoplasmosis or coccidioidomycosis must be considered.
  D. The remaining 2–3% of benign solitary nodules are bronchogenic cysts, hydatid cysts, pseudolymphomas, or AV malformations.

223. The answer is **D** [Pulmonology].
  A. This blood gas is consistent with an increase in bicarbonate with hypoxia as a result of airway obstruction that occurs much later in the attack.
  B. This blood gas is a result of respiratory acidosis, a build-up of $PaCO_2$ that indicates a partial failure of gas exchange. It occurs later in the attack.
  C. This blood gas indicates poor gas exchange and respiratory acidosis.
  D. During the initial stage of an asthma attack, the patient is still able to move air in and out with an increase in respiratory rate. **A** normal or elevated $PaCO_2$, in a patient with asthma, is an indication of poor gas exchange, resulting in an increase of $PaCO_2$ and a decrease in PaO_2.

224. The answer is **B** [Psychiatry/Behavioral Medicine].
  A. Trials of fluoxetine (Prozac, an SSRI) have yielded positive results, but this would not be the first treatment.
  B. The first consideration in the treatment of anorexia nervosa is to restore the patient's nutritional state.
  C. Depressive symptoms may coexist with anorexic nervosa; however, treatment of the nutritional deficiency should be the first step.
  D. Cognitive-behavioral therapy is important in the management of patients with eating disorders, but restoration of nutritional status must be the initial priority.

225. The answer is **B** [Psychiatry/Behavioral Medicine].
  A. Catatonic schizophrenia is characterized by marked disturbance of motor function.
  B. Paranoid schizophrenia is characterized by delusions of persecution.
  C. Disorganized schizophrenia is characterized by marked regression to primitive, disinhibited, unorganized behavior without meeting criteria for catatonic type.
  D. Undifferentiated schizophrenia is reserved for those individuals who have schizophrenia but who do not fit into a specified type.

226. The answer is **C** [Cardiovascular].
  A. Thrills associated with murmurs are almost always clinically significant.
  B. Congestive heart failure rarely causes a thrill.
  C. Thrills most often accompany loud, harsh, or rumbling murmurs of at least grade IV/VI, such as those of aortic stenosis, patent ductus arteriosus, ventricular septal defect, and mitral stenosis.
  D. Finger pads are best used for feeling impulses. Thrills are felt best through bone. The suggested technique is pressing the ball of the hand firmly on the chest.

227. The answer is **C** [Obstetrics/Gynecology].
  A. Colposcopy is used in the diagnosis of cervical dysplasia/cancer.
  B. KOH preparations are used in the diagnosis of candidiasis and bacterial vaginosis.
  C. The diagnosis of infection with *Trichomonas vaginalis* is made by observing motile protozoa on wet-prep smear.
  D. Dark-field microscopy is used in the diagnosis of infection with *Treponema pallidum*.

228. The answer is **B** [Gastrointestinal/Nutritional].
  A. Milk is not a contributing factor to heartburn.
  B. Smoking is known to aggravate heartburn.
  C. Exercise has not been shown to affect heartburn, although weight reduction (in overweight patients) is encouraged.
  D. Although fatty foods, chocolate, coffee, alcohol, mint, and high-acid foods can contribute to heartburn, a high-protein meal has not been associated with heartburn.

229. The answer is **C** [Cardiovascular].
  A. Pain with prolonged standing is common with varicose veins and should be managed conservatively with elastic support stockings and elevation when possible.
  B. Multiple varicosities may cause greater cosmetic concern but are not an indication for surgery.
  C. Surgical intervention is indicated when superficial phlebitis complicates the presence of varicose veins.
  D. The patient's age does not affect the treatment options.

230. The answer is **B** [Eyes/Ears/Nose/Throat].
  A. Artificial tears are somewhat helpful in conditions leading to dry eyes, such as sicca syndrome.
  B. Botulinum toxin injections are used for temporary correction of the lower lid entropion of older people. Surgery is indicated when lashes rub the cornea.
  C. Pilocarpine is an older antiglaucoma drug that is not often used today because of pupillary constriction in patients who are already visually challenged.
  D. Topical antibiotics are reserved for conjunctivitis or corneal abrasions complicated by bacterial infection.

231. The answer is **B** [Endocrinology].
  A. Oral hypoglycemic agents are indicated for treatment of type 2 diabetes mellitus that cannot be controlled by dietary management.
  B. Weight loss through diet and exercise may be sufficient by itself to manage a patient with type 2 diabetes mellitus. Lifestyle modification is the first step in managing new-onset type 2 diabetes unless the patient is in crisis.
  C. Insulin is not indicated for treatment of diabetes mellitus type 2 unless diet and/or oral hypoglycemic agents fail.
  D. See **C** for explanation.

232. The answer is **B** [Eyes/Ears/Nose/Throat].
  A. Although indicated, antibiotics alone are not enough for initial management.
  B. Incision and drainage is the treatment of choice and should be followed by antibiotic therapy.
  C. The abscess must be adequately drained. An MRI is not indicated during initial management.
  D. Supportive care only could lead to a worsening of symptoms.

233. The answer is **A** [Urology/Renal].
  A. Acute cystitis in women may occur following sexual intercourse. Frequency, urgency, and dysuria are common. Gross hematuria is found in some women.
  B. Urinary stones present with colicky flank pain, nausea, and vomiting. Hematuria may be microscopic or gross.
  C. Painless gross or microscopic hematuria is the most common presentation of bladder cancer. Most patients are otherwise asymptomatic.
  D. In acute pyelonephritis, urgency, frequency, and dysuria are accompanied by fever, flank pain, and shaking chills. Patients also may have nausea and vomiting.

234. The answer is **D** [Neurology].
  A. Migraines are recurrent, typically unilateral headaches. Patients may develop nausea and vomiting, but consciousness is not altered.
  B. Meningitis produces a fever and stiff neck with meningeal signs on examination.
  C. Although atypical seizures can present in many ways, the given description is more likely to be of an acute event.
  D. Subarachnoid hemorrhages typically are described as the worst headache of one's life. Patients develop nausea, vomiting, and loss or impairment of consciousness, which can be transient or can progress to deepening coma.

235. The answer is **C** [Dermatology].
  A. A first-degree or minor burn is characterized by erythema, swelling, and pain. It involves only the epidermis, and blistering is not present.
  B. A second-degree burn involves injury to the entire epidermis and a variable amount of the dermis. Vesicle and blister formation are characteristic of second-degree burns. The skin is very sensitive and painful.
  C. A third-degree burn involves destruction of the entire epidermis and dermis. The surface may appear dry with a leathery eschar or white, waxy, sooty stain. It is insensitive to pain.
  D. See **A** for explanation.

236. The answer is **D** [Endocrinology].
  A. See **D** for explanation.
  B. See **D** for explanation.
  C. See **D** for explanation.
  D. All routes of administration of desmopressin are acceptable, but the intranasal preparation has become the most commonly used and recommended route for administration.

237. The answer is **B** [Neurology].
  A. Phenobarbital is one of the safest drugs for treating seizure disorders. Side effects are mild, and a trial of mild stimulant therapy is indicated before changing to a potentially more toxic drug, such as carbamazepine.
  B. Steady state is achieved by 10–21 days in most patients started on a standard phenobarbital dose. It is reasonable to check a level at this point both to assure a therapeutic level and to determine if the dose can be decreased, minimizing the sedating effects.
  C. If seizures are well controlled, there is no indication to add a second seizure medication at this time.
  D. Bone marrow depression and hepatic toxicity are not side effects associated with use of phenobarbital.

238. The answer is **C** [Orthopedics/Rheumatology].
  A. A high WBC count is indicative of pyogenic bacterial infection.
  B. A glucose of less than 25 mg/dL typically is a pyogenic bacterial infection.

C. Uric acid crystals in the joint space are indicative of gouty arthritis.

D. A PMN count of less than 25% typically is indicative of a noninflammatory condition; however, it is not diagnostic.

239. The answer is **A** [Neurology].
    A. Short-acting anticholinesterases transiently improve symptoms of myasthenia gravis; this response often is diagnostic.
    B. Multiple sclerosis often is treated with corticosteroids; the response is variable.
    C. Hypokalemic periodic paralysis syndrome results from a transient shift of potassium into the cells.
    D. Electrophysiologic stimulation is used for the diagnosis of myasthenic syndrome (Lambert-Eaton syndrome), which usually is associated with carcinoma or autoimmune disease.

240. The answer is **C** [Eyes/Ears/Nose/Throat].
    A. Acute sinusitis typically is associated with cheek pain and pressure as well as with discolored nasal discharge.
    B. Vasomotor rhinitis, associated with clear nasal discharge, is triggered by cold and emotions.
    C. Viral rhinitis (the common cold) presents as in this scenario and is characterized by absence of fever or purulent nasal discharge.
    D. Nasal vestibulitis commonly results from folliculitis of the hairs lining the orifice and also may be associated with a furuncle.

241. The answer is **D** [Orthopedics/Rheumatology].
    A. In trauma, the fluid analysis would reveal a WBC count of less than 200 cells/μL.
    B. In osteoarthritis, fluid analysis reveals transparent joint fluid and a WBC count of 200–300 cells/μL.
    C. In septic arthritis, analysis reveals opaque joint fluid and a WBC count of greater than 50,000 cells/μL, and the culture usually is positive.
    D. Inflammatory arthritis, such as rheumatoid arthritis, causes an opaque joint fluid with elevated volume. The culture will be negative, and WBC count will be less than 50,000 cells/μL.

242. The answer is **D** [Endocrinology].
    A. Hyperthyroidism induces skin moistness, hair loss, restlessness, and heat intolerance.
    B. See **A** for explanation.
    C. See **A** for explanation.
    D. The principal symptoms of hypothyroidism are constipation, cold intolerance, dryness of skin, and myalgia.

243. The answer is **A** [Endocrinology].
    A. This patient is hypoglycemic and must receive glucose immediately. β-Blockers are known to precipitate and mask symptoms of hypoglycemia in patients with diabetes.
    B. Although the propranolol must be discontinued, this will not correct the underlying problem.
    C. The patient's presentation does not initially suggest meningitis. This test may need to be done if initial measures are not successful.
    D. Dopamine administration in a normotensive patient may lead to an unwanted hypertensive state.

244. The answer is **D** [Eyes/Ears/Nose/Throat].
    A. Chalazion is a common granulomatous inflammation of the meibomian gland. It is characterized by a hard, nontender swelling on the lower lid.
    B. Conjunctivitis usually includes injection of the conjunctiva with or without purulent discharge.
    C. Dacryocystitis presents with pain, swelling, tenderness, and redness of the tear sac area.
    D. Pterygiums are either unilateral or bilateral, painless, fleshy, triangular lesions.

245. The answer is **B** [Orthopedics/Rheumatology].
    A. Osteocytes are bone-forming units surrounded by calcified bone matrix.
    B. Osteoclasts are cells that resorb previously formed bone.
    C. Osteoblasts are bone-forming cells before being surrounded by calcified bone matrix.
    D. Osteophytes are bony outgrowths.

246. The answer is **B** [Pulmonology].
    A. Patients with asthma present with episodic wheezing, dyspnea, cough, and chest tightness, which often is worse at night. Patients may have a dry cough.
    B. The presentation described is classic for chronic bronchitis. Patients also may have central cyanosis in advanced disease.
    C. The patient with emphysema has absent or mild cough, minimal sputum production, and a thin or wasted appearance without plethora. Breath sounds are diminished. As in chronic bronchitis, smoking usually is a factor.
    D. Only 10–25% of patients have symptoms at the time lung cancer is diagnosed. Symptoms include cough, dyspnea, hemoptysis, anorexia, and weight loss. Cigarette smoking is the most important cause.

247. The answer is **D** [Eyes/Ears/Nose/Throat].
    A. The current recommendation is to treat children younger than 2 years with antibiotics, because they are more likely to develop complications.
    B. Oral ciprofloxacin is contraindicated in patients younger than 18 years.
    C. Otitis externa would be treated with a wick and topical medication.

D. The history and physical examination findings are most consistent with otitis media. Amoxicillin is an appropriate choice for an initial episode.

248. The answer is **A** [Infectious Disease].
   A. Roseola infantum (exanthema subitum, herpes virus 6) is a benign viral illness that manifests in young children as a 2- to 4-day history of moderate to high fever that abruptly ends. Within 24 hours of the end of the fever, the child breaks out in a fine, pink, maculopapular rash diffusely on the trunk and then on the neck, face, and extremities.
   B. Measles (morbillivirus) begins with a fever and coryza. On about day 4, a deep red maculopapular rash begins on face and neck and then spreads downward. The fever continues well into the period of the rash.
   C. Rubella (a togavirus) is a mild illness with absent or mild fever that may appear before or concurrent with the faint macular erythema on face and neck spreading inferiorly.
   D. Chickenpox (varicella virus) progresses from macules to papules, vesicles, and crusts. The rash is pruritic, appears in "crops," and is accompanied by moderate fever.

249. The answer is **B** [Eyes/Ears/Nose/Throat].
   A. Oral antihistamines control nasal discharge, sneezing, itching, and rhinitis with minimal decongestant effect. They are most effective if taken before exposure and are good first-line therapy, especially if combined with an intranasal corticosteroid.
   B. An intranasal corticosteroid is the mainstay of treatment for seasonal allergic rhinitis.
   C. Oral decongestants work well in conjunction with antihistamines but should not be used alone in allergic rhinitis.
   D. Intranasal cromolyn sodium may be used to prevent mild to moderate allergic rhinitis not adequately relieved by antihistamines and decongestants but is ineffective once symptoms have begun.

250. The answer is **D** [Hematology].
   A. Virchow's node is a left supraclavicular lymph node, indicating metastatic spread of GI cancer.
   B. See **D** for explanation.
   C. Dyspnea develops into Hodgkins if the mass is large; this is uncommon compared to painless lymphadenopathy.
   D. Most patients with Hodgkin's disease present because of a painless mass, most commonly in the neck.

251. The answer is **C** [Obstetrics/Gynecology].
   A. Threatened abortion is characterized by painless bleeding before the 20th week of pregnancy and a closed cervix.
   B. Inevitable abortion is characterized by vaginal bleeding and crampy lower abdominal pain. The cervix often is partially dilated.

C. Incomplete abortion is characterized by vaginal bleeding, cramping, cervical dilation, and passage of products of conception.
   D. Complete abortion is characterized by abatement of vaginal bleeding and uterine contractions, a closed cervix, and a uterus smaller than expected for the date of the last menstrual period.

252. The answer is **A** [Infectious Disease].
   A. The findings strongly suggest secondary syphilis. Nontreponemal tests, such as the VDRL or RPR, are positive at this stage.
   B. A KOH prep of the skin lesions is not appropriate, because the presentation does not suggest a fungal infection.
   C. This patient should have an HIV test, especially if she exchanges sex for drugs or has other risk factors for HIV infection; however, it will not help to establish this diagnosis of secondary syphilis.
   D. This patient should have a Pap smear if she has not had one within the recommended time frame for her age and health status; HPV testing will not help to diagnose the physical findings.

253. The answer is **B** [Orthopedics/Rheumatology].
   A. Laxity of the knee with valgus stressing is indicative of injury to the medial collateral ligament.
   B. A positive Lachman's sign is indicative of rupture of the anterior cruciate ligament. The bulge sign indicates effusion.
   C. Laxity of the knee with varus stressing is indicative of lateral collateral ligament injury.
   D. A positive posterior drawer sign is indicative of a rupture of the posterior cruciate ligament.

254. The answer is **C** [Orthopedics/Rheumatology].
   A. Lettuce, tomatoes, milk products, and refined cereals are low-purine foods.
   B. See **A** for explanation.
   C. High-purine foods may induce hyperuricemia and increase the frequency and recurrences of gouty attacks. High-purine foods include red meats, alcohol, yeast, beans, and lentils.
   D. See **A** for explanation.

255. The answer is **B** [Cardiovascular].
   A. Regular exercise and a reduced sodium diet aid in reducing the number of risk factors for coronary artery disease.
   B. In several trials, antihypertensive therapy, particularly when directed at the systolic blood pressure, has been effective in reducing the incidence of new-onset heart failure by 40–60%.
   C. See **A** for explanation.
   D. Aggressive lipid-lowering therapy in these patients has resulted in significant reduction (30%) in the incidence of heart failure.

256. The answer is **B** [Dermatology].
- **A.** Dietary restrictions will not decrease the risk of postoperative wound complications.
- **B.** Wound healing is impaired in smokers. Smoking cessation before surgery decreases the risk of wound complications.
- **C.** If not contraindicated, prophylactic therapy with aspirin should be withheld to decrease the risk of bleeding problems.
- **D.** Prophylactic antibiotics may be used during, but not before, abdominal surgery to prevent wound complications.

257. The answer is **B** [Gastrointestinal/Nutritional].
- **A.** Women of childbearing age are most likely to be deficient in folate. The classic deficiency syndrome is megaloblastic anemia.
- **B.** Pellagra is the classic niacin deficiency syndrome and often is seen in populations where corn is the major source of energy; it is still endemic in parts of China, Africa, and India. Diarrhea, dementia, and a pigmented dermatitis that develops in sun-exposed areas are typical features. Glossitis, stomatitis, vaginitis, vertigo, and burning dysesthesias are early signs.
- **C.** Beriberi is the classic syndrome of thiamine deficiency; it is common in Asian populations who consume a polished rice diet. Alcoholism and chronic renal dialysis also are common precipitants. Mild deficiency produces irritability, fatigue, and headaches.
- **D.** Vitamin K deficiency is rare except in breast-fed infants, adults with fat malabsorption, or persons taking large doses of vitamin E or anticoagulant drugs. Excessive hemorrhage is the usual manifestation.

258. The answer is **B** [Dermatology].
- **A.** See **B** for explanation.
- **B.** Fair-skinned people who burn easily (phototype I or II) are at increased risk for all types of skin cancer.
- **C.** See **B** for explanation.
- **D.** See **B** for explanation. Diet is not considered to be a factor in the development of acne.

259. The answer is **D** [Endocrinology].
- **A.** CT of the neck/thyroid is not definitive or routinely used for evaluation of the thyroid.
- **B.** Fine-needle aspiration (FNA) is indicated for evaluation of a "cold" nodule on radionuclide scan. The FNA might reveal a fluid collection suggesting a cyst but is not the method of choice to distinguish a cystic from a solid lesion. If the lesion is solid or complex on ultrasonography, it must undergo further evaluation by FNA.
- **C.** Radioactive iodine uptake is used to determine a hot from a cold nodule or toxic adenoma from Graves' disease.

- **D.** Ultrasonography of the thyroid is the procedure of choice to distinguish between a cystic and a solid lesion. It is non-invasive and highly sensitive in this regard.

260. The answer is **A** [Cardiovascular].
- **A.** Prinzmetal's angina is a form of ischemia that shows ST-segment elevations instead of the usual ST-segment depressions found in angina pectoris.
- **B.** Transient ST-segment depressions are seen in non-Prinzmetal's angina.
- **C.** ST-segment depression without Q waves is classically found with subendocardial infarction.
- **D.** ST-segment elevation with Q waves is classically found with transmural infarction.

261. The answer is **A** [Infectious Disease].
- **A.** Erythema infectiosum (fifth disease) is characterized by a "slapped cheeks" appearance, followed by a lacy rash on the trunk, neck, and extremities 1–4 days later. Mild prodrome of fever, headache, coryza, and malaise often precedes the facial rash by 2 days.
- **B.** Vesicles are a very rare and uncharacteristic progression of erythema infectiosum.
- **C.** Mucosal lesions are uncommon in erythema infectiosum.
- **D.** Arthralgias are uncommon in children with erythema infectiosum; however, they are quite common in adults (especially women) who contract this viral infection caused by parvovirus B19.

262. The answer is **C** [Cardiovascular].
- **A.** Coarctation is not associated with atrial fibrillation.
- **B.** Tachycardia is not a common finding in coarctation of the aorta.
- **C.** Left ventricular hypertrophy results from increased pressure on the left ventricle to move blood through the decreased aortic lumen.
- **D.** Coarctation is associated with left-sided cardiac changes.

263. The answer is **B** [Psychiatric/Behavioral Medicine].
- **A.** Borderline personality disorder is characterized by anger, sarcasm, anxiety, and intense and labile affect. Patients also suffer from chronic loneliness and boredom, may report numerous suicide attempts and self-mutilation, and are hypersensitive to abandonment.
- **B.** Initially, histrionic patients are charming and likeable. They also can be seductive. These patients demand attention but have a limited ability to maintain intimate relationships.
- **C.** Narcissistic persons require constant admiration, have unrealistic self-expectations, are impulsive, and lack empathy.
- **D.** A schizoid personality is a seclusive person with little desire to form interpersonal relationships or take pleasure in activities.

264. The answer is **A** [Neurology].
  A. Cluster headaches are more common in men and generally present during the third decade of life. The severe, knife-like pain is localized to the periorbital or temporal area and is accompanied by autonomic signs.
  B. Paroxysmal hemicrania presents with symptoms similar to cluster headaches. Attacks usually are more frequent but of shorter duration.
  C. Symptoms of sinus neoplasia are vague and slowly progressive. They include nasal congestion, epistaxis, nasal discharge, and local edema.
  D. Typical presentation of trigeminal neuralgia consists of sharp, short, electric shock pain in one or more divisions of the trigeminal nerve.

265. The answer is **C** [Eyes/Ears/Nose/Throat].
  A. Otitis media is not associated with purulent nasal discharge or facial pain.
  B. Dental abscess is not associated with purulent nasal discharge.
  C. The symptoms and physical findings are consistent with acute sinusitis.
  D. Allergic rhinitis is associated with clear mucoid discharge.

266. The answer is **B** [Dermatology].
  A. Stage I decubiti consist of nonblanching erythema of intact skin.
  B. Stage II decubiti involve skin loss of the epidermis and/or dermis. They may resemble a blister, abrasion, or shallow ulcer. Necrotic tissue may overlie the ulcer.
  C. Stage III decubiti are deep crateriform ulcers with full-thickness skin loss. Damage or necrosis extends down to, but not through, the fascia.
  D. Stage IV decubiti are full-thickness ulcerations with damage involving muscle, bone, or supporting structures.

267. The answer is **D** [Gastrointestinal/Nutritional].
  A. An anorectal fissure causes severe, tearing pain during defecation.
  B. Fistulas are associated with purulent discharge, itchiness, tenderness, and pain.
  C. A perianal abscess causes throbbing and continuous perianal pain.
  D. Bright red blood associated with internal hemorrhoids may range from streaks of blood on toilet paper to blood that drips into the toilet after a bowel movement. Discomfort or pain is unusual.

268. The answer is **D** [Psychiatry/Behavioral Medicine].
  A. Antianxiety medications may help with infrequent exposures to phobic stimuli but should be for short-term use only.
  B. Some data support the use of SSRIs, but these drugs are reserved for refractory cases.
  C. Hypnosis may be helpful as an adjunct to desensitization.
  D. Desensitization, biofeedback, imagery, relaxation, and other forms of behavior modification are effective primary treatment of phobias. Systematic desensitization is the most effective form of behavior therapy in patients with specific phobias.

269. The answer is **C** [Psychiatry/Behavioral Medicine].
  A. Carbamazepine and clonidine may be as effective to block withdrawal symptoms, but they are not as effective against alcohol withdrawal seizures as diazepam.
  B. See **A** for explanation.
  C. Diazepam given IV is the recommended treatment for alcohol withdrawal seizures, delirium, anxiety, tachycardia, hypertension, diaphoresis, and tremor.
  D. Antiseizure medications are not warranted when the cause is known to be alcohol withdrawal.

270. The answer is **D** [Obstetrics/Gynecology].
  A. See **D** for explanation.
  B. In general, infections caused by *Trichomonas vaginalis* and *Chlamydia trachomatis* may result in inflammatory changes on the Pap smear. They are not correlated with dysplasia.
  C. See **B** for explanation.
  D. Although herpes simplex virus was once implicated in the occurrence of cervical dysplasia, human papilloma virus has been found to have a stronger link.

271. The answer is **C** [Gastrointestinal/Nutritional].
  A. Increased pain when the patient flexes the hip against resistance is called the psoas sign and is consistent with acute appendicitis.
  B. Rebound tenderness may be elicited if the course of acute appendicitis progresses to inflame the peritoneum. The left upper quadrant is not a classic location. Appendicitis is more likely to cause rebound in the right lower quadrant.
  C. Localized tenderness with guarding in the right lower quadrant can be elicited with gentle palpation with one finger (McBurney's point).
  D. Valsalva maneuvers, such as coughing or bearing down, may help to precisely localize the inflamed area, a sign of peritoneal irritation.

272. The answer is **C** [Eyes/Ears/Nose/Throat].
  A. Internal digital compression is imprecise and not socially acceptable.
  B. If external compression, intranasal cocaine, and cautery all fail to control the bleeding, nasal packing is recommended.
  C. This is the recommended next step if external compression fails.
  D. Gelfoam packing soaked with thrombin is recommended in patients with hypercoagulability.

273. The answer is **D** [Endocrinology].
  A. IV fluids and monitoring glucose alone are inadequate therapy.
  B. Bicarbonate replacement only occasionally is used when life-threatening hyperkalemia or cardiac arrhythmias are present. If administered, it should never be given as an IV bolus to avoid driving down serum potassium levels and causing hyperosmolarity.
  C. Dextrose-containing fluids are not started until blood glucose is less than 250 mg/dL.
  D. This patient has diabetic ketoacidosis. IV fluids are started immediately, because without adequate fluid replacement, insulin will not work. Insulin must be provided in adequate quantities and administered by IV infusion initially. Once the ketoacidosis has resolved and the patient is able to drink fluids, subcutaneous insulin should be started.

274. The answer is **B** [Psychiatric/Behavioral Medicine].
  A. Lithium causes leukocytosis, not anemia.
  B. Lithium does not bind to plasma proteins and is not metabolized by the liver; it is almost entirely eliminated by the kidneys. It may cause renal concentrating defects, reduced glomerular filtration rate, nephrotic syndrome, and renal tubular acidosis.
  C. Lithium typically does not affect liver function.
  D. Lithium can cause cardiac conduction defects and ECG changes. An ECG, not an echocardiogram, is indicated.

275. The answer is **C** [Pulmonology].
  A. Bronchiolitis is more commonly found in younger patients and is characterized by rapid respiration, chest retractions, and wheezing.
  B. Pneumonia may have a similar presentation but also is likely to have rales and dullness to percussion on physical examination.
  C. Acute bronchitis classically presents with fever, malaise, cough, blood-streaked sputum, and rhonchi.
  D. Patients with tuberculosis may present with fever, malaise, cough, and blood-tinged sputum. The time course here is more consistent with acute tracheobronchitis.

276. The answer is **A** [Eyes/Ears/Nose/Throat].
  A. Vertical nystagmus is associated with central lesions.
  B. The auditory system generally is spared in conditions that cause central vertigo.
  C. Horizontal nystagmus is associated with peripheral lesions.
  D. See **B** for explanation.

277. The answer is **C** [Urology/Renal].
  A. Angiotensin-converting enzyme inhibitors, calcium channel blockers, and direct vasodilators are not helpful for symptoms of benign prostatic hyperplasia.

  B. See **A** for explanation.
  C. The α-blockers have dual therapeutic actions, on blood pressure and on bladder neck function.
  D. See **A** for explanation.

278. The answer is **D** [Obstetrics/Gynecology].
  A. See **D** for explanation.
  B. See **D** for explanation.
  C. See **D** for explanation.
  D. She has had five previous pregnancies, is currently pregnant, and thus, is G6. She has had two term deliveries, no premature deliveries, and three abortions (one spontaneous, one elective, and one ectopic) and has two living children.

279. The answer is **B** [Urology/Renal].
  A. Obstruction causes roughly proportionate rises of BUN and creatinine.
  B. Congestive heart failure characteristically increases the BUN:creatinine ratio to greater than 20:1.
  C. Trimethoprim/sulfamethoxazole and cefoxitin may cause an isolated creatinine elevation.
  D. See **C** for explanation.

280. The answer is **C** [Eyes/Ears/Nose/Throat].
  A. Acute laryngitis often presents following a viral upper respiratory infection and lasts for about a week. Chronic laryngitis is associated with vocal abuse, inhalation of irritants, gastroesophageal reflux, and chronic allergies; lymphadenopathy does not occur.
  B. Thyroid cancer may present with anterior cervical lymphadenopathy but does not present with progressive hoarseness. Most commonly, it presents with painless swelling in the thyroid region.
  C. Tobacco abuse is a common predisposing factor in cancer of the larynx. Cancer of the larynx affects men more often than women (9:1 ratio). Persistent hoarseness in this population should raise suspicion of cancer. As many as 50% of patients with laryngeal cancer present with palpable lymphadenopathy in the anterior cervical lymph nodes.
  D. Progressive hoarseness is commonly caused by vocal cord nodules. These are found in patients who exhibit vocal abuse, as occurs with singing. Tobacco abuse is not associated with vocal cord nodules.

281. The answer is **B** [Gastrointestinal/Nutritional].
  A. See **B** for explanation.
  B. Eradication of *Helicobacter pylori* has proved to be difficult. Combination regimens that use two antibiotics with a proton-pump inhibitor or bismuth are required to achieve adequate rates of eradication and to reduce the number of failures caused by antibiotic resistance. The preferred regimen is a 10- to 14-day course of a proton-pump inhibitor plus amoxicillin and clarithromycin twice daily.

C. See **B** for explanation.

D. See **B** for explanation.

282. The answer is **D** [Eyes/Ears/Nose/Throat].

A. Tympanostomy tubes would be considered a medical intervention, but they can be prophylactic.

B. To date, no studies demonstrate that humidification or using decongestants prevents otitis media.

C. See **B** for explanation.

D. Avoiding smoking near the child and in the home can decrease the incidence of recurrent episodes of otitis media.

283. The answer is **A** [Pulmonology].

A. Classic pneumonia presents with bronchial breath sounds, egophony, increased tactile fremitus, and dullness to percussion. Fever may be absent, and confusion may be the only presenting symptom in elderly patients.

B. Pulmonary edema usually is bilateral and most pronounced at the bases.

C. Pulmonary embolism rarely presents with abnormal lung findings.

D. Pulmonary hypertension rarely is associated with abnormal lung findings on physical examination.

284. The answer is **A** [Eyes/Ears/Nose/Throat].

A. Most retinal detachment begins with a tear in the superior temporal quadrant. Vitreous then passes through the tear and becomes lodged behind the sensory retina. The pull of gravity results in progressive detachment.

B. See **A** for explanation.

C. See **A** for explanation.

D. See **A** for explanation.

285. The answer is **C** [Eyes/Ears/Nose/Throat].

A. Acute lye ingestion would cause a more uniform destruction and sloughing of oral mucosa. The child would be more uncomfortable. Nausea and vomiting would occur after eating.

B. Drug eruption generally does not cause lymphadenopathy.

C. This is the typical presentation of herpetic gingivostomatitis.

D. Coxsackievirus causes herpangina, which manifests as grayish-white tonsillar and palatal papules that become shallow ulcers. High fever, malaise, and vomiting frequently are found.

286. The answer is **A** [Pulmonology].

A. Cromolyn and nedocromil sodium inhaled medications are mast cell stabilizers that are very effective in the prevention of asthma when there is a known precipitant, such as exercise.

B. β_2-Agonists provide quick symptomatic relief in mild to moderate asthma. Their use before exercise is an effective choice, but treatment should begin before exercise to prevent symptoms.

C. Theophylline has a long half-life and delayed onset of action. This drug must get to a steady state in the bloodstream to be effective in management. It is not indicated for acute symptoms as needed.

D. Conditioning will not relieve these symptoms. Exercise-induced asthma is a clinical syndrome and not a manifestation of poor cardiopulmonary conditioning.

287. The answer is **D** [Gastrointestinal/Nutritional].

A. Hepatic adenomas typically cause right upper quadrant pain; typically, they are not an incidental finding.

B. Hepatoblastoma is the most common malignant liver tumor during early childhood.

C. Mixed hamartoma is a rare benign lesion that usually is cystic in nature.

D. Most patients with hepatic hemangioma are asymptomatic; the tumors are discovered incidentally.

288. The answer is **B** [Dermatology].

A. Molluscum contagiosum in an otherwise healthy young person need not be treated.

B. Liquid nitrogen, electrocautery, or curettage are the recommended treatment choices for molluscum contagiosum, a viral skin infection commonly seen in patients with AIDS. When this disorder occurs in children, the lesions often resolve without treatment, but it is difficult to eradicate in patients with AIDS.

C. Warts appear as verrucous papules without umbilication and may be treated with paring and salicylic acid treatments.

D. Corns are found over pressure points and are treated with warm water soaks and paring.

289. The answer is **A** [Obstetrics/Gynecology].

A. Rh immune globulin is most effective if given within 72 hours after delivery. It may be given beyond that, but its effectiveness may be less certain.

B. See **A** for explanation.

C. See **A** for explanation.

D. See **A** for explanation.

290. The answer is **A** [Obstetrics/Gynecology].

A. A simple mass smaller than 6 cm most often is an ovarian follicle cyst. These usually resolve with the subsequent menses. Observation and repeat pelvic examination in 6–8 weeks is appropriate in reproductive-age women with such cysts.

B. Manual decompression is not appropriate for any ovarian mass.

C. Laparotomy is reserved for painful or solid masses, those larger than 6 cm, or certain masses in postmenopausal women. Surgery carries the risks of bleeding and infection as well as those inherent in anesthesia.

D. The role of transvaginal sonography with directed fine-needle aspiration in treatment of ovarian cysts currently is under investigation. It may be an option in patients with multiple cysts and a history of rupture.

291. The answer is **B** [Urology/Renal].
A. Gross hematuria is associated with significant genitourinary disease and should be investigated to rule out malignancy.
B. Evaluation of painless hematuria should begin with urinalysis and culture. Results will help to guide further workup.
C. Cystoscopy is a component of second-line evaluation. It is indicated if, based on urinalysis findings, bladder neoplasm or benign prostatic hyperplasia is suspected as the cause.
D. Gross hematuria rarely is the sole manifestation of urinary tract infection, especially in male patients.

292. The answer is **A** [Hematology].
A. The history of an autoimmune disorder (systemic lupus erythematosus) with acute anemia and a high reticulocyte count is indicative of autoimmune hemolytic anemia.
B. The anemia in congenital spherocytosis is variable but typically mild.
C. G6PD deficiency is associated with hemolysis but not with spherocytosis.
D. Hemolytic-uremia syndrome presents as hemolytic anemia with low platelets, bleeding, proteinuria, and hematuria. Jaundice and splenomegaly do not occur.

293. The answer is **D** [Infectious Disease].
A. Hairy leukoplakia is found in patients with HIV disease or other causes of immunodeficiency.
B. A petechial rash on the conjunctiva, pharynx, and extremities is typical of endocarditis.
C. A pharyngeal pseudomembrane is found in diphtheria.
D. Characteristic embolic findings in endocarditis include splinter hemorrhages, petechiae, Janeway lesions, and Osler nodes.

294. The answer is **A** [Hematology].
A. A positive direct Coombs' test in autoimmune hemolytic anemia indicates the presence of autoantibodies that have saturated the bindings sites in the RBCs.
B. Elevated indirect bilirubin occurs in hemolysis.
C. Hemoglobin electrophoresis is abnormal in hemoglobinopathies, such as sickle-cell disease.
D. The osmotic fragility test is abnormal in hereditary spherocytosis because of the loss of some RBC surface, leaving the cells vulnerable to swelling.

295. The answer is **A** [Gastrointestinal/Nutritional].
A. In a patient with clinical features of acute hepatitis, anti-HCV is the initial screening test for hepatitis

C. In some patients, detectable levels of anti-HCV are delayed for weeks or months, so retesting for anti-HCV during convalescence or direct test for HCV RNA may be necessary.
B. HCsAg titers do not exist.
C. HCV RNA by PCR and anti-HCV by Immunoblot are supplemental or confirmatory tests.
D. See **C** for explanation.

296. The answer is **D** [Pulmonology].
A. Consolidation is associated with pneumonia.
B. Kerley B lines are associated with congestive heart failure.
C. Air bronchograms are associated with pneumonia.
D. Visceral pleural lines, especially on expiration, are diagnostic of pneumothorax.

297. The answer is **B** [Eyes/Ears/Nose/Throat].
A. Vertigo triggered by head movement occurs in positional vertigo.
B. Meniere's disease is characterized by hearing loss and episodic vertigo usually accompanied by tinnitus.
C. Labyrinthitis usually presents suddenly with severe vertigo that may last for weeks.
D. Unilateral hearing loss with vertigo is the common pattern of an acoustic neuroma.

298. The answer is **B** [Gastrointestinal/Nutritional].
A. Women who are single because of divorce or death are at slightly higher risk of eating disorders; middle-aged men are not.
B. The age of onset for eating disorders is bimodal, with peaks around ages 14 and 18. The disorder is more common among women in higher socioeconomic groups and among whites.
C. Adolescents are at higher risk, but that risk is significantly greater in the middle to upper classes.
D. Children from goal- or achievement-oriented families are at higher risk, but the risk in male children is much lower than that in female children.

299. The answer is **C** [Gastrointestinal/Nutritional].
A. See **C** for explanation.
B. Transient, mild hyperglycemia is common in pancreatitis, but this is nonspecific.
C. During acute pancreatitis, serum lipase levels increase in parallel with serum amylase levels. The lipase level remains elevated longer and may help to diagnose pancreatitis after an attack has ended.
D. Serum triglyceride levels of greater than 1,000 mg/dL may precipitate attacks of acute pancreatitis but are not diagnostic.

300. The answer is **D** [Urology/Renal].
A. Calcium is given as an antagonist and stabilizes cardiac conduction abnormalities.
B. Sodium polystyrene sulfonate (Kayexalate) binds with potassium; it is a cation-exchange resin.

C. Sodium bicarbonate shifts the potassium back into the cells.

D. Amiloride (Midamor) inhibits potassium excretion and should be avoided in patients with hyperkalemia.

301. The answer is **D** [Obstetrics/Gynecology].

A. See **D** for explanation.

B. See **D** for explanation.

C. See **D** for explanation.

D. Indications for admission to the hospital of patients with PID include failure to respond to outpatient therapy, inability to tolerate outpatient therapy (e.g., from nausea and vomiting), fever greater than 39.0°C, those with guarding and rebound tenderness in lower quadrants, or patients who look toxic. This patient meets several of these criteria and should be admitted for IV antibiotics.

302. The answer is A [Urology/Renal].

A. Anorexia, fatigue, and weakness are early symptoms of renal failure.

B. Late symptoms of renal failure include oliguria, dyspnea, chest pain, nausea, vomiting, and abdominal pain.

C. Polyuria and polydipsia are common manifestations of diabetes, and back pain is reported in pyelonephritis.

D. Nausea, anorexia, pruritus, and abdominal pain suggest hepatobiliary tract obstruction.

Ophthalmology and Otolaryngology

Nancy E. Orr

I. DISORDERS OF THE EYES

A. Disorders of the globe

  1. Trauma

    a. General characteristics

      (1) Traumatic disorders affecting the globe include blunt or penetrating trauma, foreign bodies, and chemical burns.

      (2) All management steps should be taken as soon as possible, especially with penetrating trauma and foreign bodies. The first step of the history is to find out when and how the accident, trauma, or burn occurred.

    b. Physical examination

      (1) Observe: Inspect, noticing any abnormalities:

        (a) Orbit: for edema or hematoma.

        (b) Lids: for laceration, hematomas, edema, and foreign bodies.

        (c) Pupils: for irregularity—alert suspicion for ruptured globe.

        (d) Extraocular muscles: for unequal, limited, or decreased movement—indicate laceration or entrapment of eye muscles.

        (e) Anterior chamber: for hyphema.

        (f) Interior of eye with funduscope: for ruptured retinal vessels, which may indicate physical abuse, such as shaken baby syndrome.

      (2) Palpate orbital rim: for irregularity, which may indicate a fracture. If rupture of the globe is suspected, do not palpate.

    c. Measurements

      (1) Visual acuity is tested using the Snellen chart. This is important to establish a baseline; any decrease indicates serious trauma.

      (2) Pupillary reactions should be checked. Unequal reactions might indicate severe trauma to the globe, head trauma, or nerve palsies.

      (3) Check for intraocular pressure. After appropriate anesthesia, carefully use the Schiötz tonometer.

    d. Treatment

      (1) Penetrating trauma

        (a) The object should not be removed.

        (b) The patient should be transported to the emergency room for consult with an ophthalmologist and for CT.

      (2) Foreign body

        (a) The eyelids should be carefully everted, stained with a fluorescein strip, and observed with a Wood's lamp.

        (b) Gently attempt to remove the foreign body using a moistened, cotton-tipped swab.

        (c) Patching may be beneficial. If a large corneal abrasion occurs. Patching should be limited to 24 hrs. Reexamine the nextday.

        (d) A rust ring on the cornea indicates metallic foreign bodies. These may be removed with a rotating burr, or the patient may be referred to an ophthalmologist.

      (3) Chemical burns (acid or alkali)

        (a) The eye should be irrigated with water or normal saline for at least 30 minutes. Use sterile solution if available. A chemical burn can continue to cause damage even after flushing.

(b) An eye shield should be placed on the eye.

(c) Because an acid or alkali burn is severe, transport the patient to the emergency room, and refer to an ophthalmologist.

2. Blow-out fracture

a. General characteristics

(1) The orbital floor is composed of maxillary, palatine, and zygomatic bones. These bones are very thin.

(2) Blunt trauma, such as that from a fist or a ball, causes the floor to fracture, trapping the orbital structures.

b. Clinical features

(1) Patients present with swelling and misalignment. Movement of the globe is restricted, specifically an inability to look up due to entrapment of the infraorbital nerve and the musculature.

(2) Double vision is common.

(3) Subcutaneous emphysema and exophthalmos are present.

c. Treatment

(1) Prompt referral to an ophthalmologist is important.

(2) Patients should be kept calm and avoid sneezing or anything that would increase pressure.

(3) Nasal decongestants, ice packs or cold compresses, and antibiotics are started during transport.

3. Corneal abrasion

a. General characteristics. It usually is caused by minor trauma, such as that from a fingernail, contact lens, eyelash, or small foreign body.

b. Clinical features

(1) Pain and sensation of a foreign body can be accompanied by photophobia, tearing, injection, and blepharospasm.

(2) Record visual acuity before examining or treating.

(3) A slit-lamp examination or fluorescein staining will reveal an epithelial defect but a clear cornea. A search for foreign bodies is required.

c. Treatment

(1) Topical anesthetic will provide immediate relief; however, it should be used only to assist in confirming the diagnosis and should not be prescribed.

(2) Antibiotic ointment, such as polymyxin/bacitracin, should be applied. Acetaminophen is given for analgesia.

(3) Patching for no longer than 24 hours is recommended only for large abrasions (>5–10 mm) to promote healing.

(4) Follow-up of all abrasions within 1–2 days is essential.

4. Retinal disorders

a. Retinal detachment

(1) General characteristics

(a) The underlying pathogenesis is a separation of the retina from the pigmented epithelial layer, causing the detached tissue to appear as flapping in the vitreous humor.

(b) The tear usually begins at the superior temporal retinal area.

(c) The tear can happen spontaneously or be secondary to trauma or extreme myopia.

(2) Clinical features

(a) The patient may report acute onset of blurred or blackened vision that occurs over several hours and progresses to complete or partial monocular blindness.

(b) It is classically described as a curtain being drawn over the eye from top to bottom.

(c) The patient may sense floaters or flashing lights at the initiation of symptoms.

(3) There will be a relative afferent pupillary defect. Funduscopic examination may reveal the rugous retina flapping in the vitreous humor.

(4) Treatment

(a) An emergency consult with an ophthalmologist regarding possible laser surgery or cryosurgery is needed.

(b) Patients with retinal detachment should remain supine, with the head turned to the side of the retinal detachment.

(c) Prognosis is good: 80% will recover without recurrence, 15% will require retreatment, and 5% will never reattach.

b. Macular degeneration

(1) This disorder may be age-related or secondary to the toxic effects of drugs, such as chloroquine or phenothiazine. It is the leading cause of irreversible central visual loss.

(2) Drusen deposits are found in Bruch's membrane, leading to degenerative changes, loss of nutritional supply, atrophy, and neovascularization.

(3) It usually has an insidious onset, and its chief clinical feature is gradual loss of vision. Metamorphopsia is the phenomenon of wavy or distorted vision and can be measured with an Amsler grid.

(4) Mottling, serous leaks, and hemorrhages commonly develop on the retina.

(5) There is no effective treatment. If detected early, laser therapy or intravitreal injections of monoclonal antibody drugs may slow the progression of macular degeneration.

c. Central retinal artery occlusion

(1) General characteristics

(a) This disorder is considered to be an ophthalmic emergency; prognosis is poor, even with immediate treatment.

(b) Common causes are emboli, thrombotic phenomenon, and vasculitides.

(2) Clinical features

(a) It is characterized by sudden, painless, and marked unilateral loss of vision.

(b) Funduscopy reveals arteriolar narrowing, separation of arterial flow (box-carring), retinal edema, and perifoveal atrophy (cherry red spot). Ganglionic death leads to optic atrophy and a pale retina.

(3) Treatment

(a) Emergency referral to an ophthalmologist is necessary. Vessel dilation and paracentesis are attempted to save the eye.

(b) A workup for atherosclerotic disease is warranted to prevent recurrence.

d. Central retinal vein occlusion

(1) This usually occurs secondary to a thrombotic event.

(2) Patients present with sudden, unilateral, painless blurred vision or complete visual loss.

(3) Examination reveals an afferent pupillary defect and a "blood and thunder" retina (dilated veins, hemorrhages, edema, and exudates).

(4) Vision typically is resolved with time, at least partially. A workup for further thrombosis is warranted.

e. Retinopathy

(1) Systemic disorders, including diabetes, hypertension, preeclampsia–eclampsia, blood dyscrasias, and HIV disease, may affect the retina.

(2) Diabetic retinopathy

(a) This is the leading cause of blindness in adults in the United States. Patients with diabetes should have yearly dilated ophthalmoscopic examinations.

(b) Nonproliferative: venous dilation, microaneurysms, retinal hemorrhages, retinal edema, hard exudates.

(c) Proliferative: neovascularization, vitreous hemorrhage.

(3) Treatment includes optimized glucose control, regulation of blood pressure, laser photocoagulation, and vitrectomy. Severe disease is permanent.

5. Cataract

a. General characteristics

(1) A cataract is any opacity of the natural lens of the eye. It may involve a small part of the lens or the entire lens. The degree of opacification also is variable.

(2) Cataracts may develop secondary to the natural aging process, trauma, congenital causes, or medication use (e.g., corticosteroids, lovastatin).

(3) Excess sun exposure predisposes to cataract development.

b. Clinical features

(1) The insidious onset of decreased vision is the main clinical feature.

(2) A gradual diminution of vision is characteristic. Patients also may complain of double vision, fixed spots, or reduced color.

(3) On examination, there is a translucent, yellow discoloration in the lens. On funduscopy, the cataract appears black on a red background.

c. Treatment

(1) Treatment is warranted to improve activities of daily living, prevent secondary glaucoma, and permit visualization of the fundus.

(2) Treatment involves intracapsular or extracapsular extractions of the cataract with lens replacement.

(3) Prognosis is excellent; postoperative bleeding occurs in less than 0.1%.

6. Glaucoma

a. General characteristics

(1) This condition is defined as increased intraocular pressure with optic nerve damage. Any impediment to the flow of aqueous humor through the trabecular meshwork and canal of Schlemm will increase pressure in the anterior chamber.

(2) Glaucoma may be acute or chronic. Types include angle-closure glaucoma and open-angle glaucoma.

(3) Open-angle glaucoma affects people older than 40 years and is more common in African Americans and in patients with a family history of glaucoma.

b. Clinical features

(1) Angle-closure glaucoma is an ophthalmic emergency.

(a) Painful eye and loss of vision are important clinical features.

(b) Physical examination reveals circumlimbal injection, steamy cornea, fixed mid-dilated pupil, and decreased visual acuity.

(c) The anterior chamber is narrowed; intraocular pressure is acutely elevated.

(d) Nausea, vomiting, and diaphoresis are common.

(2) Open-angle glaucoma

(a) This is a chronic, asymptomatic, and potentially blinding disease defined as increased intraocular pressure, defects in the peripheral visual field, and increased cup-to-disc ratios.

c. Treatment

(1) Angle-closure glaucoma

(a) These patients must be referred immediately to an ophthalmologist. Start IV carbonic anhydrase inhibitor, topical β-blocker, and osmotic diuresis.

(b) Mydriatics should not be administered to these patients.

(c) Treatment is via laser or surgical iridotomy.

(2) Open-angle glaucoma

(a) Patients need to be referred to an ophthalmologist.

(b) Treatment consists of topical or systemic medications to decrease the pressure by decreasing aqueous production and increasing outflow.

7. Orbital cellulitis

a. General characteristics

(1) Orbital cellulitis is more common in children than in adults.

(2) Orbital cellulitis has several possible causes, including sinusitis, dental infections, facial infections, infection of the globe or eyelids, and infections of the lacrimal system. Less often, it results from trauma.

(3) Causative agents in children younger than 4 years include *Haemophilus influenzae* and *Streptococcus pneumoniae*. In older children and adults, it occurs secondary to acute or chronic sinusitis and has many possible causative agents.

b. Clinical features

    (1) Orbital cellulitis presents with ptosis, eyelid edema, exophthalmos, purulent discharge, and conjunctivitis.

    (2) Examination will reveal fever, decreased range of motion in the eye muscles, and a sluggish pupillary response.

c. Laboratory studies

    (1) Workup includes CBC, blood cultures, and cultures of any drainage.

    (2) Sinus radiography and CT may help to determine the cause and extent of disease. CT will show broad infiltration of the orbital soft tissue.

d. Treatment

    (1) Orbital cellulitis constitutes a medical emergency requiring hospitalization and IV antibiotics.

    (2) Antibiotics should be broad spectrum until the causative agent is identified.

B. Disorders of the adnexa

  1. Disorders of the lacrimal system

    a. Dacryostenosis is common in the newborn after the first month of life and occurs when the duct does not open.

      (1) The obstruction usually resolves by 9 months of age.

      (2) Treatment includes warm compresses and massage; if no *resolution,* surgical probe is indicated.

    b. Dacryocystitis is an inflammation of the lacrimal gland caused by obstruction. Common pathogens include *Staphylococcus aureus,* β-hemolytic streptococci, *Staph epidermidis,* and *Candida* sp.

      (1) Pain, swelling, tenderness, redness, and purulent discharge are characteristic.

      (2) Treatment is warm compresses and antibiotics.

  2. Eyelids

    a. Blepharitis is chronic inflammation of the lid margins.

      (1) Causes include seborrhea, staphylococcal or streptococcal infection, or dysfunction of the meibomian glands.

      (2) Clinical features

        (a) Rims are red, and eyelashes adhere.

        (b) Dandruff-like deposits (scurf) and fibrous scales (collarettes) may be seen.

        (c) The conjunctiva is clear or slightly erythematous.

      (3) Treatment

        (a) Lid scrubs using diluted baby shampoo on cotton-tipped swabs are helpful.

        (b) Topical antibiotics can be used if infection is suspected. Systemic antibiotics are reserved for recalcitrant cases.

    b. Hordeolum

      (1) General characteristics

        (a) A hordeolum is an acute development of a small, painful nodule or abscess within a gland in the upper or lower eyelid.

        (b) Types

          (i) Internal hordeola: Caused by inflammation and infection of a meibomian gland, with abscess formation in that gland. They are situated deep from the palpebral margin.

          (ii) External hordeola (commonly referred to as a sty): Caused by the inflammation and infection of the glands of Moll or Zeis, with abscess formation in those glands. They are situated immediately adjacent to the edge of the palpebral margin.

        (c) Causal pathogen for either type of hordeolum is typically *Staphylococcus aureus.*

        (d) Hordeolum is not contagious.

      (2) Clinical features

        (a) Hordeolum is characterized by acute onset of pain and edema of the involved eyelid.

        (b) There is a palpable, indurated area in the involved eyelid, which has a central area of purulence with surrounding erythema.

      (3) Treatment
        (a) Warm compresses should be applied several times per day for 48 hours.
        (b) Topical antibiotics should be used if secondary infection develops.
        (c) Incision and drainage may be indicated if it does not resolve.

c. Chalazion
      (1) General characteristics
        (a) This is a relatively painless, indurated lesion deep from the palpebral margin.
        (b) It often is secondary to a chronic inflammation of an internal hordeolum of the meibomian gland.
      (2) Clinical features
        (a) The chalazion is characterized by insidious onset with minimal irritation.
        (b) It can become pruritic and cause erythema of the involved lid.
      (3) Treatment involves warm compresses and referral to an ophthalmologist for an elective excision.

d. Entropion and ectropion
      (1) Entropion: The lid and lashes are turned in secondary to scar tissue or a spasm of the orbicularis oculi muscles.
      (2) Ectropion: The edge of the eyelid everts secondary to advanced age, trauma, infection, or palsy of the facial nerve.
      (3) Treatment: Involves surgical repair if the condition causes trauma, excessive tearing, exposure keratitis, or cosmetic distress.

C. Disorders of the conjunctiva

1. Viral conjunctivitis

  a. General characteristics
      (1) Viral infection in the conjunctiva usually is caused by adenovirus type 3, 8, or 19.
      (2) Viral conjunctivitis is highly contagious. Transmission is by direct contact, usually via the fingers, to the contralateral eye or other persons.
      (3) Viral conjunctivitis can be transmitted in swimming pools (epidemic keratoconjunctivitis), and it is most common in midsummer to early fall.

  b. Clinical features. Viral conjunctivitis is characterized by acute onset of unilateral or bilateral erythema of the conjunctiva, copious watery discharge, and ipsilateral tender preauricular lymphadenopathy.

  c. Treatment
      (1) Therapy includes eye lavage with normal saline twice a day for 7–14 days; vasoconstrictor-antihistamine drops also may have beneficial effects.
      (2) Hot compresses reduce discomfort.
      (3) Ophthalmic sulfonamide drops may prevent secondary bacterial infection but are not routinely prescribed.

2. Bacterial conjunctivitis

  a. General characteristics. Bacterial infection in the conjunctiva may occur with common or rare pathogens.
      (1) Common pathogens include *Streptococcus pneumoniae, Staphylococcus aureus, Haemophilus aegyptius*, and *Moraxella* sp..
        (a) Transmission is via direct contact or via fomites. Autoinoculation, from one eye to the other, usually via the fingers, is typical.
        (b) The natural history of an infection caused by these common pathogens usually is self-limiting, but a secondary keratitis can develop.
      (2) Rare pathogens include *Chlamydia trachomatis* and *Neisseria gonorrhea*.
        (a) Transmission is by direct contact or fomites, including nonchlorinated swimming sources. It also can be transmitted via sexual contact or to a neonate via vaginal delivery.
        (b) The natural history of an infection caused by these rare pathogens is a severe conjunctivitis and keratitis with development of permanent visual impairment.

  b. Clinical features
      (1) Bacterial conjunctivitis is characterized by the acute onset of copious, purulent discharge from both eyes.

(2) Patients may have a mild decrease in visual acuity and mild discomfort. The eyes may be "glued" shut on awakening.

c. Laboratory studies

(1) Common pathogens: Gram stain should show the presence of polymorphonuclear cells (PMNs) and a predominant organism.

(2) Rare pathogens: Gram stain and Giemsa stain should show PMNs.

(a) When *Chlamydia trachomatis* is the pathogen, no organisms will be seen.

(b) When *Neisseria gonorrhea* is the pathogen, intracellular Gram-negative diplococci will be present.

d. Treatment

(1) Specific therapy includes application of topical antibiotics.

(2) For the rare pathogens, treatment also may require concurrent systemic antibiotics.

3. Pinguecula

a. General characteristics. It is caused by chronic actinic exposure, repeated trauma, and dry and windy conditions.

b. Clinical features

(1) Elevated, yellowish, fleshy conjunctival mass found on the sclera adjacent to the cornea.

(2) Painless inflammation may occur.

c. Treatment

(1) No treatment is necessary.

(2) If it is cosmetically undesirable or chronically inflamed, it can be resected.

4. Pterygium

a. General characteristics

(1) Slowly growing thickening of the bulbar conjunctiva.

(2) It can be unilateral or bilateral.

b. Clinical features

(1) A highly vascular, triangular mass grows from the nasal side toward the cornea.

(2) It occasionally encroaches on the cornea and interferes with vision.

c. Treatment

(1) Excision is warranted if it interferes with vision.

(2) Recurrence is common.

D. Optic nerve and visual pathways

1. Papilledema

a. This condition is defined as an increase in intracranial pressure.

b. Causes are numerous but may include malignant hypertension, hemorrhagic strokes, acute subdural hematoma, and pseudotumor cerebri.

c. The disc appears swollen, and the margins are blurred, with an obliteration of the vessels.

d. The patient may be asymptomatic or may complain of transient visual alterations that last for seconds.

e. Treatment consists of therapy for the underlying cause.

2. Blurred vision and decreased visual acuity

a. The location of the lesion determines the effect on vision.

(1) Lesions anterior to the optic chiasm will affect only one eye.

(2) Lesions at the optic chiasm will affect both eyes partially.

(3) Lesions posterior to the chiasm will yield corresponding defects in both visual fields.

b. The quality of visual loss helps to determine the diagnosis.

(1) Transient visual loss may be secondary to a transient ischemic attack, an emboli (amaurosis fugax), or temporal (giant cell) arteritis.

(a) Temporal arteritis (giant cell arteritis) is one of the more common causes and is characterized by a tender temporal artery, fever, malaise, and a strikingly increased erythrocyte sedimentation rate.

(b) Prompt treatment with systemic corticosteroids is necessary to prevent permanent blindness.

   (2) Sudden visual loss may be secondary to central retinal vein or branch vein occlusion, optic neuropathy, papillitis, and retrobulbar neuritis.

   (3) Gradual visual loss may be secondary to macular degeneration, tumors, cataracts, or glaucoma.

3. Strabismus

   a. Strabismus is a condition in which binocular fixation is not present.

   b. Strabismus may occur in one eye or both. A cover test or corneal light reflex test will reveal this abnormality.

   c. It may be corrected with eye exercises or, in severe cases, with surgery.

4. Amblyopia

   a. Amblyopia is reduced visual acuity not correctable by refractive means.

   b. It may be caused by strabismus, uremia, or toxins, such as alcohol, tobacco, lead, and other toxic substances.

5. Icterus or jaundice, which is a yellowing of the sclera, is caused by the retention of bilirubin.

6. Blue or cyanotic sclera may be normal or seen in infants with osteogenesis imperfecta.

II. DISORDERS OF THE EARS

A. Hearing impairment (hearing loss) may be of acute or chronic onset.

1. General characteristics

   a. Hearing loss may result from either conductive or sensorineural physiologic causes.

   b. The Weber and Rinne tests are used to help differentiate conductive from sensorineural hearing loss.

   (1) Lateralization to the affected ear on the Weber test indicates conductive hearing loss. Conductive loss also will result in air conduction greater than bone conduction on the affected side.

   (2) Sensorineural defects will have impairment of both air conduction and bone conduction, but air conduction will remain greater.

2. Conductive hearing loss is caused by impaired transmission of sound along the external canal, across the ossicles, and through the oval window. It is often temporary.

   a. There is an increased threshold for perceived sound intensity.

   b. Possible causes of conductive hearing loss

   (1) Cerumen impaction may require removal either by irrigation or by use of a wire loop or cerumen spoon.

   (2) Acute otitis externa also may cause a conductive hearing loss because of the exudate in the external canal.

   (3) Otosclerosis, which is caused by abnormal new bone formation in the oval window, causes conductive hearing loss and is amenable to surgery.

   (4) Otitis media also may cause conductive hearing loss.

3. Sensorineural hearing loss is any hearing loss secondary to a disruption in the nerves or the mechanics of hearing. It has many causes (e.g., neural degeneration, decreased cilia, problems in the ossicles).

   a. Presbycusis

   (1) General characteristics

   (a) Presbycusis is the most common cause of sensorineural hearing loss.

   (b) It occurs with age in most people; men are affected more often than women.

   (c) There is probably a genetic predisposition; it may be caused or exacerbated by noise exposure.

   (2) Clinical features

   (a) It usually involves the higher frequencies and may be associated with tinnitus.

   (b) The patient or family members may complain that there is difficulty in sound discrimination.

   (3) Treatment. This type of loss may or may not be helped by hearing aids.

   b. Meniere's disease

   (1) General characteristics

   (a) This is a recurrent and usually progressive group of symptoms, including acquired chronic hearing loss, tinnitus, and dizziness or vertigo.

   (b) The cause is unknown; symptoms result from distention of the endolymphatic compartment of the inner ear.

(2) Clinical features

    (a) Hearing loss is accompanied by episodes of tinnitus, vertigo, and nausea and vomiting. The attacks may last from minutes to hours, but unsteadiness may last longer.

    (b) The hearing loss may abate with each attack, but hearing rarely returns to the pre-attack level.

(3) Treatment

    (a) Most cases can be managed with diuretics and salt restriction.

    (b) Surgical intervention may be indicated if symptoms progress.

c. Acoustic trauma (e.g., an explosion, a shotgun blast) or chronic noise exposure can cause sensorineural hearing loss.

d. Acoustic neuroma (vestibular schwannoma) is a neoplastic cause of hearing loss.

    (1) It is more predominant in females and usually is unilateral.

    (2) The patient may present with insidious hearing loss; with progressive growth, a patient may develop tinnitus, vertigo, ataxia, and brainstem dysfunction.

    (3) It is diagnosed via CT or MRI, and the treatment is surgical.

4. Drug-induced hearing loss

    a. It may be caused by streptomycin, kanamycin, neomycin, ethacrynic acid, chloramphenicol, and other drugs.

    b. The onset is insidious, and tinnitus may be the first symptom.

    c. Hearing loss usually is high frequency.

    d. It may or may not be reversible with cessation of the drug.

5. Infancy and childhood hearing loss

    a. Congenital causes: Include asphyxia, erythroblastosis, and maternal rubella.

    b. Acquired causes: Include measles, mumps, pertussis, meningitis, influenza, and labyrinthitis.

    c. Clinical features: Include inattentiveness to mother or lack of reaction to noise.

    d. Treatment: Involves correction of underlying causes.

B. Otitis media (infection of the middle ear)

1. General characteristics

    a. The pathophysiology involves underlying poor drainage from the eustachian tubes because of age (i.e., the tubes may be straight in children), inflammation and edema, or a congenital deformity (e.g., Down's syndrome, cleft palate, adenoidal hypertrophy).

    b. Otitis media is most common in children 4–24 months of age but can occur at any age.

    c. It is caused by bacteria in 70–90% of cases; the most common organisms are *Streptococcus pneumoniae, Haemophilus influenzae, Moraxella catarrhalis, Streptococcus pyogenes*, and *Staphylococcus aureus*.

    d. Recurrent cases often are associated with allergies or exposure to secondhand smoke.

2. Clinical features

    a. The patient may present with fever, pressure, pain, and hearing loss.

    b. The eardrum will be immobile and may appear erythematous and bulging. Bullae suggest mycoplasmal infection.

    c. Rupture of the tympanic membrane results in otorrhea and decreased pain; typically, chronic otitis media ensues.

    d. Inadequate treatment of otitis media may cause mastoiditis. Patients will exhibit spiking fevers, postauricular pain, and erythema.

3. Treatment

    a. First-line antibiotics include amoxicillin, erythromycin/sulfonamide, clavulanic acid/amoxicillin, trimethoprim/sulfamethoxazole, and cefaclor. If the patient is allergic to penicillin, erythromycin or clarithromycin is indicated.

    b. When medication fails to heal the otitis media, the patient may need myringotomy, tympanostomy, adenoidectomy, or a combination of these procedures.

    c. Mastoiditis is treated with IV antibiotics; if medication fails, mastoidectomy is indicated.

C. Otitis externa

1. General characteristics

    a. Otitis externa, generally known as swimmer's ear, is common in the teenage years.

      b. The cause is a combination of mechanical obstruction that inhibits drainage of water from the external ear canal and an infectious agent.

      c. Certain conditions may predispose to otitis externa (e.g., eczema, seborrheic dermatitis, psoriasis). The causative organisms include Pseudomonas sp., Enterobacteriaceae, Proteus sp., and, rarely, fungi.

  2. Clinical features

      a. Physical signs include pain in the ear and tenderness with manipulation of the tragus or the auricle.

      b. Otoscopic examination reveals a canal that is edematous and obscured with purulent debris.

  3. Treatment

      a. Use of otic antibacterial drops and keeping the canal dry usually are effective.

      b. In diabetic or immunocompromised patients, malignant otitis externa may develop, which is a necrotizing infection extending to the blood vessels, bone and cartilage; this requires hospitalization and parenteral antibiotics.

D. Vertigo

  1. General characteristics

      a. True vertigo is the sensation of movement (spinning, tumbling, or falling) or a person's sensation of objects spinning around him or her.

      b. Peripheral vertigo is caused by labyrinthitis, Meniere's disease, positional vertigo, vestibular neuronitis, migrainous vertigo, and obstructing anatomic abnormalities.

      c. Central vertigo is caused by brainstem vascular disease, arteriovenous malformations, tumors of the brainstem or cerebellum, multiple sclerosis, or vertebrobasilar migraine syndrome.

  2. Clinical features

      a. Vertigo usually is accelerated with movement.

      b. It may be accompanied by nystagmus.

        (1) Peripheral vertigo is characterized by sudden onset, nausea and vomiting, tinnitus, and decreased hearing. Nystagmus is horizontal with a rotary component, fast-phase beats away from the diseased side, and fixation inhibition.

        (2) Central vertigo is characterized by a slower onset, nonfatiguable nystagmus, vertical greater than horizontal plane, and no latency or suppression by fixation. There usually are accompanying motor, sensory, or cerebellar deficits.

      c. The condition may last from days to weeks.

  3. Laboratory studies.

      a. The Hallpike or Nylen-Barany maneuver (i.e., quickly turning the patient's head 90° while the patient is in the supine position) is used to reproduce the vertigo. This test is more likely to be positive with peripheral causes.

      b. Audiometry, caloric stimulation, electronystagmography, CT, MRI, and evoked potentials are performed as indicated by history and physical examination findings.

  4. Treatment is per underlying cause.

      a. Acute attacks can be treated with diazepam.

      b. Mild vertigo may respond to meclizine, cyclizine, or dimenhydrinate.

      c. Severe vertigo may be treated with scopolamine.

      d. Bed rest may be necessary during acute attacks; however, patients with chronic vertigo should be encouraged to move about.

      e. Interventional and surgical therapies are available for recalcitrant cases.

E. Labyrinthitis is a phenomenon of severe acute vertigo, hearing loss, and tinnitus. The cause is unknown, but it may occur after an otitis or viremia. It may be treated meclizine, promethazine or dimenhydrinate.

F. Barotrauma is the inability to equalize barometric stress on the middle ear, resulting in pain.

  1. Barotrauma is caused by auditory tube dysfunction. This can result from congenital narrowing or acquired mucosal edema.

  2. Symptoms are most likely to occur during airplane descent, rapid altitude change, or underwater diving.

  3. Patients should be instructed to swallow or yawn to autoinflate the tube. Systemic or topical decongestants also may help. If the pressure is not equalized, the tympanic membrane may rupture. A middle ear infection often follows this trauma.

4. If symptoms persist after removal of the offending agent, then decongestants, autoinflation, or myringotomy can be tried.

G. Tympanic membrane rupture: Small ruptures in the tympanic membrane usually will close on their own in time. Larger ruptures may require a tympanoplasty for closure. It is important to not allow any water into the ear until the rupture is closed.

III. DISORDERS OF THE NOSE, SINUS, AND THROAT

A. Sinusitis

1. General characteristics

a. Sinusitis refers to any inflammation of the sinus cavities.

b. It usually follows an upper respiratory tract infection (URI).

c. The causative agents are the same as for otitis media (see II.B).

d. Specific risk factors for the development of acute sinusitis include a recent URI, chronic rhinitis, cigarette smoking, history of trauma or presence of a foreign body, any of which can obstruct drainage and increase the risk of infection.

2. Clinical features

a. Patients complain of headache and pain in the face that worsens when leaning forward, green purulent drainage, fever, and malaise.

b. Physical examination reveals tenderness to palpation over the sinuses or opacification of the sinus with trans-illumination.

3. Laboratory studies

a. A radiograph using the Waters view will reveal opacification, air–fluid levels, or an abnormally thick mucosa.

b. CT is indicated only in the case of recurrence or other complications or if the host is immunocompromised.

c. Osteomyelitis, cavernous sinus thrombosis, or an orbital cellulitis are among the complications of sinusitis.

4. Treatment

a. Treatment of sinusitis includes antibiotics, saline nasal spray, decongestants, and hot packs or steam.

b. Treatment should last for 10–14 days; patients should be carefully monitored for any signs of complications.

B. Rhinitis

1. General characteristics

a. Rhinitis refers to any inflammation of the nasal mucosa.

b. There are three basic types: allergic rhinitis, vasomotor rhinitis, and rhinitis medicamentosa.

(1) Allergic rhinitis is an immunoglobulin E–mediated reactivity to airborne antigens (e.g., pollen, molds, danders, dust). It commonly occurs in people who have other atopic diseases (e.g., asthma, eczema, atopic dermatitis) and with a family history.

(2) Vasomotor rhinitis is rhinorrhea caused by increased secretion of mucus from the nasal mucosa. It may be precipitated by changes in temperature or humidity, odors, alcohol, or result from a neurovascular imbalance.

(3) Rhinitis medicamentosa is caused by the overzealous use of decongestant drops or sprays. This causes a rebound congestion, which prompts increased use of the agent, creating a vicious cycle.

2. Clinical features

a. Allergic rhinitis

(1) Symptoms may be confused with those of a common cold.

(2) Signs may include allergic shiners (bluish discoloration below the eyes), scratchy eyes, rhinorrhea, itchy or watery eyes, sneezing, nasal congestion, dry cough, and pale, boggy, or bluish mucosa.

(3) The discharge usually is clear and watery.

b. Vasomotor rhinitis

(1) In its purest form, vasomotor rhinitis consists of bogginess of the nasal mucosa associated with a complaint of stuffiness and rhinorrhea.

(2) The symptoms are labile and can clear quickly.

    c. Rhinitis medicamentosa

      (1) Patients experience severe congestion and pain.

      (2) Discharge is typically minimal.

  3. Treatment

    a. Allergic rhinitis: Avoid any known allergens and use antihistamines, cromolyn sodium, nasal or systemic corticosteroids, nasal saline drops, and immunotherapy.

    b. Vasomotor rhinitis: Avoid the irritant.

    c. Rhinitis medicamentosa: Discontinue the irritant. It may be quite uncomfortable for the patient; sometimes the use of topical corticosteroids is warranted through the withdrawal period.

C. Pharyngitis

  1. General characteristics

    a. Sore throat is one of the most common reasons for outpatient visits.

    b. The causes of pharyngitis are bacterial and viral; differentiation between the two types of causes is important to direct treatment.

  2. Clinical features

    a. The overall manifestations of pharyngitis include sore throat, difficulty swallowing, fever, erythema of the tonsils and posterior pharynx, lymph node enlargement, rhinitis, and cough, all in varying degrees.

    b. Infection that penetrates the tonsillar capsule leads to cellulitis and peritonsillar abscess, a medical emergency.

  3. Common types of pharyngitis and their management

    a. Streptococcal pharyngitis

      (1) Clinical features

        (a) Acute onset, fever, exudate in posterior pharynx or on tonsils, and cervical adenopathy. In children, it may present as abdominal pain secondary to adenopathy in the abdomen.

        (b) Rapid Strep screening; if negative and the diagnosis is still suspicious, throat culture should be obtained to confirm.

      (2) Treatment

        (a) Treat with a penicillin or erythromycin.

        (b) Complications of improper or incomplete treatment include rheumatic fever, Ludwig's angina, and tonsillar abscess.

    b. Viral pharyngitis

      (1) Clinical features

        (a) Insidious onset, often with coryza, and usually lacking exudate. Fever is low grade; lymphadenopathy may or may not be present.

        (b) Obtain a rapid strep screen or throat culture to rule out streptococcal infection.

      (2) Treatment. Treatment is supportive in nature.

    c. Peritonsillar cellulitis and abscess

      (1) Clinical features include severe sore throat, pain on swallowing or opening the mouth wide, deviation of the soft palate and uvula, and a muffled voice.

      (2) Treatment requires either aspiration or incision and drainage followed by a course of antibiotics. Tonsillectomy may be indicated in about 10% of cases.

D. Laryngitis

  1. General characteristics. It typically is viral and follows an upper respiratory tract infection.

  2. Clinical features. Hoarseness is the hallmark; there is little to no pain with loss of voice.

  3. Treatment is supportive; patients should not overuse their voice (e.g., shouting, singing) to prevent the formation of vocal nodules.

E. Aphthous ulcers (canker sores) and other oral lesions

  1. General characteristics. Canker sores can be idiopathic or associated with herpes virus.

  2. Clinical features. They are found on the buccal mucosa, can be single or multiple, and manifest as painful, round ulcers with red halos. Typically, they are recurrent.

3. Treatment is nonspecific; symptomatic treatment includes topical steroids or anti-inflammatories.

4. Candidiasis causes burning pain in areas of the tongue, inside the cheek, or in the throat. It can be scraped off, which leaves the underlying area raw, erythematous, and friable. It often is seen in immunocompromised patients and in the use of broad-spectrum antibiotics. It is treated with antifungals in the form of a liquid, with which the patient performs a "swish and swallow" technique, or in a troche that is allowed to dissolve in the mouth.

5. Leukoplakia is a painless white area on the tongue, inside the cheek, on the lower lip, or on the floor of the mouth. It usually is seen in patients who use chewing tobacco, smokers, those with AIDS, and with ETOH abuse. Unlike candidiasis, it cannot be scraped off. The area should be biopsied to rule out cancer; however, less than 5% of these areas have been shown to be malignant. Malignancies are more likely in an erythroplastic lesion.

F. Epiglottitis

  1. General characteristics

    a. Epiglottitis is a life-threatening infection of the epiglottis and surrounding tissues that leads to obstructive respiratory disease.

    b. It is most commonly caused by *Haemophilus influenzae* type B; other causes include group A streptococci, pneumococci, or staphylococci.

    c. It is more common in children but can occur at any age. It has become more common in adults, because most children have received the vaccine against. Haemophilus influenzae.

  2. Clinical features. Onset is abrupt, with high fever, difficulty swallowing, sore throat, drooling, and in children, sitting in the tripod or sniffing position.

  3. Laboratory studies

    a. A lateral soft-tissue neck radiograph reveals a thumb-like projection (the classic thumb sign).

    b. Controlled intubation should be performed, and the patient should not be left alone until intubation has occurred.

    c. Examination should be limited, causing no undue distress until the airway is maintained.

  4. Treatment

    a. Patients need IV fluids and antibiotics for 24–72 hours, followed by oral antibiotics to complete a 10-day course.

    b. All unimmunized close contacts should be given prophylaxis with rifampin.

G. Epistaxis (nosebleed)

  1. Kiesselbach's plexus on the anterior aspect of the nose is the most common site of epistaxis.

  2. Epistaxis may be caused by minor trauma, dry mucosa, nasal trauma, or an acquired or genetic coagulopathy.

  3. Treatment

    a. Begin with the patient sitting or standing upright, apply firm pressure to the nares for 10–15 min, and then identify the bleeding site. Visualization is aided by use of a light source and a nasal speculum.

    b. If a bleeding site can be identified, anesthetize with cocaine or lidocaine, and cauterize with a silver nitrate stick.

    c. Recauterize and pack if necessary. The packing is left in place for 24 hours.

    d. The patient should be told to return if bleeding recurs.

  4. Posterior bleed (Woodruff's plexus) is uncommon and significant, requiring emergency evaluation and treatment.

    a. It usually is caused by acute trauma, and the bleeding generally is arterial. Often, blood is seen in the posterior pharynx.

    b. The bleeding may compromise the airway, and a posterior pack must be placed. This usually requires an ear, nose, and throat consult.

    c. The patient is at risk for toxic shock syndrome secondary to retained packing.

H. Polyps

  1. Polyps are pedunculated tumors found on the nasal mucosa.

  2. They often are seen in patients with allergic rhinitis, and they often are easily visualized. There is a somewhat common triad of asthma, nasal polyps, and aspirin sensitivity.

  3. Patients may have nasal phonations and complain of feeling congested all the time.

  4. In most cases, polyps are benign. They should be removed if corticosteroid treatment fails to diminish their size.

Pulmonology

Matthew A. McQuillan

I. INFECTIOUS DISORDERS

A. Pneumonia

1. Pneumonia denotes inflammation in the alveoli or interstitium of the lung caused by microorganisms.

2. Pneumonia ranks as the primary cause of mortality from infectious diseases.

3. Classic community-acquired pneumonia (CAP)

  a. General characteristics

    (1) Acquired in the home or nonhospital environment.

    (2) In most cases of CAP, the causative agent is not identified. However, in those cases where an agent is identified, bacteria are more commonly found.

    (3) Causative agents include *Streptococcus pneumoniae, Haemophilus influenzae, Moraxella catarrhalis, Staphylococcus aureus, Klebsiella pneumoniae,* and other Gram-negative bacilli. Viral causes include influenza virus, respiratory syncytial virus (RSV), adenovirus, and parainfluenza.

  b. Clinical features

    (1) Typical presentation is a 1- to 10-day history of increasing cough, purulent sputum, shortness of breath, tachycardia, pleuritic chest pain, fever or hypothermia, sweats, and rigors.

    (2) Physical examination may reveal altered breath sounds and crackles, dullness to percussion if an effusion is present, and bronchial breath sounds over an area of consolidation.

    (3) Table 2-1 provides classic descriptions of pneumonias caused by specific organisms. Although these characteristics may help in attempting to identify specific pathogens, exceptions and less typical presentations are common.

    (4) Table 2-2 lists the pathogens more likely to occur in certain patient groups. *Streptococcus pneumoniae* remains the most common cause of pneumonia in all groups.

  c. Laboratory findings

    (1) Organisms may be detected with conventional stain or sputum culture, although typically, this is not done before starting treatment. The most common bacterial pathogen identified is *Streptococcus pneumoniae.*

    (2) Chest radiography (CXR) shows lobar or segmental infiltrates, air bronchograms, and pleural effusions. There is no pathognomonic radiographic presentation.

  d. Treatment

    (1) The patient who is otherwise healthy and free of respiratory distress or complications may be treated as an outpatient with oral antibiotics and appropriate supportive care.

    (2) Doxycycline, macrolides (clarithromycin, azithromycin), or fluoroquinolones are appropriate choices for outpatient treatment.

    (3) Neutropenia, involvement of more than one lobe, or poor host resistance indicates a need for hospitalization. Also, consider hospitalization for patients older than 50 years with comorbidities, altered mental status, or hemodynamic instability.

    (4) If inpatient treatment is necessary, consider coverage of *Streptococcus pneumoniae* and *Legionnella* sp. with ceftriaxone or cefotaxine plus azithromycin or a fluoroquinolone.

4. Atypical community-acquired pneumonia

  a. General characteristics

    (1) As the term *atypical* implies, this form of pneumonia has a clinical presentation different from that of classic community-acquired pneumonia.

    (2) *Mycoplasma pneumoniae* is the most common cause of atypical pneumonias. Other causes include viruses (influenza types A and B and adenoviruses), *Chlamydia pneumoniae, Legionella* sp., and *Moraxella* sp.

TABLE 2-1 **Typical Manifestations of Pneumonia per Pathogen**

Organism	Typical Manifestations
Mycoplasma pneumoniae	Low-grade fever Cough Bullous myringitis Cold agglutinins
Pneumocystis jiroveci (nee *carinii*)	Slower onset, immunosuppression Increased lactate dehydrogenase More hypoxemic than appears on chest radiography Interstitial infiltrates
Legionella pneumoniae	Chronic cardiac or respiratory disease Hyponatremia Diarrhea, other systemic symptoms
Chlamydia pneumoniae	Longer prodrome Sore throat, hoarseness
Streptococcus pneumoniae	Single rigor Rust-colored sputum
Klebsiella pneumoniae	Currant jelly sputum Chronic illness, including alcohol abuse

b. Clinical features
  (1) The typical presentation of atypical pneumonia is a low-grade fever with relatively mild pulmonary symptoms, which are self-limited, occurring in young, otherwise healthy adults. A nonproductive cough, myalgia, and fatigue are common.
  (2) *Legionella* infection is associated with exposure to contaminated water droplets from cooling and ventilation systems. Acute development of high fever, dry cough, dyspnea, and systemic symptoms are common.
  (3) Viral pneumonias are variable in presentation but often are associated with epidemics and upper respiratory symptoms.
c. Laboratory findings
  (1) Organisms usually are not detected with conventional stain or culture of sputum.
  (2) The WBC count is normal or only slightly elevated.
  (3) Radiography shows segmental unilateral lower lung zone infiltrates or diffuse infiltrates.

TABLE 2-2 **Pathogens More Likely to Cause Pneumonia in Certain Patient Groups**

Patient Characteristic	Pathogen More Likely Seen in this Group
Alcohol abuse	*Klebsiella pneumoniae*
COPD	*Haemophilus pneumoniae*
Cystic fibrosis	*Pseudomonas* sp.
Young adults, college settings	*Mycoplasma pneumoniae* *Chlamydia pneumoniae*
Air conditioning/aerosolized water	*Legionella pneumoniae*
Postsplenectomy	Encapsulated organisms *Streptococcus pneumoniae* *Haemophilus pneumoniae*
Leukemia, lymphoma	Fungus
Children, <1 year	Respiratory syncytial virus
Children, >2 years	Parainfluenza virus

d. Treatment

(1) Antibiotic treatment is started empirically based on the clinical features. Regimens include erythromycin (for suspected *Mycoplasma pneumoniae* and *Legionella* infection) and tetracycline (for suspected *Chlamydia* infection).

(2) Viral pneumonias are treated with supportive measures (analgesics, fluids, cough suppressants) unless influenza is suspected. Amantidine and rimantadine are no longer recommended in the treatment of influenza because of increasing resistance. Neuraminidase inhibitors (inhaled zanamivir or oral oseltamivir) may be used if antiviral therapy is indicated.

5. Hospital-acquired (nosocomial) pneumonia

   a. General characteristics

   (1) Hospital-acquired pneumonia is caused by organisms that colonize ill patients, staff, and equipment, producing clinical infection more than 48 hours after admission to the hospital. Those at highest risk are ICU patients on mechanical ventilation.

   (2) Pneumonia is the second most common cause of hospital-acquired infection.

   (3) The causative organisms are unique and the mortality rate is 20–50%.

      (a) The usual organisms are *Staphylococcus aureus* and Gram-negative bacilli, which are easy to recover from respiratory secretions.

      (b) *Pseudomonas aeruginosa* is the most likely pathogen in intensive care units and carries the worst prognosis. Others include *Staphylococcus aureus*, *Klebsiella* sp., *Escherichia coli*, and *Enterobacter* sp.

   b. Laboratory findings. Diagnosis is clinical and supported with Gram's stain and culture of sputum and blood.

   c. Treatment includes use of appropriate empirical antibiotics. If an organism is isolated, therapy can be based on the culture results. Patients may need aggressive supportive measures, including mechanical ventilation as appropriate.

6. Pneumonia: HIV Related

   a. General characteristics

   (1) *Pneumocystis jiroveci* (formerly *P. carinii*) is the most common opportunistic infection in patients with HIV disease, typically with CD4 counts of less than 200.

   (2) *Pneumocystis* infection also occurs in patients with cancer, malnourished states, immunosuppression.

   (3) Other pathogens common in patients with HIV and pneumonia include *Streptococcus*, *Haemophilus*, *Pseudomonas*, and *Mycobacterium* sp.

   b. Clinical features

   (1) Pneumocystis pneumonia typically presents with fever, tachypnea, dyspnea, and nonproductive cough.

   (2) Nonpneumocystis pneumonia typically follows a more fulminant course than in non-HIV-infected persons.

   c. Laboratory findings

   (1) CXR is the cornerstone of diagnosis. The radiograph typically shows diffuse or perihilar infiltrates; no effusions are seen.

   (2) Lymphopenia and a low CD4 count are typical.

   (3) Sputum staining, via either induced sputum or bronchoalveolar lavage, will establish the diagnosis in more than 90% of patients.

   d. Treatment

   (1) Trimethoprim/sulfamethoxazole (Bactrim) is the treatment of choice.

   (2) There is an extremely high mortality rate (near 100%) if not treated.

   (3) Prophylaxis is recommended in all patients with a CD4 count of less than 200 or with a history of *Pneumocystis* infection. Trimethoprim/sulfamethoxazole is the antibiotic of choice.

B. Tuberculosis (TB)

   1. General characteristics

   a. *Mycobacterium tuberculosis* infection is acquired by inhaling organisms within aerosol droplets expelled during coughing by people with active disease.

   b. Most exposed people mount an immune response sufficient to prevent progression from primary infection to clinical illness. Approximately 5% of exposed people fail to contain the primary infection and progress to active TB within 2 years; this is known as progressive primary TB.

c. Overall, 10% of persons infected with TB will develop the disease. This is called primary TB.

d. Approximately 95% of infected persons contain the bacterium. This is known as latent TB infection (LTBI). These patients are not considered to be infectious, nor can they spread TB. They are asymptomatic but have inactive TB in their body. Reactivation TB develops from LTBI.

e. Outbreaks have been seen since the emergence of organisms resistant to multiple antituberculous drugs.

2. Clinical features

a. Cough is the most common symptom. It begins as a dry cough and progresses to a productive cough, with or without hemoptysis, typically over 3 weeks or longer.

b. The classic symptom complex includes fever, drenching night sweats, anorexia, and weight loss. Other common pulmonary symptoms are cough, pleuritic chest pain, dyspnea, and hemoptysis. Posttussive rales are classic.

c. On examination, the patient may appear chronically ill and malnourished.

3. Laboratory findings

a. Radiography

(1) Primary TB: homogeneous infiltrates, hilar/paratracheal lymph node enlargement, segmental atelectasis, cavitations with progressive disease.

(2) Reactivation TB: fibrocavitary apical disease, nodules, infiltrates, posterior and apical segments of the right upper lobe, apical-posterior segments of left upper lobe, superior segments of the lower lobes.

(3) Ghon complexes (calcified primary focus) and Ranke complexes (calcified primary focus and calcified hilar lymph node) represent healed primary infection.

b. The tuberculin skin test identifies individuals who have been infected, but it does not differentiate between active and latent infection. Tuberculin skin testing, such as PPDs (Purified protein derivative) are reported according to diameter of induration, not erythema (Table 2-3).

c. Definitive diagnosis requires the identification of *Mycobacterium tuberculosis* from cultures or by DNA or RNA amplification techniques. Demonstration of acid-fast bacilli on sputum supports, but does not confirm, a diagnosis of TB.

4. Treatment

a. Antituberculous drugs, including isoniazid (INH), rifampin (RIF), pyrazinamide (PZA), and ethambutol (EMB), are the cornerstone of therapy. The Centers for Disease Control recommend multiple drug regimens such as:

(1) LTBI: Treat only after active TB is ruled out; INH for 9 months and RIF for 4 months (only if in contact with TB-resistant persons).

(2) Active TB: INH/RIF/PZA/EMB for 2 months, followed by INH/RIF for 4 months.

(3) For more information and alternative treatment regimens see www.cdc.gov

TABLE 2-3	**Classification of Positive Tuberculin Skin Test Reactions**
Reaction Size	**Group**
≥5 mm	HIV-positive persons Recent contacts of those with active tuberculosis Persons with evidence of tuberculosis on chest radiography Immunosuppressed patients on steroids
≥10 mm	Recent immigrants from countries with high rate of tuberculosis HIV-negative injection drug users Mycobacteriology laboratory personnel Residents/employees of high-risk congregate settings Persons with certain medical conditions: diabetes mellitus, silicosis, chronic renal failure, etc. Children <4 years Infants, children, adolescents exposed to adults at high risk
≥15 mm	Persons with no risk factors for tuberculosis

    b. Antituberculous class-specific side effects

        (1) INH: hepatitis, peripheral neuropathy; coadminister vitamin B_6 (pyridoxine) to reduce risk.

        (2) RIF: hepatitis, flu syndrome, orange body fluid (e.g., orange urine).

        (3) EMB: optic neuritis (red-green vision loss).

    c. Patients with active disease require combination chemotherapy for 6–9 months; patients infected with HIV require therapy for at least 1 year.

    d. INH for 6–12 months is indicated for prophylaxis in patients who have tested negative in the past but are now positive with known or unknown exposure (converters).

    e. The bacillus Calmette-Guérin vaccine can be administered to a tuberculin-negative person in cases with a high risk for intense, prolonged exposure to untreated or ineffectively treated cases of infectious TB. This practice is not recommended in the United States, but it is common in areas with endemic TB.

C. Acute bronchitis

  1. General characteristics

    a. More than 90% of cases are caused by viruses including rhinovirus, coronavirus, and respiratory syncytial virus (RSV).

    b. Bronchitis is defined as inflammation of the airways (trachea, bronchi, bronchioles) characterized by cough.

    c. In patients with chronic lung disease, causes also include *Haemophilus influenzae, Streptococcus pneumoniae,* and *Moraxella catarrhalis.*

  2. Clinical features

    a. Signs and symptoms include cough (with or without sputum), dyspnea, fever, sore throat, headache, myalgias, substernal discomfort, and expiratory rhonchi or wheezes.

    b. Bronchitis can be difficult to distinguish from pneumonia, so the examination should be conducted to identify comorbid conditions that may influence treatment.

  3. Laboratory findings. Generally, no laboratory evaluation is required unless there is a strong need to differentiate bronchitis from pneumonia.

  4. Treatment

    a. Supportive measures include hydration, expectorants, analgesics, β_2-agonists, and cough suppressants.

    b. For acute exacerbations of chronic bronchitis, in which bacterial causes are more likely, empiric first-line treatment is a second-generation cephalosporin; second-line treatment is a second-generation macrolide or trimethoprim/sulfamethoxazole.

    c. Antibiotics are indicated for the following: elderly patients, those with underlying cardiopulmonary diseases and a cough for more than 7–10 days, and any patient who is immunocompromised.

    d. For acute exacerbations in otherwise healthy adults, no empiric treatment is needed.

D. Acute bronchiolitis

  1. General characteristics

    a. Bronchiolitis primarily is an illness of young children and infants.

    b. RSV is the most common cause; other agents include parainfluenza, adenovirus, and rhinovirus.

  2. Clinical features

    a. Signs and symptoms include rhinorrhea, sneezing, wheezing, and low-grade fever.

    b. Nasal flaring, tachypnea, and retractions indicate respiratory distress.

  3. Laboratory findings

    a. The CBC usually is normal. Nasal washings for RSV culture and antigen assay often are done in infants.

    b. CXR is normal but can show air-trapping and peribronchial thickening.

  4. Treatment

    a. If RSV is present, consider hospitalization and administration of ribavirin.

    b. Supportive measures, such as nebulized albuterol, IV fluids, antipyretics, and humidified oxygen, are important.

E. Acute epiglottiditis

  1. General characteristics

    a. This is a severe, life-threatening infection of the epiglottis.

    b. The most frequent pathogen is *Haemophilus influenzae* type b.

c. It may occur at any age, but is most common between ages 2 and 7 years.

d. The more recent administration of the H. influenzae type B (Hib) vaccine has decreased the incidence of epiglottiditis in children. Most adults, however, have not been immunized, therefore, the incidence has increased in this population.

2. Clinical findings

a. Signs and symptoms include sudden onset of high fever, respiratory distress, severe dysphagia, drooling, and muffled voice.

b. Examination may reveal mild stridor with little or no coughing; patients usually are upright with the neck extended.

3. Laboratory findings

a. Direct visualization of the epiglottis is diagnostic, but manipulation may initiate sudden, fatal airway obstruction.

b. Once the airway is secured, obtain a CBC and blood and epiglottic cultures.

c. A lateral neck radiograph shows swollen epiglottis (thumb sign).

4. Treatment

a. Secure airway. Do not move or upset the child unless ready to manage the airway.

b. Administer cefotaxime or ceftriaxone for 7–10 days.

II. NEOPLASTIC DISEASE

A. Bronchogenic carcinoma

1. Bronchogenic carcinoma is the leading cause of cancer deaths in men and women. There are more deaths from lung cancer than from colon, breast, and prostate combined.

2. The overall 5-year survival rate is 15%.

3. Bronchogenic carcinoma is divided into two major categories based on staging and treatment options: small cell lung cancer (SCLC), and non-SCLC (NSCLC).

a. SCLC is more likely to spread early and rarely is amenable to surgery (mean survival is 6–18 weeks).

b. NSCLC is grows more slowly.

4. NSCLC includes squamous cell carcinoma (SCC), adenocarcinoma, and large cell carcinoma.

a. Squamous cell carcinoma

(1) General characteristics

(a) SCC represents 25–35% of cases.

(b) SCC tends to originate in the central bronchi and to metastasize to regional lymph nodes. It is prone to early metastasis and an aggressive clinical course; assume micrometastases at presentation.

(2) Clinical features include cough, chest pain, weight loss, dyspnea, and hemoptysis.

(3) Laboratory findings

(a) Anteroposterior and lateral radiographs may show hilar masses, peripheral masses, atelectasis, infiltrates, cavitation (10% of patients), and pleural effusions.

(b) Cytologic examination of sputum, if adequate cells are obtained, permits definitive diagnosis of a specific cell type in many cases.

(c) Bronchoscopy, examination of pleural fluid, and biopsy also are used to establish a diagnosis by looking at specific cell types through direct visualization.

(4) Treatment

(a) Options include surgery, radiation therapy, and chemotherapy.

(b) Surgery remains the treatment of choice. The 5-year survival rate after resection is 35–40%.

b. Adenocarcinoma

(1) General characteristics

(a) Adenocarcinoma is the most common type of bronchogenic carcinoma, accounting for 35–40% of cases.

(b) These cancers typically metastasize to distant organs.

      (c) These tumors arise from mucus glands, usually appear in the periphery of the lung, and are not amenable to early detection through sputum examination.

      (d) Bronchoalveolar cell carcinoma, a subtype of adenocarcinoma, is a low-grade carcinoma.

   (2) Clinical features. Patients may exhibit lymphadenopathy, hepatomegaly, and clubbing, along with cough and weight loss

   (3) Laboratory findings

      (a) Carcinoembryonic antigen usually is positive, because adenocarcinomas express low-molecular-weight cytokeratins and epithelial membrane antigen.

      (b) Small peripheral masses usually can be seen with radiography and often in relation to focal scars or regions of interstitial fibrosis.

   (4) Treatment

      (a) The interval between development of the first lung cancer cell and clinical presentation of the disease has been estimated at 5–10 years. This delay in recognition usually allows ample time for metastasis.

      (b) Symptomatic lung cancer usually is advanced and often is not resectable.

      (c) If resectable, solid tumor with mucin production is associated with the poorest prognosis and bronchoalveolar tumor with the most favorable.

  c. Large cell carcinoma

   (1) Large cell carcinoma is a heterogeneous group of undifferentiated types that do not fit elsewhere.

   (2) Cytology typically shows large cells.

   (3) Doubling time is rapid, and metastasis is early.

   (4) They may be central or peripheral masses.

5. Small (oat) cell carcinoma

  a. General characteristics

   (1) Small cell carcinomas account for 20–25% of lung cancers.

   (2) This is the most aggressive type of carcinoma and tends to metastasize early.

  b. Clinical features

   (1) Paraneoplastic syndromes occur in 15–20% of patients with lung cancer (Table 2-4).

   (2) There is little or no atelectasis, but there is early lymphatic and hematogenous spread (i.e., brain, liver, bones, kidney, adrenal glands).

  c. Laboratory findings

   (1) CXRs commonly show a hilar mass and mediastinal widening.

   (2) Cavitation is exceedingly rare.

TABLE 2-4 Paraneoplastic Syndromes		
Classification	**Syndrome**	**Histological Type**
Endocrine/metabolic	Cushing's syndrome	Small cell
	SIADH	Small cell
	Hypercalcemia	Squamous cell
	Gynecomastia	Large cell
Neuromuscular	Peripheral neuropathy	Small cell
	Myesthenia (Eaton-Lambert)	Small cell
	Cerebellar degeneration	Small cell
Cardiovascular	Thrombophlebitis	Adenocarcinoma
Hematologic	Anemia	All
	DIC	All
	Eosinophilia	All
	Thrombocytosis	All
Cutaneous	Acanthosis nigricans	All

DIC, disseminated intravascular coagulation; *SIADH*, syndrome of inappropriate anti-diuretic hormone.

TABLE 2-5	Sphere of Lung Cancer Complications
SVC syndrome	Compression of superior vena cava (SVC): plethora, headache, mental status changes
Pancoast's tumor	Tumor of the lung apex Causes Horner's syndrome and shoulder pain Affects brachial plexus & cervical sympathetic nerve
Horner's syndrome	Unilateral facial anhidrosis, ptosis, miosis
Endocrine	Carcinoid syndrome: flushing, diarrhea, telangiectasias
Recurrent laryngeal nerve	Hoarseness
Effusions	Exudative

     (3) The majority of SCLCs are located centrally, arise in the peribronchial tissues, and infiltrate the bronchial submucosa.

    d. Treatment. Combination chemotherapy is the treatment of choice for patients with small cell carcinoma and results in improved median survival, although patients rarely live for more than 5 years after the diagnosis is established.

  6. Complications common to all types of bronchogenic carcinoma are listed in Table 2-5.

B. Solitary pulmonary nodule

  1. General characteristics

    a. Pulmonary nodules also are known as coin lesions. If the lesion measures greater than 3 cm, it is referred to as a mass.

    b. Most solitary nodules are infectious granulomas from old or active TB, fungal infection, and foreign body reaction. Approximately 40% are malignant and represent carcinoma, hamartoma, or metastasis (but these are usually multiple) as well as bronchial adenoma (95% are carcinoid tumors).

    c. Malignancy is rare in patients younger than 30 years. Smokers have an increased risk of malignancy; this increased risk rises with the number of pack-years smoked.

  2. Clinical features. Most pulmonary nodules are found unexpectedly at radiography and are asymptomatic.

  3. Laboratory findings

    a. A solitary pulmonary nodule (coin lesion) is a round or oval, sharply circumscribed, pulmonary lesion (up to 5 cm in diameter) surrounded by normal lung tissue.

    b. Central cavitation, calcification, or surrounding (satellite) lesions may occur.

    c. A lesion that has not enlarged in more than 2 years suggests a benign cause. Most are infectious granulomas.

    d. Malignant lesions occasionally are symptomatic, tend to occur in patients older than 45 years, usually are greater than 2 cm in diameter, often have indistinct margins, exhibit rapid progression in size, and rarely are calcified.

  4. Treatment

    a. Lesions with a low probability of malignancy can be watched. Patients should undergo CT every 3 months for a year; if stable, frequency of CT can be reduced to every 6 months for the next 2 years.

    b. Lesions with a high probability of malignancy should be resected as soon as possible. An interim biopsy is not recommended.

    c. Lesions with intermediate probability of malignancy should be biopsied; use transthoracic needle biopsy or bronchoscopy if peripheral. False-positive rates can be as high as 25%. High-resolution CT or position-emission tomography may aid in establishing the diagnosis. High-resolution CT is best to delineate the mass and detect adenopathy or the presence of multiple nodules.

C. Carcinoid tumors

  1. General characteristics

    a. Also known as carcinoid adenomas or bronchial gland tumors, these are well-differentiated neuroendocrine tumors that affect men and women equally. Patients usually are younger than 60 years.

    b. Carcinoid tumors are low-grade malignant neoplasms. They grow slowly and rarely metastasize.

2. Clinical features

a. Hemoptysis, cough, focal wheezing, and recurrent pneumonia. Bleeding and obstruction are common.

b. Carcinoid syndrome (flushing, diarrhea, wheezing, hypotension) is rare.

3. Laboratory findings

a. Bronchoscopy reveals a pink or purple central lesion that is well vascularized. They can be pedunculated or sessile.

b. CT and octreotide scintigraphy localize the disease. CT will localize the lesion as well as monitor for growth.

4. Treatment. Surgical excision carries a good prognosis. The lesions are resistant to radiation therapy and to chemotherapy.

III. OBSTRUCTIVE PULMONARY DISEASE

A. Asthma

1. General characteristics

a. Asthma is characterized by three components: obstruction to airflow, bronchial hyperreactivity, and inflammation of the airway. It is a disease of chronic inflammation leading to airway narrowing and increased mucus production.

b. Asthma affects 5% of the population. Prevalence, hospitalization, and mortality have risen during the past 20 years.

c. Many asthma syndromes have been identified: extrinsic allergic, allergic bronchopulmonary aspergillosis, intrinsic asthma, extrinsic nonallergic, aspirin sensitivity, exercise induced, and asthma associated with chronic obstructive pulmonary disease (COPD).

d. The strongest predisposing factor to asthma is atopy. Atopic triad: wheeze, eczema, seasonal rhinitis.

e. Exacerbations often are correlated with common precipitants: allergens (especially dust and dust mites, dander, cockroaches, and pollen), exercise, upper respiratory tract infections, postnasal drip, gastroesophageal reflux disease, drugs (β-blockers, angiotensin-converting enzyme inhibitors, aspirin, NSAIDs), stress, cold air or change in the weather, environmental irritants, and others.

2. Clinical features

a. Patients have an intermittent occurrence of cough, chest tightness, breathlessness, and wheezing. One-third of children have no wheeze.

b. Patients undergo asymptomatic periods between these attacks.

c. Asthma is classified according to frequency of symptoms and pulmonary function testing (Table 2-6).

TABLE 2-6	**Classification of Severity of Chronic Stable Asthma**		
Severity	**Symptoms**	**Nighttime Symptoms**	**Lung Function**
Mild intermittent	Symptoms ≤2 times/week Asymptomatic and normal PEF Exacerbations brief (few hours to few days); intensity may vary	≤2 times/month	FEV$_1$ or PEF ≥80% predicted PEF variability ≤20%
Mild persistent	Symptoms >2 times/week but <1/day	>2 times/month Exacerbations may affect activity	FEV$_1$ or PEF ≥80% predicted
Moderate persistent	Daily symptoms Daily use of inhaled short-acting β$_2$-agonist Exacerbations ≥2 times/week; may last days	>1 time/week	FEV1 or PEF >60% to <80% predicted PEF variability >30%
Severe persistent	Continual symptoms Limited physical activities Frequent exacerbations	Frequent	FEV$_1$ or PEF ≤60% predicted PEF variability >30%

FEV$_1$, forced expiratory volume in 1 second; PEF, peak expiratory flow rate.
Source: National Asthma Education and Prevention Program Expert Panel Report 2: Guidelines for the Diagnosis and Management of Asthma. Publication 97-4051. Bethesda, MD: National Institutes of Health, 1997.

3. Laboratory findings

   a. Airflow obstruction is indicated by decreased ratio of forced expiratory volume in 1 second to forced vital capacity (FEV_1 to FVC; <75%). A greater than 10% increase in FEV_1 after bronchodilator therapy is supportive of the diagnosis.

   b. Arterial blood gas (ABG) measurements may be normal in mild cases, but in severe cases, they can reveal hypoxemia and hypocapnia, with a Pao_2 of less than 60 mm Hg and a $Paco_2$ of more than 40 mm Hg.

   c. CXR may show hyperinflation. Radiography is only indicated if pneumonia is suspected, the asthma is complicated, or another disorder is suspected.

   d. Handheld peak expiratory flow meters estimate variability and quantify severity of attacks. Use of this objective device should be encouraged in patients with chronic disease.

   e. A histamine or methacholine challenge test (bronchial provocation test) may help to establish the diagnosis of asthma when spirometry is nondiagnostic. The FEV_1 decreases by more than 20%.

4. Treatment

   a. The goals of treatment are to minimize chronic symptoms; prevent recurrent exacerbations and, thus, minimize the need for urgent care visits; and maintain near-normal pulmonary function.

   b. Asthma medications can be divided into long-term control (corticosteroids, cromolyn, nedocromil, long-acting bronchodilators, leukotriene modifiers, and theophylline) and quick-relief medications (short-acting inhaled β_2-agonists, ipratropium bromide, and systemic corticosteroids).

   c. Treatment algorithms are based on both the severity of the patient's baseline asthma and the severity of asthma exacerbations (Table 2-7).

   d. β-Adrenergic agonists should be available to induce bronchodilation during acute symptoms.

   e. Inhaled corticosteroids are the most effective anti-inflammatory medications for management of chronic asthma.

   f. Patients should be educated about their disease and the use of peak flow monitoring. Daily evaluation of pulmonary function with a peak flow meter is an important component of optimal asthma management. This type of monitoring warns of changes in disease status and allows for adjustments on a daily basis if needed.

B. Bronchiectasis

1. General characteristics

   a. Bronchiectasis is defined as an abnormal, permanent dilatation of the bronchi and destruction of bronchial walls. It can be congenital (cystic fibrosis) or acquired from recurrent infections (TB, fungal infection, lung abscess) or obstruction (tumor).

   b. Bronchiectasis results from bronchial injury subsequent to severe infection and/or inflammation.

   c. Cystic fibrosis causes half of all cases.

2. Clinical features

   a. Symptoms include chronic purulent sputum (often foul smelling), hemoptysis, chronic cough, and recurrent pneumonia.

   b. Physical examination may reveal localized chest crackles and clubbing.

3. Laboratory findings

   a. High-resolution chest CT is the imaging modality of choice; it reveals dilated, tortuous airways.

   b. CXR in patients with clinically significant bronchiectasis is abnormal. The degree of abnormality depends on the extent and severity of disease. Crowded bronchial markings and basal cystic spaces are characteristic. CXR may reveal tram-track lung markings, honeycombing, and atelectasis.

   c. Bronchoscopy is warranted to evaluate hemoptysis, remove secretions, and rule out obstructing lesions.

4. Treatment

   a. A productive cough should be managed with the appropriate antibiotic, bronchodilators, and chest physiotherapy.

   b. Antibiotics are prescribed for 10–14 days for acute symptoms; suppressive therapy may be helpful in severe disease or in patients with rapid recurrence. Amoxicillin, amoxicillin/clavulanate, trimethoprin/sulfamethoxazole, and tetracyclines are effective choices.

   c. Bronchodilators are helpful for maintenance and for curing acute exacerbations.

   d. Patients with disabling symptoms or progressive bronchiectasis can be considered for surgery; however, surgery has little long-term benefit.

TABLE 2-7	Stepwise Approach for Managing Asthma		
Step	**Daily Medication**	**As-Needed Medication**	**Comments**
Step 1: mild intermittent	None needed	Short-acting bronchodilator: inhaled β_2-agonists as needed for symptoms Intensity of treatment depends on severity of exacerbation Use of short-acting inhaled β_2-agonists >2 times/week may indicate the need for long-term control therapy	Teach basic facts about asthma Teach inhaler-inhalation chamber technique Discuss role of medications Develop self-management and action plans Discuss appropriate environmental-control measures
Step 2: mild persistent	One daily medication Anti-inflammatory: either inhaled corticosteroid (low dose) or cromolyn or nedocromil Less desirable alternatives: sustained-release theo-phylline or leukotriene modifier	Short-acting bronchodilator: inhaled β_2-agonists as needed for symptoms Intensity of treatment depends on severity of exacerbation Use of short-acting inhaled β_2-agonists on a daily basis or with increasing frequency indicates the need for addi-tional long-term control therapy	Step 1 actions plus the following: Teach self-monitoring Refer to group education, if available Review and update self-management plan
Step 3: moderate persistent	Either: 1) inhaled coricosteroid (medium dose) or 2) inhaled coricosteroid (low-medium dose) and a long-acting bronchodilator (long-acting inhaled β_2-agonist, sustained-release theophylline or long-acting β_2-agonist tablets) If needed: inhaled corticosteroid (medium-high dose) and long-acting bronchodilator (long-acting inhaled β_2-agonist, sustained-release theophylline or long-acting β_2-agonist tablets)	Short-acting bronchodilator: inhaled β_2-agonists as needed for symptoms Intensity of treatment depends on severity of exacerbation Use of short-acting inhaled β_2-agonists on a daily basis or with increasing frequency indi-cates the need for additional long-term control therapy	Step 1 actions plus the following: Teach self-monitoring Refer to group education, if available Review and update self-man-agement plan
Step 4: severe persistent	Add systemic corticosteroid	Short-acting bronchodilator: inhaled β_2-agonists as needed for symptoms Intensity of treatment depends on severity of exacerbation Use of short-acting inhaled β_2-agonists on a daily basis or with increasing frequency indi-cates the need for additional long-term control therapy	Refer for eduction and counseling

FEV$_1$, forced expiratory volume in 1 second; PEF, peak expiratory flow rate.
Source: National Asthma Education and Prevention Program Expert Panel Report 2: Guidelines for the Diagnosis and Management of Asthma. Publication 97-4051. Bethesda, MD: National Institutes of Health, 1997.

C. Chronic obstructive pulmonary disease (COPD)

1. General characteristics

a. COPD is a clinical and pathophysiologic syndrome that includes emphysema and chronic bronchitis. These disorders have overlapping features, and because patients often have characteristics of more than one disorder, both are classified together as COPD (Table 2-8).

TABLE 2-8	COPD Comparisons	
	Emphysema Predominant	**Bronchitis Predominant**
Patient type	"Pink puffers"	"Blue bloaters"
Clinical findings	Exertional dyspnea Cough is rare Quiet lungs No peripheral edema Thin; recent weight loss Barrel chest Pursed lips breathing Hyperventilation	Mild dyspnea Chronic productive cough Noisy lungs: rhonchi and wheeze Peripheral edema Overweight and cyanotic
Chest radiography	Decreased lung markings at apices Flattened diaphragms Hyperinflation Parenchymal bullae and blebs Small, thin-appearing heart	Increased interstitial markings at bases Diaphragms not flattened

     (1) Emphysema is a condition in which the air spaces are enlarged as a consequence of destruction of alveolar septae.

     (2) Chronic bronchitis is a disease characterized by a chronic cough that is productive of phlegm occurring on most days for 3 months of the year for 2 or more consecutive years without an otherwise-defined acute cause.

  b. Smoking is the most important cause of COPD. Other causes include environmental pollutants, recurrent upper respiratory infections, eosinophilia, and bronchial hyper-responsiveness.

2. Clinical features

  a. Patients present with a history of progressive shortness of breath, excessive cough, and sputum production. Patients with predominantly emphysematous COPD may have dry cough and weight loss.

  b. The physical examination of a patient with advanced COPD may reveal asthenia, dyspnea, pursed lip breathing, and grunting expirations.

  c. Chest examination

     (1) Signs of hyperinflation with increase in the anteroposterior dimension are noted.

     (2) Percussion yields increased resonance.

     (3) Auscultation reveals decreased breath sounds and early inspiratory crackles.

     (4) Wheezing may not be present at rest but can be evoked with forced expiration or exertion.

     (5) The duration of expiration is prolonged.

  d. In patients with chronic bronchitis, rhonchi reflect secretions in the airways, and breathing typically is raspy and loud.

3. Laboratory findings

  a. Chest radiograph

     (1) CXR may show hyperinflation of the lungs and flat diaphragms. Although suggestive, a CXR is not sensitive or specific enough to serve as a diagnostic or screening tool.

     (2) If emphysema is the main clinical feature, parenchymal bullae or subpleural blebs are pathognomonic.

     (3) In chronic bronchitis, nonspecific peribronchial and perivascular markings may be present.

  b. Pulmonary function testing

     (1) Airflow obstruction demonstrated on forced expiratory spirometry is suggestive.

     (2) The FEV_1 to FVC ratio is decreased.

  c. The CBC may show polycythemia caused by chronic hypoxemia.

4. Treatment

  a. In symptomatic patients, the goal of treatment is to improve functional state and to relieve symptoms.

  b. Smoking cessation is the single most important intervention.

  c. Anticholinergic inhalers (ipratropium or tiotropium) are superior to β-adrenergic agonists in achieving bronchodilation.

d. Short-acting bronchodilators should be prescribed for acute exacerbations of dyspnea.

e. These patients are at high risk for acute infections; therefore, oral antibiotics frequently are necessary.

f. Supplemental oxygen is the only therapy that alters the course of COPD in patients with resting hypoxemia (PaO_2 <55 mm Hg or SaO_2 <88%).

g. Graded aerobic physical exercise should be encouraged.

h. Steroids are effective but should be used with caution.

i. Patients should receive the pneumococcal vaccine and yearly influenza vaccine.

D. Cystic fibrosis

1. General characteristics

　a. Cystic fibrosis is an autosomal recessive disorder that results in the abnormal production of mucus by almost all exocrine glands, causing obstruction of those glands and ducts.

　b. Patients are at increased risk of malignancies of the GI tract, osteopenia, and arthropathies.

　c. Median survival is about 31 years of age.

2. Clinical features

　a. The diagnosis should be suspected in any young patient who presents with a history of chronic lung disease, pancreatitis, or infertility.

　b. Symptoms include cough, excess sputum, decreased exercise tolerance, sinus pain, purulent nasal discharge, steatorrhea, diarrhea, and abdominal pain.

　c. Signs include clubbing, increased anteroposterior chest diameter, and apical crackles.

3. Laboratory findings

　a. ABG studies reveal hypoxemia and, in advanced disease, a chronic, compensated respiratory acidosis.

　b. Pulmonary function tests reveal a mixed obstructive and restrictive pattern.

　c. CXR may reveal hyperinflation; peribronchial cuffing; mucous plugging; bronchiectasis; increased interstitial markings; small, round peripheral opacities; focal atelectasis; or pneumothorax.

　d. Thin-section CT may confirm the presence of bronchiectasis.

　e. An elevated quantitative sweat chloride test (>60 mEq/L) performed on two different days can be diagnostic; however, a normal result does not exclude the diagnosis. If the diagnosis is strongly suspected, DNA testing can provide definitive evidence of cystic fibrosis.

4. Treatment

　a. Comprehensive multidisciplinary therapy improves the control of symptoms and the chances of survival.

　b. Therapies focus on the following areas: clearance of airway secretions, reversal of bronchoconstriction, treatment of respiratory infections, replacement of pancreatic enzymes, and nutritional and psychosocial support.

IV. PLEURAL DISEASES

A. Pleural Effusion

1. General characteristics

　a. Pleural effusions (the accumulation of significant volumes of pleural fluid) may result from inflammation of structures adjacent to the pleural space or lesions within the chest.

　b. Small effusions may not cause symptoms and may be first discovered on a routine radiograph.

　c. 25% of effusions are associated with malignancy.

　d. There are four types of effusions.

　　(1) Exudates are associated with "leaky capillaries"; examples include infection, malignancy, and trauma.

　　(2) Transudates ("intact capillaries") are associated with increased hydrostatic or decreased oncotic pressure; examples include congestive heart failure, atelectasis, and renal or liver disease (cirrhosis).

　　(3) An empyema is an infection within the pleural space.

　　(4) A hemothorax indicates bleeding into the pleural space, commonly as a result of trauma or malignancy.

2. Clinical features

    a. With a small inflammatory effusion, pleural pain (pleurisy) often is present, and a friction rub may be heard.

    b. Large or bilateral pleural effusions may lead to dyspnea, but orthopnea is uncommon in the absence of congestive heart failure.

    c. A dull to flat percussion note over the area of fluid may be heard with reduced or absent breath sounds.

    d. The mediastinum usually is shifted away from the side of the large effusion.

3. Laboratory findings

    a. Radiographic findings include blunting of the costophrenic angle, loss of sharp demarcation of the diaphragm and heart, and mediastinal shift to the uninvolved side.

    b. Lateral decubitus radiographs can help to identify small effusions and differentiate free flowing versus loculated fluid.

    c. CT may be useful if plain-film radiography cannot separate parenchymal and pleural densities.

    d. Thoracentesis is the gold standard; the fluid is sent for protein, lactate dehydrogenase (LDH), pH, total WBC and differential cell counts, glucose, cytology, and Gram's stain with culture and sensitivity.

    e. Transudates versus exudates (Light's criteria): Fluid is considered to be an exudate if meets any *one* of the following:

        (i)   Pleural fluid protein to serum protein ratio of greater than 0.5

        (ii) Pleural fluid LDH to serum LDH ratio of greater than 0.6

        (iii) Pleural fluid LDH greater than two-thirds the upper limit of normal for serum LDH

4. Treatment

    a. Unless the cause has been clearly established, the presence of fluid is an indication for thoracocentesis. Removal of fluid via thoracocentesis allows fluid examination, radiographic visualization of the lung parenchyma, and relief of symptoms.

    b. Transudate pleural effusions resolve when underlying causes are treated.

    c. Malignant effusions may require drainage and pleurodesis. The most commonly used irritants are doxycycline and talc.

    d. Empyema requires drainage and antibiotic therapy.

B. Pneumothorax

1. General characteristics

    a. Pneumothorax is the accumulation of air in the pleural space.

    b. The cause may be spontaneous (primary pneumothorax), traumatic, or iatrogenic.

    c. Tall, thin males between 10 and 30 years of age are at greatest risk of primary pneumothorax.

    d. Tension pneumothorax is secondary to a sucking chest wound or a pulmonary laceration that allows air to enter the chest with inspiration but does not allow it to leave on expiration.

2. Clinical features

    a. Pneumothorax is characterized by the acute onset of ipsilateral chest pain and dyspnea. Physical findings depend on the size of the pneumothorax and may include unilateral chest expansion, decreased tactile fremitus, hyperresonance, and diminished breath sounds.

    b. Tension pneumothorax is associated with a mediastinal shift to the contralateral side and impaired ventilation, leading to cardiovascular compromise.

3. Laboratory findings

    a. Expiratory CXR reveals the presence of pleural air. A visceral pleural line may be the only evidence of a small pneumothorax.

    b. ABG analysis, if done, reveals hypoxemia.

4. Treatment depends on the severity.

    a. Small pneumothoraces resolve spontaneously.

    b. For severely symptomatic or large pneumothoraces, chest tube placement is performed.

    c. If tension pneumothorax is suspected, a large-bore needle should be inserted to allow air to move out of the chest.

    d. Patients should be followed with serial CXR every 24 hours until resolved.

V. PULMONARY CIRCULATION

A. Pulmonary embolism

1. General characteristics

a. Pulmonary embolism (PE) arises from thrombi in the venous circulation or the right side of the heart, from tumors that have invaded the venous circulation, and from other sources. More than 90% of pulmonary emboli originate as clots in the deep veins of the lower extremities; others include air emboli from central lines, amniotic fluid from active labor, and fat from long bone (femur) fracture.

b. Risk factors revolve around Virchow's triad: hypercoagulable state, venous stasis, and vascular intimal inflammation or injury. Specific risks include surgical procedures (orthopedic, pelvic, abdominal), cancer, oral contraceptives, and pregnancy.

c. Approximately 50–60% of patients with deep vein thrombosis will experience a PE; half of these will be asymptomatic, often being found only on autopsy. Symptomatic PE is a serious and potentially fatal condition.

2. Clinical features

a. Symptoms include pleuritic chest pain, dyspnea, apprehension, cough, hemoptysis, and diaphoresis.

b. Signs include tachycardia, tachypnea, crackles, accentuation of the pulmonary component of the second heart sound, and a low-grade fever.

3. Laboratory findings

a. ABG measurements show acute respiratory alkalosis secondary to hyperventilation.

b. An electrocardiogram shows tachycardia and nonspecific ST-T wave changes. The classic $S_1Q_3T_3$ pattern, indicating cor pulmonale, is seen in fewer than 20% of patients with symptomatic PE.

c. CXR may show nonspecific abnormalities. The main purpose of obtaining CXR is to rule at other abnormalities and aid in interpreting a ventilation-perfusion scan.

d. A ventilation–perfusion lung scan shows perfusion defects with normal ventilation. A normal scan rules out clinically significant thromboembolism. Nondiagnostic scans warrant further testing.

e. Pulmonary angiography remains the definitive test for diagnosis but is reserved for cases in which the diagnosis is uncertain after noninvasive testing.

f. Spiral CT is gaining popularity as an initial method of identifying pulmonary embolus.

4. Treatment

a. Anticoagulation therapy is initiated; heparin is the anticoagulant of choice. Low-molecular-weight heparin or warfarin is continued after the acute phase.

b. Duration of therapy depends on the clinical situation. A minimum of 3 months is advised.

c. Vena cava interruption (filter) is helpful in patients at high risk of recurrence who are unable to tolerate anticoagulants.

d. Prevention is the key. For high-risk patients, consider the following: early ambulation, intermittent pneumatic compression stockings; low dose heparin and low-molecular-weight heparin, or a combination of mechanical and pharmacological measures.

B. Pulmonary hypertension

1. General characteristics

a. Pulmonary hypertension is present when the pulmonary arterial pressure rises to a level inappropriate for a given cardiac output. Once present, it is self-perpetuating.

b. Primary (idiopathic) pulmonary hypertension is rare and has a fatal outcome.

c. Secondary pulmonary hypertension has many causes that develop as a result of obliteration and obstruction of the pulmonary arterial tree.

d. Hypoxia is the most important and potent stimulus of pulmonary arterial vasoconstriction. Other causes include acidosis and veno-occlusive conditions.

2. Clinical features

a. Clinical manifestations may include dyspnea, weakness, fatigue, edema, ascites, cyanosis, and syncope.

b. Signs may include narrow splitting and accentuation of the second heart sound and a systolic ejection click.

3. Laboratory findings

    a. CXR may show enlarged pulmonary arteries, and the electrocardiogram shows right ventricular hypertrophy, atrial hypertrophy, and right ventricular strain.

    b. Echocardiography may be useful in estimating pulmonary arterial pressure, but right heart catheterization offers more precise hemodynamic monitoring.

4. Treatment

    a. Treatment of primary pulmonary hypertension may include chronic oral anticoagulants, calcium channel blockers to lower systemic arterial pressure, and prostacyclin (a potent pulmonary vasodilator). Despite these measures, heart–lung transplantation usually is needed.

    b. Treatment of secondary pulmonary hypertension consists of treating the underlying disorder in addition to those mentioned above.

VI. RESTRICTIVE PULMONARY DISEASE

A. Idiopathic fibrosing interstitial pneumonia (formerly idiopathic pulmonary fibrosis)

    1. General characteristics

        a. This is the most common diagnosis among patients with interstitial lung disease.

        b. There are three histopathologic patterns, with different natural histories and treatments: usual interstitial pneumonia; respiratory bronchiolitis–associated interstitial lung disease; and acute interstitial pneumonitis.

    2. Clinical features

        a. Symptoms include an insidious, dry cough; exertional dyspnea; and constitutional symptoms (fatigue, malaise, etc.).

        b. Examination may reveal clubbing and inspiratory crackles.

    3. Laboratory findings

        a. CXR demonstrates evidence of progressive fibrosis over several years.

        b. CT shows diffuse, patchy fibrosis with pleural-based honeycombing.

        c. Pulmonary function tests may show a restrictive pattern (decreased lung volume with a normal to increased FEV/FVC ratio).

    4. Treatment remains controversial, because none has been shown to improve survival or quality of life compared to no treatment.

B. Pneumoconioses

    1. General characteristics

        a. Pneumoconioses are chronic fibrotic lung diseases caused by the inhalation of coal dust or various inert, inorganic, or silicate dusts.

        b. Clinically important pneumoconioses include coal workers' pneumoconiosis, silicosis, and asbestosis.

TABLE 2-9	**Comparison of Pneumoconioses**		
Disease	**Occupation**	**Diagnosis**	**Complications**
Asbestosis	Insulation, demolition, construction	Bx: asbestos bodies CXR: linear opacities at bases and pleural plaques	Increased risk of lung cancer and mesothelioma, especially if a smoker
Coal worker's pneumonoconiosis	Coal miner	CXR: nodular opacities at upper lung fields	Progressive massive fibrosis
Silicosis	Miners, sand blasters, quarry workers, stone workers	CXR: nodular opacities at upper lung fields	Increased risk of tuberculosis; progressive massive fibrosis
Berryliosis	High technology fields: aerospace, nuclear power, ceramics, foundries, tool & die manufacturing	CXR: diffuse infiltrates and hilar adenopathy	Requires chronic steroids

Bx, biopsy; *CXR*, chest radiography.

2. Clinical features

  a. In simple cases, pneumoconioses usually are asymptomatic.

  b. In complicated cases, patients have dyspnea, inspiratory crackles, clubbing, and cyanosis.

  c. Table 2-9 provides a comparison of the most common pneumoconioses.

3. Laboratory findings

  a. Pulmonary function tests show restrictive dysfunction and reduced diffusing capacity.

  b. Chest radiographs

    (1) Coal workers' pneumoconiosis: Small opacities are prominent in the upper lung fields.

    (2) Silicosis: Small, rounded opacities are seen throughout the lung, and hilar lymph nodes may be calcified.

    (3) Asbestosis: Interstitial fibrosis, thickened pleura, and calcified plaques appear on the diaphragms or lateral chest wall.

4. Treatment is primarily supportive.

  a. No effective treatment is available. Supportive therapy includes oxygen, vaccinations (pneumovax, influenza vaccine), and rehabilitation.

  b. Corticosteroids may relieve the chronic alveolitis in silicosis.

  c. Smoking cessation is especially important for patients with asbestosis, because smoking interferes with short asbestos fiber clearance from the lung. Smoking and asbestos are synergistically linked to lung cancer.

C. Sarcoidosis

  1. General characteristics

    a. Sarcoidosis is a multiorgan disease of idiopathic cause. It is characterized by noncaseating granulomatous inflammation in affected organs (e.g., lungs, lymph nodes, eyes, skin, liver, spleen, salivary glands, heart, nervous system).

    b. Approximately 90% of patients have lung involvement.

    c. The incidence is highest in North American blacks (especially women) and in northern European whites.

  2. Clinical features

    a. Common respiratory symptoms include cough, dyspnea of insidious onset, and chest discomfort.

    b. Patients may present with malaise, fever, and symptoms consistent with the involvement of various organs.

    c. Extrapulmonary findings are common and include erythema nodosum or enlargement of parotid glands, lymph nodes, liver, or spleen.

  3. Laboratory findings

    a. Serum blood tests may show leukopenia, eosinophilia, elevated erythrocyte sedimentation rate, hypercalcemia, and hypercalciuria.

    b. Angiotensin-converting enzyme levels are elevated in 40–80% of patients.

    c. Radiographic findings demonstrate symmetric bilateral hilar and right paratracheal adenopathy and bilateral diffuse reticular infiltrates.

    d. Transbronchial biopsy of the lung or fine needle node biopsy confirms the diagnosis. Biopsy shows noncaseating granulomas.

  4. Treatment. Approximately 90% of cases are responsive to corticosteroids and can be controlled with modest maintenance doses.

VII. OTHER PULMONARY DISEASES

  A. Acute (adult) respiratory distress syndrome (ARDS)

  1. General characteristics

    a. Three clinical settings account for 75% of ARDS cases: sepsis syndrome (the single most important), severe multiple trauma, and aspiration of gastric contents. Other causes include shock, toxic inhalation, near-drowning, and multiple transfusions.

    b. The underlying abnormality in ARDS is increased permeability of the alveolar capillary membranes, which leads to development of protein-rich pulmonary edema.

2. Clinical features

    a. Physical examination shows tachypnea, frothy pink or red sputum, and diffuse crackles.

    b. Many patients are cyanotic with increasingly severe hypoxemia that is refractory to administered oxygen.

3. Laboratory findings

    a. CXR may be normal at first. Infiltrates tend to be peripheral (spares the costophrenic angles) with air bronchograms in 80% of patients. The heart is normal in size.

    b. Pulmonary capillary wedge pressure is normal.

    c. Multiple organ failure is common.

4. Treatment

    a. Treatment includes identification and specific treatment of the underlying precipitating and secondary conditions.

    b. Supportive care also is required to compensate for the severe respiratory dysfunction. Oxygen should be delivered via endotracheal intubation with positive pressure ventilation. Hypoxia often is refractory to treatment.

    c. The mortality rate associated with ARDS is high, which reflects the severity of the predisposing conditions.

    d. One-third of deaths occur within 3 days of the onset of symptoms. The remaining deaths occur within 2 weeks of diagnosis and are caused by infection and multiple organ failure.

B. Aspiration of foreign bodies

  1. General characteristics

    a. Knowledge of the Heimlich maneuver is lifesaving.

    b. Aspiration may be of gastric contents, inert material, toxic material, or poorly chewed food. The degree of injury depends on the substance aspirated.

  2. Clinical features

    a. An episode of choking and coughing or unexplained wheezing or hemoptysis should raise the suspicion of foreign body aspiration.

    b. Asphyxia may result from the aspiration of obstructing material.

    c. Pneumonia may develop secondary to aspiration of toxic materials.

    d. Acute gastric aspiration is one of the most common causes of ARDS.

  3. Laboratory studies. Expiratory radiography may reveal regional hyperinflation caused by a check-valve effect.

  4. Treatment

    a. Bronchoscopy may help to establish the diagnosis but also can be the treatment of choice for removal of the object.

    b. Cultures should be obtained if postobstructive pneumonia is suspected.

C. Hyaline membrane disease

  1. General characteristics

    a. Hyaline membrane disease is the most common cause of respiratory disease in the preterm infant.

    b. It is caused by a deficiency of surfactant.

  2. Clinical features. The infant will demonstrate typical signs of respiratory distress.

  3. Laboratory findings. CXR demonstrates air bronchograms, diffuse bilateral atelectasis causing a ground-glass appearance, and doming of the diaphragm.

  4. Treatment

    a. Synchronized intermittent mandatory ventilation should be used.

    b. Administration of exogenous surfactants can be used in the delivery room as prophylaxis or as rescue in established hyaline membrane disease.

Cardiology

Rebecca Lovell Scott

I. MAJOR PRINCIPLES OF CARDIAC CARE

A. Three factors are needed to maintain adequate pressure in the cardiovascular system.

   1. A functioning pump

   2. Sufficient fluid volume

   3. Resistance

B. All cardiac pathologies result from abnormalities of electrical or contractile functions of the heart muscle, fluid load, or vascular resistance.

II. SHOCK

A. General characteristics

   1. Shock is severe cardiovascular failure caused by poor blood flow or inadequate distribution of flow.

   2. Inadequate oxygen delivery to body tissues results in shock, which may lead to organ failure and death.

   3. The physical responses to shock are mediated by catecholamines, renin, antidiuretic hormone, glucagon, cortisol, and growth hormone.

   4. Shock may result from multiple causes.

   a. Hypovolemic shock is caused by hemorrhage, loss of plasma, or loss of fluid and electrolytes, resulting in decreased intravascular volume. This may be caused by obvious loss or "third space" sequestration.

   b. Cardiogenic shock may arise from myocardial infarction (MI), arrhythmias, heart failure, defects in the valves or septum, hypertension, myocarditis, cardiac contusion, or myocardiopathies.

   c. Causes of obstructive shock include tension pneumothorax, pericardial tamponade, obstructive valvular disease, and pulmonary problems, including massive pulmonary embolism.

   d. Shock caused by poorly regulated distribution of blood volume includes septic shock, systemic inflammatory response syndrome (signs of systemic inflammation without end-organ damage), anaphylaxis, and neurogenic shock.

   (1) Septic shock is the most common of these and has a mortality rate of 40–80%.

   (2) Causes of neurogenic shock include spinal cord injury or adverse effects of spinal or epidural anesthetic.

B. Clinical features

   1. Signs and symptoms of shock include low blood pressure, orthostatic changes, tachycardia, peripheral hypoperfusion, altered mental status, oliguria or anuria, insulin resistance, and metabolic acidosis.

   2. The actual blood pressure reading in shock is not as important as the decrease in blood pressure compared to the usual blood pressure for the individual patient.

   3. End-organ hypoperfusion usually results in cool or mottled extremities and weak or absent peripheral pulses.

   4. Mental status may remain normal, or the patient may be agitated, restless, confused, obtunded, or comatose.

C. Laboratory studies

   1. All patients require a CBC, blood type and cross-match, and coagulation parameters.

   2. Electrolytes, glucose, urinalysis, and serum creatinine will aid in determining the cause of shock.

   3. Pulse oximetry or serial arterial blood gases are needed to monitor oxygenation.

D. Treatment must address both the specific cause and the manifestations of shock.

   1. The first step in treatment is attention to basic life support.

   2. Specific treatments depend on the cause of shock.

   3. The Trendelenburg or supine position with legs elevated maximizes blood flow to the brain.

   4. Oxygen and IV fluids are essential.

   5. Urine flow should be monitored via indwelling catheter and sustained at 0.5 mL/kg/hr or more.

6. Continuous cardiac monitoring is preferable to intermittent. Central venous pressure monitoring or capillary wedge pressure is helpful.
7. Pressors will increase glomerular filtration rate, contractility, and heart rate.

III. ORTHOSTASIS/POSTURAL HYPOTENSION

A. General characteristics
1. Postural hypotension may be related to reduced cardiac output, paroxysmal cardiac dysrhythmias, low blood volume, medications, and various endocrine and metabolic disorders.
2. Postural hypotension is a reversible cause of syncope and a major cause of falls in the elderly.

B. Clinical features
1. Postural hypotension is a greater than 20 mm Hg drop in systolic blood pressure between supine and sitting and/or standing measurements.
2. If accompanied by a rise in pulse of more than 15 bpm, depleted blood volume is the probable cause.
3. If no change in pulse occurs, medications or peripheral neuropathies are the probable cause.

C. Laboratory studies are directed at the suspected cause.

D. Treatment is directed at the suspected cause.

IV. HYPERTENSION

A. General characteristics
1. Primary (essential) hypertension causes 95% of cases of elevated blood pressure. It has no specific identifiable cause; pathogenesis is multifactorial.
   a. Genetic predisposition is an important factor.
   b. Environmental factors also are important and include salt intake and obesity.
   c. Other hypothesized factors are related to sympathetic nervous system hyperactivity, the renin-angiotensin system, defects in sodium excretion, and abnormalities in sodium and potassium exchange at the cellular level.
   d. Exacerbating factors include excessive use of alcohol, cigarette smoking, lack of exercise, polycythemia, use of nonsteroidal anti-inflammatory drugs, and low potassium intake.
   e. The metabolic syndrome (upper body obesity, hyperinsulinemia and insulin resistance, hypertriglyceridemia, and hypertension) is associated with development of diabetes and increased risk of cardiovascular complications.
2. Secondary causes of hypertension (5%) include sleep apnea, estrogen use, pheochromocytoma, coarctation of the aorta, pseudotumor cerebri, renal disease, renal artery stenosis, chronic steroid therapy, Cushing's syndrome, thyroid and parathyroid disease, and primary hyperaldosteronism.
3. Essential hypertension is exacerbated in males, blacks, sedentary individuals, and smokers.
4. Hypertension plays a major role in the genesis and exacerbation of other forms of cardiovascular disease and causes numerous secondary disorders.
5. Hypertensive urgencies reflect blood pressures that must be reduced within hours.
6. Hypertensive emergencies reflect blood pressure that must be reduced within 1 hour to prevent end-organ damage or death.
7. Malignant hypertension is defined as elevated blood pressure associated with papilledema and either encephalopathy or nephropathy; if untreated, progressive renal failure occurs.
8. Complications of untreated hypertension include cardiovascular disease, cerebrovascular disease, dementia, renal disease, aortic dissection, and atherosclerotic complications.

B. Clinical features (Table 3-1)
1. The essential diagnostic criterion is a systolic pressure of greater than 140 mm Hg or a diastolic pressure of greater than 90 mm Hg on three occasions.
2. Most patients with mild to moderate hypertension are asymptomatic; the most commonly voiced symptom is nonspecific headache.

TABLE 3-1	Classification of Blood Pressure for Adults 18 Years of Age and Older	
Category	Systolic Pressure (mm Hg)	Diastolic Pressure (mm Hg)
Normal	<120	<80
Prehypertension	120–139	80–99
Hypertension		
Stage 1	140–159	90–99
Stage 2	≥160	≥100

Source: The Seventh Report of the Joint National Committee on Prevention, Detection, Evaluation, and Treatment of High Blood Pressure: The JNC7 Report. JAMA 2003;289:2560–2572.

3. End-organ damage in untreated hypertension includes heart failure, renal failure, stroke, dementia, aortic dissection, atherosclerosis, and retinal hemorrhage.

4. In hypertensive urgencies, the systolic pressure usually is greater than 220 mg Hg, or the diastolic pressure is greater than 125 mm Hg. Optic disc edema and progressive end-organ complications also are seen.

5. In hypertensive emergencies, the diastolic pressure usually is greater than 130 mm Hg, with hypertensive encephalopathy, nephropathy, intracranial hemorrhage, aortic dissection, preeclampsia or eclampsia, pulmonary edema, unstable angina, or MI.

C. Laboratory studies

1. Electrocardiography (ECG) may reveal left ventricular hypertrophy or heart failure (Fig. 3-1).

2. Chest radiograph may show ventricular hypertrophy (Fig. 3-2); however, chest radiography is not considered to be necessary in the evaluation of uncomplicated hypertension.

3. Decreased hemoglobin or hematocrit or elevations in blood urea nitrogen (BUN), creatinine, and glucose (serum or urine) may indicate related renal disease or diabetes. Other parameters that should be measured include serum uric acid, plasma aldosterone concentration, plasma renin activity, calculation of plasma aldosterone:renin ratio, and serum potassium.

4. A lipid profile is important for ascertaining the associated risk of atherosclerosis.

5. In hypertensive urgencies and emergencies, diagnostic testing targets end-organ function.

D. Treatment

1. Nonpharmacologic therapies of essential hypertension should be stressed and include following the DASH (**D**ietary **A**pproaches to **S**top **H**ypertension) diet (low saturated fat, cholesterol, and total fat; increased fruits, vegetables, fat-free or low-fat milk or milk products, and fiber), weight loss, exercise, cessation of smoking, limitation of alcohol, and in some cases, limitation of sodium.

2. Initial therapy or monotherapy may be initiated with a number of agents.

a. Diuretics initially reduce plasma volume and chronically reduce peripheral resistance. Potassium supplements may be needed for some patients.

b. β-Adrenergic antagonists are used to decrease heart rate and cardiac output.

c. Angiotensin-converting enzyme (ACE) inhibitors, which also inhibit bradykinin degradation and stimulate synthesis of vasodilating prostaglandins, are the initial drug of choice for hypertensive patients with diabetes. The major side effect of ACE inhibitors is cough.

FIGURE 3-1 Electrocardiographic findings in left ventricular hypertrophy. **A,** Deep S waves in V_1 and V_2. **B,** Tall R waves in V_5 and V_6. (From Stein E. Rapid analysis of electrocardiograms: a self-study program. 3rd ed. Philadelphia: Lippincott Williams & Wilkins, 2000.)

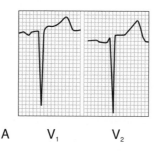

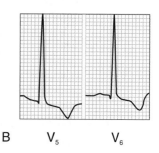

A V_1 V_2 B V_5 V_6

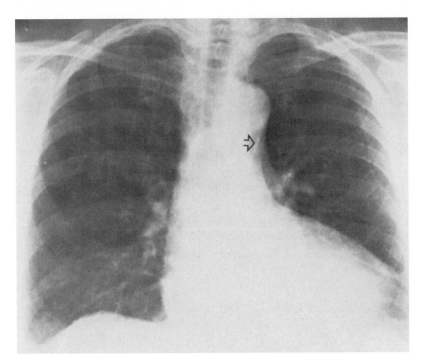

FIGURE 3-2 Hypertensive cardiovascular disease, frontal view. Note the left ventricular prominence and a slight increase in the tortuosity of the aorta at its arch. There is calcification in the descending aorta (arrow).
(From Daffner RH. Clinical radiology: the essentials. 2nd ed. Baltimore: Williams & Wilkins, 1999.)

   d. Angiotensin II receptor–blocking agents block the interaction of angiotensin II on receptors. They do not increase bradykinins and, therefore, do not cause cough.

   e. Calcium channel blockers for peripheral vasodilation may be preferable in African-American and elderly patients.

3. Other agents for use in refractory cases or special situations.

   a. α-Adrenergic antagonists to lower peripheral vascular resistance may be the initial drug of choice in men with symptomatic prostatic hyperplasia.

   b. Central sympatholytics, arteriolar dilators, and peripheral sympathetic inhibitors also may play a role in treatment.

4. Treatment of secondary causes of hypertension targets the underlying cause.

5. Hypertensive urgencies and emergencies are treated with parenteral agents; care must be taken not to decrease the blood pressure too rapidly.

   a. Preferred agents include sodium nitroprusside and, if myocardial ischemia is present, nitroglycerin or a β-blocker. Aortic dissection calls for nitroprusside and a β-blocker, usually labetalol.

   b. Other acceptable agents include nicardipine, enalapril, diazoxide, hydralazine, trimethaphan, fenoldopam, and loop diuretics.

   c. Oral agents for less severe emergencies include clonidine, captopril, and nifedipine.

V. CONGESTIVE HEART FAILURE (CHF)

A. General characteristics

   1. CHF is a clinical syndrome characterized by dyspnea and abnormal retention of water and sodium.

   2. CHF results from changes in one or more of the following: contractile ability of the heart muscle, preload and afterload of the ventricle, and heart rate.

   3. Alterations may result from multiple causes, including myocardial and pericardial disorders as well as valvular and congenital abnormalities. High output failure has noncardiac causes (e.g., thyrotoxicosis, severe anemia).

   4. CHF adversely affects left atrial pressure and cardiac output.

B. Clinical features

   1. Left-sided failure causes exertional dyspnea plus cough, fatigue, orthopnea, paroxysmal nocturnal dyspnea, basilar rales, and gallops.

   2. Right-sided failure is characterized by distended neck veins, tender or nontender hepatomegaly, nausea, and dependent pitting edema; it often is caused by left-sided failure. Predominant features are edema and hepatomegaly.

    3. Cardiac signs include parasternal lift, enlarged apical impulse, diminished first heart sound, and an S_3 gallop. An S_4 gallop may be heard in diastolic failure.

    4. A hallmark of CHF is paroxysmal nocturnal dyspnea.

    5. Sympathetic activity produces pallor and clammy skin.

    6. Nocturia is a common symptom.

    7. Hypotension and a narrow pulse pressure are typical.

C. Laboratory studies

    1. Patients may have anemia, renal insufficiency, hyperkalemia, hyponatremia, and elevated liver enzymes; those on diuretics may develop hypokalemia.

    2. Chest radiography may show cardiomegaly and bilateral or right-sided pulmonary effusions, perivascular or interstitial edema, venous dilation, and alveolar fluid (Fig. 3-3).

    3. ECG may show nonspecific changes (e.g., low voltage), underlying arrhythmia, intraventricular conduction defects, left ventricular hypertrophy, nonspecific repolarization changes, or MI.

    4. Echocardiography is useful to determine size and function of the chambers, valve abnormalities, pericardial effusion, shunting, and segmental wall abnormalities.

    5. Serum B-type natriuretic peptide (BNP) or amino terminal pro-BNP may be elevated.

    6. Stress imaging, radionuclide angiography, and cardiac catheterization may be indicated.

    7. Older patients should have thyroid function testing.

D. Treatment

    1. Correction of reversible causes is key to management.

    2. Preventive and rehabilitative nonpharmacologic measures include progressive aerobic exercise, low sodium diet, and stress reduction.

    3. Diuretic therapy reduces fluid volume and produces relief of symptoms.

    4. Initial therapy in most patients is a thiazide or loop diuretic and an angiotensin-converting enzyme inhibitor. Other drugs include potassium-sparing diuretics, angiotensin II–receptor blockers, β-blockers, direct inotropic agents (digitalis), and arterial and venous vasodilators.

    5. Calcium channel blockers, preferably amlodipine, are used only to treat associated angina or hypertension.

    6. Patients may require anticoagulants or antiarrhythmics, as dictated by the underlying disease.

    7. Increasingly, implantable cardioverter-defibrillators and biventricular pacing are being used.

    8. Coronary revascularization or cardiac transplantation may be indicated.

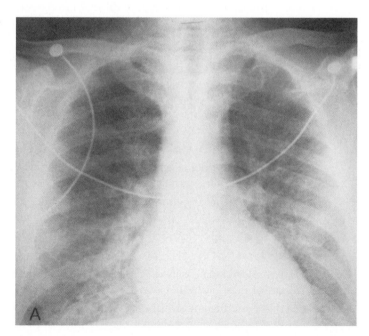

FIGURE 3-3 Congestive heart failure, frontal view. Note the mild pulmonary edema and pulmonary venous engorgement.
(From Daffner RH. Clinical radiology: the essentials. 2nd ed. Baltimore: Williams & Wilkins, 1999.)

VI. ATHEROSCLEROTIC OCCLUSIVE DISEASE

A. General characteristics

1. Atherosclerosis is characterized by lipid deposition, fibrosis, calcification, and plaque formation in the intima of large and medium vessels.

2. Atherosclerosis is associated with premature coronary and peripheral vascular morbidity and mortality.

   a. Atherosclerotic heart disease is the most common cause of cardiac-related death and disability.

   b. Men are affected fourfold more often than women; however, by the age of 70 years, the ratio is 1:1.

3. The cause is closely related to smoking and elevated (>200 mg/dL) cholesterol levels because of diet or familial dyslipidemias. C-reactive protein is an important marker.

4. Management of both blood glucose and blood pressure is essential to the control of vascular disease.

5. Obesity, sedentary lifestyle, and homocystinuria must be addressed.

B. Clinical features. These depend on the location of the vessels involved (e.g., cerebral occlusions lead to cognitive disorders, renal artery blockage leads to kidney failure).

C. Treatment

1. Smoking cessation is essential.

2. Dietary modifications and other treatment of dyslipidemias are important.

3. Areas under investigation include the use of macrolide antibiotics and various forms of gene therapy.

VII. ISCHEMIC HEART DISEASE

A. General characteristics

1. Ischemic heart disease is characterized by insufficient oxygen supply to cardiac muscle, most commonly caused by atherosclerotic narrowing and less often caused by constriction of coronary arteries. Rare causes include congenital anomalies, emboli, arteritis, and dissection.

2. Risk factors include male sex, increased age, low-estrogen state, cigarette smoking, family history, hypertension, diabetes mellitus, obesity, inactivity, and dyslipidemias.

3. Metabolic syndrome is a major contributor to coronary heart disease and includes three or more of the following: abdominal obesity, triglycerides ≥150 mg/dL, HDL <40 for men and <50 for women, fasting glucose ≥110 mg/dL, and hypertension.

4. Cocaine use is an important cause of myocardial ischemia and infarction.

B. Clinical features

1. Ischemia causes angina pectoris. Angina is characterized by paroxysmal chest "squeezing" or pressure, often accompanied by a sensation of smothering and a fear of impending death.

   a. Stable angina is exacerbated by physical activity and is relieved by rest.

   b. Prinzmetal's, or variant, angina is caused by vasospasm at rest, with preservation of exercise capacity.

   c. Unstable angina is an increasing pattern of pain in previously stable patients. It is less responsive to medication, lasts longer, and occurs at rest or with less exertion.

2. Levine's sign, which is a clenched fist over the sternum and clenched teeth when describing chest pain, may be seen in patients with ischemia.

3. Angina pectoris usually is midsternal but may radiate to the jaw, shoulders, arms, wrists, back of the neck, or some combination of these, usually on the left.

4. Angina pectoris usually lasts for less than 3 minutes. Angina pectoris lasting for more than 30 minutes suggests unstable angina, MI, or another diagnosis.

5. Angina is relieved by sublingual nitroglycerin.

C. Laboratory studies

1. Horizontal or down-sloping ST-segment depression on ECG during an anginal attack is among the most sensitive clinical signs, although the ECG will be normal in 25% of those with angina.

2. Exercise testing is the most useful noninvasive test. An ST-segment depression of 1 mm (0.1 mV) is considered to be a positive test.

3. Myocardial perfusion scintigraphy, radionuclide angiography, positron-emission tomography, and ambulatory ECG monitoring may be indicated.

4. Echocardiography is used to evaluate left ventricular function, an important prognostic indicator.

5. Newer testing modalities are ultrafast or cine CT and cardiac MRI.

6. Coronary angiography is the definitive diagnostic procedure but should be used selectively because of cost and invasiveness.

D. Treatment

1. Preventive and rehabilitative treatment includes exercise, weight reduction, diet low in fat and cholesterol, smoking cessation, and aggressive control of diabetes, hypertension, and hyperlipidemias.

2. Aggravating factors (e.g., hypertension) must be identified and treated.

3. Sublingual or translingual spray nitroglycerin or sublingual isosorbide dinitrate is the primary pharmacotherapy for acute anginal attacks.

4. Long-acting nitrate (oral, ointment, or transdermal patches) therapy should include a daily 8- to 10-hour, treatment-free interval to prevent drug tolerance. Major adverse effects of nitrates include headache, nausea, and hypotension.

5. β-Blockers prolong life in patients with coronary disease and are first-line therapy for chronic angina.

6. Calcium channel blockers decrease cardiac muscle oxygen demand.

7. Platelet-inhibiting agents (e.g., aspirin, clopidogrel, ticlopidine) reduce the possibility of infarction because of emboli.

8. Revascularization provides long-term relief of ischemia in suitable patients.

VIII. ACUTE CORONARY SYNDROME (ACS)

A. General characteristics

1. ACS includes a spectrum of problems, ranging from unstable angina to MI.

2. These conditions are classified simply as ST-elevated or non-ST-elevated events rather than as unstable angina, Q-wave infarction, or non-Q-wave infarction.

   a. Based on initial findings, patients are able to be triaged to acute reperfusion therapy if indicated.

   b. Determination of the occurrence of acute MI is based on evolution of cardiac markers.

   (1) MI is a result of prolonged myocardial ischemia, usually as a result of thrombus formation on a preexisting atherosclerotic plaque. Other causes include prolonged vasospasm, reduced myocardial blood flow, excessive metabolic demand, embolic occlusion, vasculitis, aortitis, coronary artery dissection, and cocaine use.

   (2) Signs and symptoms, prognosis, and complications depend on the size and location of the infarct.

3. One-fifth of patients with acute MI will die, usually of ventricular fibrillation, before reaching a hospital.

4. About one-third of acute MIs are "silent" or accompanied by minor pain only. Older people, women, and those with diabetes mellitus are more likely to present atypically.

B. Clinical features

1. Chest pain is the common presenting factor in ACS.

2. The patient with MI usually develops increasingly severe, prolonged (>30 min) anterior chest pain at rest and during the early morning hours, which can lead to arrhythmias, hypotension, shock, and heart failure.

3. Diaphoresis, weakness, anxiety, restlessness, light-headedness, syncope, cough, dyspnea, orthopnea, nausea, vomiting, and abdominal bloating often are present in patients with MI.

4. Patients may be bradycardic or tachycardic as well as hypotensive or hypertensive.

5. Low-grade fever may develop after 12 hours and last for several days.

6. Lung fields may be clear, or rales and wheezing may be present.

7. The cardiovascular examination may be quite normal, or it may reveal jugular venous distention, soft heart sounds, murmur of mitral regurgitation, and an S_4 gallop.

8. Pericardial friction rubs may appear after 24 hours.

9. Dressler's syndrome (post-MI syndrome) includes pericarditis, fever, leukocytosis, and pericardial or pleural effusion, usually 1–2 weeks post-MI.

C. Laboratory studies

1. ECG changes form the basis of an initial and ongoing evaluation of ACS.

   a. In acute MI, progression from peaked T waves to ST-segment elevations (or depressions) to Q waves to T-wave inversions classically occurs over hours to days but is not present in all cases (Fig. 3-4).

   b. The location of cardiac damage may be determined by examining changes on the ECG (Table 3-2).

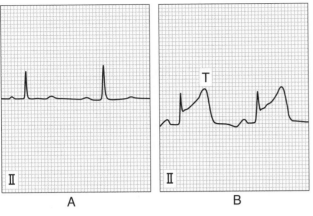

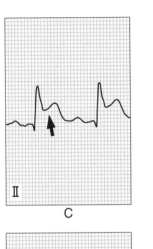

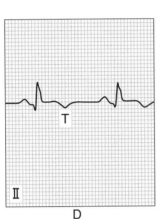

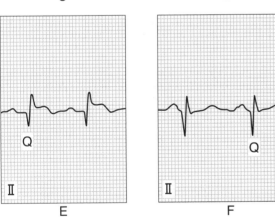

FIGURE 3-4 Evolutionary changes of a Q-wave infarction as seen from lead II. Examples are not necessarily from the same patient. **A**, Normal. **B** and **D**, T wave becomes tall, then inverts symmetrically. **C**, ST segment elevates (arrow). **E**, Significant Q waves develop. **F**, Healed infarction. Q waves persist, but ST segment and T wave return to normal.
(From Mulholland GC, Brewer BB. Improving your skills in 12-lead ECG interpretation. Baltimore: Williams & Wilkins, 1990.)

TABLE 3-2	**Determining Location of Cardiac Damage by Examining ECG Changes**
ECG Location	**Localization of Acute MI Found in ECG Leads**
Inferior	II, III, aVF
Posterior	V_1, V_2
Anteroseptal	V_1, V_2
Anterior	V_1, V_2, V_3
Anterolateral	V_4, V_5, V_6

ECG, electrocardiogram; *MI*, myocardial infarction.

TABLE 3-3	Cardiac Markers in Acute Myocardial Infarction			
Marker	**Timing of Initial Elevation (hr)**	**Peak Elevation (hr)**	**Return to Normal**	**Sampling Schedule**
Myoglobin	1–4	6–7	24 hr	Often beginning 1–2 hr after onset of chest pain
Cardiac troponin I	3–12	24	5–10 days	12 hr after onset of chest pain
Cardiac troponin T	3–12	12–48	5–14 days	12 hr after onset of chest pain
Total CK	3–5	24	28–72 hr	May not be drawn owing to many false positives; CK-MB more sensitive
CK-MB	3–12	24	48–72 hr	Three times, 12 hr apart
LDH	10	24–48	10–14 days	Once, at least 24 hr after onset of chest pain

CK, creatine kinase; *CK-MB*, isoenzyme of CK containing M and B subunits; *LDH*, lactate dehydrogenase.

2. Serial cardiac enzymes—isoenzyme of creatine kinase containing M and B subunits (CK-MB), troponin T, and troponin I—demonstrate characteristic elevations (Table 3-3).

3. Echocardiography may show abnormalities of cardiac wall motion; Doppler studies may show postinfarction ventricular septal defect or mitral regurgitation.

4. Chest radiography may indicate congestive failure or signs of aortic dissection.

5. MRI with gadolinium contrast is one of the most sensitive tests to quantify the extent of an infarction.

6. Scintigraphy and radionuclide angiography may be helpful in establishing the diagnosis; hemodynamic studies may be useful in the management of cases with cardiogenic shock.

D. Treatment

1. All patients with suspected ACS should receive IV fluids, oxygen, nitroglycerin, and pain management. Serial ECG and pulse oximetry are important components of monitoring. Some patients may require sedation with a benzodiazepine.

2. In patients with ST-segment elevations, anticoagulation and antiplatelet therapy should include aspirin and heparin, either low-molecular-weight or unfractionated. Clopidogrel may be used in non-ST-segment elevation ACS.

3. β-blockers should be initiated in the absence of contraindications.

4. Calcium channel blockers are used only in patients who cannot take nitrates and β-blockers or in those with contraindications to these drugs.

5. Patients with an acute ST-segment elevation should undergo interventions to promote reperfusion.

   a. Thrombolytic therapy within the first 3 hours of the onset of pain reduces mortality and limits the size of infarction. Some benefit may occur if therapy is initiated within the first 12 hours. In the United States, alteplase, reteplase, and tenecteplase are the most commonly used agents.

   b. Immediate coronary angiography and primary percutaneou coronary intervention are superior to thrombolysis in high-volume centers with experienced operators.

6. Patients with non-ST-segment elevation must undergo risk stratification. Rating systems aid in deciding which patients should undergo aggressive treatment. Several scoring systems are available based on the risk of reinfarction or death.

   a. The TIMI (**T**hombolysis **I**n **M**yocardial **I**nfarction) system is the quickest and easiest scoring system and can be completed easily at the bedside. One point is given for each of the following factors: age >65 years, three or more risk factors for coronary artery disease, use of aspirin within the last 7 days, known coronary artery disease with stenosis >50%, more than one episode of rest angina within the last 24 hours, ST-segment deviation, and elevated cardiac markers. Scores of three or more are considered to be high risk.

   b. PURSUIT (**P**latelet Glycoprotein IIb/IIIa in **U**nstable Angina: **R**eceptor **S**uppression **U**sing **I**ntegritin) and GRACE (**G**lobal **R**egistry of **A**cute **C**oronary **E**vents) are somewhat more complex scoring methods. Age, gender, vital signs, ST-segment changes, and historical factors are included to predict risk.

   c. It is essential to carefully monitor patients with non-ST-segment elevation and to intervene in cases of patients likely to progress to infarction.

IX. CONGENITAL HEART ANOMALIES

A. General characteristics

1. Congenital heart anomalies are classified as either cyanotic or noncyanotic.

a. Cyanotic types all involve right-to-left shunts.

(1) Tetralogy of Fallot consists of a subaortic septal defect, right ventricular outflow obstruction, overriding aorta, and right ventricular hypertrophy.

(2) Pulmonary atresia most often occurs with an intact ventricular septum.

(a) The pulmonary valve is closed.

(b) An atrial septal opening and patent ductus arteriosus are present.

(3) Hypoplastic left heart syndrome actually is a group of defects with a small left ventricle and normally placed great vessels.

(4) Transposition of the great vessels most commonly is a complete transposition of the aorta and pulmonary artery.

b. Noncyanotic types

(1) Atrial septal defect is an opening between the right and left atria. Of the four types, ostium secundum is the most common.

(2) Ventricular septal defects may be muscular, perimembranous, or outlet openings between the ventricles.

(3) Patent (persistent) ductus arteriosus is a failure to close or a delay in closure of the channel bypassing the lungs, which allows placental gas exchange during the fetal state.

(4) Coarctation of the aorta involves narrowing in the proximal thoracic aorta.

2. Congenital heart anomalies are the most common congenital structural malformations.

B. Clinical features. See Table 3-4.

C. Laboratory studies to evaluate cardiac anomalies may include chest radiography, ECG, echocardiography, Doppler ultrasound, MRI, radionuclide flow studies, cardiac catheterization and angiography.

D. Treatment of most congenital heart anomalies is surgical.

X. VALVULAR DISORDERS

A. Aortic and mitral valve disorders

1. General characteristics

a. Aortic stenosis narrows the valve opening, impeding the ejection function of the left side of the heart.

b. Aortic insufficiency (regurgitation) results in volume overloading of the left ventricle.

c. Mitral stenosis impedes blood flow between the left atrium and ventricle.

d. Mitral insufficiency causes backflow and volume overload of the left atrium.

e. Mitral valve prolapse usually is asymptomatic, but it may cause mitral regurgitation.

f. Valve-related progressive heart failure leads to pulmonary hypertension and congestion.

g. The most frequent causes of mitral and aortic valve disorders are congenital defects; others include rheumatic heart disease, connective tissue disorders, infection, and senile degeneration.

h. Most patients present as adults after extended periods of asymptomatic conditions.

2. Clinical features (Table 3-5)

a. The most common presenting symptoms include dyspnea, fatigue, and decreased exercise tolerance.

b. Patients also may have cough, rales, paroxysmal nocturnal dyspnea or hemoptysis, and hoarseness.

c. Carotid pulses typically are thready in aortic stenosis; aortic insufficiency produces widened pulse pressures.

d. Most patients with mitral valve prolapse are thin females with minor chest wall deformities, midsystolic clicks, and late systolic murmur.

3. Laboratory studies

a. ECG is not useful in establishing the diagnosis.

b. Chest radiography

TABLE 3-4	**Comparison of Findings in Various Congenital Defects**			
Anomaly	**Frequency**	**Murmur**	**Other Physical Findings**	**Important Clinical Information**
CYANOTIC DEFECTS				
Tetralogy of Fallot	6–10% of significant congenital heart defects	Crescendo-decrescendo holosystolic at LSB, radiating to back	Cyanosis; clubbing; increased RV impulse at LLSB; loud S_2	Polycythemia usually present; TET (hyper-cyanotic) spells include extreme cyanosis, hyper-pnea, and agitation—a medical emergency
Pulmonary atresia	1–3% of congenital heart disease	Depends on presence of tricuspid regurgitation	Cyanosis with tachypnea at birth; tachypnea without dyspnea; hyperdynamic apical impulse; single S_1 and S_2	Sudden onset of severe cyanosis and acidosis requires emergency treatment
Hypoplastic left heart syndrome	7–9% of significant congenital heart defects	Variable; not diagnostic	Shock; early heart failure; respiratory distress; single S_2; presentation varies with specific syndrome	Occurs more often in males; accounts for 25% of cardiac deaths before age 7 days
Transposition of the great vessels	5–7% of all congenital heart defects; 2nd most common in neonates	Systolic murmur if associated VSD; systolic ejection murmur if pulmonary stenosis	Cyanosis in newborn is most common sign; tachypnea without respiratory distress; if large VSD, symptoms of CHF and poor feed-ing; single loud S_2; absent LE pulses if aortic arch obstruction	
NONCYANOTIC DEFECTS				
Atrial septal defect	~7% of congenital heart disease; 2nd most common	Systolic ejection murmur 2nd LICS; early to mid-dle systolic rumble	Failure to thrive; fatiga-bility; RV heave; wide fixed split S_2	
VSD	Most common of all congenital heart defects	Systolic murmur at LLSB; others depend on severity of defect	Depends on size of defect—from asympto-matic to signs of CHF	Outlet VSDs more com-mon in Japanese and Chinese
PDA	12–15% of significant congenital heart dis-ease; higher in pre-mature infants	Continuous (machinery) murmur in patients with isolated PDA	Wide pulse pressure, hyperdynamic apical pulse	
Coarctation of the aorta		Systolic, LUSB and left interscapular area; may be continuous	Infants may present with CHF; older children may have systolic hyper-tension or murmur	Differences between arterial pulses and blood pressure in UE and LE pathognomonic

CHF, congestive heart failure; *LE*, lower extremity; *LICS*, left intercostal space; *LLSB*, left lower sternal border; *LSB*, left sternal border; *LUSB*, left upper sternal border; *PDA*, patent ductus arteriosus; *RV*, right ventricle; *UE*, upper extremity; *VSD*, ventricular septal defect.

(1) With aortic valve disorders, chest radiograph may show left-sided atrial enlargement and ventricular hypertrophy.

(2) With mitral valve disorders, chest radiography may show atrial enlargement alone.

c. Echocardiography, particularly transesophageal, and cardiac catheterization are the only definitive methods of identifying structural and functional abnormalities. Doppler ultrasound is particularly useful for pressure gradient study.

4. Treatment

a. The only effective long-term treatments are surgical repair, replacement of the defective valve, and balloon valvuloplasty.

TABLE 3-5	Comparison of Findings in Aortic and Mitral Valve Disorders						
Valve Disorder	**Murmur Location**	**Radiation**	**Intensity**	**Pitch/ Quality**	**Aids to Hearing**	**Associated Findings**	**Timing**
Aortic stenosis	2nd RICS	To neck and LSB	Often loud with a thrill	Medium pitch; harsh	Patient sitting and leaning forward	Midsystolic	
Aortic regurgitation	2nd–4th LICS	To apex and RSB	Grade 1–3	High pitch; blowing	Patient sitting and leaning forward; full exhalation	Midsystolic or Austin Flint murmur suggests large flow; arterial pulses large and bounding	Systolic (soft) and diastolic decrescendo
Mitral stenosis	Apex	Little or none	Grade 1–4	Low pitch	Patient in left lateral position; full exhalation	S_1 accentuated; opening snap follows S_2	Mid-diastolic
Mitral regurgitation	Apex	To left axilla	Soft to loud	Medium to high pitch; blowing		S_2 often decreased; apical impulse prolonged	Pansystolic

LICS, left intercostal space; *LSB,* left sternal border; *RICS,* right intercostal space; *RSB,* right sternal border.

    b. Patients with good exercise tolerance may be treated medically with diuretics and vasodilators for pulmonary congestion and with digoxin or β-blockers for dysrhythmias.

    c. Anticoagulant therapy is recommended for the prevention of thromboemboli, particularly if atrial fibrillation occurs.

    d. Antibiotics may be indicated for prevention of endocarditis and recurrent rheumatic fever.

  B. Tricuspid and pulmonic valve disorders

    1. General characteristics

      a. Patients with congenital anomalies of these valves usually present during infancy or childhood; adults may present with stenosis resulting from rheumatic scarring or connective tissue disease.

      b. Tricuspid regurgitation may be intrinsic or functional.

      c. In all cases, right-sided pressure overload leads to right-sided cardiomegaly, systemic venous congestion, and right-sided heart failure.

    2. Clinical features (Table 3-6)

TABLE 3-6	Comparison of Findings in Tricuspid Regurgitation and Pulmonic Stenosis						
Valve Disorder	**Murmur Location**	**Radiation**	**Intensity**	**Pitch/ Quality**	**Aids to Hearing**	**Associated Findings**	**Timing**
Tricuspid regurgitation	LLSB; holosystolic	To right sternum and xiphoid area	Variable	Medium; blowing	Increases slightly with inspiration	JVP often elevated	Pansystolic
Pulmonic stenosis	2nd–3rd LICS; midsystolic crescendo-decrescendo	To left shoulder and neck	Soft to loud, possibly associated with thrill	Medium; harsh		Early pulmonic ejection sound common	Systolic

JVP, jugular venous pressure; *LICS,* left intercostal space; *LLSB,* left lower sternal border.

a. Patients usually present with exercise intolerance.

b. Jugular venous distention, peripheral edema, and hepatomegaly reflect systemic venous congestion.

3. Laboratory studies

   a. Chest radiography may show a prominent right heart border with dilation of the superior vena cava.

   b. ECG findings may show right-axis deviation, P-wave abnormalities associated with right atrial enlargement, or the prominent R and deep S waves of right ventricular hypertrophy.

   c. Echocardiography or cardiac catheterization are the only definitive methods of identifying structural or functional abnormalities.

4. Treatment

   a. Sodium restriction and diuretic therapy decrease fluid volume and right atrial filling pressure.

   b. Underlying conditions causing pulmonary hypertension are treated with arterial vasodilators or positive inotropic agents.

   c. Definitive treatment includes surgical repair, valvuloplasty, or replacement with porcine or synthetic prostheses.

XI. RATE AND RHYTHM DISORDERS

A. Overview of Arrhythmias

1. General Characteristics

   a. How dangerous an arrhythmia is depends on how much it impairs cardiac output or how likely it is to deteriorate into a more serious disturbance.

   b. Susceptibility is based on genetic abnormalities and acquired structural heart disease.

   c. Electrolyte abnormalities, hormonal imbalances, hypoxia, drug effects, and myocardial ischemia increase susceptibility.

   d. Classification of arrhythmias includes those caused by disorders of impulse formation or automaticity, abnormalities of conduction, reentry, and triggered activity.

2. Clinical features

   a. Presentation ranges from asymptomatic to symptomatic to lethal.

   b. Specific features depend on the individual arrhythmia (see below).

3. Laboratory studies include ECG monitoring, measurements of heart rate variability, signal-averaged ECG, electrophysiologic testing, and autonomic testing.

4. Treatment: antiarrhythmic drugs are divided into four classes based on mechanism of action (Table 3-7).

B. Supraventricular arrhythmias

1. General characteristics

   a. Sinus bradycardia (heart rate, <60 bpm) may be normal in athletes; in others, it usually represents sinus node pathology, with increased risk for ectopic rhythms.

   b. Sinus tachycardia (heart rate, >100 bpm) occurs with fever, exercise, pain, emotion, shock, thyrotoxicosis, anemia, heart failure, and use of many drugs.

   c. Atrial premature beats frequently are found in normal hearts and do not alone constitute heart disease.

   d. Paroxysmal supraventricular tachycardia (PSVT) is the most common paroxysmal tachycardia and usually occurs in persons without structural problems.

   e. Atrial fibrillation is the most common chronic arrhythmia, and both incidence and prevalence increase with age. It is called "holiday heart" when caused by excessive alcohol use or withdrawal.

   f. Atrial flutter usually occurs in patients with chronic obstructive pulmonary disease, CHF, atrial septal defect, or coronary artery disease.

   g. Junctional rhythms occur in patients with normal hearts or those with myocarditis, coronary artery disease, or digitalis toxicity.

2. Clinical features

   a. Patients may present with palpitations, angina, fatigue, and other symptoms of heart failure.

   b. Patients may be completely asymptomatic.

TABLE 3-7	Antiarrhythmic Drugs		
Class	Action	Indications	Examples
Ia	Sodium channel blockers; depress phase 0 depolarization; slow conduction; prolong repolarization	Supraventricular tachycardia; V tach; prevention of V fib; symptomatic ventricular premature beats	Guanidine, procainamide, disopyramide, moricizine
Ib	Shorten repolarization	V tach; prevention of V fib; symptomatic ventricular premature beats	Lidocaine, mexiletine, phenytoin
Ic	Depress phase 0 repolarization; slow conduction	Life-threatening V tach; refractory supraventricular tachycardia	Flecainide, propafenone
II	β-Blockers; slow AV conduction	Supraventricular tachycardia	Esmolol, propranolol, acebutolol
III	Prolong action potential	Refractory V tach; supraventricular tachycardia; prevention of V tach; V fib	Amiodarone, bretylium (indicated for V fib and V tach only)
IV	Slow calcium channel blockers	Supraventricular tachycardia	Verapamil, diltiazem
V	Adenosine: slows conduction time through AV node, interrupts reentry pathways; digoxin: direct action on cardiac muscle and indirect action on cardiovascular system via ANS	Supraventricular tachycardia	Adenosine, digoxin

ANS, autonomic nervous system; *AV*, atrioventricular; *V fib*, ventricular fibrillation; *V tach*, ventricular tachycardia.

3. Laboratory studies. Characteristic ECG findings assist in the diagnosis of supraventricular arrhythmias (Fig. 3-5).

4. Treatment depends on the specific arrhythmia.

a. Mechanical measures to interrupt acute PSVT include Valsalva maneuver, coughing, breath holding, stretching, putting the head between the knees, and unilateral carotid sinus massage.

b. Nonpharmacologic interventions may include surgical or radiofrequency ablation of abnormal sites, cardioversion, and electrical pacing. Synchronized cardioversion nearly always is successful, but it should not be used in cases of suspected digitalis toxicity.

c. Pharmacotherapy may be used to terminate or prevent supraventricular arrhythmias.

(1) IV administration of adenosine or IV or oral administration of verapamil terminates most episodes of PSVT. Other possibilities include esmolol, edrophonium, metaraminol, phenylephrine, digoxin, and procainamide.

(2) Prevention usually is initiated with digoxin and/or verapamil or a β-blocker.

d. Treatment of acute atrial fibrillation depends on the presentation and includes electric cardioversion, treatment of underlying disease, and control of rate. Treatment of chronic atrial fibrillation includes control of rate and prevention of thromboembolism.

e. Chemical conversion with ibutilide or electric cardioversion usually is successful in the treatment of atrial flutter. Amiodarone is the treatment of choice for chronic atrial flutter. Radiofrequency ablation is recommended for refractory conditions.

C. Ventricular arrhythmias

1. General characteristics

a. Ventricular premature beats may be benign or may lead to sudden death in persons with underlying heart disease.

b. Ventricular tachycardia (V tach)

(1) V tach is defined as three or more consecutive ventricular premature beats.

(2) It may be sustained or unsustained.

(3) It is a frequent complication of acute MI.

c. Torsades de points is a V tach in which the QRS complex twists around the baseline.

d. In ventricular fibrillation, no effective pumping action exists; without intervention, death ensues.

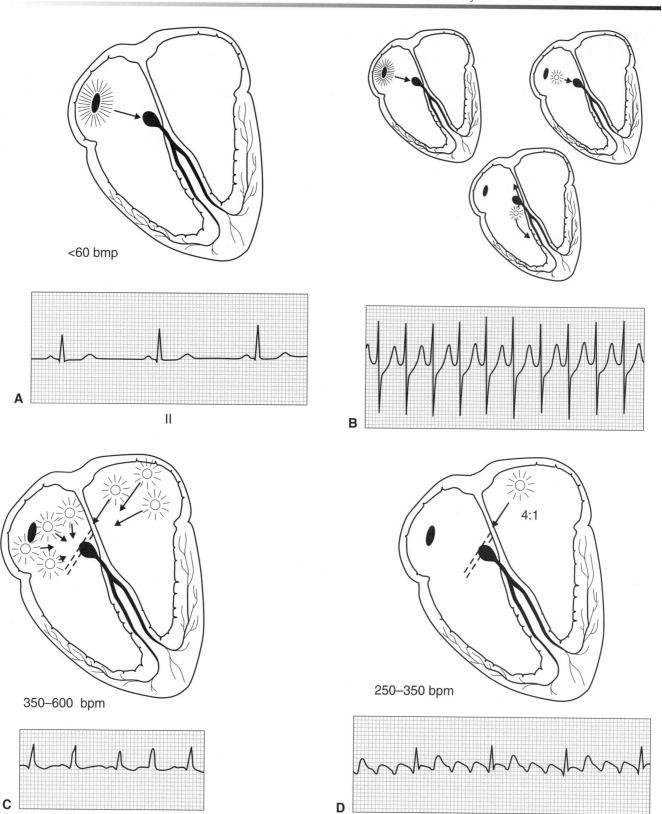

<60 bmp

A

II

B

350–600 bpm

C

250–350 bpm

4:1

D

FIGURE 3-5 (continued)

FIGURE 3-5 Electrocardiographic findings in supraventricular arrhythmias. **A**, Sinus bradycardia. **B**, Supraventricular tachycardia. **C**, Atrial fibrillation. **D**, Atrial flutter. **E**, Junctional rhythm, P waves. (From Stein E. Rapid analysis of electrocardiograms: a self-study program. 3rd ed. Philadelphia: Lippincott Williams & Wilkins, 2000.)

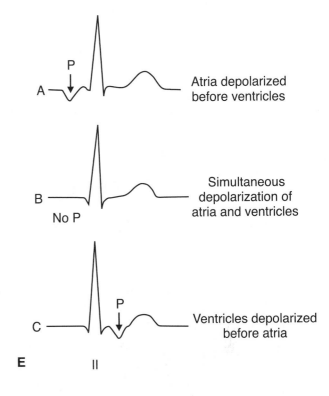

2. Clinical features

    a. Patients with ventricular premature beats may be asymptomatic or aware of skipped beats.

    b. Patients with V tach may be asymptomatic or experience dizziness and syncope.

    c. Ventricular fibrillation is associated with sudden death, most often occurring in the early morning.

3. Laboratory studies. Characteristic ECG findings assist in diagnosing ventricular arrhythmias (Fig. 3-6).

4. Treatment

    a. Ventricular premature beats may be treated with β-blockers only if the patient is symptomatic; class I and III agents may be used with caution only in symptomatic individuals.

    b. In V tach with severe hypotension or loss of consciousness, cardioversion may be necessary; ventricular over-drive pacing may help.

    c. The preferred pharmacologic interventions for V tach include lidocaine, procainamide, amiodarone, and bretylium (Table 3-7). Empiric magnesium may help.

    d. In many types of ventricular arrhythmias, patients with an identifiable site of arrhythmic origin may benefit from radiofrequency ablation.

    e. Some patients may be appropriate for implantable cardioverter-defibrillators.

XII. CONDUCTION DISTURBANCES

A. General characteristics

    1. Sick sinus syndrome

        a. Sick sinus syndrome most often is found in the elderly, but it may occur even in infants.

        b. It may be caused or exacerbated by digitalis, calcium channel blockers, β-blockers, sympatholytic agents, and antiarrhythmic drugs. It may result from underlying collagen vascular or metastatic disease, surgical injury, or rarely, coronary disease.

        c. It is reversible if caused by digitalis, quinidine, β-blockers, or aerosols.

    2. Atrioventricular (AV) block is characterized by refractory conduction of impulses from the atria to the ventricles through the AV node and/or bundle of His and is divided into first-degree, second-degree (subdivided into Mobitz type I [Wenckebach] and Mobitz type II), and complete or third-degree block.

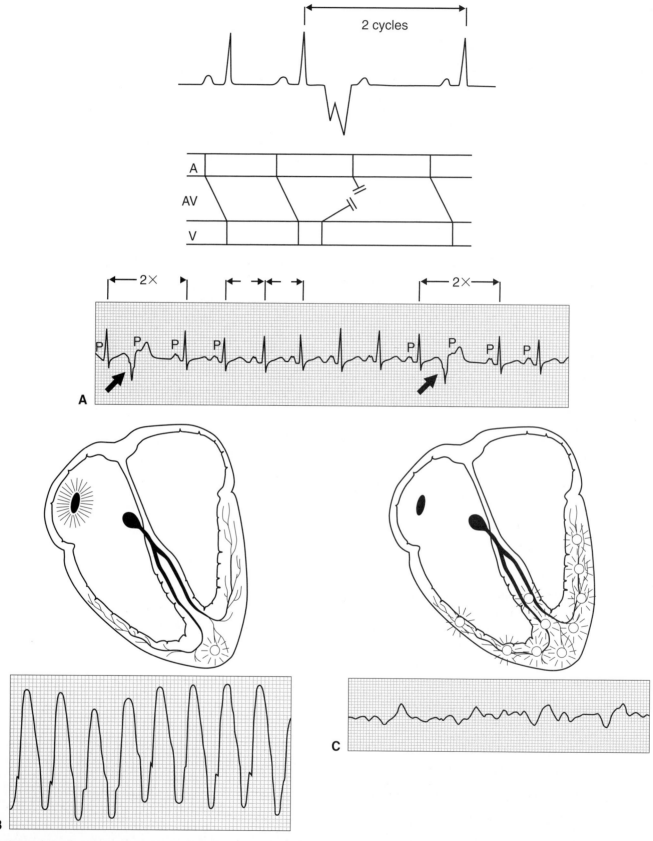

FIGURE 3-6 Electrocardiographic findings in ventricular arrhythmias. **A**, Premature ventricular contractions (arrows) frequently are identified by the accompanying compensatory pause. **B**, Ventricular tachycardia showing sustained tachycardia (it can also be intermittent). **C**, Ventricular fibrillation.
(From Stein E. Rapid analysis of electrocardiograms: a self-study program. 3rd ed. Philadelphia: Lippincott Williams & Wilkins, 2000.)

B. Clinical features

    1. Most patients with sick sinus syndrome are asymptomatic, but patients may have syncope, dizziness, confusion, heart failure, palpitations, or angina.

    2. AV conduction block may produce weakness, fatigue, light-headedness, and syncope.

C. Laboratory studies. ECG changes associated with conduction disturbances are shown in Figure 3-7.

D. Treatment

    1. Most symptomatic patients with sick sinus syndrome require permanent pacing.

    2. The only effective long-term treatment for AV conduction disorders is cardiac pacing.

XIII. CARDIOMYOPATHIES

A. General characteristics

    1. Cardiomyopathies are categorized by their presentation and their pathophysiology.

    2. Dilated cardiomyopathy

        a. Dilated cardiomyopathies are the most common type (95%) and are associated with reduced strength of ventricular contraction, resulting in dilation of the left ventricle.

        b. Causes are genetic abnormalities (25–30%), idiopathic, excessive alcohol consumption, postpartum state, chemotherapy toxicity, endocrinopathies, and myocarditis.

        c. It is more common in men (especially African American men).

    3. Hypertrophic obstructive cardiomyopathy

        a. This cardiomyopathy (4%) has massive hypertrophy, particularly of the septum; small left ventricle; systolic anterior mitral motion; and diastolic dysfunction.

        b. It is almost exclusively transmitted genetically. The apical variety is more common in persons of Asian descent; hypertrophic cardiomyopathy in the elderly is a distinct form.

        c. Sudden cardiac death occurs in patients younger than 30 years at a rate of 2–3% yearly.

    4. Restrictive cardiomyopathy

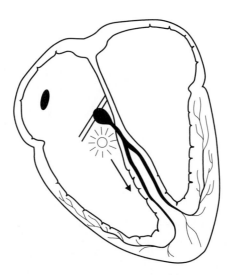

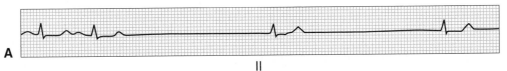

A

II

FIGURE 3-7 (*continued*)

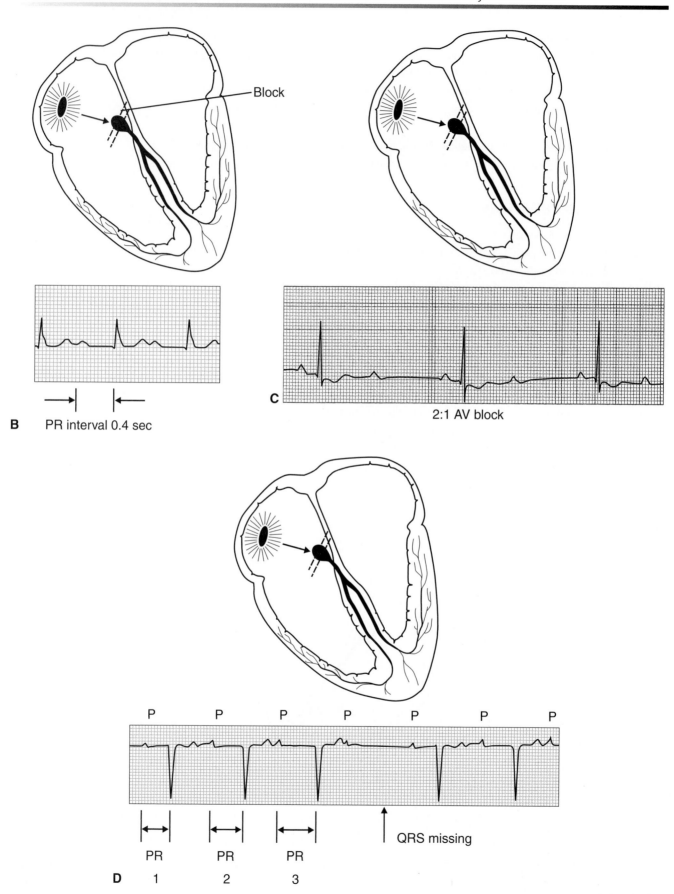

B PR interval 0.4 sec

C 2:1 AV block

D 1 2 3

QRS missing

FIGURE 3-7 (continued)

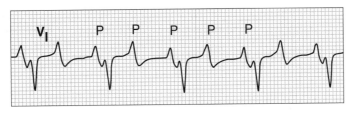

2:1

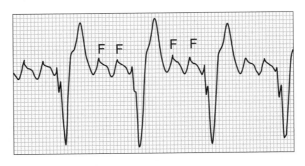

4:1

E   3:1

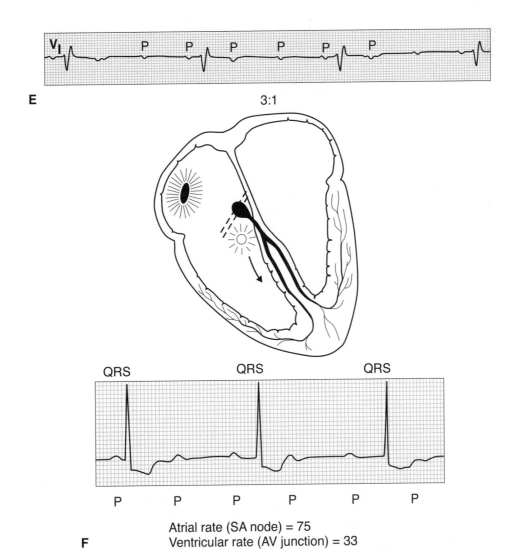

Atrial rate (SA node) = 75
F   Ventricular rate (AV junction) = 33

FIGURE 3-7 Electrocardiographic findings in conduction disturbances. **A**, Sinus arrest. **B**, First-degree atrioventricular (AV) block. **C**, Second-degree AV block. **D**, Second-degree AV block (Mobitz I block). **E**, Second-degree AV block. **F**, Third-degree (complete) AV block. *SA*, sinoatrial.
(From Stein E. Rapid analysis of electrocardiograms: a self-study program. 3rd ed. Philadelphia: Lippincott Williams & Wilkins, 2000.)

      a. Restrictive cardiomyopathy (1%) results from fibrosis or infiltration of the ventricular wall because of collagen-defect diseases, most commonly amyloidosis; radiation; postoperative changes; diabetes; and endomyocardial fibrosis.

      b. The left ventricle is small or normal, with mildly reduced function.

B. Clinical features

  1. Dilated cardiomyopathies result in signs and symptoms of left or biventricular congestive failure; the most common presentation is dyspnea.

  2. Hypertrophic obstructive cardiomyopathy

      a. Patients most commonly present with dyspnea and angina. Syncope and ventricular arrhythmias are common. It may be asymptomatic.

      b. Physical examination may show sustained point of maximal impulse or triple apical impulse, loud S_4 gallop, variable systolic murmur, and a bisferiens carotid pulse.

  3. Restrictive cardiomyopathy

      a. Patients present with decreased exercise tolerance; in advanced disease, patients develop right-sided congestive failure.

      b. Pulmonary hypertension usually is present.

C. Laboratory studies

  1. Dilated cardiomyopathies

      a. ECG may show nonspecific ST- and T-wave changes, conduction abnormalities, and ventricular ectopia.

      b. Chest radiography in long-standing disease shows cardiomegaly and pulmonary congestion.

      c. Echocardiography, nuclear studies, and cardiac catheterization show left ventricular dilation and dysfunction, with high diastolic pressures and low cardiac output.

  2. Hypertrophic obstructive cardiomyopathy

      a. Chest radiography often is not remarkable.

      b. ECG abnormalities include nonspecific ST- and T-wave changes, exaggerated septal Q waves, and left ventricular hypertrophy.

      c. Echocardiography, Doppler ultrasound, myocardial perfusion studies, cardiac MRI, and cardiac catheterization show left ventricular hypertrophy, asymmetric septal hypertrophy, small left ventricle, and diastolic dysfunction.

  3. Restrictive cardiomyopathy

      a. Chest radiography may show a mildly to moderately enlarged cardiac silhouette.

      b. Echocardiography is the key to diagnosis; other low-voltage changes on ECG are typical. Cardiac MRI is distinctive, and cardiac catheterization may demonstrate normal or mildly reduced left ventricular function.

      c. Endomyocardial biopsy may be necessary to differentiate restrictive disease from other forms of cardiomyopathy or pericarditis.

D. Treatment

  1. Dilated cardiomyopathies

      a. Abstinence from alcohol is essential.

      b. Underlying disease should be treated.

      c. CHF requires supportive treatment.

  2. Hypertrophic cardiomyopathies

      a. Initial treatment employs β-blockers or calcium channel blockers; disopyramide is used for its negative inotropic effects.

      b. Surgical or nonsurgical ablation of the hypertrophic septum may be required.

      c. Dual-chamber pacing, implantable defibrillators, or mitral valve replacement may be indicated.

  3. Diuretics and steroids may help patients with restrictive cardiomyopathies

XIV. PERICARDIAL DISORDERS

A. General characteristics

  1. Pericarditis most often occurs as the result of infection (viral or bacterial), autoimmune disease, neoplasms, radiation therapy, or chemotherapy toxicity; tuberculous pericarditis is common outside of developed nations.

2. Pericardial effusion (secondary to pericarditis, uremia, or cardiac trauma) produces restrictive pressure on the heart.

3. Cardiac tamponade occurs when fluid compromises cardiac filling and impairs cardiac output.

B. Clinical features

1. The primary presenting symptom of acute pericarditis is pleuritic chest pain relieved by sitting upright and leaning forward; a friction rub is characteristic.

2. Constrictive pericarditis presents with slowly progressive dyspnea, fatigue, and weakness, accompanied by edema, hepatomegaly, and ascites.

3. Pericardial effusions may be painful or painless, often accompanied by cough and dyspnea.

4. In infectious conditions, patients may be febrile.

5. Cardiac tamponade typically presents with tachycardia, tachypnea, narrow pulse pressure, and pulsus paradoxus.

C. Laboratory studies

1. Elevated WBC indicates infection, necessitating blood and pericardial fluid cultures.

2. Chest radiography or echocardiography is useful to determine the extent of cardiac effusion (Fig. 3-8) and calcification.

3. ECG changes include nonspecific T-wave changes and low QRS voltage. Electrical alternans is pathognomonic of effusion.

4. Echocardiography, Doppler ultrasound, and MRI may be helpful for more accurate diagnosis or before invasive procedures.

D. Treatment

1. In the presence of hemodynamic compromise, pericardiocentesis is necessary to relieve fluid accumulation.

2. Strictly inflammatory conditions may be treated with steroids or nonsteroidal anti-inflammatory drugs.

3. Infectious conditions require antibiotic therapy only if bacterial infection is suspected.

4. Constrictive conditions require diuresis.

XV. INFECTIVE ENDOCARDITIS

A. General characteristics

1. Most cases of infective endocarditis are caused by *Streptococcus viridans*, *Staphylococcus aureus*, and enterococci.

2. In IV drug users, *Staphylococcus aureus* is the most common cause, and the tricuspid valve frequently is involved.

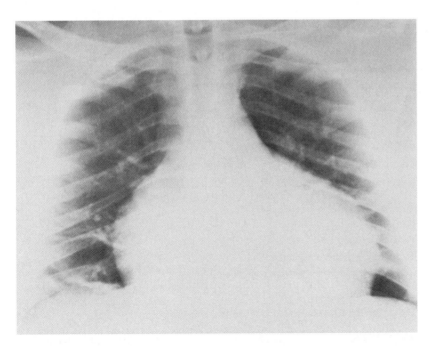

FIGURE 3-8 Pericardial effusion, frontal view. Note the massive enlargement of the patient's cardiac silhouette (water bottle heart).
(From Daffner RH. Clinical radiology: the essentials. 2nd ed. Baltimore: Williams & Wilkins, 1999.)

3. Prosthetic valve endocarditis most often is caused by staphylococci, Gram-negative organisms, and fungi during the first 2 months after implantation.

4. Most patients with endocarditis have an underlying cardiac defect that provides a nidus for disease.

5. Infection may result from direct intravascular contamination or from bacteremia, which is common during dental, upper respiratory, urologic, and lower GI procedures and, possibly, suction abortions.

B. Clinical features

1. Most patients present with fever (although this may be absent in the elderly) and nonspecific symptoms (e.g., cough, dyspnea, arthralgias, back or flank pain, GI complaints).

2. Approximately 90% of patients will have a stable murmur, but this may be absent in right-sided infections. A changing murmur is diagnostically significant.

3. Classic features occur in 25% of patients and include palatal, conjunctival, or subungual petechiae; splinter hemorrhages; Osler nodes (painful, violaceous, raised lesions of the fingers, toes, or feet); Janeway lesions (painless red lesions of the palms or soles); and Roth spots (exudative lesions in the retina).

4. Pallor and splenomegaly are common.

C. Laboratory studies

1. Three sets of blood cultures at least 1 hour apart should be obtained, ideally before starting antibiotics.

2. Chest radiography may demonstrate underlying cardiac abnormality or reveal pulmonary infiltrates if the right side of the heart is involved.

3. The ECG has no specific diagnostic features.

4. Echocardiography is useful to identify the specific valves involved; transesophageal echocardiography is particularly useful.

5. The Duke criteria (Table 3-8) are used to establish the diagnosis of infective endocarditis.

D. Treatment

1. Antibiotic prophylaxis before dental work or surgical procedures should be used in patients with predisposing cardiac abnormalities.

2. Empiric antibiotic treatment should include coverage of staphylococci, streptococci, and enterococci, pending blood culture results.

3. Valve replacement, especially of the aortic valve, may be necessary if the condition does not resolve with antibiotic therapy, if an abscess develops, or if a fungal infection is the cause.

4. Anticoagulants are contraindicated in patients with native valve infection and are controversial in patients with prosthetic valves.

TABLE 3-8	**Clinical Criteria for Infective Endocarditis**

Patient must have (1) two major, (2) one major and one minor, or (3) three minor criteria for the diagnosis to be made on clinical grounds.

Major Criteria

- Two positive blood cultures of a typically causative microorganism
- Evidence of endocardial involvement on echocardiography
- Development of a new regurgitant murmur

Minor Criteria

- Predisposing factor
- Fever ≥100.4°F (38°C)
- Vascular phenomena (e.g., embolic disease or pulmonary infarction)
- Immunologic phenomena (e.g., glomerulonephritis, Osler nodes, Roth spots)
- Positive blood culture not meeting major criteria

For details, see Bayer AS, Bolger AF, Taubert KA, et al. Diagnosis and management of infective endocarditis and its complications. Circulation 1998;98:2936–2948.

XVI. RHEUMATIC HEART DISEASE

A. General characteristics
  1. Rheumatic fever is a systemic immune response following β-hemolytic streptococcal pharyngitis.
  2. It is most common in recent immigrants, but new U.S. outbreaks have occurred. Children from 5 to 15 years of age most often are affected.
  3. Rheumatic valve disease may be self-limited or lead to progressive deformity of the valve.
  4. The mitral valve most often is involved (75–80%), followed by the aortic valve (30%).

B. Clinical features
  1. Two major or one major and two minor Jones criteria are required to establish the diagnosis of rheumatic fever.
    a. Major criteria: carditis, erythema marginatum, subcutaneous nodules, chorea, and polyarthritis.
    b. Minor criteria: fever, polyarthralgias, reversible prolongation of the PR interval, rapid erythrocyte sedimentation rate or C-reactive protein.
  2. Supportive evidence includes positive throat culture or Rapid Strep test and elevated or rising streptococcal antibody titer.

C. Treatment
  1. Strict bed rest is essential until the patient is stable.
  2. Salicylates reduce fever and relieve joint problems; corticosteroid use relieves joint symptoms but does not seem to prevent cardiac disease.
  3. IM penicillin is used for documented streptococcal infection; in patients who are allergic to penicillin, erythromycin is used.
  4. Prevention includes early treatment of streptococcal pharyngitis. Prevention of recurrence is essential.

XVII. PERIPHERAL VASCULAR DISORDERS

A. Peripheral arterial disease
  1. General characteristics
    a. Peripheral arterial disease usually is a result of atherosclerosis and is a significant independent risk factor for cardiovascular morbidity and mortality.
    b. Lower extremity disease results in ischemia and pain, causing significant limitation of activity or disability.
    c. Acute arterial occlusion may be caused by thrombosis or embolism.
    d. Thrombotic disease also may be a result of trauma, hypovolemia, inflammatory arteritis, polycythemia, dehydration, repeated arterial punctures, and hypercoagulable states.
    e. Three patterns of disease exist.
      (1) Type 1: 15–20% of patients, limited to the aorta and common iliac artery, most commonly found in men and women 40–55 years of age who smoke heavily or have hyperlipidemia.
      (2) Type 2: 25% of patients; involves the aorta, common iliac artery, and external iliac artery.
      (3) Type 3: most common, 60–70% of patients; multilevel disease affecting the aorta and the iliac, femoral, popliteal, and tibial arteries.
    f. Patients with type 2 and 3 peripheral arterial disease have typical risk factors for atherosclerotic disease and, usually, high incidence of cerebrovascular and coronary artery disease.
  2. Clinical features
    a. Lower leg pain with exercise, which is relieve by rest (intermittent claudication), usually is the first symptom of peripheral disease. Later, pain at rest occurs.
    b. Erectile dysfunction occurs with iliac artery disease.
    c. Severe, chronic disease results in numbness, tingling, and ischemic ulcerations, which may lead to gangrene.
    d. Symptoms of occlusion depend on the artery, the area it supplies, and the collateral circulation.
    e. Extremity occlusion usually results in pain, pallor, pulselessness, paresthesias, poikilothermia, and paralysis.
  3. Laboratory studies
    a. Doppler flow studies are used to determine systolic pressures in the posterior tibial and dorsalis pedis arteries.

      b. An ankle-brachial index of less than 0.8 indicates significant disease.

      c. Catheter or magnetic resonance angiography is used for locating stenotic sites and for accurate diagnosis of thrombosis or embolism.

  4. Treatment

      a. Cigarette smoking is contraindicated. Progressive exercise is recommended. Lipid-lowering medications reduce the risk for new-onset or worsening claudication.

      b. Cilostazol is the main drug treatment. Aspirin should be used routinely in all patients without a contraindication. Clopidogrel or warfarin may be selected postoperatively. Propinonyl-L-carnitine and ginko biloba may improve walking distance.

      c. Erectile dysfunction may require revascularization or treatment with a phosphodiesterase, such as sildenafil.

      d. Lower extremity revascularization must be preceded by a thorough cardiac and carotid evaluation.

      e. Thromboendarterectomy, embolectomy, thrombolytic therapy, and endovascular surgery may be indicated.

B. Varicose veins

  1. General characteristics

      a. Approximately 15% of adults, particularly women who have been pregnant, develop varicosities. Other risk factors include family history, prolonged standing, and history of phlebitis.

      b. The main mechanisms are superficial venous insufficiency and valvular incompetence; inherited defects in vein walls or valves also play a role.

  2. Clinical features

      a. Dilated, tortuous veins develop superficially in the lower extremities, particularly in the distribution of the long saphenous vein. *Smaller blue-green, flat reticular veins, telangiectasias,* and *spider* veins are further evidence of venous dysfunction.

      b. Varicosities may be asymptomatic or associated with aching and fatigue.

      c. Chronic distal edema, abnormal pigmentation, fibrosis, atrophy, and skin ulceration may occur.

      d. The Brodie-Trendelenburg test differentiates saphenofemoral valve incompetence from perforator vein incompetence.

  3. Laboratory studies are not necessary; however, Doppler sonography locates incompetent valves before surgery.

  4. Treatment

      a. Graduated elastic stockings give external support.

      b. Leg elevation and regular exercise provide symptomatic relief.

      c. Small venous ulcers heal with leg elevation and compression bandages; larger ulcers may require compression boot dressing or skin grafts.

      d. Interventional techniques include stab avulsion, endovenous radiofrequency ablation, compression sclerotherapy, and rarely, surgical stripping of the saphenous tree.

C. Thrombophlebitis and deep venous thrombosis (DVT)

  1. General characteristics

      a. Thrombophlebitis involves partial or complete occlusion of a vein and inflammatory changes. Virchow's triad of stasis, vascular injury, and hypercoagulability predispose a vein to development of thrombophlebitis.

      b. Superficial thrombophlebitis may occur spontaneously or following trauma.

      c. DVT most often occurs in the lower extremities and pelvis.

      d. DVT is associated with major surgical procedures (especially total hip replacement), prolonged bed rest, use of oral contraceptives and hormone replacement therapy, and inherited and cancer-associated hypercoagulable states. Increasingly, air travel is being recognized as a cause.

      e. Other risk factors include advanced age, type A blood, obesity, multiparity, inflammatory bowel disease, and lupus erythematosus.

  2. Clinical features

      a. Superficial thrombophlebitis may present with erythema, tenderness, and induration of the involved vein or with no symptoms. It is most common in the long saphenous vein.

      b. Half of patients with DVT have no early signs or symptoms; classic findings of DVT include swelling of the involved calf, heat and redness over the site, and a positive Homans' sign.

   3. Diagnostic studies

    a. Duplex ultrasound is the preferred study for DVT. Negative results in a patient with a high suspicion for DVT indicates the need for further study.

    b. Venography is the most accurate method for definitive diagnosis of DVT, but it is associated with increased risk and rarely is used.

    c. D-Dimer is a fibrin degradation product that is elevated in the presence of thrombus. An elevated D-dimer does not sufficiently diagnose thrombophlebitis; most hospitalized patients will have an elevated level. A negative D-dimer test (<500 ng/dL), however, suggests that ultrasound may be omitted.

   4. Treatment

    a. Superficial disease is treated with bed rest, heat, elevation of the extremity, and nonsteroidal anti-inflammatory drugs.

    b. Prevention of DVT in bedridden patients is accomplished by elevation of the foot of the bed, leg exercises, and compression hose; in high-risk patients, anticoagulation may be appropriate.

    c. Prevention of perioperative and travel-associated DVT includes early or frequent ambulation, leg exercises, and compression hose.

    d. Preferred treatment is anticoagulation with low-molecular-weight heparin or with heparin followed by warfarin.

D. Chronic venous insufficiency

   1. General characteristics

    a. Chronic venous insufficiency is characterized by loss of wall tension in veins, which results in stasis of venous blood and often is associated with a history of DVT, leg injury, or varicose veins.

    b. Prevention is accomplished by early aggressive treatment of venous reflux states, such as acute thrombophlebitis or varicose veins.

   2. Clinical features

    a. Progressive edema starting at the ankle is followed by skin and subcutaneous changes.

    b. Itching, dull pain with standing and pain with ulceration is common.

    c. Skin is shiny, thin, and atrophic with dark pigmentary changes and subcutaneous induration.

    d. Ulcers most commonly occur just above the ankle (stasis ulcer).

   3. Treatment

    a. General therapeutic measures include elevation of the legs, avoidance of extended sitting or standing, and compression hose.

    b. Stasis dermatitis should be treated with wet compresses and hydrocortisone cream; chronic dermatitis may require addition of zinc oxide with ichthammol and an antifungal cream.

    c. Ulcerations may be treated with wet compresses, compression boots or stockings, and occasionally, skin grafting.

XVIII. GIANT CELL ARTERITIS

A. General characteristics

   1. Giant cell arteritis is a systemic inflammatory condition of medium and large vessels. It primarily affects those older than 50 years and frequently coexists with polymyalgia rheumatica.

   2. It most frequently involves the temporal artery and other extracranial branches of the carotid artery.

   3. If not treated aggressively, it can cause blindness.

   4. Large vessel problems (e.g., thoracic aortic aneurysm) occur in 15% of patients within 7 years.

B. Clinical features

   1. Patients have headache, scalp tenderness, jaw claudication, throat pain, and visual abnormalities.

   2. Symptoms of polymyalgia rheumatica (pain and stiffness mainly of shoulder and pelvic girdle) are present in 50% of patients.

   3. Nonclassic symptoms include: respiratory tract problems, mononeuritis multiplex, fever of unknown origin, or unexplained neck and head pain.

   4. The temporal artery examination can be normal, nodular, enlarged, tender, or pulseless.

FIGURE 3-9 A CT scan through the abdomen showing a large abdominal aortic aneurysm (arrows). Note the central enlarged lumen (L), the more peripheral hematoma (H), and the calcification of the wall on the left side.
(From Daffner RH. Clinical radiology: the essentials. 2nd ed. Baltimore: Williams & Wilkins, 1999.)

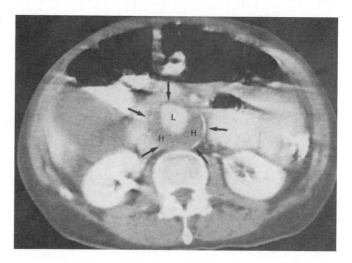

   C. Laboratory studies

      1. Erythrocyte sedimentation rate and C-reactive protein are markedly elevated.

      2. Most patients have a normochromic normocytic anemia and thrombocytosis; some have elevated alkaline phosphatase.

      3. Temporal artery biopsy should be performed promptly.

   D. Treatment is high-dose prednisone (1–2 months before tapering) and low-dose aspirin.

XIX. AORTIC ANEURYSMS

   A. General characteristics

      1. An aortic aneurysm is a weakness and subsequent dilation of the vessel wall, usually caused by genetic defect or atherosclerotic damage to the intima.

      2. Atherosclerosis is the most common cause, although some exist as congenital defects or as a result of syphilis, giant cell arteritis, vasculitis, or trauma.

      3. Aneurysms may occur in the abdominal (90%) or thoracic (10%) aorta.

      4. Rupture (dissection) leads to rapid death in 90% of patients.

   B. Clinical features

      1. Abdominal aortic aneurysm may be asymptomatic or present as a pulsating abdominal mass, sometimes accompanied by abdominal or back pain.

      2. Renal or lower extremity occlusive disease is present in 25% of patients.

      3. Thoracic aortic aneurysms may be asymptomatic or cause substernal, back, or neck pain; dyspnea, stridor, and cough; dysphagia; hoarseness; or symptoms of superior vena cava syndrome.

      4. Symptoms often indicate dissection.

      5. Rupture causes severe back, abdominal, or flank pain and hypotension and shock.

   C. Laboratory studies

      1. Abdominal ultrasound is the study of choice for abdominal aneurysms; this may be followed by contrast-enhanced CT or MRI (Fig. 3-9). Angiography is most often used before elective repair.

      2. Thoracic aneurysms may require aortography for diagnosis; CT and MRI are preferred over ultrasound.

   D. Treatment

      1. The only effective treatment is endovascular or open surgical repair.

      2. Five year survival after repair is greater than 60%.

Hematology

Rebecca Lovell Scott

I. ANEMIAS

A. General characteristics

1. Anemias are conditions involving hemoglobin concentrations or packed RBC concentrations at levels below normal (Table 4-1).

2. Anemias may be caused by increased red cell destruction, decreased red cell production, or bleeding, or they may be secondary to a systemic disease.

3. Congenital anemia may be suggested by personal or family history.

4. Anemias present in many forms, including hypochromic microcytic anemias (iron deficiency anemia, thalassemia, sickle-cell anemia, and long-standing anemia of chronic disease), normochromic normocytic anemias, and macrocytic anemias (Fig. 4-1). Macrocytic anemias may develop from megaloblastic or nonmegaloblastic causes.

   a. In microcytic anemias with mean corpuscular volume (MCV) of less than 70 fL, the cause is iron deficiency or thalassemia.

   b. Macrocytic anemias with MCV of greater of >125 fL almost always are megaloblastic, except for those associated with myelodysplastic syndromes.

5. Anemias also may be classified on a pathophysiologic basis: diminished production or increased rate of loss of RBCs (Table 4-2).

B. Clinical features

1. Many patients have few signs or symptoms. The most common are fatigue, headache, and exertional dyspnea.

2. Acute anemia of rapid onset may cause tachycardia, orthostatic hypotension, faintness, and pale, cold extremities.

3. Chronic anemia may cause findings associated with hyperkinetic circulation (e.g., large pulse volume, tachycardia).

4. Pronounced anemia may cause pallor, cheilosis, jaundice, beefy red tongue, and koilonychia.

5. Smooth tongue and other mucosal changes suggest nutritional deficiencies (iron, folate, vitamin B12).

6. Signs of primary hematologic disease (lymphadenopathy, hepatosplenomegaly, bone tenderness) may be present.

C. Laboratory studies (Table 4-3)

1. Hemoglobin, hematocrit (Hct), red cell indices, and red cell distribution width

2. Peripheral smear

3. Corrected reticulocyte count

D. Hypochromic microcytic anemias (MCV <80 fL)

1. Iron deficiency anemias

   a. General characteristics

      (1) Iron deficiency anemias result from an inadequate supply of iron for synthesis of hemoglobin. Iron deficiency is the most common cause of anemia in the world.

      (2) In adults, blood loss, particularly from the GI tract, almost universally is the cause of the iron deficiency. Chronic aspirin or nonsteroidal anti-inflammatory drug (NSAID) use also may be the cause.

      (3) Although menstrual blood loss plays a major role, menstruation should not automatically be assumed to cause a woman's iron deficiency.

      (4) Low dietary intake of iron may occur in children and in pregnant women.

      (5) Other causes include decreased absorption of iron, increased requirements, hemoglobinuria, blood donation, iron sequestration, trauma, and intravascular hemolysis.

   b. Clinical features

      (1) Lack of iron causes few specific complaints. General complaints in severe iron deficiency (Hct <25%) include pallor, easy fatigability, irritability, anorexia, tachycardia, tachypnea on exertion, and poor weight gain in infants.

      (2) Pica is a hallmark of iron deficiency.

TABLE 4-1	Values for Normal Adult Blood	
Parameter	Males	Females
Hemoglobin	13.6–17.5 g/dL	12.0–15.5 g/dL
Hematocrit	39–49%	35–45%
Red blood cells	4.6–6.3 million/mL	4.2–5.4 million/mL

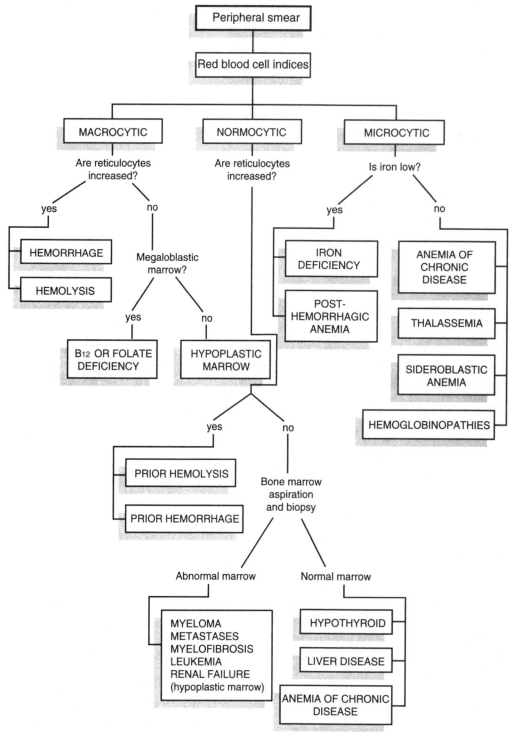

FIGURE 4-1 Diagnostic approach to anemias.
(From Nirula R. High-Yield Internal Medicine. Baltimore: Lippincott Williams & Wilkins, 2003.)

TABLE 4-2 Pathophysiologic Classification of Anemias

Decreased Production	Increased Production
Hemoglobin synthesis	Blood loss
Iron deficiency	Intrinsic hemolysis
Thalassemia	Hereditary spherocytosis
Anemia of chronic disease	Elliptocytosis
DNA synthesis	Sickle cell
Megaloblastic anemia	Unstable hemoglobin
Stem cell	G6PD deficiency
Aplastic anemia	Extrinsic hemolysis
Myeloproliferative leukemia	Warm and cold antibody
Bone marrow infiltration	TTP-HUS
Carcinoma	Mechanical cardiac valve
Lymphoma	Clostridial infection
Pure red cell aplasia	Hypersplenism

G6PD, glucose-6-phosphate dehydrogenase; *TTP-HUS*, thrombotic thrombocytopenic purpura–hemolytic-uremic syndrome.

(3) Severe deficiency may cause brittle nails, cheilosis, smooth tongue, and formation of esophageal webs (Plummer-Vinson syndrome).

(4) Iron deficiency anemia responds promptly to iron therapy.

 c. Laboratory findings

  (1) Hemoglobin and hematocrit are decreased.

  (2) Peripheral smear

   (a) Initially, there are no changes in red cell size.

   (b) Later, the peripheral smear shows hypochromic microcytic red cells. Smear shows anisocytosis and poikilocytosis.

   (c) Severe anemia causes severely hypochromic cells, target cells, and nucleated red cells.

  (3) A plasma ferritin level of less than 30 μg/L reliably indicates iron deficiency anemia.

  (4) Serum iron is decreased to less than 30 μg/dL, and total iron-binding capacity is elevated. Transferrin saturation decreases to less than 15%.

  (5) MCV is normal early on but falls later in the course of the disease.

  (6) Platelet count is elevated in severe anemia.

 d. Treatment

  (1) Ferrous sulfate, 325 mg t.i.d., should be given in a slowly escalating dose. It is best absorbed on an empty stomach, but is frequently given with meals due to intolerability. Orange juice may enhance absorption.

  (2) Although hematocrit will be within the normal range in 2 months, therapy should be continued for up to 6 months or longer to replenish tissue stores.

TABLE 4-3 Red Blood Cell Studies

Parameter	Normal Range
Mean corpuscular hemoglobin	26–34 pg
Mean corpuscular volume	80–100 fL
Mean corpuscular hemoglobin concentration	31–36 g/dL
Red cell distribution width	11.5–14.5%
Corrected reticulocyte count	0.5–2.5%

        (3) Supplementation during pregnancy and lactation is essential.

        (4) Parenteral iron is appropriate for patients with intolerance to oral iron, GI disease, and continuing blood loss. Sodium ferric gluconate is less likely than iron dextran to cause anaphylaxis.

        (5) Identification of sources of occult blood loss is imperative.

        (6) Treatment failures may be caused by nonadherence, poor absorption, incorrect diagnosis, or ongoing blood loss.

2. Thalassemia syndromes

    a. General characteristics

        (1) Thalassemia syndromes are hereditary anemias in which synthesis of α- or β-globin chains is reduced, resulting in defective hemoglobinization of RBCs.

            (a) α-Thalassemia results from gene deletion; β-thalassemia results from point mutations.

            (b) α-Thalassemia most commonly is seen in persons of Southeast Asian or Chinese origin; β-thalassemia more commonly is seen in Mediterranean populations.

        (2) The most prominent feature is microcytosis out of proportion to the degree of anemia.

        (3) Thalassemia should be suspected in a person with a positive family history or a personal history of lifelong microcytic anemia, especially if unresponsive to iron therapy.

        (4) Thalassemias also may be classified as hypoproliferative anemias, hemolytic anemias, or anemias related to abnormal hemoglobin.

    b. Clinical features

        (1) Deficits range from silent carrier status to profound anemia.

        (2) α-Thalassemia

            (a) Patients may have mild symptoms or none (thalassemia trait; carriers). Patients often are diagnosed after a nonresponse to treatment for a prescribed iron deficiency.

            (b) Patients with one α-globin chain have hemoglobin H disease, which is variably symptomatic; when all four chains are deleted, stillbirth occurs from hydrops fetalis.

        (3) β-Thalassemia major

            (a) Problems begin at 4–6 months, when the switch from fetal hemoglobin (hemoglobin F) to adult hemoglobin occurs. These problems include severe anemia, growth retardation, abnormal facial structure, pathologic fractures, osteopenia, bone deformities, hepatosplenomegaly, and jaundice.

            (b) Before effective iron chelation and allogeneic stem cell transplantation, patients usually died from cardiac failure by age 30.

    c. Laboratory findings

        (1) Table 4-4 differentiates the thalassemias per typical hematocrit, hemoglobin electrophoresis, reticulocyte count, and peripheral smear.

        (2) Serum iron and ferritin levels characteristically are normal or elevated.

        (3) Hemoglobin level usually is between 3 and 6 g/dL.

TABLE 4-4   **Differentiation of Thalassemias per Laboratory Parameters**

Type	Hematocrit	Hemoglobin Electrophoresis	Peripheral Smear	Reticulocyte Count
α-Thalassemia minor (trait)	28–40%	Normal	Target cells Acanthocytes	Normal
α-Thalassemia H	22–32%	Hemoglobin H	Target cells Poikilocytes	Increased
β-Thalassemia minor	28–40%	Hemoglobin A_2 Hemoglobin F	Target cells Basophilic stippling	Normal or increased
β-Thalassemia major	As low as 10%	Hemoglobin F Hemoglobin A_2	Target cells Poikilocytes Basophilic stippling Nucleated RBCs	Increased

(4) Thalassemia produces more marked microcytosis for degree of anemia than iron deficiency does; red cell morphologic changes occur earlier.

(5) Diagnosis is confirmed by hemoglobin electrophoresis.

d. Treatment

(1) Patients with mild disease should not receive iron because of the risk of iron overload.

(2) Persons with hemoglobin H disease need folic acid supplements and should avoid iron supplements and oxidative drugs (e.g., dapsone, primaquine, quinidine, sulfonamides, nitrofurantoin).

(3) Treatment for β-thalassemia major consists of transfusions to keep hemoglobin concentrations at least 12 g/dL; however, iron overload may result in hemosiderosis, heart failure, cirrhosis, endocrinopathies. Deferoxamine is used to avoid or postpone hemosiderosis.

(4) Allogeneic bone marrow transplantation also is used with increasing success; splenectomy may be required.

(5) Genetic counseling, testing, and prenatal diagnosis for severe forms are essential.

3. Other hypochromic microcytic anemias

a. Sideroblastic anemias are acquired disorders with reduced hemoglobin synthesis causing iron accumulation, especially in the mitochondria.

(1) Prussian blue staining of bone marrow cells shows ringed sideroblasts.

(2) Causes include myelodysplasia, chronic alcoholism, and lead poisoning.

(3) Laboratory findings

(a) Hematocrit usually is 20–30%.

(b) MCV varies.

(c) Peripheral smear shows normal and hypochromic cells.

(d) In lead poisoning, basophilic stippling of red cells is present.

(e) Bone marrow evaluation is necessary to establish the diagnosis.

(4) Treatment

(a) Treat the underlying cause.

(b) Transfusion may be required.

(c) Patients do not respond to erythropoietin.

b. Hypochromic microcytic anemia may be associated with systemic or chronic disease.

c. Hypochromic microcytic anemia may be associated with copper deficiency.

E. Normochromic normocytic anemias (MCV = 80–100 fL)

1. General characteristics. These anemias are caused by organ failure or impaired marrow function resulting from systemic disease.

a. The organ failure causing these anemias may be associated with kidney, endocrine, thyroid, or liver disease; anemia of renal disease usually is more severe.

b. Significant anemia in patients with chronic disease usually indicates coexisting iron or folate deficiency.

c. The impaired marrow function causing these anemias may be associated with chronic infection, aplastic anemia, infiltrative marrow disease (myelophthisic syndromes), and pure red cell aplasia.

d. Aplastic anemia arises from injury or abnormal expression of the pluripotent hematopoietic stem cell.

e. T cell–mediated autoimmune suppression of hematopoiesis is the most common cause; other causes are radiation, chemotherapy, toxins, pharmaceuticals, and systemic lupus erythematosus.

2. Clinical features

a. Anemia associated with chronic disease usually is mild and remits with treatment of the disease.

b. Clinical features are consistent with any underlying disease.

c. Patients with aplastic anemia have weakness, fatigue, vulnerability to infection, pallor, purpura, and petechiae. Hepatosplenomegaly, lymphadenopathy and bone tenderness suggest an alternative diagnosis.

3. Laboratory studies are ordered according to the underlying disease.

a. Anemia of chronic disease usually is normochromic normocytic or mildly hypochromic microcytic.

b. Anemia of chronic disease has normal or increased bone marrow iron stores and serum ferritin and normal or low total iron-binding capacity.

      c. Red cell morphology and reticulocyte count are unremarkable or mildly abnormal.

      d. Serum iron and transferrin saturation may be extremely low, but serum ferritin should be normal or elevated, except in cases of coexisting iron deficiency.

      e. Pancytopenia is the hallmark of aplastic anemia; bone marrow is hypocellular.

   4. Treatment

      a. In anemia of chronic disease, the underlying disease must be treated.

      b. Erythropoietin is effective in treating anemia of renal failure, cancer, and inflammatory disorders.

      c. Mild aplastic anemia is treated supportively with transfusions of red cells and platelets; severe disease is treated with bone marrow transplantation or immunosuppression.

F. Macrocytic anemias (MCV >100 fL)

   1. General characteristics

      a. These include anemias caused by acute hemorrhage and hemolysis.

      b. Macrocytic anemias also include deficiencies leading to megaloblastic states.

   2. Folic acid deficiency anemia

      a. General characteristics

         (1) Folic acid deficiency most often is caused by poor dietary intake; other causes include defective absorption, pregnancy, hemolytic anemias, alcohol abuse, and consumption of folic acid antagonists.

         (2) Inadequate intake is the most common cause in alcoholics, persons with anorexia, and those whose diet is low in fruits and vegetables.

         (3) Malabsorption is a rare cause.

         (4) The daily requirement of folic acid is 50–100 mg/dL and usually is met by the diet.

         (5) Pregnancy, hemolytic anemias, and exfoliative skin disease increase requirements.

      b. Clinical features

         (1) Sore tongue (glossitis)

         (2) Vague GI symptoms.

         (3) No neurologic symptoms (in contrast to vitamin B_{12} deficiency)

      c. Laboratory findings

         (1) Macro-ovalocytes and hypersegmented polymorphonuclear cells are pathognomonic.

         (2) Howell-Jolly bodies are typical.

         (3) RBC folate level of less than 150 ng/mL is diagnostic.

         (4) Serum vitamin B_{12} level is normal.

      d. Treatment

         (1) Oral replacement (1 mg/day) with folic acid is the first line of treatment.

         (2) Avoid alcohol and folic acid metabolism antagonists.

   3. Vitamin B_{12} deficiency (cobalamin)

      a. General characteristics

         (1) Pernicious anemia is the most common cause and leads to atrophic gastritis and increased risk of gastric carcinoma. Other autoimmune diseases may be present.

         (2) Other causes include strict vegan diet, gastric surgery, and Crohn's disease.

         (3) Irreversible neurologic damage can be caused by uncorrected deficiency. Folate administration can mask the deficiency but does not correct it.

         (4) Foods of animal origin supply vitamin B_{12}.

         (5) Absorption occurs in the terminal ileum and storage in the liver.

      b. Clinical features

         (1) The physical examination will be unremarkable in most patients; glossitis and vague GI symptoms may be present.

         (2) Neurologic findings include stocking-glove paresthesias, loss of position, fine touch and vibratory sensation, clumsiness, dementia, and ataxia.

c. Laboratory studies

(1) Anemia may be severe, and MCV usually is markedly elevated but may be normal.

(2) Anisocytosis, poikilocytosis, macro-ovalocytosis, and hypersegmented neutrophils are seen.

(3) Reticulocyte count is reduced.

(4) Serum lactate dehydrogenase (LDH) and indirect bilirubin are elevated.

(5) Serum vitamin B_{12} is abnormally low.

(6) Schilling test (a 24 hr urine collection of radioactive vitamin B_{12}) is rarely used today.

d. Treatment

(1) Lifelong supplemental vitamin B_{12} usually is given IM for pernicious anemia.

(2) Daily oral cobalamin may be used.

(3) Reversible causes of malabsorption should be treated.

(4) Strict vegans, persons who have undergone gastrectomy or resection of the ileum, and those with blind loop syndrome require supplementation to prevent anemia.

(5) Neurologic signs and symptoms are reversible if treated within 6 months.

4. Hemolytic anemias

a. General characteristics

(1) Hemolytic anemias are those characterized by episodic or continuous RBC destruction.

(2) Classification usually is based on intrinsic red cell defects or extracellular causes.

(a) Intrinsic causes include hereditary spherocytosis and elliptocytosis, paroxysmal nocturnal hemoglobinuria, glucose-6-phosphate dehydrogenase (G6PD) deficiency, methemoglobinemia, and sickle-cell syndromes.

(b) Causes external to the erythrocyte include autoimmune and lymphoproliferative diseases, drug toxicity, thrombotic thrombocytopenic purpura, hemolytic-uremic syndrome, disseminated intravascular coagulation (DIC), valvular hemolysis, metastatic adenocarcinoma, vasculitides, infections, hypersplenism, and burns.

b. Clinical features

(1) Anemia from both causes may present with jaundice, gallstones, pallor, and symptoms related to decreased oxygen delivery to the tissues.

(2) Infection with parvovirus B19 can lead to a transient aplastic crisis. Risk for infection with *Salmonella* and *Pneumococcus* sp. is increased.

c. Laboratory findings

(1) An elevated reticulocyte count in the presence of a falling or stable hematocrit is the hallmark of hemolytic anemia.

(2) Peripheral smear may reveal immature red cells, nucleated red cells, or morphologic changes.

(3) Transient hemoglobinemia indicates intravascular hemolysis and may be accompanied by hemoglobinuria.

(4) Unconjugated (indirect) bilirubin is elevated; total bilirubin may rise to 4 mg/dL.

(5) Serum LDH indicates microangiopathic hemolysis.

d. Treatment depends on the underlying disorder.

5. Sickle-cell anemia

a. General characteristics

(1) Sickle-cell anemia is an autosomal recessive hemolytic anemia.

(2) RBCs containing primarily hemoglobin S sickle under deoxygenated conditions.

(3) In the United States, this disease most often is seen in blacks (1 in 400 births); 8% carry the hemoglobin S gene as the sickle cell trait.

b. Clinical features

(1) Problems begin in infancy, when hemoglobin F levels fall.

(2) By childhood or adolescence, vascular occlusions produce painful crises, lasting for hours to days, with organ swelling and dysfunction and infarction.

(3) Sickling is increased by red cell dehydration, acidosis, and hypoxemia.

(4) Patients with sickle-cell anemia are at increased risk for cholelithiasis, splenomegaly, poorly healing ulcers, infection with encapsulated organisms (e.g., *Streptococcus pneumoniae*), strokes, priapism, retinopathies leading to blindness, and osteomyelitis.

(5) Hemolytic or aplastic crises may be life-threatening.

(6) Avascular necrosis of the femoral head is common.

(7) Life expectancy is 40–50 years.

(8) Sickle cell trait may result in difficulty concentrating urine.

c. Laboratory findings

(1) Electrophoresis shows hemoglobin S in red cells.

(2) Peripheral smear reveals sickled cells (5–50%) and target cells, nucleated RBCs, and Howell-Jolly bodies

(3) Reticulocyte count is elevated.

(4) WBC count is elevated; thrombocytosis may be present.

(5) Indirect bilirubin may be elevated.

d. Treatment

(1) Symptomatic treatment includes administration of analgesics, fluids, and oxygen.

(2) Vaso-occlusive crises may require exchange transfusion.

(3) Patients should receive pneumococcal vaccine and folate supplementation.

(4) Genetic counseling for patients with either the disease or trait is recommended. Prenatal testing is available.

6. G6PD deficiency

a. General characteristics

(1) G6PD deficiency is an X-linked recessive disorder commonly seen in American black males (10–15%) and in some Mediterranean populations.

(2) G6PD activity declines as erythrocytes age beyond 40 days.

(3) Oxidant drugs (e.g., dapsone, primaquine, quinidine, sulfonamides, nitrofurantoin) and infection cause episodic hemolysis.

(4) Severe deficiency may cause chronic hemolysis.

b. Clinical features

(1) Patients with episodic hemolysis usually are healthy and have no splenomegaly.

(2) Female carriers rarely are affected.

c. Laboratory findings

(1) During hemolytic episodes, reticulocytes and serum indirect bilirubin increase.

(2) Peripheral smear reveals bite cells and Heinz bodies.

(3) G6PD levels will be low between hemolytic episodes; in severe cases, G6PD levels will always be low.

d. Treatment

(1) In most cases, hemolytic episodes are self-limited as red cells are replaced.

(2) Oxidative drugs should be avoided.

II. POLYCYTHEMIA VERA

A. General characteristics

1. Polycythemia vera is a slowly progressive bone marrow disorder characterized by increased numbers of RBCs and increased total blood volume.

2. Unregulated expansion of red cell mass causes hyperviscosity, which leads to decreased cerebral blood flow.

3. Secondary causes of erythrocytosis include chronic hypoxia, often caused by cigarette smoking, and renal tumors.

4. Morbidity and mortality most commonly result from thrombosis; other complications include bleeding, peptic ulcer disease, and GI bleeding.

5. Median age at presentation is 60 years, and 60% of patients are male. Median survival time for patients with polycythemia vera is 11–15 years.

B. Clinical features

   1. Diagnostic criteria include splenomegaly, normal arterial oxygen saturation, and an elevated red cell mass.

   2. Patients may present with symptoms of increased blood viscosity and volume (i.e., headache, dizziness, fullness in the head and face, weakness, fatigue, tinnitus, blurred vision); burning, pain, and redness of the extremities; and rarely, stroke.

   3. Generalized pruritus after bathing is characteristic.

   4. Epistaxis may be the presenting complaint.

   5. Incidence of peptic ulcer disease is high.

   6. Plethora, systolic hypertension, engorged retinal veins, and splenomegaly may be found on physical examination.

   7. Thrombosis is the most common complication and cause of most morbidity and mortality; increased bleeding also occurs.

   8. Absence of splenomegaly suggests secondary polycythemia.

C. Laboratory findings

   1. At sea level, hematocrit levels in polycythemia vera are greater than 54% in males and greater than 51% in females.

   2. Patients without splenomegaly must have two of the following to establish the diagnosis: thrombocytosis, leukocytosis, elevated leukocyte alkaline phosphatase, elevated serum vitamin B_{12}, or elevated vitamin B_{12}-binding capacity.

   3. Peripheral smear shows neutrophilic leukocytosis, increased basophils and eosinophils, and increased numbers of large, bizarre platelets.

   4. Red cell morphology usually is normal; erythropoietin levels generally are low.

   5. The bone marrow is hypercellular in all cell lines; iron stores usually are absent.

   6. Hyperuricemia also develops.

D. Treatment

   1. Phlebotomy is the treatment of choice.

   2. Myelosuppressive therapy with hydroxyurea may be indicated; anagrelide may be added or substituted.

   3. Low-dose aspirin reduces the risk of thrombosis without increasing the risk of bleeding.

III. MALIGNANCIES

A. Leukemias

   1. General characteristics

      a. Leukemias are diseases characterized by unrestrained growth of leukocytes and leukocyte precursors in the tissues.

      b. Leukemias are classified according to cell type and may be myeloid or lymphoid.

      c. They also are classified as either acute or chronic.

      d. Risk factors include a positive family history, exposures to ionizing radiation, benzene, and certain alkylating agents.

   2. Acute leukemias

      a. General characteristics

         (1) There are two types of acute leukemias: acute lymphocytic leukemia (ALL), and acute myelogenous leukemia (AML).

         (2) The incidence increases with age. In children, ALL (80%) is more common than AML. Most diagnoses are made in children between 3 and 7 years of age.

         (3) AML primarily is a disease of adulthood (median age at onset is 60 years).

      b. Clinical features

         (1) Most clinical findings are related to replacement of normal bone marrow with malignant cells.

         (2) Gingival bleeding, epistaxis, and menorrhagia may be the presenting complaint; DIC is less common.

         (3) Infections from neutropenia commonly are caused by Gram-negative bacteria or fungi; common presentations include cellulitis, pneumonia, and perirectal infection. Death may occur if treatment is delayed.

(4) Children and young adults present with fatigue, abrupt onset of fever, lethargy, headache, and bone and/or joint pain.

(5) Older adults have a slow, progressive onset, with lethargy, anorexia, and dyspnea.

(6) Symptoms of anemia, thrombocytopenia, gingival hyperplasia, rashes, or cranial nerve palsies occur in most patients.

(7) Lymphadenopathy and hepatosplenomegaly are more common with ALL than in AML.

c. Laboratory findings

(1) The hallmark of acute leukemia is pancytopenia with circulating blasts; blasts make up at least 20% of nucleated cells in the bone marrow.

(2) Hyperuricemia is present.

(3) Auer rods (rod-shaped structures in cell cytoplasm) signify myeloid leukemia.

(4) WBC counts usually are high.

(5) Bone marrow biopsy confirms the diagnosis.

(6) In ALL, a mediastinal mass may be seen on chest radiography.

(7) Terminal deoxynucleotidyl transferase is present in 95% of ALL cases.

(8) Cytogenetic studies are the most powerful prognostic factors; presence of the Philadelphia chromosome is unfavorable in ALL.

d. Treatment

(1) Induction (remission-inducing) chemotherapy is targeted toward eradication of most of the leukemic cells.

(2) Consolidation therapy destroys the remainder of the leukemic cells.

(3) Increased serum urate levels may be caused by the treatment. Allopurinol and diuretics may be needed to prevent uric acid stones.

(4) Allogeneic bone marrow transplantation is used in patients with adverse cytogenetics or poor response to treatment.

(5) Greater than 50% of children with ALL can be cured with chemotherapy (induction plus consolidation therapy). Prognosis is related to age and WBC count at diagnosis.

(6) Greater than 70% of adults younger than 60 years achieve complete remission with treatment for AML; further chemotherapy leads to cure in 30–40% of patients.

3. Chronic leukemias

a. General characteristics

(1) Chronic lymphocytic leukemia (CLL) is a clonal malignancy of B lymphocytes.

(2) CLL is the most prevalent of all leukemias. It is twice as common in men as in women. Incidence increases with advancing age; median age at presentation is 65 years.

(3) The B-cell form accounts for 95% of CLL cases.

(4) Prognostic staging uses the Rai system.

(5) Chronic myelocytic leukemia (CML) is a myeloproliferative disorder.

b. Clinical features

(1) CML

(a) CML presents in young to middle-aged adults (median age at presentation is 55 years).

(b) It occurs in three phases: chronic, accelerated, and acute (blast crisis).

(c) It inevitably transforms into acute disease.

(d) Symptoms

(i)   Fatigue, anorexia, weight loss, low-grade fever, and excessive sweating are common.

(ii) Most patients also have abdominal fullness caused by splenomegaly.

(iii) Rare presentations include blurred vision, respiratory distress, and priapism.

(e) The symptoms of CML develop gradually. It generally runs a mild course until the blast-crisis phase.

(2) CLL

(a) CLL usually has an indolent course, with a median survival time of 6 years. It often is harmless but is resistant to cure. A variant, polylymphocytic leukemia, is more aggressive.

       (b) Clinical manifestations of CLL include peripheral lymphocytosis and lymphocytic invasion of bone marrow, liver, spleen, and lymph nodes.

       (c) Patients may have recurrent infections, splenomegaly, and lymphadenopathy.

       (d) Richter's syndrome occurs in 5% of cases; an isolated node transforms into aggressive, large-cell lymphoma.

   c. Laboratory findings

     (1) The hallmark of CLL is isolated lymphocytosis, with a leukocytosis of greater than 20,000 cells/mL.

     (2) The hallmark of CML is leukocytosis, with a median WBC count of 150,000 cells/mL. The Philadelphia chromosome is identified in 95% of cases.

     (3) Identification of the BCR-ABL gene by polymerase chain reaction has replaced the search for the Philadelphia chromosome to establish the diagnosis.

     (4) Peripheral smear

       (a) CML may show anemia and thrombocytosis.

       (b) CLL shows increased mature small lymphocytes; smudge cells are pathognomonic.

     (5) Bone marrow is hypercellular with a left shift.

   d. Treatment

     (1) CML

       (a) STI571 (imitanib mesylate) has replaced the former standard therapy. It is very effective during the chronic phase.

       (b) Hydroxyurea is used for imitanib intolerance.

       (c) Allogeneic bone marrow transplantation may be the initial treatment and is the only therapy proven to be curative.

     (2) CLL. Treatment of CLL usually is palliative once the disease is symptomatic.

B. Hodgkin's disease

  1. General characteristics

    a. Hodgkin's disease refers to a group of cancers characterized by enlargement of lymphoid tissue, spleen, and liver and the presence of Reed-Sternberg cells.

    b. The Epstein-Barr virus also appears to be an important factor, because it can be found in 40–50% of cases.

    c. Hodgkin's disease usually arises in a single area and spreads to contiguous nodes.

    d. It is most common between the ages of 15 and 45 years, peaking in the 20s, and again after age 50. It is rare in children under the age of 5.

    e. Among adults 15–45 years of age, it is more common in men.

  2. Clinical features

    a. Patients usually present with painless cervical, supraclavicular, and mediastinal lymphadenopathy. Pain in the affected node after ingestion of alcohol may occur.

    b. The nodular sclerosis subtype commonly is seen in young women; other subtypes are lymphocyte predominant, mixed cellularity, and lymphocyte depletion.

    c. Stage A designation indicates a lack of constitutional symptoms. One-third of patients present with constitutional (stage B) symptoms (fever, night sweats, weight loss, pruritus, and fatigue), which are associated with a poorer prognosis.

  3. Laboratory studies

    a. The Ann Arbor system is used to stage Hodgkin's and non-Hodgkin's lymphoma (Table 4-5).

    b. Basic staging includes CT of neck, chest, abdomen, and pelvis as well as biopsy of the bone marrow; laparotomy is no longer routine.

    c. Reed-Sternberg cells confirm the diagnosis.

  4. Treatment

    a. Combination chemotherapy cures more than 50% of patients, even those with advanced-stage disease.

    b. Radiation therapy is the initial treatment of choice for patients with low-risk stage IA and IIA disease; the 10-year survival rate exceeds 80%.

TABLE 4-5	Staging for Hodgkin's Disease: The Ann Arbor Criteria
Stage	**Criteria**
I	Single LNR (I) or a single ELS (IE)
II	Two or more LNRs on the same side of the diaphragm (II) or one solitary ELS and one or more LNRs on the same side of the diaphragm (IIE)
III	LNR on both sides of the diaphragm (III)
	With spleen involvement (IIIS) or solitary involvement of an ELS (IIIE) or both (IIIES)
	III_1 = upper abdomen; III_2 = lower abdomen
IV	Diffuse involvement of ELS with or without node involvement
A, B	Presence of constitutional symptoms (fever, night sweats, loss of 10% of body weight) = B; absence = A

ELS, extralymphatic site; *LNR,* lymph node region.

    c. Most other patients receive adriamycin, bleomycin, vinblastine, and dacarbazine (ABVD) chemotherapy; shorter, intensive treatments are under study.

C. Non-Hodgkin's lymphoma

  1. General characteristics

    a. Lymphomas are a group of malignancies that arise from lymphocytes; pathogenesis is related to cytogenetic abnormalities.

    b. About 90% of cases are derived from B lymphocytes.

    c. The incidence of B-cell lymphomas is higher in patients with HIV disease and other immunodeficiencies.

    d. Peak incidence occurs between 20 and 40 years of age.

    f. These lymphomas are divided into clinically indolent and aggressive groups.

      (1) Indolent lymphomas tend to convert to aggressive disease.

      (2) One-third of aggressive lymphomas are curable with chemotherapy.

  2. Clinical features

    a. Diffuse or isolated, painless, persistent lymphadenopathy is the most common presentation; bone marrow involvement is frequent.

    b. Common extralymphatic sites are the GI tract, skin, bone, and bone marrow. Burkitt's lymphoma is likely to present with abdominal fullness.

    c. Fever, night sweats, weight loss, pruritus, and fatigue are less likely than with Hodgkin's disease but do occur in intermediate- and high-grade disease.

  3. Laboratory studies

    a. Persistent, unexplained, enlarged nodes should be biopsied.

    b. Staging is accomplished by chest radiography, CT of the abdomen and pelvis, bone marrow biopsy, and possibly lumbar puncture.

    c. Serum LDH is a useful prognostic marker.

    d. Molecular profiling is under study.

  4. Treatment

    a. No clear consensus exists regarding treatment because of multiple new modalities. In some cases, spontaneous remission may occur.

    b. Aggressive lymphomas require aggressive combination chemotherapy or autologous stem cell transplantation.

D. Multiple myeloma

  1. General characteristics

    a. Multiple myeloma is a malignancy of plasma cells, possibly caused by a herpes virus.

    b. Replacement of bone marrow leads to failure; bone destruction leads to pain, osteoporosis, lytic lesions, and pathologic fractures. Plasmacytomas may cause spinal cord compression.

     c. Patients are prone to recurrent infections, particularly with encapsulated organisms, because of neutropenia and failure of antibody production in response to antigen challenge.

     d. Paraprotein levels are increased (IgG or IgA may cause hyperviscosity; light-chain components may lead to renal failure).

  2. Clinical features

     a. Median age at diagnosis is 65 years.

     b. The most common presenting complaints include anemia, bone pain (particularly in the low back or ribs), and infection. Less common presenting complaints include renal failure, spinal cord compression, and hyperviscosity syndrome.

     c. Some cases are found simply through abnormal laboratory studies, including hypercalcemia, proteinuria, and elevated erythrocyte sedimentation rate; follow-up electrophoresis will be abnormal.

  3. Laboratory studies

     a. Patients will be anemic, with normal cell morphology; rouleau formation is common.

     b. The hallmark of myeloma is a monoclonal spike on serum electrophoresis.

     c. Lytic lesions are present on radiography of the axial skeleton; generalized osteoporosis may be the only finding.

     d. Bone scans are not helpful, because multiple myeloma does not have an osteoblastic component. The usefulness of positron-emission tomography is being evaluated.

     e. Prognosis is evaluated based on bone marrow cytogenetic characteristics.

  4. Treatment options are changing rapidly and include thalidomide derivatives. Bisphosphonates are important adjuncts.

IV. BLEEDING DISORDERS

A. General characteristics

  1. Bleeding disorders involve excessive or repetitive bleeding or bleeding at unusual sites.

     a. If the bleeding is caused by problems with platelets, the mucosa and skin usually are involved (e.g., epistaxis, gum bleeding, menorrhagia). Petechiae are seen almost exclusively in thrombocytopenia rather than in platelet dysfunction.

     b. If the bleeding is caused by coagulation problems, the skin and muscles are involved; spontaneous hemarthroses are found only in severe hemophilia.

     c. Bleeding disorders may be classified as either congenital or acquired.

B. Clinical features vary with the cause of the bleeding.

  1. Congenital disorders usually involve single defects related to vascular integrity, platelet function, coagulation, or fibrinolytic systems.

  2. Acquired disorders involve more than one system (liver, kidneys, collagen vascular system, or immune system).

     a. Abnormal bleeding is seen with neoplasia, infection, malabsorption, shock, and obstetric complications.

     b. Drugs associated with bleeding include NSAIDs, aspirin, certain antibiotics, anticoagulants, thiazides, gold, and heparin.

     c. Systemic lupus erythematosus and CLL are common causes of secondary thrombocytopenic purpura.

C. Laboratory studies

  1. Initial assessment

     a. Platelet count, peripheral smear, and bleeding time should be analyzed in patients with suspected coagulation disorders.

     b. Prothrombin time (PT), partial thromboplastin time (PTT), and/or activated PTT are helpful in differentiating cause.

     c. Thrombin clotting time measures the rate of conversion of fibrinogen to fibrin in the presence of thrombin.

  2. Special studies should be done as indicated.

D. Thrombocytopenia

  1. General characteristics

     a. Thrombocytopenia is an abnormal decrease in the number of platelets in the blood. It is the most common cause of abnormal bleeding.

    b. It may be caused by impaired production, increased destruction, splenic sequestration, or dilution.

        (1) Acute idiopathic thrombocytopenic purpura (ITP) is a self-limited, autoimmune (IgG) disorder found most commonly in children of both sexes and is associated with a preceding viral upper respiratory infection.

        (2) Chronic ITP may occur at any age (peak incidence is 20–50 years) and is more common in women; it often coexists with other autoimmune diseases.

2. Clinical features

    a. Acute ITP is characterized by the abrupt appearance of petechiae, purpura, and hemorrhagic bullae on the skin and mucous membranes.

    b. Chronic ITP patients develop petechiae on the skin and mucous membranes.

    c. Patients are otherwise well and rarely febrile; other common presenting complaints are epistaxis, oral bleeding, and menorrhagia.

    d. Splenomegaly usually is not present.

    e. Heparin is the drug that most commonly causes an ITP-like reaction in hospitalized patients. Others include sulfonamides, quinine, thiazides, cimetidine, and gold. Other causes of secondary thrombocytopenia are systemic lupus erythematosus and CLL.

3. Laboratory findings

    a. Acute ITP shows decreased platelets (10,000–20,000 mcL), eosinophilia, and mild lymphocytosis.

    b. Chronic ITP shows platelet count of 25,000–75,000 mcL.

    c. Mild anemia may be present, unless autoimmune hemolytic anemia coexists (10%).

    d. Peripheral smear shows megathrombocytes; coagulation studies are normal.

4. Treatment

    a. Acute ITP usually resolves spontaneously; some patients require corticosteroids or splenectomy.

    b. Chronic ITP rarely resolves spontaneously; initial treatment is high-dose prednisone. For treatment failures, IV immunoglobulin, danazol, immunosuppressive therapy, and stem cell transplantation are used. Splenectomy is definitive and often required. Platelet transfusions may be used for life-threatening bleeding.

    c. Platelet antagonists (e.g., aspirin) should be avoided.

E. Platelet consumption syndromes

1. General characteristics. There are three major types of platelet consumption syndromes.

    a. Thrombotic thrombocytopenic purpura (TTP) is rare but often fatal. It is found in previously healthy people, most commonly between the ages of 20 and 50. It occurs more often in women than men and in patients with HIV disease. TTP may be precipitated by estrogen use, pregnancy, and drugs, such as quinine and ticlopidine.

    b. Hemolytic-uremic syndrome (HUS) is similar to TTP but is found primarily in children. Pregnancy and estrogen use may precipitate HUS in adults.

    c. DIC causes generalized hemorrhage in patients with severe underlying systemic illness, such as sepsis, tissue injury, obstetric complications, cancer, and in severe transfusion reactions.

2. Clinical features

    a. TTP is characterized by severe thrombocytopenia with purpura, petechiae, pallor, abdominal pain, microangiopathic hemolytic anemia, fever, abnormal neurologic signs, renal failure, and possibly, pancreatitis. Neurologic symptoms may wax and wane over minutes.

    b. HUS is similar to TTP but does not have associated neurologic findings. It has more renal problems than TTP. It affects primarily children younger than 10 years, particularly after infection with *Escherichia coli* 0157:H7, *Shigella* sp., *Salmonella* sp., and various viruses.

    c. In DIC, skin and mucous membrane bleeding (particularly at puncture/wound sites) and shock are more common; thrombosis (commonly digital ischemia and gangrene) less often predominates.

3. Laboratory findings

    a. TTP and HUS

        (1) Anemia, red cell fragmentation, normal leukocytes, polychromatophilia, reticulocytosis, and thrombocytopenia (less severe in HUS than in TTP) are found; Coombs' test is negative. ADAMTS 13 (a metalloprotease enzyme) is low.

        (2) LDH is markedly elevated; indirect bilirubin increases.

        (3) Coagulation tests are normal.

        (4) Renal insufficiency may be found.

    b. DIC

        (1) Evidence of coagulopathy includes hypofibrinogenemia, elevated fibrin degradation products (D-dimer is most sensitive), thrombocytopenia, and prolonged PT. ADAMTS 13 usually is absent.

        (2) Microangiopathic hemolytic anemia with fragmented red cells is present in 25% of cases.

  4. Treatment

    a. TTP

        (1) TTP requires emergency large-volume plasmapheresis.

        (2) Prednisone and antiplatelet agents have also been used.

    b. HUS

        (1) In children, conservative management usually is all that is required. Fluids and management of electrolyte imbalance are important.

        (2) Treatment of adults is plasmapheresis.

    c. DIC

        (1) Treatment primarily is prompt and aggressive therapy for the underlying cause.

        (2) Component blood transfusions are important, particularly the replacement of fibrinogen through the administration of cryoprecipitate. The role of heparin is controversial.

F. Disorders of platelet function

  1. General characteristics

    a. Congenital abnormalities are varied; most result in normal counts and morphology but prolonged bleeding time.

    b. Acquired platelet dysfunction are more common than congenital.

        (1) The most common causes of acquired platelet dysfunction are aspirin and other NSAIDs.

        (2) Acquired platelet dysfunction also is seen with the use of certain other drugs, uremia, alcoholism, myeloproliferative diseases, hypothermia, various vitamin deficiencies, and other conditions.

  2. Clinical features are prolonged bleeding time and skin and mucosal bleeding.

  3. Laboratory findings indicate a normal number of platelets, but platelet function study results are abnormal.

  4. Treatment

    a. In drug-related cases, the drug should be discontinued.

    b. Dialysis may help patients with uremia.

    c. Transfusion with platelets is necessary for serious bleeding.

G. Disorders associated with coagulation protein defects

  1. Von Willebrand's disease

    a. General characteristics

        (1) Von Willebrand's disease is an autosomal dominant, congenital bleeding disorder. It is the most common congenital coagulopathy. Most cases are mild.

        (2) It is characterized by reduced levels of factor VIII antigen or ristocetin cofactor.

        (3) Both men and women may be affected.

        (4) It occurs in six major types, all characterized by deficient or defective von Willebrand factor (vWF). Type I accounts for 75–80% of cases.

    b. Clinical features

        (1) Bleeding occurs in nasal, sinus, vaginal, and GI mucous membranes.

        (2) Spontaneous hemarthrosis and soft-tissue bleeds are less common than in hemophilia A.

        (3) Bleeding is exacerbated by aspirin and decreases with use of estrogen or pregnancy.

    c. Laboratory findings

        (1) Bleeding time is usually prolonged, particularly following aspirin use.

        (2) vWF is low.

    d. Treatment varies according to the type of disease.

        (1) Desmopressin acetate is useful in type I.

        (2) Factor VIII concentrates are preferred if factor replacement is necessary.

2. Hemophilia A (factor VIII deficiency or classic hemophilia)

   a. General characteristics

   (1) Hemophilia A is a hereditary disease characterized by excessively prolonged coagulation time.

   (2) It is the most severe bleeding disorder and the most common congenital coagulopathy after von Willebrand's disease.

   (3) It is X-linked recessive and occurs in about 1/10,000 male births.

   (4) Recent genetic mutation causes one-third of all cases of hemophilia A.

   (5) Many patients are seropositive for HIV because of infected factor VIII transfusions.

   b. Clinical features

   (1) Severely affected patients have repeated spontaneous hemorrhagic episodes with hemarthroses, epistaxis, intracranial bleeding, hematemesis, melena, microscopic hematuria, and bleeding into the soft tissue and gingiva.

   (2) Less severely affected patients may experience excessive bleeding following trauma or surgery.

   c. Laboratory findings

   (1) PTT is prolonged.

   (2) PT, bleeding time, fibrinogen level, and platelet count are normal.

   (3) Factor assay shows reduced factor VIII:C levels; vWF is normal.

   (4) Low platelet count suggests HIV-related immune thrombocytopenia.

   (5) Female carriers will have low or normal factor VIII:C and normal factor VIII antigen.

   d. Treatment

   (1) Infusion of heat-treated or recombinant factor VIII concentrates is standard treatment.

   (2) Desmopressin may elevate factor VIII levels in patients with mild to moderate disease.

   (3) Patients should avoid aspirin.

3. Hemophilia B, also known as factor IX deficiency or Christmas disease, is a heterogeneous group of disorders similar to hemophilia A but occurring less frequently. It is an X-linked recessive disorder affecting males.

4. Factor XI deficiency is a usually mild, autosomal recessive disorder seen primarily in Ashkenazi Jews. It is treated with fresh-frozen plasma.

5. Vitamin K–dependent factor deficiencies

   a. General characteristics

   (1) These are the most common acquired coagulopathies.

   (2) Deficiencies may be secondary to poor diet, liver failure, malabsorption, malnutrition, and use of some drugs, especially broad-spectrum antibiotics.

   b. Clinical features

   (1) The typical patient is postoperative, not eating well, and receiving broad-spectrum antibiotics that suppress colonic bacteria.

   (2) Features of the underlying cause are evident.

   (3) Soft-tissue bleeding may occur.

   c. Laboratory findings

   (1) PT is prolonged, and PTT may be prolonged.

   (2) Fibrinogen, thrombin time, and platelet count are normal.

   (3) Liver enzymes may be elevated.

   (4) Levels of vitamin K and factors II, VII, IX, and X are decreased.

   d. Treatment

   (1) Treatment is directed at the underlying cause.

   (2) Parenteral vitamin K rapidly restores factor production.

   (3) Treat hemorrhage with fresh-frozen plasma.

   (4) Prevention includes a diet high in leafy vegetables and treatment of malabsorption.

V. THROMBOTIC DISORDERS AND HYPERCOAGULABLE CONDITIONS

A. General characteristics

    1. Predisposing factors in patients who present with thrombus include:

        a. Age older than 40 years

        b. Venous thrombosis in the neck, arms, abdomen, or central nervous system; arterial thrombosis may result in large vessel or microvascular events.

        c. Recurrent thrombosis

        d. Family history of thrombosis

        e. Repeated thrombosis despite adequate anticoagulation, which suggests a neoplasm

    2. Congenital disorders associated with thrombotic states typically are autosomal dominant.

    3. Acquired hypercoagulable states are associated with malignancy (Trousseau's syndrome), pregnancy, nephrotic syndrome, ingestion of certain medications (especially oral contraceptive agents and pure estrogen compounds), immobilization, myeloproliferative disease, ulcerative colitis and Crohn's disease, Behçet's syndrome, intravascular devices, DIC, hyperlipidemia (particularly familial type II hyperbetalipoproteinemia), paroxysmal nocturnal hemoglobinuria, TTP-HUS, hyperviscosity syndrome, anticardiolipin antibodies, heparin-induced thrombocytopenia, and antiphospholipid syndrome.

    4. Heparin use is a rare but important cause and is not dose dependent. Thrombocytopenia also is associated with heparin-induced thrombosis.

    5. Congenital causes include antithrombin III deficiency, factor V Leiden, protein C deficiency, protein S deficiency, dysfibrogenemia, abnormal plasminogen, and activated protein C resistance.

    6. Lupus anticoagulant

        a. An IgM or IgG immunoglobulin is seen in 5–10% of patients with systemic lupus erythematosus but is more common in persons without lupus or in those taking phenothiazines.

        b. It causes bleeding in conjunction with an additional bleeding disorder and is associated with risk of thrombosis and spontaneous abortion.

B. Clinical features include typical signs and symptoms of arterial or venous thrombus formation.

C. PTT is prolonged; Russell viper venom time is specific to lupus anticoagulant.

D. Treatment

    1. Prednisone usually eliminates lupus anticoagulant.

    2. Treatment for thrombosis is standard anticoagulation; low-molecular-weight heparin may be preferred.

    3. If caused by heparin, all heparin must be withheld from the patient.

    4. No prophylaxis is indicated in an at-risk person who has not had a previous thrombotic event.

    5. At-risk persons with previous thrombotic events should be anticoagulated for prolonged periods.

Gastroenterology

Susan LeLacheur

I. DISEASES OF THE ESOPHAGUS

A. Gastroesophageal reflux disease (GERD; reflux esophagitis)

1. General characteristics

a. Reflux esophagitis is the recurrent reflux of gastric contents into the distal esophagus because of mechanical or functional abnormality of the lower esophageal sphincter.

b. GERD is present in an estimated 10% of the population; up to 60% of the population experiences heartburn at some point in their lives. In infants, about 50% have reflux, but less than 10% have evidence of esophagitis.

c. In a minority of patients, reflux causes erosion of the esophagus that leads to Barrett esophagitis (replacement of normal squamous epithelium with metaplastic columnar epithelium), which can predispose to malignancy.

d. Factors that protect the esophagus include gravity, lower esophageal sphincter tone, esophageal motility, salivary flow, gastric emptying, and tissue resistance.

2. Clinical features

a. Heartburn is the most common presenting feature, generally is worse after meals and when lying down, and often is relieved with antacids. Regurgitation or dysphagia may occur.

b. Hoarseness, halitosis, cough, hiccupping, and atypical chest pain are less common symptoms of reflux.

3. Laboratory studies

a. Barium swallow is indicated in patients with dysphagia; it may identify an associated large hiatal hernia (small hernias generally do not contribute to the disease).

b. Endoscopy is indicated when symptoms are severe or do not respond to medical therapy.

c. Endoscopy with biopsy describes the presence and extent of mucosal damage.

d. pH monitoring (to monitor reflux) can be done with an intraesophageal electrode. This can confirm and quantify pathology and is indicated in patients who do not respond to treatment, who have recurrence after treatment, or who need surgical treatment.

4. Treatment

a. Lifestyle modifications should be implemented on presumptive diagnosis, with further workup if symptoms persist. Appropriate lifestyle modifications include cessation of smoking, avoidance of eating at bedtime, avoidance of large meals, and avoidance of foods that cause irritation.

b. Pharmacotherapy

(1) Antacids or alginic acid (Gaviscon) may be used for mild symptoms.

(2) Histamine (H_2) blockers may be used, but generally in larger doses than for peptic ulcer disease. H_2-blockers are first-line treatment for mild GERD.

(3) An acid-suppressant proton-pump inhibitor (PPI; omeprazole, lansoprazole, rabeprazole, pantoprazole, or esomeprazole) is the most powerful anti-GERD medication. PPIs are first-line treatment in moderate to severe disease or in patients who are unresponsive to H_2-blockers or have evidence of erosive gastritis.

(4) A combination of an H_2-blocker at bedtime and a PPI in the daytime may be helpful in patients with significant nighttime symptoms.

(5) Anticholinergic, β-adrenergic, and calcium channel–blocking agents decrease lower esophageal sphincter pressure and, therefore, should be avoided.

c. Surgical and endoscopic techniques are available for refractory cases but have not been shown to prevent complications of the disease.

B. Infectious esophagitis

1. General characteristics

a. Infectious esophagitis is rare, except in immunocompromised persons.

b. Causes

    (1) Fungal. *Candida* sp. should be considered, especially if oral thrush is present.

    (2) Viral. Cytomegalovirus (CMV) and herpes simplex virus are common causes.

    (3) HIV, *Mycobacterium tuberculosis*, Epstein-Barr virus, and *Mycobacterium avium intracellulare* are additional but uncommon causes of infectious esophagitis.

2. Clinical features. The main clinical feature is odynophagia (painful swallowing) or dysphagia (difficult swallowing) in an immunocompromised patient.

3. Laboratory findings

    a. Endoscopy in patients with CMV or HIV reveals large, deep ulcers. Infection with herpes simplex virus is characterized by multiple shallow ulcers. Candidal infection shows white plaques.

    b. Cytology or culture from endoscopic brushings is needed for definitive diagnosis.

4. Treatment

    a. Treatment is specific to the type of infection.

    b. Fluconazole or ketoconazole for *Candida* sp.

    c. Acyclovir for herpes simplex virus.

    d. Ganciclovir for CMV.

C. Esophageal dysmotility

1. General characteristics

    a. Disorders of esophageal motility include neurogenic dysphagia, Zenker's diverticulum, esophageal stenosis, achalasia, diffuse esophageal spasm, and scleroderma.

    b. Dysmotility can be caused by neurologic factors, intrinsic or external blockage, or malfunction of esophageal peristalsis.

2. Clinical features

    a. Dysphagia is the most common presenting symptom for all motility disorders. Its presentation can help to determine the underlying cause.

    b. Neurogenic dysphagia causes difficulty with both liquids and solids and is caused by injury or disease of the brainstem or the cranial nerves involved in swallowing.

    c. Zenker's diverticulum is an outpouching of the posterior hypopharynx that can cause regurgitation of undigested food and liquid into the pharynx several hours after eating.

    d. Esophageal stenosis causes dysphagia for solid foods. Slow progression of solid food dysphagia indicates a more benign process (e.g., webs or rings), and rapid progression indicates malignancy.

    e. Achalasia is a global esophageal motor disorder in which peristalsis is decreased and lower esophageal sphincter tone is increased, causing slowly progressive dysphagia with episodic regurgitation and chest pain.

    f. Diffuse esophageal spasm is characterized by dysphagia or intermittent chest pain that may or may not be associated with eating.

    g. Scleroderma eventually progresses to involve the esophagus in most patients with the disease, causing decreased esophageal sphincter tone and peristalsis, predisposing the patient to the symptoms and complications of reflux esophagitis.

3. Laboratory findings

    a. Barium swallow can reveal both structural and motor abnormalities of the esophagus that may cause dysphagia. Achalasia typically has a "parrot-beaked" appearance (i.e., a dilated esophagus tapering to the distal obstruction) on barium swallow.

    b. Pharyngoscopy or esophagoscopy must be done (generally by an otolaryngologist) to clarify the nature of a structural lesion.

    c. Esophageal manometry can be used to assess the strength and coordination of peristalsis.

4. Treatment

    a. Neurogenic dysphagia must be managed by treating the underlying disease.

    b. Strictures

        (1) Most benign strictures can be managed by dilation.

        (2) Malignant strictures must be resected.

D. Esophageal neoplasms

    1. General characteristics

        a. About 95% of esophageal neoplasms are squamous cell carcinomas.

        b. Local spread to the mediastinum is common, because the esophagus has no serosa.

        c. The majority of esophageal cancers in the United States are related to cigarette smoking and chronic alcohol use. Contributing factors include exposure to other caustic agents (e.g., nitrosamines, fungal toxins, other carcinogens), hot foods, mucosal abnormalities, poor oral hygiene, and human papilloma virus.

    2. Clinical features. The main clinical feature of esophageal cancer is progressive dysphagia for solid food associated with marked weight loss.

    3. Laboratory findings

        a. Endoscopy with brushings is used for diagnosis.

        b. Endoscopic sonography and CT may be used for staging.

    4. Treatment

        a. Treatment of esophageal cancer is surgical.

        b. Because the disease often is advanced on discovery, it is associated with a low (5–10%) 5-year survival rate.

E. Mallory-Weiss tear

    1. A Mallory-Weiss tear is a linear mucosal tear in the esophagus, generally at the gastroesophageal junction, that occurs with forceful vomiting or retching causing hematemesis.

    2. A Mallory-Weiss tear often is associated with alcohol use, but it should be considered in all cases of upper GI bleed.

    3. Diagnosis is established by endoscopy.

    4. Most episodes resolve without treatment, but endoscopic injection of epinephrine or thermal coagulation may be required.

F. Esophageal varices

    1. General characteristics

        a. Esophageal varices are dilations of the veins of the esophagus, generally at the distal end.

        b. The underlying cause in adults is portal hypertension, most commonly caused by cirrhosis either from alcohol abuse or from chronic viral hepatitis. Use of nonsteroidal anti-inflammatory drugs (NSAIDs) can exacerbate bleeding (hepatic vein obstruction).

        c. Budd-Chiari syndrome may cause thrombosis of the portal vein, leading to esophageal varices.

    2. Diagnosis

        a. Diagnosis generally is established clinically when a patient with signs of cirrhosis presents with hematemesis.

        b. Varices generally are asymptomatic until they bleed, at which point they frequently are life-threatening.

    3. Treatment

        a. Hemodynamic support with high-volume fluid replacement and vasopressors and immediate control of bleeding is necessary, because bleeding varices have high mortality (~approximately 30% with first bleed and 50% within 6 weeks).

        b. Endoscopic therapy and pharmacologic vasoconstriction (e.g., octreotide) are the preferred therapy.

II. DISEASES OF THE STOMACH

A. Gastritis and duodenitis

    1. General characteristics

        a. Gastritis and duodenitis can be defined as inflammation of the stomach or duodenum.

        b. Protective factors

            (1) Protective factors include mucus, bicarbonate, mucosal blood flow, prostaglandins, alkaline state, hydrophobic layer, and epithelial renewal.

            (2) Any imbalance in protective factors can lead to inflammation.

        c. Causes

            (1) Autoimmune disorders (e.g., pernicious anemia) and other noninfectious factors cause type A gastritis, which involves the body of the stomach.

     (2) *Helicobacter pylori* (HP) is a Gram-negative, spiral-shaped bacillus. It is implicated in almost all non–NSAID–induced GI mucosal inflammation.

       (a) HP causes type B gastritis, which involves the antrum and body of the stomach.

       (b) HP tolerates well the acidity of a normal stomach and also is associated with peptic ulcer, gastric adenocarcinoma, and gastric lymphoma.

     (3) NSAIDs can cause gastric injury by diminishing local prostaglandin production in the stomach or duodenum.

     (4) Stress from central nervous system injury, burns, sepsis, or surgery can lead to erosion of the stomach or duodenum.

     (5) Alcohol use is another leading cause of gastritis.

  2. Clinical features

    a. The clinical features of gastritis generally reflect the underlying syndrome rather than the gastric injury itself.

    b. Dyspepsia and abdominal pain are common indicators of gastritis.

  3. Laboratory studies

    a. Endoscopy with biopsy reveals the location and extent of gastritis as well as the presence of HP.

    b. A urea breath test can be used to detect HP, because urea is a product of the bacterial metabolism. Fecal antigen testing or serology for HP also are helpful.

    c. Specific tests for underlying conditions (e.g., vitamin B_{12} level, CBC for pernicious anemia) should be used as indicated by history.

  4. Treatment

    a. Remove the causative factor (e.g., NSAID, alcohol).

    b. Treat the underlying cause.

B. Delayed gastric emptying

  1. General characteristics

    a. Delayed gastric emptying can be defined as an alteration in gastric motility.

    b. Causes include myopathic diseases of the smooth muscles and neurologic dysfunction.

  2. Clinical features include nausea and a feeling of excessive fullness after meals.

  3. Treatment. Prokinetic medications (e.g., cisapride, metoclopramide) can sometimes help to speed the movement of food through the stomach.

C. Peptic ulcer disease (PUD)

  1. General characteristics

    a. PUD describes any ulcer of the upper digestive system (e.g., gastric ulcer, duodenal ulcer).

    b. Causes. Any discreet break in mucosa caused by injury, NSAIDs, stress, ethanol, or other irritants will lead to an ulcer.

     (1) HP is the most common cause of PUD.

     (2) When HP is the cause, the ulcer disease can be eradicated with treatment.

    c. The lifetime risk of ulcer disease is 5–10%.

    d. Men and women are equally affected.

    e. Both gastric ulcers and HP are highly associated with gastric malignancy. Although most patients with HP or a gastric ulcer will not get gastric cancer, almost all patients with cancer have had HP or a gastric ulcer.

  2. Differential diagnosis. Dyspepsia, abdominal pain, discomfort, or nausea often is associated with gastric or duodenal ulcers but also can occur in a variety of other conditions, including gastritis, malignancy, and ischemic heart disease.

  3. Clinical features

    a. Abdominal pain or discomfort is the primary clinical feature.

     (1) The pain may be described as burning or gnawing and often radiates to the back.

     (2) The pain of a duodenal ulcer often improves with food, whereas the pain of a gastric ulcer typically worsens, causing associated weight loss.

    b. Dyspepsia (belching, bloating, distention, heartburn) or nausea also is reported.

    c. Complications include bleeding, perforation, and penetration.

       (1) Bleeding typically manifests as melena.

       (2) PUD is the most common cause of non-hemorrhagic GI bleeds.

4. Laboratory studies

    a. Endoscopy is best for detecting small or healing ulcers. It differentiates gastritis from ulcer disease and allows immediate biopsy of gastric or suspicious ulcers to rule out malignancy.

    b. Barium radiography was once widely used and cheaper, but it is less sensitive, with a 30% false-negative rate. Endoscopy is more sensitive and definitive.

    c. Rapid urease test via endoscope is test of choice for HP. If negative and still suspicious, histopathologic studies and culture can be done at large academic centers.

    d. Nonendoscopic tests for HP include HP antibodies (serum, plasma, or whole blood), urea breath test, or fecal antigens.

5. Treatment

    a. Irritating factors (smoking, NSAIDs, alcohol) should be avoided.

    b. Antacids, H_2-blockers, and sucralfate generally heal duodenal ulcers within 4–6 weeks and gastric ulcers within 8 weeks.

    c. Combination therapy for HP accelerates healing and prevents recurrence. Regimen options include:

       (1) PPI with clarithromycin and amoxicillin

       (2) Bismuth subsalicylate plus tetracycline, metronidazole, and PPI

       (3) Ranitidine bismuth citrate, clarithromycin and amoxicillin, tetracycline, or metronidazole

    d. Prophylactic treatment with misoprostol or a PPI should be considered in patients with a history of ulcer who require daily NSAID use; a history of complications, such as a bleed; a need for chronic steroids or anticoagulants; or significant other comorbidities.

D. Gastric neoplasm

    1. Zollinger-Ellison syndrome (ZES)

       a. General characteristics

         (1) In ZES, a gastrin-secreting tumor (gastrinoma) causes hypergastrinemia, which results in refractory PUD.

         (2) Only 1% of cases of PUD are caused by ZES.

         (3) Most gastrinomas are found in the pancreas or duodenum, but they may be found anywhere or may metastasize.

         (4) About 20% of gastrinomas are part of a syndrome known as multiple endocrine neoplasia, type I.

       b. Clinical features

         (1) Most commonly, the clinical presentation is indistinguishable from that of PUD, although ZES usually is more advanced or refractory to treatment.

         (2) Abdominal pain may be accompanied by a secretory diarrhea that improves with H_2-blockers (ranitidine, cimetidine) or PPIs (omeprazole, lansoprazole).

         (3) Occult or frank bleeding, causing anemia, may be present.

       c. Laboratory findings

         (1) A fasting gastrin level of greater than 150 pg/mL indicates hypergastrinemia.

         (2) A secretin test is needed to confirm the presence of ZES.

           (a) Patients are given secretin, 2 U/kg IV.

           (b) In most patients with ZES, the gastrin levels will increase by more than 200 pg/mL.

         (3) Endoscopy, CT, or MRI may help to localize the tumor.

       d. Treatment

         (1) Use of PPIs controls gastrin secretion.

         (2) Surgical resection of the gastrinoma should be attempted when possible.

    2. Gastric adenocarcinoma

       a. General characteristics

         (1) Gastric adenocarcinoma is among the most common types of cancer worldwide but is less common in the United States.

(2) Gastric adenocarcinoma is almost twice as common in men as in women.

(3) It almost never occurs in a patient younger than 40 years.

(4) With early diagnosis, an 80% cure rate can be accomplished. If the muscularis propria is involved, the cure rate is 50%, but if there is lymphatic spread, the cure rate is 10%.

(5) There is a strong association of gastric adenocarcinoma with HP.

b. Clinical features

(1) Dyspepsia and weight loss associated with anemia and occult GI bleeding in a patient older than 40 years are the common presenting complaints.

(2) Progressive dysphagia may be caused by a neoplasm impinging on the esophagus.

(3) Postprandial vomiting may be caused by a neoplasm near the pylorus.

(4) Signs of metastatic spread include left supraclavicular lymphadenopathy (Virchow's node) and an umbilical nodule (Sister Mary Joseph nodule).

c. Laboratory studies

(1) Iron deficiency anemia is the most common finding.

(2) Liver enzymes may be elevated with hepatic metastases.

(3) Endoscopy with cytology should be done on any patient older than 40 years with dyspepsia who is unresponsive to therapy.

(4) After the diagnosis has been established, abdominal CT is used to determine the extent of disease.

d. Treatment

(1) Treatment is either curative or palliative resection of the tumor.

(2) Chemotherapy or radiation may provide some palliative benefit.

3. Carcinoid tumors of the stomach rarely occur in response to hypergastrinemia and generally are benign and self-limited.

4. Gastric lymphoma

a. General characteristics

(1) Gastric lymphomas account for less than 2% of gastric malignancies, but the stomach is the most common extranodal site for non-Hodgkin's lymphoma.

(2) The risk of gastric lymphoma is greater by sixfold if HP infection is present.

b. Clinical features. Clinical features are the same as those for gastric adenocarcinoma.

c. Laboratory findings. Findings differ from those of gastric adenocarcinoma only in the pathology of the lesion.

d. Treatment. Treatment is resection with or without radiation or chemotherapy.

III. DISEASES OF THE SMALL INTESTINE AND COLON

A. Diarrhea

1. Diarrhea is increased frequency or volume of stool (e.g., three or more liquid or semisolid stools daily for at least 2–3 consecutive days).

2. Causes of diarrhea may be infectious (Table 5-1), toxic, dietary (e.g., laxative use), or other GI disease.

3. Patient history. The history should include all current medications as well as illness among others who have shared meals with the patient.

4. Clinical features

a. Secretory diarrhea (large volume without inflammation) indicates pancreatic insufficiency, ingestion of preformed bacterial toxins, or laxative use.

b. Inflammatory diarrhea (bloody diarrhea with fever) indicates invasive organisms or inflammatory bowel disease.

c. Antibiotic-associated diarrhea almost is always caused by *Clostridium difficile* colitis, which in the most severe cases causes the classic pseudomembranous colitis.

5. Laboratory findings

a. WBCs in stool denote an inflammatory process.

b. Cultures for bacterial agents, microscopy for parasites, or toxin identification (if enterotoxic *Escherichia coli* or *Clostridium difficile* is suspected) can identify infectious agents in stool.

TABLE 5-1	Foodborne and Waterborne Causes of Diarrhea						
Agent	**Source**	**Onset**	**Nausea and Vomiting**	**Diarrhea**	**Fever**	**Duration**	**Therapy**
Norwalk virus	Food, water	1–3 days	Yes	Watery	Low grade	1–2 days	Hydration
Rotavirus	Person to person	1–3 days	Yes	Watery	Low grade	5–8 days	Hydration
Staphylococcus aureus (toxin)	Food, after cooking	1–7 hr	Yes, rapid onset	Cramping, some diarrhea	Uncommon	Acute (4–6 hr); total (1–2 days)	Supportive
Clostridium perfringens (toxin)	Food, before cooking	8–14 hr	Uncommon	Cramping, watery	Rare	<24 hr	Supportive
Vibrio spp. (cholera)	Water	2–3 days	Some	Profuse, watery	Rare	Days	Hydration
Enterotoxic *Escherichia coli*	Food	5–15 days	Some	Cramping, watery	Low grade	1–5 days	Hydration, bismuth/loperamide
Giardia lamblia	Water, person to person	5–25 days	Nausea	Diarrhea, bloating	None possible	Until treated	Metronidazole, 250 mg twice a day for 10 days
Cryptosporidia	Water, outbreaks	2–10 days	Yes	Watery	Possible	30 days (unless HIV)	Supportive, HIV treatment
Cyclospora	Imported, uncooked foods	7 days	Nausea, anorexia	Watery	Low grade	Weeks	Trimethoprim/sulfamethoxazole twice a day for 7 days
Salmonella (invasive)	Poultry	6–72 hr	Nausea, some vomiting	Purulent	Yes, septicemia common	4–7 days	Hydration
Enterohemorrhagic *Escherichia coli* (invasive)	Undercooked ground beef	12–60 hr	No	Purulent, bloody, cramping	Yes	5–10 days	Supportive unless severe
Shigella (invasive)	Fecal–oral	1–6 days	No	Purulent, bloody, cramping	Yes	1–7 days	Supportive
Campylobacter (invasive)	Undercooked poultry	2–5 days	Some	Purulent, bloody, cramping	Yes	2–5 days	Supportive

ASA, acetylsalicylic acid.

6. Treatment
   a. Supportive therapy is sufficient for most patients with viral or bacterial diarrhea.
   b. Antibiotics may be indicated for patients with severe diarrhea and systemic symptoms (e.g., *Shigella* sp., *Campylobacter* sp., severe cases of *Clostridium difficile*).
   c. Treatment of the underlying cause is required for noninfectious diarrhea.
B. Constipation
   1. General characteristics
      a. Normal bowel function ranges from three stools per day to three stools per week. Constipation is a decrease in stool volume and an increase in stool firmness accompanied by straining.
      b. Patients older than 50 years with new-onset constipation should be evaluated for colon cancer.

2. Treatment
   a. In most cases, an increase in fiber (to 10–20 g daily) and fluid intake (up to 1.5–2 L/day), and increased exercise will resolve the problem.
   b. A patient with constipation lasting for more than 2 weeks or with constipation refractory to modifications in diet, exercise, and fluid intake should undergo further investigation to detect the underlying cause. If a treatable underlying cause is found, constipation will resolve with treatment of the disease process.

C. Small bowel obstruction
   1. Clinical features
      a. Obstruction presents with abdominal pain, distention, vomiting of partially digested food, and obstipation.
      b. Bowel sounds are high-pitched and come in rushes. Upright radiographs may illustrate air–fluid levels.
   2. Treatment is surgical, with large bowel obstruction being more urgent than small bowel obstruction.

D. Malabsorption
   1. General characteristics
      a. Malabsorption may involve a single nutrient, as with pernicious anemia (vitamin B_{12}) or lactase deficiency (lactose), or it may be global, as with celiac disease or AIDS.
      b. Malabsorption may be caused by problems in digestion, absorption, or impaired blood and lymph flow.
   2. Clinical features
      a. Diarrhea usually is the primary complaint and may be accompanied by bloating and abdominal discomfort.
      b. Weight loss and edema also may be present.
      c. Steatorrhea may occur.
      d. Specific deficiencies may cause bone demineralization, tetany, bleeding, or anemia.
   3. Laboratory findings
      a. If a 72-hour fecal fat test is normal, specific defects, such as pancreatic insufficiency and abnormal bile salt metabolism, should be considered.
      b. A D-xylose test will distinguish maldigestion (e.g., pancreatic insufficiency, bile salt deficiency) from malabsorption.
      c. Specific tests may be used to detect vitamin B_{12}, calcium, or albumin deficiency.
   4. Therapeutic trials of the following can help in both diagnosis and treatment.
      a. Lactose-free diet for lactase deficiency.
      b. Gluten-free diet for celiac disease.
      c. Pancreatic enzyme replacement for pancreatic insufficiency.
      d. Antibiotics may be indicated for specific bacterial infections if the agent is known.

E. Crohn's disease (regional enteritis)
   1. General characteristics
      a. Crohn's disease is an inflammatory bowel disease for which there is some genetic predisposition, although the cause is unknown. Crohn's disease must be differentiated from ulcerative colitis (Table 5-2).
      b. Crohn's disease may involve both the small and large bowels as well as the mouth, esophagus, and stomach. Most commonly, the terminal ileum and right colon are involved, but the rectum frequently is spared.
      c. Complications include fistulas, abscesses, aphthous ulcers, renal stones, and predisposition to colonic cancer.
      d. The success or failure of treatment is variable. The disease usually waxes and wanes throughout life.

TABLE 5-2 **Differentiation of Crohn's Disease and Ulcerative Colitis**

Characteristic	Crohn's Disease	Ulcerative Colitis
Onset	Gradual	Sudden or gradual
Distribution	Mouth to anus, predominantly, right-sided; skips areas	Distal to proximal, continuous
Symptoms	Diarrhea and pain	Bloody, pus-filled diarrhea, tenesmus
Complications	Fistulas (common), toxic megacolon, colon cancer	Toxic megacolon, colon cancer

2. Clinical features

    a. Abdominal cramps and diarrhea in a patient younger than 40 years are the most common presenting complaints.

    b. Low-grade fever, polyarthralgia, anemia, and fatigue frequently are encountered.

    c. Blood often is present in stool.

3. Laboratory findings

    a. A double-contrast barium enema or CT will show cobblestone-pattern filling defects with segmental areas of involvement (skip lesions). Fistulas and strictures also may be found.

    b. Colonoscopy is valuable in establishing the correct diagnosis, determining the extent and severity of disease, and guiding treatment. Contrast studies and endoscopic procedures should be avoided in patients with fulminant disease because of the possibility of inducing toxic megacolon.

    c. Biopsy will reveal involvement of the entire bowel wall in Crohn's disease. Granulomas are frequent.

    d. Blood tests may include increased sedimentation rate, anemia, and nutritional and electrolyte imbalances during exacerbations.

4. Treatment

    a. Aminosalicylates (sulfasalazine, mesalamine, others; available in oral, enema, or suppository forms) are the first step in medical treatment. Metronidazole or ciprofloxacin is added in perianal disease, fissures, or fistulae.

    b. Oral corticosteroids may be added if needed; they are highly effective in reducing symptoms but should be used for short-term treatment only. Steroids should be tapered as soon as possible to reduce the risk of long term side effects.

    c. If disease is refractory or frequent flare-ups require corticosteroids, consider immunomodulatory agents (6-mercaptopurine or azathioprine). These agents have a slower onset and can be quite toxic. Infliximab, a monoclonal antibody against tumor necrosis factor α, also is approved for use in severe Crohn's disease but is very expensive.

    d. Surgery is not curative in Crohn's disease and is reserved for treatment of complications. Segmental resection is the approach of choice.

F. Ulcerative colitis

  1. General characteristics

    a. Ulcerative colitis must be differentiated from inflammatory infectious conditions (Table 5-1) and from Crohn's disease (Table 5-2).

    b. The disease generally starts distally, at the rectum, and progresses proximally. Disease is continuous, skip areas are not seen.

    c. Onset generally is gradual but also can be abrupt.

  2. Clinical features

    a. Tenesmus and bloody, pus-filled diarrhea are the most common symptoms.

    b. Pain is less common but may occur, typically in the lower left quadrant.

    c. Weight loss, malaise, and fever may occur in more severe disease.

    d. Toxic megacolon and malignancy are more likely in ulcerative colitis than in Crohn's disease.

    e. Other complications include scleritis and episcleritis, arthritides, sclerosing cholangitis, and skin manifestations (erythema nodosum and pyoderma gangrenosum).

  3. Laboratory findings

    a. Anemia, increased sedimentation rate, and decreased serum albumin are common.

    b. Abdominal plain-film radiography may show colonic dilatation. Sigmoidoscopy or colonoscopy is the best method of establishing the diagnosis.

    c. Colonoscopy and barium enema should be avoided in acute disease because of the risks of perforation and toxic megacolon.

  4. Treatment

    a. Topical or oral aminosalicylates and corticosteroids are the mainstays of medical treatment. Immunomodulators are indicated for refractory disease.

    b. Surgery can be curative in ulcerative colitis. Segmental resection is possible, but total proctocolectomy is the most common surgical cure.

G. Irritable bowel syndrome (IBS)

  1. General characteristics

  a. IBS is a functional disorder without a known pathology. It is thought to be a combination of altered motility, hypersensitivity to intestinal distention, and psychological distress.

  b. IBS is the most common cause of chronic or recurrent abdominal pain in the United States.

  c. IBS generally remains an intermittent, lifelong problem. Symptoms typically begin during early to mid adulthood.

  d. IBS is more common in women than in men. Exacerbations may be associated with menses.

  e. IBS is a diagnosis of exclusion. The differential diagnosis includes lactose intolerance, cholecystitis, chronic pancreatitis, intestinal obstruction, chronic peritonitis, and carcinoma of the pancreas or stomach.

  2. Clinical features

  a. Physical examination generally is normal but may include a tender, palpable sigmoid colon and hyperresonance on percussion over the abdomen.

  b. Abdominal pain may occur anywhere or may be localized to the hypogastrium or left lower quadrant.

  (1) Pain may be worsened by food intake and typically is relieved with defecation.

  (2) Pain may be associated with bowel distention from accumulation of gas and associated spasm of the smooth muscle; postprandial urgency is common.

  c. IBS is strongly identified with changes in stool frequency and character. Constipation, diarrhea, or alternating constipation and diarrhea may occur.

  d. Dyspepsia is common.

  e. Urinary frequency and urgency are common in women.

  3. Laboratory findings generally are normal.

  a. The stool should be tested for blood, bacteria, parasites, and lactose tolerance.

  b. Barium enema, ultrasonography, or CT should be performed to rule out other pathology.

  c. Endoscopic studies are indicated in patients with persistent symptoms, weight loss or anorexia, bleeding, or history of other GI pathology.

  4. Treatment

  a. Reassurance and a strong provider–patient relationship are key. Avoidance of any known triggers is important.

  b. A high-fiber diet and bulking agents, such as psyllium hydrophilic mucilloid, are the mainstays of treatment.

  c. Antispasmodics, antidiarrheals, prokinetics, or antidepressants can be used if indicated by the patient's symptoms or course of illness.

H. Intussusception

  1. General characteristics

  a. Intussusception is the invagination of a proximal segment of the bowel into the portion just distal to it.

  b. It occurs most commonly in children (95% of cases), generally following a viral infection.

  c. In adults, intussusception almost always is caused by a neoplasm.

  2. Clinical features

  a. Children will exhibit signs of severe, colicky pain. Stool, if passed, will contain mucus and blood (currant jelly stools). A sausage-like mass may be felt on abdominal examination.

  b. Adults may present with a more indolent course of crampy abdominal pain. Bloody stool and abdominal mass are rare.

  3. Laboratory findings

  a. For children, barium or air enema may be both diagnostic and therapeutic.

  b. For adults, barium enema should not be used, and abdominal plain-film radiography shows nonspecific obstruction. CT is the best means of establishing the diagnosis, but many cases are diagnosed only at surgery.

  4. Treatment

  a. Barium enema may be curative for children; if not, surgery is needed.

  b. Adults generally require surgery.

I. Diverticular disease

  1. General characteristics

  a. Diverticulosis can be described as large outpouchings of the diverticula in the colon.

    b. Diverticulitis is defined as inflammation of the diverticula caused by obstructing matter.

    c. Approximately 60% of people older than 60 years have diverticula, or outpouchings from the colon; of these, 20% become symptomatic.

    d. Approximately 20% of patients with acute diverticulitis are younger than 40 years.

    e. In patients with diverticulosis, diverticulitis and its complications can be prevented with a high-fiber diet and avoidance of obstructing foods.

  2. Clinical features

    a. Diverticulitis

      (1) It generally presents with sudden-onset abdominal pain, usually in the left lower quadrant or suprapubic region, with or without fever.

      (2) Symptoms may range from mild disease to severe infection with peritonitis.

      (3) Altered bowel movement as well as nausea and vomiting are common.

    b. Diverticular bleeding generally presents as sudden-onset, large-volume hematochezia. It resolves spontaneously, although continuous or recurrent bleeding are indications for surgery.

  3. Laboratory findings

    a. Occult blood in the stool and mild to moderate leukocytosis may occur with diverticulitis.

    b. Plain-film radiography should be done to rule out free air.

    c. CT is warranted if patients do not respond to therapy.

    d. Barium enema should be avoided during an acute episode, because it may lead to perforation and peritonitis.

  4. Treatment

    a. Low-residue diet and broad-spectrum antibiotics are appropriate for patients with mild diverticulitis.

    b. Hospitalization for IV administration of antibiotics, bowel rest, and analgesics often is required. A nasogastric tube is inserted if ileus develops.

    c. Surgical management may be necessary in severe cases including peritonitis, large abscesses, fistulas, or obstruction.

J. Ischemic bowel disease

  1. General characteristics

    a. Mesenteric ischemia can be acute (AMI) or chronic (CMI). In chronic ischemia, the blood supply is present but insufficient to meet the needs of the intestine.

    b. For both AMI and CMI, patients generally will be older than 50 years and have other signs of cardiovascular or collagen vascular disease.

    c. AMI

      (1) AMI may be caused by arterial embolus, arterial thrombosis, or venous thrombosis, with differing risk factors and prognosis for each.

      (2) AMI represents an emergency. Mortality remains high despite advances in treatment.

    d. Intestinal infarction is more common in the small bowel than in the large bowel. Shock is common.

  2. Clinical features

    a. CMI presents as abdominal angina, with pain occurring 10–30 min after eating that is relieved somewhat by squatting or lying down.

    b. AMI presents with sudden onset of severe abdominal pain out of proportion to examination findings. Later in the process, involuntary guarding, rebound, and heme-positive stool may develop.

  3. Laboratory findings.

    a. Plain-film radiography and CT are performed to rule out other causes of abdominal pan.

    b. CT also can delineate extent of ischemia.

    c. Angiography may be helpful if the diagnosis is in question.

  4. Treatment for AMI or CMI is surgical revascularization.

K. Toxic Megacolon

  1. General characteristics

    a. Toxic megacolon is extreme dilatation and immobility of the colon and represents a true emergency.

    b. Hirschsprung's disease is a congenital aganglionosis of the colon, leading to functional obstruction in the newborn.

    c. In adults, toxic megacolon occurs as a complication of ulcerative colitis, Crohn's colitis, pseudomembranous colitis, and specific infectious causes (particularly amebiasis, *Shigella* sp., *Campylobacter* sp., and *Clostridium difficile*).

  2. Clinical features

    a. Symptoms include fever, prostration, severe cramps, and abdominal distention.

    b. A rigid abdomen and localized, diffuse or rebound abdominal tenderness is found on physical examination.

  3. Laboratory findings. Abdominal plain-film radiography will show colonic dilatation.

  4. Treatment

    a. Decompression of the colon is required. In some cases, colostomy or even complete colonic resection may be required.

    b. Careful attention must be paid to fluid and electrolyte balance.

L. Colonic polyps

  1. General characteristics

    a. Colonic polyps are common in the industrialized world and can be either benign or malignant.

    b. Removal of polyps can reduce the occurrence of colon cancer.

    c. Familial polyposis syndrome is a genetic predisposition to multiple colonic polyps and a high risk of colonic cancer.

  2. Clinical features

    a. Polyps generally are asymptomatic, although constipation, flatulence, and rectal bleeding may occur.

    b. Bleeding polyps may cause iron deficiency anemia.

  3. Laboratory findings

    a. Heme-positive stool is common.

    b. Barium enema, flexible sigmoidoscopy, and colonoscopy can detect polyps.

    c. Histologic evaluation is needed to determine dysplasia.

    d. Family members of those with familial polyposis syndrome should be evaluated every 1–2 years beginning at 10–12 years of age.

  4. Treatment depends on the size and histology of polyps. Larger and dysplastic polyps should be removed and frequent follow-up arranged.

M. Colorectal cancer

  1. General characteristics

    a. Colorectal cancer is the third leading cause of cancer death in the United States after lung cancer and skin cancers.

    b. Approximately 90% of cases occur in people older than 50 years.

    c. Prognosis

      (1) Prognosis is good in early disease.

      (2) When the cancer involves only the mucosa (Dukes A), the 5-year survival rate is greater than 90%.

      (3) Penetration through the wall or involvement of regional lymph nodes (Dukes B) has a 5-year survival rate of 70–80%.

      (4) When there are distant metastases (Dukes C), the 5-year survival rate drops to 5%.

  2. Clinical features

    a. Colorectal cancer is slow growing, and symptoms often appear late in the disease. Abdominal pain, change in bowel habits, occult bleeding, and intestinal obstruction are common presentations.

    b. Fatigue and weakness may occur if chronic blood loss has led to anemia.

    c. Changes in stool size and shape may be noted, as may frank blood in the stool.

  3. Laboratory findings

    a. Occult blood in the stool can be an early marker and is used for screening adults older than 40 years. Flexible colonoscopy is recommended in those older than 40 or 50 years. Debate continues regarding specific screening schedules, but overall, the data support screening for the general population after age 50.

    b. Carcinoembryonic antigen may be used to monitor, although not to detect, colorectal cancer.

    c. Sigmoidoscopy, colonoscopy, or barium enema may all be used to visualize suspected colonic masses, whereas chest radiography and CT are used to detect metastases.

  4. Treatment

    a. Treatment is by surgical resection, which is accompanied by chemotherapy in patients with any extension through the serosa or with lymphatic spread.

    b. Radiation may be given before surgery to reduce size of tumor.

IV. DISEASES OF THE RECTUM AND ANUS

A. Anorectal abscesses/fistula

  1. General characteristics

    a. Anorectal abscess is a result of infection, whereas fistula is a chronic complication of abscess.

    b. Fistula is an open tract between two epithelium-lined areas and most commonly is associated with deeper anorectal abscesses.

  2. Clinical features

    a. Perirectal and perianal abscesses are most common and produce painful swelling at the anus as well as painful defecation. Examination reveals localized tenderness, erythema, swelling, and fluctuance; fever is uncommon.

    b. Deeper abscesses may produce buttock or coccyx pain and rectal fullness; fever is more likely.

    c. Fistula will produce anal discharge and pain when the tract becomes occluded. The tract should not be explored on examination, because this may open new tracts.

  3. Treatment

    a. Treatment of abscess requires surgical drainage, followed by warm-water cleansing, analgesics, stool softeners, and high-fiber diet (WASH regimen).

    b. Fistulas must be treated surgically.

B. Anal fissure

  1. Anal fissures are linear lesions in the rectal wall, most commonly found on the posterior midline.

  2. Patients describe severe, tearing pain on defecation, often accompanied by hematochezia; bright red blood often is noted on the stool or tissue paper.

  3. Treatment includes bulking agents and increased fluids to avoid straining. Sitz baths will relieve acute pain. Topical nitroglycerin ointment or topical styptic, such as silver nitrate (1–2%) or Gentian Violet solution (1%), may help with healing.

C. Hemorrhoids

  1. General characteristics. Hemorrhoids are varices of the hemorrhoidal plexus.

  2. Clinical features

    a. External hemorrhoids are visible perianally.

    b. Stage I internal hemorrhoids are confined to the anal canal and may bleed with defecation.

    c. Stage II internal hemorrhoids protrude from the anal opening but reduce spontaneously. Bleeding and mucoid discharge may occur.

    d. Stage III internal hemorrhoids require manual reduction after bowel movements. Patients may develop pain and discomfort.

    e. Stage IV internal hemorrhoids are chronically protruding and risk strangulation.

  3. Treatment

    a. Stage I and II disease can be managed with a high-fiber diet and increased fluids. Bulk laxatives are helpful.

    b. Higher stage hemorrhoidal disease may benefit from suppositories with anesthetic and astringent properties.

    c. Surgical treatment is indicated for those unresponsive to conservative treatment and all stage IV hemorrhoids. Choices include injection, rubber band ligation, or sclerotherapy.

D. Pilonidal disease

  1. General characteristics

    a. Pilonidal cyst is an abscess in the sacrococcygeal cleft associated with subsequent sinus tract development.

    b. They are four times more likely in males than in females, are more common in hirsute and obese individuals, and are rare in those older than 40 years.

2. Clinical presentation is a painful, fluctuant area at the sacrococcygeal cleft.

3. Treatment

    a. Treatment is surgical drainage, which may be supplemented with antibiotics.

    b. Follicle removal may be required, with unroofing of sinus tracts.

E. Fecal impaction

  1. General characteristics

    a. Fecal impaction is a large mass of hard, retained stool. It generally occurs in the rectum, but it also may occur higher in the colon.

    b. Complications

      (1) Complications include urinary tract obstruction and infection, spontaneous perforation of the colon, and stercoral ulcer where the mass has pressed on the colon.

      (2) Fecaliths may develop and cause appendicitis.

    c. More proximal impaction generally indicates neoplasm.

  2. Clinical features

    a. Abdominal pain, rectal discomfort, anorexia, nausea, and vomiting are common but nonspecific.

    b. Headache and a general sense of illness are common, and acute confusional states may appear.

    c. Incontinence of small amounts of water and semiformed stool may occur as leakage passes by a large impaction.

    d. Rock hard stool in the rectal vault on examination is diagnostic. Abdominal mass also may be palpated, and sigmoidoscopy or barium enema may be needed to confirm a more proximal impaction.

  3. Treatment

    a. Treatment involves breaking up the impaction digitally, followed by a saline or tepid-water enema.

    b. More proximal impaction can be broken up by sigmoidoscopic water irrigation and suction.

    c. Subsequent attention must be paid to bowel habits and hydration.

V. DISEASES OF THE APPENDIX AND PANCREAS

A. Appendicitis

  1. General characteristics

    a. Appendicitis occurs when obstruction of the appendix, by fecalith or other cause, leads to inflammation and infection.

    b. Patients usually are between 10 and 30 years of age.

    c. Appendicitis affects 10% of the U.S. population, making it the most common abdominal surgical emergency.

    d. Perforation and peritonitis occur in about 20% of patients with appendicitis, causing high-grade fever, generalized abdominal pain, and increased leukocytosis.

  2. Clinical features

    a. The initial symptom is intermittent periumbilical or epigastric pain.

    b. In about 12 hours, pain typically localizes to the right lower quadrant (McBurney's point), becomes constant, and is worsened by movement, leading to rebound tenderness on examination.

    c. Nausea and anorexia are common. Vomiting may occur but generally is isolated and begins subsequent to the onset of pain.

    d. Diarrhea may occur but is not common.

    e. A low-grade fever is common; a high-grade fever is unlikely.

    f. Psoas sign (patient is supine and attempts to raise the leg against resistance) and obturator sign (patient is supine and attempts to flex and internally rotate the right hip with the knee bent) generally are positive, indicating inflammation adjacent to those muscles.

    g. Variability in anatomy can cause unusual presentations of appendicitis, with symptoms reflecting the location of the appendix.

  3. Laboratory findings

    a. Leukocytosis (usually 10,000–20,000 cells/mL) is characteristic. Higher levels suggest perforation and peritonitis.

    b. Some microscopic hematuria and pyuria may be seen.

    c. Abdominal CT may be used in some cases to confirm the diagnosis and to locate an abnormally placed appendix.

  4. Treatment.

    (1) Treatment consists of appendectomy.

    (2) If there is any reason to suspect perforation, broad-spectrum antibiotics are administered before surgery.

B. Acute pancreatitis

  1. General characteristics

    a. Causes

    (1) The most common cause is alcohol abuse, but cholelithiasis, hyperlipidemia, trauma, drugs, hypercalcemia, and penetrating PUD also may cause pancreatitis.

    (2) Pancreatitis also is associated with medications especially many of the antiretroviral medications used to treat HIV.

    b. The range of presentation is wide, ranging from mild episodes of deep epigastric pain with nausea and vomiting to the sudden onset of severe pain with shock.

  2. Clinical features

    a. The classic presentation is epigastric pain radiating to the back. The pain typically lessens when the patient leans forward or lies in a fetal position.

    b. Nausea and vomiting are common.

    c. Fever, leukocytosis, and sterile peritonitis may occur.

    d. Severe hypovolemia, adult respiratory distress syndrome, and tachycardia of greater than 130 bpm indicate a grave prognosis.

  3. Laboratory studies

    a. Elevation of serum amylase occurs but may be transient and can return to normal after 48–72 hours.

    b. Serum lipase is more sensitive and specific than amylase for acute pancreatitis, but only with elevations of threefold or greater.

    c. WBC count generally is elevated, and hemoconcentration may occur with third spacing of fluid.

    d. Liver enzymes may increase as a result of biliary obstruction.

    e. Mild hyperbilirubinemia and bilirubinuria, hyperglycemia, and hypocalcemia may occur.

    f. Poor prognosis is indicated by Ranson's criteria: leukocyte count >16,000 cells/mL, blood glucose level >200 mg/dL, lactate dehydrogenase level >350 IU/dL (normal level, 20–50 IU/dL), aspartate aminotransferase (AST) >250 IU/dL (normal level, <120 IU/dL), falling hematocrit, rising BUN, arterial Po_2 <60 mm Hg, base deficit >4 mEq/L, or falling calcium level. Risk of mortality rises with each additional factor.

  4. Treatment

    a. Oral intake must be stopped to prevent continued secretion of pancreatic juices.

    b. Fluid volume must be restored and maintained. Parenteral hyperalimentation should be started early to prevent nutritional depletion.

    c. Pain is managed with meperidine. Antibiotics should be considered.

    d. The patient must be monitored closely for complications, including pancreatic pseudocyst, renal failure, pleural effusion, hypocalcemia, and pancreatic abscess.

C. Chronic pancreatitis

  1. General characteristics

    a. Almost 90% of cases of chronic pancreatitis in the United States are caused by alcohol abuse; other causes include cholelithiasis, PUD, hyperparathyroidism, and hyperlipidemia.

    b. Some chronic cases can resolve if alcohol consumption is decreased.

    c. The classic triad of pancreatic calcification, steatorrhea, and diabetes mellitus occurs in only 20% of patients.

2. Clinical features are the same as those of acute pancreatitis, with the addition of fat malabsorption and steatorrhea late in the disease. Fecal fat will be elevated if malabsorption is present.

3. Laboratory studies

    a. The amylase level may be elevated early but will decrease with each episode of pancreatitis and cease to be a useful marker.

    b. Abdominal plain-film radiography reveals calcification in 20–30% of patients.

4. Treatment

    a. Treatment is as for acute pancreatitis. A low-fat diet should be recommended at discharge.

    b. Surgical removal of part of the pancreas can control pain.

    c. The only definitive treatment for chronic pancreatitis is to address the underlying cause, which most commonly is alcohol.

D. Pancreatic neoplasm

    1. General characteristics

        a. Pancreatic cancer is the fifth leading cause of cancer death in the United States.

        b. Risk factors include increased age, obesity, tobacco, chronic pancreatitis, previous abdominal radiation, and family history.

    2. Clinical presentation

        a. Abdominal pain occurs in most patients and, depending on the location of the tumor, can radiate.

        b. Jaundice and a palpable gallbladder (Courvier's sign) may be seen in patients with cancer of the pancreatic head.

    3. Diagnostic studies include CT (to search for metastases) and angiography (to look for vascular invasion).

    4. Treatment

        a. Treatment is surgical resection (modified Whipple procedure) in those without metastases.

        b. Subsequent radiation and chemotherapy are controversial.

        c. Prognosis is poor.

VI. DISEASES OF THE BILIARY TRACT

A. Acute cholecystitis

    1. Acute cholecystitis is caused by obstruction of the bile duct, generally by a stone, leading to chronic inflammation.

    2. Clinical presentation

        a. Colicky epigastric or right upper quadrant pain becomes steady and increases in intensity. It often occurs after a high fat meal.

        b. Right shoulder or subscapular pain may occur.

        c. Nausea, vomiting, and low-grade fever are common.

        d. Constipation and mild paralytic ileus may occur.

    3. Laboratory findings

        a. After 24 hours, bilirubin levels increase in blood and urine.

        b. Leukocytosis is common.

        c. Gallstones are found in 95% of patients with cholecystitis. Although only 20% are radiopaque, the remainder generally are visible by sonography.

        d. Hepatobiliary imaging (hepato-iminodiacetic acid scan [HIDA] or others) can be used for confirmation of the diagnosis.

        e. Endoscopic retrograde cholangiopancreatography (ERCP) can identify cause, location, and extent of biliary obstruction.

B. Choledocholithiasis

    1. General characteristics

        a. By age 75, 35% of women and 20% of men have gallstones.

        b. Only 30% of people with gallstones develop symptomatic disease.

2. Treatment

   a. Generally, only the complications of choledocholithiasis should be treated, because most people with gallstones will never develop the disease.

   b. Complications include cholecystitis, pancreatitis, and acute cholangitis.

VII. DISEASES OF THE LIVER

A. Hepatitis

   1. General characteristics

      a. Hepatitis can describe acute or chronic hepatocellular damage.

      b. The most common cause of acute hepatitis is viral; toxins (e.g., alcohol) are the second most common cause.

      c. Chronic hepatitis most often results from viral infection (hepatitis B, C, D) but often is caused by inherited disorders (e.g., Wilson disease, α-antitrypsin deficiency), autoimmune disease of the liver, or hepatic effects of systemic disease.

   2. Viral hepatitis

      a. General characteristics

         (1) The severity of the disease is highly variable, ranging from asymptomatic to fulminant, generally fatal, infection.

         (2) Hepatitis A and E are transmitted by fecal–oral contamination and can be prevented by maintaining a sanitary water supply and hand washing.

         (3) Hepatitis B, C, and D are transmitted parenterally or by mucous membrane contact.

      b. Clinical features

         (1) Fatigue, malaise, anorexia, nausea, tea-colored urine, and vague abdominal discomfort are common presenting complaints.

         (2) Hepatitis A and E are self-limited and mild, without long-term sequelae.

         (3) Hepatitis B and C can have a highly variable presentation, ranging from asymptomatic to fulminant. Chronic hepatitis B or C causing liver damage may require treatment.

         (4) Hepatitis D is seen only in conjunction with hepatitis B and is associated with a more severe course.

         (5) Hepatitis C and HIV are frequent coinfections, as are hepatitis B and HIV, necessitating specialist care if treatment of the hepatitis is indicated.

      c. Laboratory findings

         (1) Aminotransferase elevations are seen in all types of acute hepatitis, indicating hepatocellular damage.

         (2) Bilirubin of greater than 3.0 mg/dL will be associated with scleral icterus, if not frank jaundice.

         (3) Immunoglobulin M antibody to hepatitis A virus (anti-HAV) can be detected with the onset of clinical disease (after a 15- to 40-day incubation period), but it disappears after several months. HAV IgG indicates resolved hepatitis A.

         (4) Hepatitis B surface antigen (HBsAg) indicates ongoing infection of any duration; antibody against hepatitis B surface antigen (anti-HBs) indicates immunity by past infection or vaccination (Fig. 5-1).

         (5) Hepatitis B core antibody (anti-HBc) is present between the disappearance of HBsAg and the appearance of anti-HBs, indicating acute hepatitis.

         (6) Hepatitis B envelope antigen (HBeAg) indicates active infection that is highly contagious, whereas anti-HBe indicates a lower viral titer.

         (7) Hepatitis C or D generally is detected by its antibody, which for hepatitis C generally indicates ongoing infection, as it does for hepatitis D if hepatitis B infection is ongoing.

         (8) Hepatitis B may exist in a carrier state or a chronic infection. Both exhibit positive HBsAG, but in chronic infection, liver damage is demonstrated by elevated AST and alanine aminotransferase and by hepatocellular damage on biopsy. In chronic infection, the viral DNA load will be greater than 10^5 copies.

         (9) Hepatitis C antibody–positive patients should be evaluated for genotype and viral load. Types 2 and 3 have a better treatment prognosis than type 1, as does a lower HCV viral load.

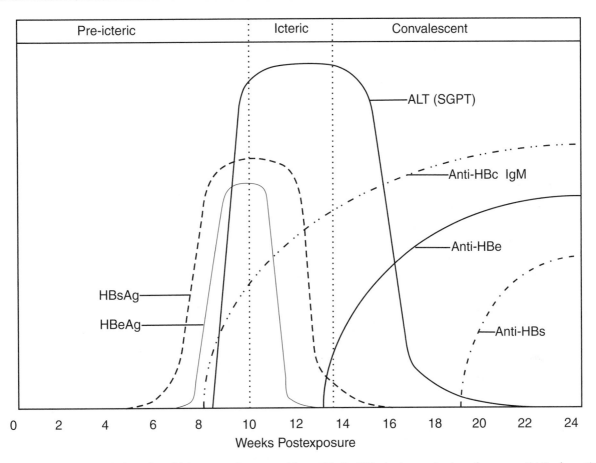

FIGURE 5-1 Relationship of clinical and laboratory features of hepatitis B. *ALT*, alanine aminotransferase; *anti-HBc*, hepatitis B core antibody; *anti-HBe*, hepatitis B envelope antigen; *anti-HBs*, hepatitis B surface antigen antibody; *HBsAg*, hepatitis B surface antigen; *IgM*, immunoglobulin M; *SGPT*, serum glutamate pyruvate transaminase.

   d. Treatment

   (1) Treatment of acute viral hepatitis is supportive. Patients with hepatitis A must be cautious about transmission to others by not sharing food or dishes and by frequent hand washing.

   (2) All patients with acute or chronic hepatitis should avoid alcohol and other hepatotoxins.

   (3) Patients with chronic hepatitis B or C may be referred to a specialist for treatment. Interferon therapies are evolving and increasing in efficacy.

   (4) Patients with hepatitis C should be vaccinated against hepatitis A and B.

3. Toxic hepatitis

   a. Toxic hepatitis may be caused by numerous agents, including alcohol, acetaminophen, carbon tetrachloride, isoniazid, halothane, phenytoin, and many others.

   b. Both diagnosis and treatment are accomplished by discontinuing the suspected agent. Acetylcysteine can be used for acetaminophen toxicity.

   c. Toxic hepatitis may be reversible, depending on the amount of the toxin. If the patient survives the acute episode, the prognosis is good.

B. Cirrhosis

1. General characteristics

   a. Cirrhosis is irreversible fibrosis and nodular regeneration throughout the liver.

   b. In the United States, more than 45% of cases are alcohol related, with the remainder associated with hepatitis B or C or with congenital disorders.

2. Clinical presentation

   a. Weakness, fatigue, and weight loss are common.

   b. Nausea, vomiting, and anorexia usually are present.

    c. Menstrual changes (generally amenorrhea), impotence, loss of libido, and gynecomastia occur.

    d. Abdominal pain and hepatomegaly generally are present.

    e. Late-stage disease includes ascites, pleural effusions, peripheral edema, ecchymoses, esophageal varices, and signs of hepatic encephalopathy (e.g., asterixis, tremor, dysarthria, delirium, and eventually, coma).

  3. Laboratory findings

    a. Laboratory values often are minimally abnormal until late in the disease.

    b. Anemia is common, as are mild elevations of AST and alkaline phosphatase, increased gamma globulin, and decreased albumin.

    c. Ultrasonography, CT, or MRI can confirm the size and number of nodules and is helpful in guiding biopsy.

  4. Treatment

    a. Abstinence from alcohol is the key feature of treatment.

    b. Salt restriction and bed rest may be sufficient treatment for ascites, although spironolactone, 100 mg daily, may be added as a diuretic.

    c. Liver transplant is indicated in selected patients.

C. Liver abscess generally is caused by *Entamoeba histolytica* or by the coliform bacteria. It may occur either after travel or secondary to an intra-abdominal infection and presents with fever and abdominal pain.

D. Liver neoplasm

  1. General characteristics

    a. Liver neoplasms may be malignant or benign, and malignant neoplasms may be primary or metastatic.

    b. Benign liver neoplasms include cavernous hemangioma, hepatocellular adenoma, and infantile hemangioendothelioma.

    c. The liver is a common site of metastasis for other primary cancers, especially lung and breast. If the primary tumor is silent, liver manifestations may be the presenting complaints.

    d. Primary hepatocellular carcinoma is associated with hepatitis B, hepatitis C, aflatoxin B1 exposure (found in foodstuffs in certain subtropical regions), and cirrhosis.

  2. Clinical characteristics

    a. Presenting complaints include malaise, weight loss, abdominal swelling, weakness, jaundice, and upper abdominal pain.

    b. Hepatomegaly, splenomegaly, hepatic bruit, ascites, jaundice, wasting, and fever may be detected on examination.

  3. Laboratory findings

    a. α-Fetoprotein may be elevated in hepatic carcinoma.

    b. Imaging with sonography, CT, MRI, or hepatic angiography can show the lesion.

    c. Needle biopsy generally should not be used if the tumor is resectable.

  4. Treatment

    a. Benign neoplasms should be treated if the tumor size indicates a danger of rupturing the hepatic capsule.

    b. Treatment of metastatic disease involves treatment of the primary lesion.

    c. Surgical resection of hepatic carcinoma may be attempted if the cancer is confined to one lobe and there is no concurrent cirrhosis. Liver transplant also can be considered. The overall prognosis is poor.

VIII. HERNIAS

A. General characteristics

  1. A hernia is a protrusion of an organ or structure through the wall that normally contains it.

  2. Hernias of various types can entrap the intestines and cause intestinal blockage.

B. Types

  1. Umbilical hernia generally is congenital and appears at birth. Many resolve on their own, but surgery may be indicated.

  2. Diaphragmatic hernia involves protrusion of the stomach through the diaphragm. It can cause gastroesophageal reflux disease. Acid reduction may suffice, and surgical repair can be used for more serious cases.

3. Incisional hernias are associated more commonly with vertical incisions, especially in patients with concurrent obesity or wound infection.

4. Inguinal hernias can be indirect (most common; passage of intestine through the internal inguinal ring down the inguinal canal, may pass into the scrotum), indirect (passage of intestine through external inguinal ring at Hesselbach's triangle, rarely enters the scrotum), or femoral (least common; passage through femoral ring).

5. Hiatal or diaphragmatic hernia is protrusion of the stomach through the esophageal hiatus.

6. Ventral hernia occurs when there is a weakening in the anterior abdominal wall and may be either incisional or umbilical.

C. Treatment of hernias is surgical.

IX. CONGENITAL ABNORMALITIES

A. Esophageal atresia commonly is associated with tracheoesophageal fistula.

1. Atresia presents in newborns as excessive saliva and choking or coughing with attempts to feed.

2. Inability to pass a nasogastric tube will establish the diagnosis.

3. Treatment is surgical, but pulmonary aspiration should be prevented in the interim by suction and withholding of oral feedings.

B. Diaphragmatic hernia causes immediate respiratory distress in the newborn, because the affected lung is compressed by pressure from abdominal contents.

1. Immediate intubation and ventilation is required, along with suction of the stomach by nasogastric tube.

2. Diagnosis can be made if bowel sounds are heard in the chest.

3. Radiography shows loops of bowel in the involved hemithorax, with displacement of the heart and mediastinal structures.

C. Hypertrophic pyloric stenosis is caused by hypertrophy of the pyloric muscle and generally develops within the first 4–6 weeks of life.

1. Projectile vomiting without bile is the presenting symptom.

2. A mobile "olive" mass may be palpated deep in the epigastrium.

3. Barium swallow will reveal delayed gastric emptying and "string sign," or the long, narrow pyloric lumen.

4. Treatment is surgical (pyloromyotomy).

D. Bowel atresia can occur in the ileum (most common), duodenum, jejunum, or colon and presents with signs of obstruction within the first few days of life.

E. Hirschsprung's disease (congenital megacolon) is caused by congenital absence of Meissner's and Auerbach's autonomic plexuses enervating the bowel wall.

1. Symptoms may include constipation or obstipation, vomiting, and failure to thrive.

2. Treatment is surgical resection of the affected bowel.

X. NUTRITIONAL DEFICIENCIES

Vitamin	Sources	Function(s)	At-risk Groups	Deficiency	Toxicity
Vitamin A	Liver Fish oils fortified milk eggs	Vision, epithelial cell maturity, resistance to infection, antioxidant	Elderly, alcoholics, liver disease	Night blindness, dry skin	Skin disorders, hair loss, teratogenicity
Vitamin D	Fortified milk	Calcium regulation, cell differentiation	Elderly, shut-ins with low sun exposure	Rickets, osteomalacia	Hypercalcemia, kidney stones, soft tissue deposits
Vitamin E	Plant oils, wheat germ, asparagus, peanuts, margarine	Retard cell aging, vascular and red cell wall integrity, antioxidant	Rare	Hemolytic anemia, degenerative nerve changes	Inhibition of vitamin K, myalgia, headache, weakness

(continued)

Vitamin	Sources	Function(s)	At-risk Groups	Deficiency	Toxicity
Vitamin K	Liver, green leafy vegetables, broccoli, peas, green beans	Clotting	Rare	Bleeding	Anemia, jaundice
Thiamin	Pork, grains, dried beans, peas, brewer's yeast	Carbohydrate metabolism, nerve function	Alcoholism, poverty	Beriberi (nervous tingling, poor coordination, edema, weakness, cardiac dysfunction)	N/A
Riboflavin	Milk, spinach, liver, grains	Energy	N/A	Oral inflammation, eye disorders	N/A
Niacin	Bran, tuna, salmon, chicken, beef, liver, peanuts, grains	Energy, fat metabolism	Poverty, alcoholism	Pellagra (diarrhea, dermatitis, dementia)	Flushing
Pantothenic acid	Liver, broccoli eggs	Energy, fat metabolism	Alcoholism	Tingling, fatigue, headache	N/A
Biotin	Cheese, egg, cauliflower, peanut butter, liver	Glucose production, fat synthesis	Alcoholism	Dermatitis, tongue pain, anemia, depression	N/A
B6 pyridoxine	Animal protein, spinach, broccoli, bananas, salmon	Protein metabolism, neurotransmitter synthesis, hemoglobin	Adolescents, alcoholism	Headache, anemia Seizures, flaky skin, sore tongue	Nerve destruction
Folate	Green leafy vegetables, orange juice, grains, organ meats	DNA synthesis	Alcoholism, pregnancy	Megaloblastic anemia, sore tongue, diarrhea, mental disorders	N/A
B12 cobalamin	Animal foods	Folate metabolism, nerve function	Elderly, vegans	Megaloblastic anemia, poor nerve function	N/A
Vitamin C	Citrus fruits, strawberries, broccoli, greens	Collagen synthesis, hormone function, neurotransmitter synthesis	Alcoholism, elderly men	Scurvy (poor wound healing, Petechiae, bleeding gums)	Diarrhea

Adapted from Wardlaw GM. Perspective in Nutrition. 4th ed., McGraw-Hill, 1999

XI. METABOLIC DISORDERS

A. Lactose intolerance

1. Lactose is digested by lactase, which is produced in the small intestine.

2. The persistence of lactase production past the age of 12 is common only in northern European populations. For most of the world's population, lactase does not persist, and lactose-containing products are not well digested.

3. Symptoms of lactose intolerance include nausea, bloating, flatulence, diarrhea, cramping, and occasionally, vomiting.

4. Lactose intolerance is easily managed by avoiding milk and dairy products or use of lactase enzyme tablets or drops.

B. Phenylketonuria

1. Phenylketonuria is a rare autosomal recessive inability to metabolize the protein phenylalanine.

2. Phenylalanine and its metabolites accumulate in the central nervous system, causing mental retardation and movement disorders.

3. Screening at birth is simple and allows early detection and management; diagnosis after age 3 will lead to irreversible brain damage.

4. Management is by a low-phenylalanine diet and tyrosine supplementation. Breast milk is low in phenylalanine, and special formulas are available. Strict control of protein intake is required for life.

Nephrology and Urology

6

Robert J. McNellis

I. RENAL FAILURE

A. Acute renal failure (ARF)

1. General characteristics

a. ARF refers to a syndrome of rapidly deteriorating kidney function with the accumulation of nitrogenous wastes. Serum creatinine acutely increases by more than 0.5 mg/dL and more than 50% over baseline levels.

b. Of the many conditions that can cause ARF, two diseases account for the majority of cases: reduced renal perfusion, and acute tubular necrosis.

c. Causes are classified into three categories: prerenal, intrinsic renal, and postrenal (Table 6-1).

d. ARF occurs in 5% of hospitalized patients and in up to 30% of critical care patients. The overall mortality rate for ARF is 50%.

2. Clinical features

a. A thorough medical history can identify possible causes of ARF, such as exposure to nephrotoxins, family history of renal disease, urologic disease, or contributing factors, such as hypertension or diabetes.

b. General symptoms include nausea, vomiting, diarrhea, pruritus, drowsiness, dizziness, hiccups, shortness of breath, anorexia, and hematochezia.

c. Signs can reflect the underlying cause.

(1) Tachycardia and hypotension may indicate prerenal causes.

(2) A distended bladder, costovertebral angle tenderness, or enlarged prostate suggest postrenal causes.

(3) Other signs include absent or decreased urine flow, change in mental status, edema, weakness, dehydration, rashes, jugular venous distention, uriniferous odor, and ecchymosis.

3. Laboratory studies

a. Urinalysis is essentially normal in prerenal and postrenal causes of ARF with only a few hyaline casts. Granular casts, WBCs and casts, RBCs and casts, proteinuria, and epithelial cells indicate intrinsic renal causes of ARF.

b. Other blood and urine studies

(1) Prerenal causes

(a) Decreased urine sodium

(b) Fractional excretion of sodium (FE_{Na}) <1%

(c) Urine osmolality >500 mOsm

(d) Elevated BUN:plasma Cr ratio (>20:1)

(2) Intrinsic renal causes

(a) Increased urine sodium

(b) FE_{Na} >2%

(c) Urine osmolality of 250–300 mOsm

(d) Decreased BUN:plasma Cr ratio (<15:1)

(3) Postrenal causes. Urine sodium, FE_{Na}, osmolality, and BUN:Cr ratio can vary, depending on how long the obstruction has been present.

c. Many other abnormal laboratory findings are associated with loss of renal function, including azotemia, decreased creatinine clearance, and hyperkalemia. Other blood chemistries and hematologic tests are abnormal, depending on the severity of disease.

4. Treatment

a. Treatment involves the correction of underlying hemodynamic abnormalities. Appropriate fluid management is critical.

b. Short-term dialysis should be implemented when serum creatinine exceeds 5–10 mg/dL. Other indications for dialysis include unresponsive acidosis, electrolyte disorders, fluid overload or uremic complications.

TABLE 6-1	**Causes of Acute Renal Failure**

Prerenal causes (60–70%)
  Hypovolemia
  Hypotension
  Ineffective circulating volume (CHF, cirrhosis, nephrotic syndrome, early sepsis)
  Aortic aneurysm
  Renal artery stenosis or embolic disease
Intrinsic renal causes (25–40%)
  Acute tubular necrosis,
  Nephrotoxins (aminoglycosides, radiologic contrast)
  Interstitial diseases (acute interstitial nephritis, SLE, infection)
  Glomerulonephritis
  Vascular diseases (polyarteritis nodosa, vasculitis)
Postrenal causes (5–10%)
  Tubular obstruction
  Obstructive uropathy (urolithiasis, BPH, bladder outlet obstruction)

BPH, benign prostatic hyperplasia; *CHF*, congestive heart failure; *SLE*, systemic lupus erythematosus.

    c. Reversible causes must be corrected by restoring circulating volume in the hypovolemic patient, improving perfusion in the hypotensive patient, or removing obstructions to renal blood flow or urine flow.

    d. Medical therapy may include IV saline, mannitol, or furosemide, depending on the cause. All medications should be adjusted for decreased renal function.

B. Chronic renal failure and insufficiency

  1. General characteristics

    a. Definitions

      (1) Chronic renal failure and insufficiency are points along the spectrum of chronic kidney disease, which is defined as decreased kidney function for 3 months or longer.

        (a) Kidney function is reflected by the glomerular filtration rate (GFR).

        (b) Normal GFR in persons older than 30 years is 125 mL/min.

        (c) Chronic kidney disease is defined as a GFR of less than 60 mL/min per 1.73 m^2 body surface area.

      (2) Chronic renal insufficiency describes mild to moderate decrease in GFR (15–60 mL/min) without the presence of uremic symptoms.

      (3) Chronic renal failure is a slowly progressive and irreversible reduction in GFR, usually with signs and symptoms of uremia. Failure is defined as GFR less than 15 ml/min per 1.73 m^2 or as the need for dialysis or kidney transplantation.

    b. Diabetes mellitus, hypertension, glomerulonephritis, and polycystic kidney disease are the most common causes (Table 6-2).

    c. Patients with chronic kidney disease generally progress to chronic renal failure.

      (1) The rate of progression depends on the underlying cause, the effectiveness of treatments, and the individual patient.

      (2) The 5-year survival rate for chronic renal failure is 35%.

  2. Clinical features

    a. Uremic symptoms develop insidiously and include fatigue, malaise, anorexia, nausea, vomiting, metallic taste, hiccups, dyspnea, orthopnea, impaired mentation, insomnia, irritability, muscle cramps, restless legs, weakness, pruritus, easy bruising, and altered consciousness.

    b. Signs include cachexia, weight loss, muscle wasting, pallor, hypertension, ecchymosis, sensory deficits, asterixis, and Kussmaul respirations.

  3. Laboratory findings

    a. Measurement of GFR is the gold standard. The Cockcroft-Gault formula or the Modification of Diet in Renal Disease (MDRD) equation will give a fairly accurate prediction of GFR, with the MDRD probably being more accurate.

    b. Proteinuria is a marker for kidney damage. Microalbuminuria appears early in the disease.

TABLE 6-2	Causes of Chronic Renal Failure

Diabetes mellitus

Hypertension

Glomerulonephritis

Polycystic kidney disease

Other causes
  Primary glomerular diseases (membranous nephropathy, minimal change disease, IgA
    nephropathy)
  Secondary glomerular diseases (sickle cell anemia, SLE)
  Tubulointerstitial renal diseases (nephrotoxins, infection, multiple myeloma, HIV)
  Chronic pyelonephritis (tuberculosis)
  Vascular diseases (renal artery stenosis or obstruction)
  Obstructive nephropathies (nephrolithiasis, prostate disease, neurogenic bladder)

HIV, human immunodeficiency virus; *SLE*, systemic lupus erythematosus.

    c. BUN and creatinine are elevated.

    d. Hemoglobin and hematocrit, serum electrolytes, and urinalysis are abnormal.

  4. Treatment

    a. Angiotensin-converting enzyme (ACE) inhibitors and angiotensin-receptor blockers slow the progression of renal dysfunction.

    b. Managing comorbid conditions improves the outcome, including hypertensive therapy, tight glycemic control, cholesterol-lowering therapy, tobacco cessation, and weight control.

    c. Erythropoietin, iron supplements, and antiplatelet therapy should be considered to maintain hemoglobin and bleeding time as needed.

    d. Medical therapy requires careful drug dosing to adjust for decreased renal function.

    e. Dietary management includes restriction of protein intake, adequate caloric intake, calcium and vitamin D supplements, and limitation of water, sodium, potassium, and phosphorus.

    f. Need for hemodialysis, peritoneal dialysis, or kidney transplantation should be coordinated with nephrology service.

II. GLOMERULONEPHROPATHIES

  A. Glomerulonephritis (GN)

    1. General characteristics

      a. GN generally refers to damage of the renal glomeruli by deposition of inflammatory proteins in the glomerular membranes as the result of an immunologic response.

      b. About 60% of cases are in children 2–12 years of age.

      c. Prognosis is excellent in children and worse in adults, especially in those with preexisting renal disease.

    2. Causes

      a. The major causes of GN are listed in Table 6-3.

      b. Causes are divided into focal GN, which is characterized by involvement of less than half the glomeruli, and diffuse GN, which affects most glomeruli.

    3. Clinical features

      a. Hematuria is present; urine often is tea colored.

      b. Oliguria or anuria is present.

      c. Edema of the face and eyes is present in the morning, and edema of the feet and ankles occurs in the afternoon and evening.

      d. Hypertension also is a common, but not an essential, clinical finding.

TABLE 6-3	**Causes of Glomerulonephritis**	
Type	**Children**	**Adults**
Focal	Benign hematuria Henoch-Schönlein purpura Mild postinfectious GN IgA nephropathy Hereditary nephritis	IgA nephropathy Hereditary nephritis SLE
Diffuse	Postinfectious GN Membranoproliferative GN	SLE Membranoproliferative GN Rapidly progressive GN Postinfectious GN Vasculitis

GN, glomerulonephritis; *IgA*, immunoglobulin A; *SLE*, systemic lupus erythematosus.

4. Laboratory findings
   a. Antistreptolysin O titer is increased in 60–80% of cases, because a common cause of GN is poststreptococcal infection.
   b. Urinalysis reveals RBC casts, RBCs and WBCs, and proteinuria.
   c. Serum complement (C3) levels are decreased.
   d. Renal biopsy may be done to determine exact diagnosis or severity of disease.
5. Treatment
   a. Steroids and immunosuppressive drugs may be used to control the immune response.
   b. Dietary management. Salt and fluid intake should be decreased.
   c. Dialysis should be performed if symptomatic azotemia is present.
   d. Medical therapy
      (1) ACE inhibitors are renoprotective in GN.
      (2) Use medications as appropriate for hyperkalemia, pulmonary edema, peripheral edema, acidosis, and hypertension.
B. Nephrotic syndrome
   1. General characteristics
      a. Nephrotic syndrome is defined as excretion of more than 3.5 g of protein per 1.73 m^2 in 24 hours. It manifests with hypoalbuminemia, lipiduria, hypercholesterolemia, and edema.
      b. It can affect adults and children, depending on the underlying cause (Table 6-4).

TABLE 6-4	**Causes of Nephrotic Syndrome**
Primary Renal Disease	**Secondary Renal Disease**
Focal GN	Poststreptococcal GN
Focal glomerulosclerosis	SLE
IgA nephropathy	Malignancy
Membranoproliferative GN	Toxemia of pregnancy
Membranous glomerulopathy	Drugs and nephrotoxins
Mesangial proliferative GN	Lymphomas and leukemias
Minimal change disease	
Rapidly progressive GN	
Congenital nephrotic syndrome	

GN, glomerulonephritis; *IgA*, immunoglobulin A; *SLE*, systemic lupus erythematosus.

    c. It commonly occurs with GN.

    d. Prognosis depends on the specific cause and degree of renal damage. Complete remission is possible if the underlying disease is treatable.

  2. Clinical features

    a. Symptoms include malaise, abdominal distention, anorexia, facial edema/puffy eyelids, oliguria, scrotal swelling, shortness of breath, and weight gain.

    b. Signs include ascites, edema, hypertension, orthostatic hypotension, retinal sheen, and skin striae.

  3. Laboratory findings

    a. Urinalysis reveals proteinuria, lipiduria, glycosuria, hematuria, and foamy urine.

    b. Microscopic examination of the urine shows RBC casts, granular casts, hyalinuria, and fatty casts.

    c. Blood chemistry shows hypoalbuminemia and azotemia.

    d. C3 levels can be low or normal, depending on the cause.

  4. Treatment

    a. Medical therapy

      (1) ACE inhibitors should be used early in the course of the disease.

      (2) Judicious use of diuretics is recommended to reduce fluid accumulations.

    b. Dietary management

      (1) Sodium and fluid intake should be restricted.

      (2) Dietary protein and potassium can be normal but not excessive.

    c. Infections should be treated aggressively.

    d. Anticoagulants should be used if thromboses are present.

    e. Excessive sunlight should be avoided, because skin photosensitivity is common.

    f. Nephrotoxic drugs (e.g., nonsteroidal anti-inflammatory drugs, aminoglycoside antibiotics) should be avoided.

    g. Some patients respond to steroid therapy.

    h. Frequent relapsers or steroid nonresponders may try cyclophosphamide or cyclosporine.

III. POLYCYSTIC KIDNEY DISEASE (PKD)

A. General characteristics

  1. PKD is a genetic disorder characterized by growth of numerous cysts in the kidneys. The cysts can replace the mass of the kidneys, reducing function and leading to kidney failure.

  2. Autosomal dominant PKD is the most common form and almost always is bilateral. Symptoms typically develop during the fourth decade of life.

  3. The less common autosomal recessive disease begins in utero and leads to fetal and neonatal death. Surviving infants have significantly reduced life expectancy.

  4. An acquired form of cystic kidney disease occurs in individuals with long-term renal disease.

B. Clinical features

  1. The most common symptoms of autosomal dominant PKD are back and flank pain and headaches.

  2. Hematuria, hypertension, recurrent urinary tract infection, weight loss, renal colic, as well as nausea and vomiting also may be present.

  3. One or both kidneys may be palpable and feel nodular or tender. Cysts also may be present on the liver, pancreas, and intestines.

C. Laboratory findings

  1. Anemia may be noted on CBC. Urinalysis shows proteinuria, hematuria, and, commonly, pyuria and bacteriuria.

  2. The diagnostic method of choice is ultrasonography, which shows fluid-filled cysts.

  3. Imaging studies

    a. Plain-film radiography of the abdomen shows enlarged kidneys.

    b. Excretory infusion urography reveals multiple lucencies.

    c. Angiography shows bending of small vessels around cysts.

    d. CT shows large renal size and multiple thin-walled cysts.

D. Treatment

    1. There is no cure for PKD; treatment is supportive to ease symptoms and prolong life.

    2. General measures should include management of pain, control of hypertension, high intake of fluids, and a low-protein diet.

    3. Infections should be treated vigorously to prevent further renal damage.

    4. Dialysis or transplantation should be considered when renal insufficiency becomes life-threatening. Transplantation has been successful, and non-PKD kidneys do not develop cysts.

IV. NEPHROLITHIASIS

A. General characteristics

    1. Nephrolithiasis (renal calculi) occur throughout the urinary tract and are common causes of pain, infection, and obstruction.

    2. Stones

        a. Caused by increased saturation of urine with stone-forming salts.

        b. Typically are formed in the proximal tract and pass distally.

        c. They lodge at the ureteropelvic junction, the ureterovesicular junction, or the ureter at the level of the iliac vessels.

    3. Nephrolithiasis commonly occurs during the third to fourth decade of life. The disease is two- to threefold more common in males than in females.

    4. Four major types of stones exist.

        a. Calcium: 75–85% of stones are formations of calcium crystals; these stones are radiopaque.

        b. Uric acid: 5–8% of stones are formed by precipitation of uric acid; these stones are radiolucent.

        c. Cystine: Less than 1% of stones are caused by an impairment of cystine transport; these stones are radiolucent.

        d. Struvite: 10–15% of stones are formed by the combination of calcium, ammonium, and magnesium and are radiopaque. Formation is increased by urinary tract infections; therefore, this type is twice as common in females than in males.

    5. Patients usually have complete return to health, but recurrences are common (up to 50% in 5 years).

B. Clinical features

    1. Nephrolithiasis generally is asymptomatic until inflammation or obstruction develops.

    2. Clinical features of nephrolithiasis include back pain and renal colic that waxes and wanes.

    3. The pain can radiate to the groin, testicles, suprapubic area, or labia.

    4. Symptoms include hematuria, dysuria, urinary frequency, fever, chills, nausea, and vomiting.

    5. Signs include diaphoresis, tachycardia, tachypnea, restlessness, costovertebral angle tenderness, and abdominal distention because of ileus.

C. Laboratory findings

    1. Urinalysis reveals microscopic or gross hematuria.

    2. Urine culture should be performed to rule out infection.

    3. Plain-film radiography of the abdomen can identify radiopaque stones.

    4. Renal ultrasonography or CT can identify stones at the ureterovesicular junction.

    5. An IV urogram is indicated if the diagnosis remains uncertain.

D. Treatment

    1. Stones measuring less than 5 mm

        a. Many are likely to pass spontaneously and, in an otherwise healthy individual, may be managed on an outpatient basis.

        b. The patient should drink plenty of fluids.

        c. Strain urine to catch the stone, and save it for analysis.

d. Use an adequate supply of oral analgesics.

e. Follow up weekly or biweekly to monitor progress. Most stones that pass do so within 2–4 weeks of onset of symptoms.

2. Stones measuring 5–10 mm

a. These are less likely to pass spontaneously; patients should be considered for early elective intervention if no other complicating factors (e.g., infection, high-grade obstruction, solitary kidney) are present.

b. Treatment. Increased fluids and analgesics are needed.

c. Elective lithotripsy or ureteroscopy with stone extraction may be used.

3. Stones measuring greater than 10 mm

a. These are not likely to pass spontaneously; these patients are more likely to have complications.

b. The patient should be treated on an inpatient basis if they are unable to maintain adequate oral intake.

c. Vigorous hydration should be maintained.

d. Antibiotics should be administered if signs of infection are present.

e. Ureteral stent or percutaneous nephrostomy should be used if renal function is jeopardized.

f. Urgent treatment with extracorporeal shock wave lithotripsy can be used for renal stones of less than 2 cm or for ureteral stones of less than 1 cm; ureteroscopic fragmentation also may be used. Percutaneous nephrolithotomy can be used for stones of greater than 2 cm.

4. Medications should be administered including morphine, meperidine, or ketorolac for pain; hydrochlorothiazide to increase urine production; and allopurinol for uric acid stones.

V. DISORDERS OF SALT AND WATER

A. Hyper- and hyponatremia reflect disturbances in water homeostasis. Serum sodium accurately reflects changes in serum osmolality and, therefore, changes in free water balance.

B. Disorders of water deficiency: hypernatremia

1. General characteristics

a. In hypernatremia, the water content of body fluid is deficient in relation to sodium content (serum sodium >145 mEq/L).

b. Hypernatremia generally results from either inadequate fluid intake or excess water loss. Causes include sodium excess, deficit of thirst, hypotonic fluid loss, urinary loss, GI loss, insensible loss, burns, diuretic therapy, osmotic diuresis, and diabetes insipidus (DI).

c. It occurs commonly in the elderly, and it may occur in infants with diarrhea.

2. Clinical features

a. Neurologic manifestations include thirst, restlessness, irritability, disorientation, delirium, convulsions, and coma.

b. Other findings include dry mouth and dry mucous membranes, lack of tears and decreased salivation, flushed skin, tachycardia, hypotension, fever, oliguria and anuria, hyperventilation, lethargy, and hyperreflexia.

3. Laboratory findings

a. By definition, plasma sodium will be greater than 145 mEq/L. Urine sodium should be decreased, and urine should be concentrated (except in DI).

b. DI

(1) Low urine sodium and polyuria usually indicate DI.

(2) Antidiuretic stimulation does not increase urine osmolality in DI (see V.D.).

c. Hyperosmolar coma may be indicated by elevated serum glucose, decreased urine output, and increased urine osmolality.

4. Treatment

a. Hypernatremia should be treated on an inpatient basis.

b. The underlying cause must be treated.

c. Free water may be administered orally, which is the preferred route, or IV, as a 5% dextrose solution.

      d. Hypovolemia should be treated first and hypernatremia second.

      e. Dialysis should be implemented if sodium is greater than 200 mEq/L.

      f. Use caution during treatment because rapid correction of hypernatremia can cause pulmonary or cerebral edema, especially in patients with diabetes mellitus.

C. Disorders of water excess: hyponatremia

  1. General characteristics

      a. Hyponatremia is defined as a plasma sodium concentration of less than 135 mEq/L. Signs and symptoms may not occur until the concentration falls below 125 mEq/L.

      b. Hyponatremia is the most common electrolyte disorder seen in the general hospital population.

      c. Types and their occurrence

        (1) Hyponatremia with hypervolemia occurs in the setting of congestive heart failure, nephrotic syndrome, renal failure, and hepatic cirrhosis.

        (2) Hyponatremia with euvolemia occurs with hypothyroidism and syndrome of inappropriate antidiuretic hormone (SIADH) release.

        (3) SIADH is defined as hypotonic hyponatremia; urine osmolality of greater than 100 mOsm/kg; normal cardiac, hepatic, thyroid, adrenal, and renal function; and absence of extracellular fluid volume deficit.

        (4) Hyponatremia with hypovolemia occurs with renal or nonrenal sodium loss.

        (5) Table 6-5 provides an approach to the causes of hyponatremia.

  2. Clinical features

      a. Symptoms may include lethargy, disorientation, muscle cramps, anorexia, hiccups, nausea, vomiting, and seizures.

      b. Signs include weakness, agitation, hyporeflexia, orthostatic hypotension, Cheyne-Stokes respirations, delirium, coma, or stupor.

TABLE 6-5   **Differential Diagnosis of Hyponatremia**

1. Is the plasma osmolality between 280 and 295 mOsm/kg?
   If yes, think isotonic hyponatremia (paraproteinemia, hypertriglyceridemia).

2. Is the plasma osmolality >295 mOsm/kg?
   If yes, think hypertonic hyponatremia (hyperglycemia).

3. Is the plasma osmolality <280 mOsm/kg?
   If yes, think hypotonic hyponatremia, and measure the urine osmolality.

4. Is the urine osmolality <100 mOsm/kg?
   If yes, think excessive water intake (primary polydipsia).

5. Is the urine osmolality >100 mOsm/kg?
   If yes, think impaired renal diluting ability, and assess the ECFV.

6. Does the ECFV appear normal?
   If yes, think endocrinopathies (hypothyroidism, glucocorticoid insufficiency), SIADH (drugs, tumors, CNS disorders, nausea, pain, stress), a reset osmostat, potassium depletion, or thiazide diuretics.

7. Is the ECFV decreased and the urine sodium increased (>20 mEq/L)?
   If yes, think renal solute loss (diuretics, osmotic diuresis, Addison's disease)

8. Is the ECFV decreased and the urine sodium decreased (<10 mEq/L)?
   If yes, think extrarenal sodium loss.

9. Is the ECFV increased and the urine sodium increased?
   If yes, think renal failure.

10. Is the ECFV increased and the urine sodium decreased?
    If yes, think edematous disorders (CHF, cirrhosis, nephritic syndrome)

CHF, congestive heart failure; *CNS*, central nervous system; *ECFV*, extracellular fluid volume; *SIADH*, syndrome of inappropriate antidiuretic hormone.

3. Laboratory findings

    a. Serum sodium of less than 135 mEq/L.

    b. Plasma osmolality usually is decreased, except in cases of fluid redistribution due to hyperglycemia or proteinemia.

    c. Urine sodium is increased or decreased, depending on the cause (Table 6-5).

    d. If SIADH is suspected, CT may be done to rule out central nervous system (CNS) disorder, and chest radiography may be done to rule out lung pathology.

4. Treatment

    a. Treat hypovolemia on an inpatient basis, especially if symptomatic or if serum sodium is less than 125 mEq/L.

    b. Treat the underlying cause, which usually requires fluid restriction.

    c. Monitor volume status.

    d. In severe symptomatic hyponatremia with sodium of less than 120 mEq/L, hypertonic saline may be used very cautiously.

        (1) Overly rapid correction can cause central pontine myelinolysis, resulting in neurologic damage.

        (2) Serum sodium levels should be checked hourly and neurologic status closely monitored.

    e. In chronic hyponatremia unresponsive to fluid restriction, demeclocycline may be used to induce nephrogenic DI.

D. Diabetes Insipidus (DI)

1. General characteristics

    a. DI is a disorder of water conservation.

    b. Neurogenic DI is caused by deficient secretion of arginine vasopressin from the posterior pituitary.

    c. Nephrogenic DI is caused by kidneys that are unresponsive to normal vasopressin levels.

    d. Nephrogenic DI may be an inherited X-linked trait or acquired as a result of lithium therapy, hypokalemia, hypercalcemia, or renal disease.

2. Clinical features

    a. Physical findings are associated with the primary cause.

    b. Polyuria, nocturia, and polydipsia are the main symptoms.

3. Laboratory findings

    a. Neurogenic and nephrogenic DI can be distinguished by water deprivation and desmopressin (deamino-8-D-arginine vasopressin) testing.

    b. Urine osmolality of less than 250 mOsm/kg despite hypernatremia indicates DI.

4. Treatment

    a. Neurogenic DI is best treated with parenteral or intranasal desmopressin.

    b. Diuretics, chlorpropamide, or carbamazepine can be used in patients with mild disease.

    c. Nephrogenic diabetes can be treated with diuretics or indomethacin.

    d. Dietary measures, such as limiting salt and protein intake, can be helpful.

E. Volume depletion

1. General characteristics

    a. Volume depletion occurs when body fluids are lost from the extracellular compartment at a rate that exceeds intake.

    b. Fluid can be lost from the GI tract, kidneys, or skin or from "third spacing" in the abdomen or injured tissues.

2. Clinical features

    a. Volume-depleted patients become thirsty, and urinary output decreases.

    b. Mild volume depletion can cause increased heart rate, fatigue, and muscle cramps.

    c. Moderate fluid loss causes dizziness and hypotension when standing.

    d. Severe hypovolemia results in general hypotension, signs of ischemia and shock, as well as lethargy and confusion.

    e. Decreased skin turgor and dry mucous membranes are unreliable signs of hypovolemia in older adults.

3. Laboratory testing

    a. Hematocrit and serum albumin are increased.

    b. Urinary sodium decreases.

    c. Urea increases, but there is little change in serum creatinine.

4. Treatment

    a. Mild hypovolemia can be treated by increasing dietary salt, which leads to increased water intake with normal thirst mechanisms.

    b. Severe volume depletion can be treated with oral fluids containing electrolytes, glucose, and amino acids.

    c. IV fluids should be used when patients cannot tolerate oral solutions. Isotonic fluids should be given until tissue perfusion has improved.

VI. ELECTROLYTE DISORDERS

A. Disorders of potassium

    1. Hyperkalemia

        a. General characteristics

            (1) Hyperkalemia refers to an elevated serum potassium level.

            (2) It may result from cellular redistribution from intracellular to extracellular compartment, potassium retention, impaired potassium excretion, or elevations caused by hemolysis or thrombocytosis.

            (3) It most commonly is associated with renal failure, ACE inhibitors, hyporeninemic hypoaldosteronism, cell death, and acidosis.

        b. Clinical features

            (1) Severe hyperkalemia can result in arrhythmia and cardiac arrest.

            (2) Neurologic symptoms include numbness, tingling, weakness, and flaccid paralysis.

        c. Laboratory findings

            (1) Serum potassium level is greater than 5 mEq/L; serum creatinine and BUN should be measured to assess renal function. Urine potassium, creatinine and osmolality can reveal decreased fractional excretion of potassium.

            (2) The electrocardiogram (ECG) changes evolve as potassium rises to greater than 6 mEq/L.

                (a) Earliest ECG manifestation is peaking of the T waves (>6.5 mEq/L).

                (b) Flattening of the P wave, prolongation of the PR interval, and widening of the QRS complex are seen with more severe hyperkalemia (>7 mEq/L).

                (c) A final event is a sine-wave pattern with cardiac arrest (>8–10 mEq/L).

        d. Treatment

            (1) Potentially life-threatening hyperkalemia should be treated first, then the underlying cause discovered. Review the clinical situation, determine the acid-base status, and consider drug-induced conditions.

            (2) Potassium-sparing drugs or dietary potassium should be discontinued.

            (3) In severe hyperkalemia with ECG changes, calcium gluconate should be given IV to antagonize the effects of hyperkalemia on the heart.

            (4) Sodium bicarbonate, glucose, and insulin may be administered to drive potassium back into the intracellular compartment. The onset of action is rapid but the duration short; therefore, serial potassium levels should be followed until correction is complete.

            (5) Sodium polystyrene sulfonate (Kayexalate), a cation-exchange resin, is used to remove potassium from the body when levels are extremely high.

    2. Hypokalemia

        a. General considerations

            (1) Hypokalemia is defined as a decreased serum potassium level.

            (2) It can result from a shift of potassium into the intracellular compartment or from potassium losses of extrarenal or renal origin.

            (3) It most commonly occurs with use of diuretics, renal tubular acidosis, or GI losses.

b. Clinical features

(1) Cardiovascular manifestations are the most important, resulting in ventricular arrhythmias, hypotension, and cardiac arrest.

(2) Neuromuscular manifestations also occur, including malaise, skeletal muscle weakness, cramps, and smooth muscle involvement, leading to ileus and constipation.

(3) Other manifestations include polyuria, nocturia, and hyperglycemia.

c. Laboratory findings

(1) Serum potassium is less than 3.5 mEq/L.

(2) ECG may reveal flattened or inverted T waves, increased prominence of U waves, depression of the ST segment, and ventricular ectopy.

(3) The most helpful tests for causal workup include blood acid-base parameters, urinary potassium, and chloride levels.

d. Treatment

(1) Hypokalemia usually is not an emergency unless cardiac manifestations are present. In nonemergent conditions, oral potassium therapy is preferred, usually with potassium chloride.

(2) For emergent situations (serum potassium <2.5 mEq/L or arrhythmias), IV replacement is indicated.

(3) Hypokalemia potentiates the effects of cardiac glycosides on myocardial conduction and may lead to digitalis intoxication. More aggressive potassium replacement may be required in this situation.

B. Disorders of calcium and phosphorus

1. General considerations

a. Mechanisms for calcium and phosphorus homeostasis are complex and carefully maintained by several interrelated and interdependent mechanisms. These involve vitamin D, the small intestine, renal tubules, parathyroid hormone (PTH), and bone.

b. Increased PTH levels result in increased serum calcium and decreased phosphorus. Conversely, decreased levels of PTH result in decreased serum calcium and increased phosphorus.

c. Parathyroid disorders, chronic renal failure, and malignancy are the most common causes of disorders of calcium and phosphorus.

2. Hypercalcemia

a. General characteristics

(1) Hypercalcemia is a significant elevation in serum calcium after adjustment for albumin level (see below).

(2) This is one of the most common disorders of calcium and phosphorus, especially in hospitalized patients with malignancy (e.g., lung cancer; squamous cell carcinoma of the head, neck, esophagus; female genital tract carcinoma; multiple myeloma; lymphoma; renal cell carcinoma).

(3) Other causes include vitamin D intoxication, hyperparathyroidism, and sarcoidosis.

b. Clinical features. Severity of symptoms depends on calcium level, rapidity of onset of hypercalcemia, state of hydration, and the underlying malignancy, if any.

(1) Symptoms include anorexia, nausea, constipation, polyuria, polydipsia, dehydration, and change in level of consciousness (lethargy, stupor, and coma).

(2) Signs of intravascular volume depletion (e.g., orthostatic hypotension and tachycardia) are frequent.

c. Laboratory studies

(1) Serum calcium is high.

(a) The calcium level must be corrected for albumin levels.

(b) Corrected calcium = measured total calcium + 0.8 *(4 − albumin).

(2) Serum phosphorus level

(a) If elevated, it suggests vitamin D intoxication.

(b) If decreased, it suggests primary hyperparathyroidism.

(3) Chest radiography may reveal an underlying pulmonary mass.

(4) Perform urinalysis for hematuria, an early sign of renal cell carcinoma.

(5) Erythrocyte sedimentation rate may be elevated in monoclonal gammopathy. Protein electrophoresis of serum or urine may be needed to confirm the diagnosis.

(6) A 24-hour urine collection for calcium determination.

(a) An elevated urine calcium suggests malignant neoplastic or paraneoplastic process.

(b) A decreased urine calcium suggests primary hyperparathyroidism.

(7) Serum vitamin D levels. Elevations are consistent with vitamin D toxicity.

d. Treatment

(1) Isotonic saline should be used for volume repletion. Loop diuretics should be used if the patient is hypervolemic after volume repletion.

(2) Manage the underlying cause.

3. Hypocalcemia

a. General characteristics

(1) Hypocalcemia may be more common than hypercalcemia, and it can be found in a significant number of critically ill patients.

(2) It commonly results from chronic disease. Although it typically presents in a mild, asymptomatic form, severe hypocalcemia can result in complete cardiovascular collapse.

b. Clinical features

(1) Symptoms include dry skin, brittle nails, pruritis, muscle cramping, shortness of breath, and numbness and tingling in the extremities. Severe cardiovascular manifestations include syncope and angina.

(2) Signs include psoriasis, dry skin, and perioral numbness. Cardiovascular signs include wheezing, bradycardia, crackles, and a third heart sound.

(3) Classic neurologic findings include the Trousseau's sign (carpal tunnel spasm after BP cuff applied for 3 min) and the Chvostek's sign (spasm of facial muscle after tapping facial nerve in front of ear). Other neurologic manifestations include irritability, confusion, dementia, and seizures.

c. Laboratory studies

(1) Hypocalcemia is defined as a corrected serum calcium level of less than 8.5 mEq/L.

(2) Ionized calcium also should be measured. Magnesium, phosphate, albumin, liver function tests, and other electrolytes should be obtained.

(3) BUN and creatinine should be measured to assess renal function.

d. Treatment

(1) Treat any emergent cardiovascular states.

(2) Severe hypocalcemia should be replaced (calcium gluconate or calcium chloride) IV.

(3) Mild hypocalcemia can be treated on an outpatient basis with oral calcium and vitamin D supplements.

C. Disorders of magnesium

1. Hypermagnesemia

a. General characteristics

(1) Hypermagnesemia is defined as plasma magnesium levels of greater than 2.1 mEq/L.

(2) Most magnesium is stored in bone and muscle.

b. Clinical features

(1) Symptomatic hypermagnesemia rarely occurs, except in patients with renal failure who are given magnesium-containing products, such as laxatives or antacids.

(2) Hypermagnesemia can be iatrogenically induced as part of treatment in eclampsia or preterm labor.

(3) Signs and symptoms reflect impaired neuromuscular transmission.

(a) Initially, deep tendon reflexes are reduced.

(b) Muscle weakness, hypotension, respiratory depression, and then cardiac arrest can follow with increasing magnesium levels.

(c) Nausea, vomiting, and flushing also can occur.

c. Laboratory tests.

(1) ECG shows widened QRS complex, prolonged PR interval, and increased T wave amplification.

(2) Bleeding and clotting times are increased.

d. Treatment

(1) Administration of 10–20 mL of 10% calcium gluconate IV over 10 min.

(2) IV furosemide may increase excretion of magnesium.

(3) Dialysis is effective in severe hypermagnesemia.

2. Hypomagnesemia

a. General characteristics

(1) Hypomagnesemia is defined as plasma magnesium levels of less than 1.4 mEq/L. Plasma levels do not reflect total body stores.

(2) Hypomagnesemia usually presents when total body stores are severely depleted. Depletion usually results from diminished intake and impaired absorption.

(3) Most commonly associated with chronic alcoholism, chronic diarrhea, hypoparathyroidism, hyperaldosteronism, diuretic therapy, osmotic diuresis, and nutritional deficiencies (e.g., prolonged parenteral feeding, malnutrition).

b. Clinical features. Signs and symptoms include lethargy, anorexia, nausea and vomiting, weakness, tetany, and seizures.

c. Laboratory tests

(1) Hypocalcemia and hypocalciuria commonly are associated with causes of magnesium depletion.

(2) ECG may show prolonged PR and QT intervals.

d. Treatment

(1) Administer oral magnesium sulfate or chloride for chronic hypomagnesemia. Administer twice the estimated deficit over several days.

(2) In severe symptomatic hypomagnesemia, a 10% magnesium sulfate solution can be administered IV.

VII. ACID-BASE DISORDERS

A. General characteristics

1. Disturbances in the acid-base equilibrium are common, especially in patients who are critically ill.

2. They may be respiratory (characterized by alterations in carbon dioxide [CO_2]) or metabolic (characterized by alterations in serum bicarbonate). Table 6-6 summarizes the relationships.

3. pH

a. The pH usually is considered to be "normal" between 7.35 and 7.45.

b. A pH of less than 7.35 represents acidemia.

c. A pH of greater than 7.45 represents alkalemia.

d. A pH of 7.2 or lower represents severe acidemia.

e. A pH of 7.6 or greater represents severe alkalemia.

4. Compensation for changes in the hydrogen ion concentration will always occur in the buffering system, the lungs or kidneys. The degree of compensation depends on the duration of the disturbance and the functioning of the organ.

TABLE 6-6 Acid-Base Disorders			
Disorder	**pH**	**Carbon Dioxide (Pco$_2$)**	**Bicarbonate (HCO$_3$)**
Respiratory acidosis	Decreased (↓)	Increased (↑)[a]	Increased (↑)
Respiratory alkalosis	Increased (↑)	Decreased (↓)[a]	Decreased (↓)
Metabolic acidosis	Decreased (↓)	Decreased (↓)	Decreased (↓)[a]
Metabolic alkalosis	Increased (↑)	Increased (↑)	Increased (↑)[a]
[a]Represents the primary disturbance			

B. Respiratory acidosis

   1. General characteristics

   a. Respiratory acidosis is defined as a primary increase in the partial pressure of CO_2 (PCO_2) in the blood and decreased blood pH.

   b. It is the result of alveolar hypoventilation leading to pulmonary CO_2 retention.

   c. The causes of respiratory acidosis include all disorders that reduce pulmonary function and CO_2 clearance, such as primary pulmonary disease, neuromuscular disease (myasthenia gravis), primary CNS dysfunction (severe brainstem injury), and drug-induced hypoventilation.

   2. Clinical features

   a. Metabolic encephalopathy with headache and drowsiness is the most characteristic change.

   b. If not corrected, initial CNS symptoms may progress to stupor and coma.

   3. Laboratory findings

   a. Acute CO_2 retention leads to an increase in blood PCO_2 with minimal change in plasma bicarbonate content. Serum electrolyte levels are close to normal.

   b. After 2–5 days, renal compensation occurs, leading to increased hydrogen ion secretion and bicarbonate production in the distal nephron, after which the plasma bicarbonate level steadily increases.

   4. Treatment

   a. The underlying disorder must be identified and corrected.

   b. A blood PCO_2 of greater than 60 mm Hg may indicate the need for assisted ventilation if CNS or pulmonary muscular depression is severe.

C. Respiratory alkalosis

   1. General characteristics

   a. Respiratory alkalosis is defined primarily by decreased blood PCO_2 and increased blood pH.

   b. Respiratory alkalosis is the result of excessive elimination of CO_2 via the lungs.

   c. The causes of respiratory alkalosis include any disorders associated with inappropriately increased ventilatory rate and CO_2 clearance.

   d. Anxiety (hysterical hyperventilation) is the most common cause of respiratory alkalosis. Other causes include salicylate intoxication, hypoxia, intrathoracic disorders, primary CNS dysfunction, Gram-negative septicemia, liver insufficiency, and pregnancy.

   2. Clinical features

   a. Obvious hyperventilation usually is present, particularly when alkalosis is caused by cerebral or metabolic disorders.

   b. The breathing pattern in the anxiety-induced syndrome varies from frequent, deep, sighing respirations to sustained and obvious rapid, deep breathing.

   c. Acute alkalemia may produce a tetany-like syndrome, which may be indistinguishable from acute hypocalcemia.

   d. Circumoral paresthesias, acroparesthesias (painful burning of hands and feet), giddiness, or light-headedness may occur.

   3. Diagnosis

   a. In acute alkalosis, increased respiratory rate leads to a loss of CO_2 via the lungs, which in turn increases the blood pH.

   b. Within hours after an acute decrease in arterial PCO_2, hydrogen ion secretion in the distal nephron decreases, leading to a decrease in plasma bicarbonate. Serum chloride level also is elevated.

   4. Treatment

   a. The primary goal of therapy is to correct the underlying disorder.

   b. Use of CO_2-enriched breathing mixtures or controlled ventilation may be required in cases of severe respiratory alkalosis (pH >7.6).

D. Metabolic acidosis

   1. General characteristics

   a. Metabolic acidosis is an elevation in the normal serum concentration of hydrogen ions that is initiated either by the loss of bicarbonate from or by the addition of hydrogen ions to the serum.

b. Several conditions may result in increased hydrogen ions in the serum.

  (1) These include lactic acidosis, diabetic ketoacidosis, starvation ketosis, and ethylene glycol, methanol, and salicylate intoxication; these conditions result in an increased anion gap.

  (2) Hydrogen ions also may be retained in renal tubular acidosis, renal insufficiency, and adrenal insufficiency.

c. Conditions that may result in the loss of bicarbonate include diarrhea, pancreatic or biliary drainage, and ureterosigmoidostomy; these conditions typically have a normal anion gap.

2. Clinical features

  a. Hyperventilation is the earliest and most recognized sign, resulting from stimulation of the respiratory drive to blow off CO_2 (pulmonary compensation).

  b. Ventricular arrhythmias may occur.

  c. Neurologic symptoms range from lethargy to frank coma.

3. Laboratory studies

  a. Arterial blood gas measurements reveal a pH <7.35, decreased plasma bicarbonate, and decreased P_{CO_2} (compensation).

  b. The anion gap should be calculated to determine levels of unmeasured anions; the normal value is 12 mEq/L.

  c. Anion gap = serum sodium − (serum bicarbonate + serum chloride).

4. Treatment

  a. Identify and, if possible, remove the primary cause of the metabolic acidosis.

  b. Insulin therapy and volume repletion are the mainstays of therapy for diabetic ketoacidosis.

  c. Bicarbonate therapy can be considered if the pH is less than 7.20. Blood pH should be carefully monitored, because ongoing acid production may increase bicarbonate requirements.

E. Metabolic alkalosis

1. General characteristics

  a. Metabolic alkalosis is defined as an increase in serum bicarbonate with no change in P_{CO_2}, causing an increase in extracellular pH to greater than 7.45.

  b. Metabolic alkalosis and increased serum bicarbonate can be caused by loss of hydrogen, addition of bicarbonate, or disproportionate loss of chloride.

  c. It is maintained by the impaired renal excretion of bicarbonate.

  d. Common causes include vomiting, nasogastric tube suctioning, villous adenoma, chloride diarrhea, diuretics, hypercalcemia, milk-alkali syndrome, and chloride and potassium depletion because of excessive steroids.

2. Clinical features

  a. Neurologic abnormalities, including paresthesias, carpopedal spasm, and light-headedness, occasionally may progress to confusion, stupor, and coma.

  b. Symptoms arising from volume depletion frequently are present; weakness, muscle cramps, and postural dizziness may develop.

  c. Abnormalities secondary to potassium depletion may lead to polyuria, polydipsia, and muscle weakness.

3. Laboratory studies

  a. Arterial blood gas measurements reveal pH greater than 7.45, increased serum bicarbonate, and increased P_{CO_2} (pulmonary compensation).

  b. Urine chloride concentrations can distinguish between hypovolemic hypochloremic patients with a decreased urine chloride concentration (<20 mEq/L) and volume-expanded patients with mineralocorticoid excess who have urine chloride concentrations of greater than 30 mEq/L.

4. Treatment

  a. Interventions to increase renal excretion of bicarbonate are the most effective therapy for metabolic acidosis.

  b. Chloride-responsive conditions (e.g., gastric fluid loss, diuretic therapy) are treated with solutions containing sodium chloride to repair the sodium and chloride deficits.

  c. Chloride-resistant conditions (e.g., mineralocorticoid excess) can be successfully treated by removing an adrenal adenoma, if present, or by using spironolactone, an aldosterone antagonist.

VIII. URINARY TRACT INFECTION

  A. Cystitis

    1. General characteristics

      a. Cystitis is an infection of the bladder most commonly caused by coliform bacteria (especially *Escherichia coli*) and occasionally Gram-positive bacteria (enterococci).

      b. The route of infection typically is ascending from the urethra.

    2. Clinical features

      a. Irritative voiding symptoms (frequency, urgency, dysuria) are common, as is suprapubic discomfort.

      b. Women may demonstrate gross hematuria. Symptoms in women often may appear following sexual intercourse.

      c. Physical examination may elicit suprapubic tenderness, but examination often is unremarkable.

    3. Laboratory studies

      a. Urinalysis shows pyuria, bacteriuria, and varying degrees of hematuria.

      b. Urine culture is positive for the offending organism.

      c. Imaging is warranted only if pyelonephritis, recurrent infections, or anatomic abnormalities are suspected.

    4. Treatment

      a. Uncomplicated cystitis in women can be treated with short-term antimicrobial therapy.

        (1) The suggested regimen is a fluoroquinolone for 3 days.

        (2) Resistant *Escherichia coli* are common, but trimethoprim/sulfamethoxazole can be used as an alternative to a quinolone in susceptible strains.

      b. Uncomplicated cystitis is rare in men.

      c. Fluids should be encouraged.

      d. Hot sitz baths or urinary analgesics (phenazopyridine) may provide symptomatic relief.

  B. Pyelonephritis

    1. General characteristics

      a. Acute pyelonephritis is an infectious inflammatory process involving the kidney parenchyma and renal pelvis.

      b. Gram-negative bacteria are the most common causative agents, including *Escherichia coli*, *Proteus* sp., *Klebsiella* sp., *Enterobacter* sp., and *Pseudomonas* sp. The infection usually ascends from the lower urinary tract.

      c. Chronic pyelonephritis is the result of progressive inflammation of the renal interstitium caused by bacterial infection, vesicoureteral reflux, or both.

    2. Clinical features

      a. Symptoms include fever, flank pain, shaking chills, and irritative voiding symptoms. Nausea, vomiting, and diarrhea are not uncommon.

      b. Young children may have fever and abdominal discomfort.

      c. Signs include fever and tachycardia. Costovertebral angle tenderness usually is pronounced.

    3. Laboratory studies

      a. CBC shows leukocytosis and left shift.

      b. Urinalysis shows pyuria, bacteriuria, and varying degrees of hematuria. WBC casts may be seen.

      c. Urine culture (if obtained before beginning antibiotics) demonstrates heavy growth of the offending agent.

      d. In complicated pyelonephritis, renal ultrasound may show hydronephrosis secondary to obstruction.

    4. Treatment

      a. In the outpatient setting, treatment with quinolones or trimethoprim/sulfamethoxazole for 1–2 weeks has shown to be effective in immunocompetent patients. Immunocompromised patients should be treated for a longer duration.

      b. Hospital admission is required for patients with severe infections or complicating factors, such as older age, comorbid conditions, or signs of obstruction.

      c. IV fluoroquinolones or ampicillin and gentamicin should be initiated while waiting for sensitivity results. IV antibiotics should be continued for 24–48 hour after the patient becomes afebrile; oral antibiotics are then given to complete a minimum of 2 weeks of therapy.

    d. Failure to respond warrants ultrasound imaging to exclude complicating factors that may require prompt intervention.

    e. Follow-up urine cultures are mandatory 1–2 weeks following treatment.

C. Prostatitis

  1. General characteristics

    a. Acute bacterial prostatitis is caused by ascending infection of Gram-negative rods into the prostatic ducts.

    b. Chronic bacterial prostatitis may be associated with evolution or recurrence of an acute bacterial infection.

    c. Chronic nonbacterial prostatitis is the most common of the prostatitis syndromes, and its cause is unknown. It may represent a noninfectious inflammatory disorder, perhaps with an autoimmune origin, and is a diagnosis of exclusion. It often is associated with the term chronic pelvic pain syndrome.

    d. Prostatic abscess is an uncommon complication of acute bacterial prostatitis.

  2. Clinical features

    a. Acute infection is characterized by sudden onset of high fever, chills, and low back and perineal pain.

    b. Chronic infection has more variable symptoms, ranging from asymptomatic to acute symptomatology.

    c. All forms of prostatitis present with irritative bladder symptoms (frequency, urgency, dysuria) and some obstruction.

    d. The prostate is swollen and tender.

  3. Laboratory studies

    a. Urinalysis reveals pyuria.

    b. Prostatic fluid culture typically is positive for *Escherichia coli* in acute infections. Chronic infection is characterized by recurrence of the same organism or enterococcus. In nonbacterial prostatitis, cultures are negative.

    c. The four-glass localization test is the classic means of distinguishing a prostate infection from another urinary tract infection. Urine samples are taken at initial void, midstream, and after prostatic massage; prostatic secretions account for the fourth sample. Assessment of the samples helps to localize the nidus of infection.

  4. Treatment

    a. Antibiotics are the most effective treatment for bacterial infections.

      (1) For men younger than 35 years, ofloxacin for 10 days or ceftriaxone, 250 mg IM, followed by 10 days of doxycycline is recommended.

      (2) In men older than 35 years, a fluoroquinolone or trimethoprim/sulfamethoxazole may be used for 10–14 days.

      (3) Some experts suggest that 3–4 weeks of treatment is necessary to effectively eradicate the acute infection.

      (4) In chronic prostatitis, ciprofloxacin for 4 weeks, ofloxacin for 6 weeks, or trimethoprim/sulfamethoxazole for 1–3 months can be used.

      (5) Antibiotics are not effective in nonbacterial prostatitis.

    b. Nonsteroidal anti-inflammatory drugs are effective analgesics.

    c. Chronic, recurrent, or resistant prostatitis with or without prostatic calculi may need transurethral resection of the prostate for ultimate resolution.

D. Orchitis

  1. General characteristics

    a. Orchitis commonly is caused by ascending bacterial infection from the urinary tract.

    b. It occurs in 25% of postpubertal males who have mumps infection.

  2. Clinical features

    a. Testicular swelling and tenderness, usually unilateral, occurs.

    b. Fever and tachycardia are common.

  3. Laboratory studies

    a. Urinalysis reveals pyuria and bacteriuria with bacterial infection.

    b. Cultures are positive for suspected organisms.

    c. Ultrasonography is useful if abscess is suspected.

    4. Treatment

        a. If mumps is the cause, symptomatic relief with ice and analgesia should be provided.

        b. If bacteria is the cause, the orchitis should be treated like epididymitis.

        c. Carefully evaluate any scrotal masses.

E. Epididymitis

    1. General characteristics

        a. Epididymitis is infection of the epididymis acquired by retrograde spread of organisms through the vas deferens.

        b. In men younger than 35 years, chlamydia and gonococci are the most common organisms.

        c. In men older than 35 years, *Escherichia coli* is the most common organism.

    2. Clinical features

        a. Epididymitis presents with heaviness and dull, aching discomfort in the affected hemiscrotum, which can radiate up the ipsilateral flank.

        b. The epididymis is markedly swollen and exquisitely tender to touch, eventually becoming a warm, erythematous, enlarged scrotal mass.

        c. The patient may have fever and chills.

        d. The Prehn's sign (relief of pain with scrotal elevation) is a classic sign, but it is not very reliable.

    3. Laboratory studies

        a. Urinalysis reveals pyuria and bacteriuria.

        b. Cultures show positive results for suspected organisms.

    4. Treatment

        a. In men younger than 35 years, ceftriaxone, 250 mg IM, plus doxycycline, 100 mg b.i.d. orally for 10 days, may be administered for gonococci or chlamydia.

        b. In men older than 35 years, ciprofloxacin 500 mg b.i.d. orally for 10–14 days may be used.

        c. Supportive care may include bed rest, scrotal elevation, and analgesics.

IX. BENIGN PROSTATIC HYPERPLASIA

A. General characteristics

    1. Proliferation of the fibrostromal tissue of the prostate can lead to compression of the prostatic urethra, creating an obstruction of the urinary outlet.

    2. Benign prostatic hyperplasia is a disease of older men; the mean age of onset is 60–65 years.

B. Clinical features

    1. The symptom complex is referred to as prostatism, which includes symptoms of obstruction and irritation.

    2. Obstructive symptoms include decreased force of urinary stream, hesitancy and straining, postvoid dribbling, and sensation of incomplete emptying.

    3. Irritative symptoms include frequency, nocturia, and urgency.

    4. Recurrent urinary tract infections and urinary retention also can occur.

    5. Digital rectal examination typically reveals an enlarged prostate.

C. Laboratory studies

    1. Prostate-specific antigen typically is slightly elevated.

    2. Other tests are done to evaluate for renal damage, infection, and prostate or bladder cancer, as suspected.

D. Treatment

    1. Men with mild to moderate symptoms may choose watchful waiting and frequent monitoring.

    2. Options for medical therapy include α-adrenergic agonists and 5α-reductase inhibitors.

    3. Procedures that may be used to relieve obstruction include use of balloon dilation, microwave irradiation, and stent placements.

    4. Surgical treatment is transurethral resection of prostate or transurethral incision of prostate.

X. INCONTINENCE

A. General characteristics

1. Urinary incontinence is defined as the unintentional leakage of urine at inappropriate times.

2. Women experience incontinence twice as often as men. Older women experience it more often than younger women.

3. Incontinence can be classified based on the underlying pathophysiologic mechanism.

   a. Urge incontinence results from bladder contractions that cannot be controlled by the brain.

   b. Stress incontinence is caused by dysfunction of the urethral sphincter, allowing urine to leak with increased intra-abdominal pressure.

   c. Overflow incontinence occurs when urinary retention leads to bladder distention and overflow of urine through the urethra.

   d. Functional incontinence is untimely urination caused by physical or cognitive disability preventing a person from reaching a toilet.

   e. Mixed incontinence is a combination of elements of both stress and urge incontinence.

B. Clinical features

1. Reversible causes of incontinence, such as medication side effects, recent prostatectomy, excess fluid intake, atrophic vaginitis, fecal impaction, urinary tract infection, impaired mobility, and glycosuria should be identified.

2. The principal symptom of urge incontinence is a strong desire to void, followed by loss of urine.

3. Overactive bladder disorder is a related symptom complex characterized by frequency of urination, urgency to urinate, and nocturia. Patients may present with or without urge incontinence.

4. The principal symptom of stress incontinence is leakage of urine with increased intra-abdominal pressure, such as with sneezing, coughing, or laughing.

5. Untreated overflow incontinence can lead to hydronephrosis and obstructive nephropathy.

6. Incontinence is common with neurologic diseases (stroke, Parkinson's disease or dementia), metabolic disorders (hypoxemia, diabetic neuropathy), and pelvic disorders (uterine prolapse).

C. Laboratory findings

1. Urinalysis can identify diabetes-related glycosuria or acute urinary tract infection.

2. Postvoid residual urine volume should be measured to identify urinary retention.

3. Simple cystometry (instillation of water into the bladder) can identify bladder contractions.

4. Stress test, ultrasonography, cystoscopy, and urodynamics also may be used.

D. Treatment

1. Pelvic floor muscle training (or Kegel exercises), electrical muscle stimulation, biofeedback, and bladder training can be used to improve the strength and control of the pelvic muscles. Pessaries or implants can help decrease stress incontinence.

2. Anticholinergic medications, such as oxybutynin or tolterodine, are effective for urge incontinence. α-Adrenergics or estrogen can be used for stress incontinence.

3. Tolterodine and oxybutynin can be used for overactive bladder.

4. Catheterization, either intermittent or indwelling, can be used for overflow incontinence.

5. Although surgical treatments often are the last resort, they are very effective for stress incontinence.

XI. NEOPLASMS OF THE URINARY TRACT

A. Prostate cancer

1. General characteristics

   a. Prostate cancer is a common, generally slow-growing, malignant neoplasm of the adenomatous cells of the prostate gland that can lead to urinary obstruction and metastatic disease.

   b. A disease of aging, it rarely is seen in men younger than 40 years.

   c. The cause is unknown. Risk factors may include genetic predisposition, hormonal influences, dietary and environmental factors, and infectious agents.

    2. Clinical features

        a. Many cases are not clinically apparent.

        b. Symptoms of urinary obstruction occur.

        c. In advanced disease, patients may present with bone pain from metastases.

        d. The prostate may be enlarged, nodular, and asymmetric.

    3. Laboratory studies

        a. Prostate-specific antigen usually is elevated in patients with prostate cancer.

        b. Pathologic examination of tissue removed for treatment of obstructive prostatic hyperplasia reveals that 10% have malignancy.

        c. Transrectal ultrasound reveals hypoechoic lesions in prostate.

        d. Biopsy confirms the diagnosis of adenocarcinoma and allows histologic grading, which can provide prognostic information.

    4. Treatment

        a. Appropriate treatment depends on the staging, which is done by abdominal and pelvic CT or MRI, pelvic lymphadenectomy, and bone scan.

        b. The Gleason score is based on the architectural pattern. Low-grade tumors that are more well differentiated may not require any treatment, whereas higher-grade tumors more typically are aggressive and, therefore, should be managed more aggressively.

        c. Stage A and B disease (tumor confined to the prostate) may be treated with radical retropubic prostatectomy, brachytherapy or external-beam radiation therapy.

        d. Stage C disease (tumor with local invasion) is treated similar to stage A and B disease, but with reduced effectiveness.

        e. Stage D disease (distant metastases) is treated with hormonal manipulation using orchiectomy, antiandrogens, luteinizing hormone–releasing hormone agonists, or estrogens. Chemotherapy has limited usefulness, and palliative treatment is given for advanced disease.

B. Bladder cancer

    1. General characteristics

        a. Causal factors for bladder cancer include exposure to tobacco; occupational carcinogens from rubber, dye, printing, and chemical industries; schistosomiasis; and chronic infections.

        b. Uroepithelial tumors account for 3% of cancer deaths in the United States. Bladder carcinoma is three times more common in men than in women, and it usually occurs in patients 40–70 years of age.

    2. Clinical features

        a. Hematuria is the most common presenting symptom.

        b. Bladder irritability and infection are other presenting symptoms.

    3. Laboratory findings

        a. CBC and blood chemistry should be done to evaluate for infection and renal function.

        b. Cystoscopy, which has an accuracy rate of nearly 100%, is the definitive diagnostic procedure. Biopsy confirms the pathologic diagnosis.

        c. Radiologic procedures include IV urogram, pelvic and abdominal CT, chest radiography, bone scan, and retrograde pyelography for renal pelvic or ureteral tumors and staging.

    4. Treatment

        a. Treatment depends on the stage.

        b. Superficial lesions are treated with endoscopic resection and fulguration, followed by cystoscopy every 3 months. Recurrent or multiple lesions can be treated with an intravesical instillation of thiotepa, mitomycin, or bacillus Calmette-Guérin.

        c. Radical cystectomy is used for recurrent cancer, diffuse transitional cell carcinoma in situ, or tumors that have invaded the muscle.

        d. Combination chemotherapy has been used in bladder-sparing trials with or without radiation therapy.

C. Renal cell carcinoma (RCC)

    1. General characteristics

    a. RCC is the most common type of renal malignancy. It accounts for 3% of all adult cancers.

    b. RCC is more common in men, usually affecting those older than 55 years. Incidence is equivalent in whites and blacks but is about one-third higher in Hispanics.

    c. The cause is unknown, but cigarette smoking is a risk factor. There is an inherited form that is autosomal dominant.

2. Clinical features

    a. RCC is associated with a wide range of presenting signs and symptoms and often is called the "internists' tumor."

    b. The most common symptom is gross or microscopic hematuria, followed by pain or an abdominal mass. The classic triad of gross hematuria, flank pain, and a palpable mass, however, occurs only in a small percentage of patients.

    c. RCC is associated with paraneoplastic syndromes, including erythrocytosis, hypercalcemia, hypertension, and hepatic dysfunction in the absence of hepatic metastases.

3. Laboratory findings

    a. Normochromic anemia occurs in nearly one-third of patients with RCC. An elevated erythrocyte sedimentation rate has been reported in up to 75% of patients.

    b. Patients presenting with hematuria should have an IV urogram, which usually identifies calcification overlying the renal shadow. Confirming studies need to be done.

    c. Patients presenting with an abdominal mass usually undergo CT, which is more sensitive than IV urogram for RCC detection. CT shows a heterogeneous, decreased density within the renal parenchyma.

    d. Ultrasonography can further identify lesions found on IV urogram. Renal angiography, radionuclide imaging, fine-needle aspiration, and tumor markers have limited usefulness in diagnosing RCC.

    e. MRI is equivalent to CT for staging of RCC.

4. Treatment

    a. Treatment depends on the stage of the tumor, so a thorough staging evaluation is required.

    b. Radical nephrectomy is the primary treatment for localized disease (stage I, II and IIIA lesions.) Neoadjuvant or adjuvant radiation therapy has not been shown to prolong survival for early stage lesions.

    c. Radiation therapy is an important method of palliation in patients with disseminated disease to the brain, bone, and lungs. Radical nephrectomy has little role in advanced disease.

    d. Hormonal therapy and chemotherapy have shown little effect.

    e. Medications, such as α-interferon and interleukin, have been successful in reducing the growth of some RCCs, including some with metastasis.

D. Wilms' tumor

1. General characteristics

    a. Wilms' tumor, also known as nephroblastoma, is the most common renal tumor of childhood.

    b. There are approximately 500 cases per year in familial and nonfamilial forms. Most occur in healthy children, but about 10% occur in children with recognized malformations.

    c. Most cases of Wilms' tumor are curable, but on histologic study, about 10% of patients have anaplasia, which is associated with a poorer prognosis.

2. Clinical features

    a. The most common sign is an asymptomatic abdominal mass found by a family member or during physical examination.

    b. Symptoms at presentation might include anorexia, nausea and vomiting, fever, abdominal pain, or hematuria.

    c. Hypertension caused by elevated renin levels can occur.

3. Laboratory findings

    a. Urinalysis may show hematuria, and anemia may be present.

    b. Ultrasonography is the initial study of choice to evaluate abdominal masses.

    c. Abdominal CT is performed in patients with suspected Wilms' tumors to assess tumor extension and regional lymph nodes. MRI also can provide information regarding tumor extension.

    d. Chest radiography is used to evaluate the presence of metastases in the lungs.

4. Treatment

    a. The goal of therapy is to provide the highest possible cure rate with the lowest treatment-related morbidity.

    b. Because of the rarity of the tumor, nearly all patients are enrolled in clinical trials. The most effective therapy is a multimodal approach that incorporates surgery, chemotherapy, and in some patients, radiation therapy.

    c. Radical nephrectomy with lymph node sampling is the treatment of choice in surgically resectable tumors. Unresectable tumors should undergo preoperative chemotherapy, followed by biopsy.

    d. Wilms' tumor is chemosensitive and responsive to dactinomycin, vincristine, and doxorubicin.

    e. Radiation therapy is added for higher-stage tumors (stage III and IV) and for tumors with focal anaplasia.

E. Testicular cancer

  1. General characteristics

    a. Testicular cancer is the most common malignancy in young men, with an average age at diagnosis of 32 years.

    b. Risk factors include history of cryptorchidism or a previous history of testicular cancer.

  2. Clinical features

    a. More than 90% of patients present with a painless, solid, testicular swelling. Occasionally, patients with painful testicular masses are erroneously diagnosed as having epididymitis or orchitis.

    b. Para-aortic lymph node involvement can present as ureteral obstruction.

    c. Patients also may present with abdominal complaints from an abdominal mass or with pulmonary symptoms from multiple nodules.

  3. Laboratory studies

    a. Scrotal ultrasonography may reveal a suspicious intratesticular echogenic focus.

    b. Radiologic studies for staging include radiography of the chest and CT of the chest, abdomen, and pelvis. Other studies that may be used to delineate pathology include excretory urography, venacavogram, bipedal lymphangiography, and bone scans.

    c. Tumors are classified pathologically as seminomatous or nonseminomatous (subtypes are embryonal carcinoma, teratoma, yolk sac carcinoma, and choriocarcinoma).

    d. Elevated blood levels of α-fetoprotein or β-human chorionic gonadotropin are diagnostic for nonseminomatous germ cell tumors; the majority of patients with seminoma have normal levels.

  4. Treatment

    a. Treatment depends on pathology and stage. Staging is based on degree of spread.

      (1) Orchiectomy is always performed for diagnostic and therapeutic reasons.

      (2) Seminomatous tumors are radiosensitive; nonseminomatous tumors are radioresistant.

    b. Nonseminomatous tumors

      (1) Stage I disease limited to the testis can be treated with nerve-sparing retroperitoneal lymph node dissection or rigorous surveillance without surgery or chemotherapy.

      (2) Stage II tumors can be treated with surgery or chemotherapy.

      (3) Stage III disease should be treated with surgery and chemotherapy.

    c. Seminomatous tumors

      (1) The mainstay of therapy for stage I disease isolated to the testis is radiation therapy to the para-aortic and ipsilateral iliac nodal areas.

      (2) Therapy for stage IIa and IIb adds increased radiation to the affected nodes.

      (3) Therapy for stage IIc and III is chemotherapy.

XII. MALE REPRODUCTIVE DISORDERS

A. Phimosis

  1. General characteristics

    a. Characterized by inability to retract the foreskin over the glans penis.

    b. Phimosis may be congenital or acquired.

      (1) Congenital phimosis is common in children and adolescents and usually is physiologic.

      (2) Acquired phimosis is more typical in adults and usually caused by poor hygiene and chronic balanitis.

2. Clinical features

    a. History of recent catheterization or forcible retraction of the foreskin.

    b. Foreskin cannot be retracted over the glans penis.

    c. Obstructed urinary stream, hematuria, or pain of the prepuce can indicate more severe constriction.

3. Laboratory findings. None usually required.

4. Treatment

    a. As long as it is asymptomatic, a congenital phimosis should be left alone.

    b. If symptomatic, referral for circumcision usually is necessary.

    c. Steroidal creams or nonsteroidal ointments may be of benefit.

B. Paraphimosis

  1. General characteristics

    a. Paraphimosis is defined as entrapment of the foreskin behind the glans penis.

    b. Frequent catheterizations without reducing the foreskin can lead to paraphimosis.

    c. Forcibly retracting a constricted foreskin (phimosis) for cleaning or catheterization can lead to paraphimosis.

    d. Vigorous sexual activity can predispose men to paraphimosis.

  2. Clinical features

    a. Pain, edema, tenderness, and erythema of the glans and foreskin are present.

    b. Identification of any encircling foreign bodies, such as hair, clothing, rubber bands, or metallic objects is important.

  3. Laboratory findings. None required.

  4. Treatment

    a. Paraphimosis should be reduced emergently.

      (1) Manual reduction should be tried initially.

      (2) Surgical techniques to incise the restricted foreskin can be used if manual reduction fails.

    b. Inability to reduce a paraphimosis requires emergent urologic referral.

    c. After reduction, referral for circumcision is necessary, because the condition is likely to recur.

C. Erectile dysfunction

  1. General characteristics

    a. Erectile dysfunction is defined as the consistent inability to maintain an erect penis with sufficient rigidity to allow sexual intercourse. It is part of a broader classification of sexual dysfunctions.

    b. Normal erections require intact parasympathetic and somatic nerve supply, unobstructed arterial inflow, adequate venous constriction, hormonal stimulation, and psychological desire. Disorders of any of these systems may result in impotence.

    c. Most cases of male erectile disorders have a primary organic rather than a psychogenic cause. Nearly all cases have a secondary psychogenic component.

    d. This condition affects millions of American men, and its incidence is age related.

    e. Erectile dysfunction in men with type 2 diabetes can be an indicator of early, silent cardiovascular disease.

  2. Clinical features

    a. The medical history must be adequately evaluated.

    b. A sexual history should be taken, including detailed information on timing and frequency of sexual relations, partners, presence of morning erections, ejaculation, and masturbation.

    c. Past medical history should document presence of hypertension, diabetes, endocrine disease, medications, pelvic surgery, or trauma.

    d. Physical examination should look for penile deformities (e.g., Peyronie's disease [fibrous plague causing penile curvative]) testicular atrophy, hypertension, peripheral neuropathy, and other signs of endocrine, vascular, or neurologic abnormalities.

  3. Laboratory findings

    a. CBC, urinalysis, lipid profile, thyroid function tests, serum testosterone, glucose, and prolactin screening should be done, depending on the suspected cause.

    b. Measurement of follicle-stimulating hormone and luteinizing hormone may be required for patients with abnormalities of testosterone or prolactin.

c. Nocturnal penile tumescence testing can be done to differentiate between organic and psychogenic impotence. Patients with psychogenic impotence have normal nocturnal erections of adequate frequency and rigidity.

d. Direct injection of vasoactive substances into the penis induces erections in men with intact vascular systems.

e. Patients who do not achieve erections with injections may undergo studies to evaluate the arterial and venous vasculature, such as ultrasonography of the cavernous arteries, pelvic arteriography, and cavernosonography.

4. Treatment

a. True psychogenic causes can be treated with behaviorally oriented sex therapy. Patients with organic causes of impotence also may benefit from counseling.

b. Phosphodiesterase-5 (PDE-5)–inhibitor therapy is now the standard treatment for erectile dysfunction. Sildenafil, vardenafil, and tadalafil are the drugs currently indicated for erectile dysfunction.

c. Side effects of PDE-5 therapy include headache, flushing, dyspepsia, rhinitis, and visual disturbances.

d. For men in whom PDE-5 therapy is ineffective or inappropriate, there are other treatments, including vacuum constriction devices, use of injected or inserted vasoactive substances, and penile prostheses. Patients with disorders of the arterial system are candidates for arterial reconstruction.

D. Scrotal masses

1. Hydrocele

a. General characteristics. A hydrocele is a mass of the fluid-filled congenital remnants of the tunica vaginalis, usually resulting from a patent processus vaginalis.

b. Clinical features

(1) A soft, nontender fullness of the hemiscrotum that transilluminates.

(2) The mass may wax and wane in size; an indirect hernia may be concurrently present.

c. Laboratory studies. Few laboratory studies are warranted for hydrocele.

(1) Urinalysis with microscopic analysis is negative.

(2) Ultrasonography rarely is indicated but can distinguish between hydrocele, spermatocele, and testicular tumors.

d. Treatment. Elective repair as clinically indicated.

2. Spermatocele

a. General characteristics

(1) A spermatocele typically is a painless cystic mass containing sperm.

(2) Most spermatoceles are less than 1 cm in size.

(3) They lie superior and posterior and are distinct from the testes.

(4) Some may simulate a solid tumor.

b. Clinical features. Palpable, round, firm cystic mass with distinct borders, free floating above the testicle, which transilluminates. It may be tender.

c. Laboratory studies

(1) Needle aspiration should not be performed.

(2) Scrotal ultrasonography provides a very accurate diagnosis.

d. Treatment.

(1) No medical treatment required.

(2) Large spermatoceles can be surgically removed or sclerosed.

E. Testicular torsion

1. General characteristics

a. The testis is abnormally twisted on its spermatic cord, thus compromising arterial supply and venous drainage of the testis, leading to testicular ischemia.

b. This condition is most common in young males (most common in those 12–18 years of age), especially with a history of cryptorchidism (late descent of the testes).

2. Clinical features

    a. Sudden onset of severe unilateral pain and scrotal swelling are present.

    b. Testis is painful to palpation; testicle and scrotum are edematous. There is no relief with elevation of the testicle (negative Prehn's sign).

3. Laboratory findings

    a. Testicular torsion is a clinical diagnosis.

    b. If the diagnosis is equivocal, do not wait for laboratory studies.

    c. Doppler ultrasonography demonstrates decreased blood flow to the affected spermatic cord and testis.

    d. Radioisotope scan demonstrates decreased uptake in the affected testes.

4. Treatment

    a. Mild analgesics may be administered once the diagnosis is made.

    b. This is a surgical emergency. Manual detorsion (twisting the testes outward and laterally) may be attempted by experienced clinicians, but whether this is successful or not, surgery will be required. Surgical detorsion and orchiopexy are the definitive therapy.

    c. Emergent surgical intervention on the affected testis must be followed by elective surgery on the contralateral testis, which also is at risk of torsion.

F. Varicocele

  1. General characteristics

    a. Varicocele is the formation of a venous varicosity in the spermatic vein.

    b. The left spermatic vein has an increased incidence of varicosity because of several anatomic factors.

  2. Clinical features

    a. A chronic, nontender mass that does not transilluminate is seen, usually on the left side.

    b. The lesion has the consistency of a "bag of worms," increases in size with Valsalva, and decreases in size with elevation of the scrotum or supine position.

  3. Laboratory studies

    a. No laboratory studies are required.

    b. If the diagnosis is inconclusive, Doppler sonography is the diagnostic method of choice.

  4. Treatment. Surgical repair can be performed if the varicocele is painful or if it appears to be a cause of infertility.

7 Gynecology

Rebecca Lovell Scott

I. MENSTRUAL DISORDERS

A. Amenorrhea

1. General characteristics

  a. Primary amenorrhea is the absence of spontaneous menstruation by age 16.

  b. Secondary amenorrhea

   (1) In a woman who has previously menstruated, secondary amenorrhea is defined as the absence of menses for 6 months or longer.

   (2) In a woman with oligomenorrhea, secondary amenorrhea is defined as the absence of menses for 12 months.

  c. The most common cause of secondary amenorrhea is pregnancy; amenorrhea not caused by pregnancy occurs in fewer than 5% of women during their lifetime.

  d. Women who fail to menstruate in the presence of estrogen stimulation of the endometrium are at increased risk for endometrial cancer.

2. Clinical features

  a. Primary amenorrhea is divided into four categories based on clinical features.

   (1) Amenorrhea in a woman with no secondary sexual characteristics suggests gonadal agenesis or dysgenesis, ovarian resistance syndrome, galactosemia, gonadotropin-releasing hormone (GnRH) deficiency, constitutional pubertal delay, a central nervous system mass lesion, stress, or hyperprolactinemia.

   (2) Amenorrhea in a woman with breast development but no pubic or axillary hair suggests androgen insensitivity.

   (3) Amenorrhea in a woman with normal secondary sexual characteristics suggests imperforate hymen, transverse vaginal septum, or cervical or mullerian agenesis.

   (4) Amenorrhea in a woman with incompletely developed sexual characteristics suggests a tumor of the hypothalamus or pituitary, hypothyroidism, premature ovarian failure, or hyperprolactinemia.

  b. Secondary amenorrhea

   (1) Pregnancy is the most common cause of secondary amenorrhea.

   (2) Signs and symptoms associated with drug use, stress, significant weight change, or excessive exercise may be present and alert the clinician to cause.

   (3) In women with normal estrogen, the cause is likely to be Asherman's syndrome (intrauterine synechlae) or polycystic ovarian syndrome.

   (4) In hypoestrogenic women, causes include central nervous system tumor, stress, hyperprolactinemia, hypophysitis, Sheehan's syndrome, and premature ovarian syndrome.

   (5) Galactorrhea may be present.

3. Laboratory studies

  a. A pregnancy test is advisable.

  b. Serum follicle-stimulating hormone (FSH), estrogen, prolactin, and testosterone levels are likely to be required.

  c. A progesterone challenge test will determine the presence or absence of sufficient estrogen.

  d. Other tests may be indicated, including thyroid studies, MRI or CT of the hypothalamus and pituitary or pelvis, genetic testing, and pelvic and transvaginal ultrasonography.

4. Treatment: Depends on the underlying cause.

B. Dysmenorrhea

  1. General characteristics

    a. Primary dysmenorrhea is painful menstruation caused by excess prostaglandin E_2 secretion in the menstrual fluid, leading to painful uterine contractions; prostaglandin E_2 causes smooth muscle contraction, leading to nausea, vomiting, and diarrhea. Onset is usually within 3–6 months of menarche.

    b. Secondary dysmenorrhea is painful menstruation caused by an identifiable clinical condition, usually a disease of the uterus or pelvis (e.g., endometriosis, adenomyosis, pelvic inflammatory disease, use of an intrauterine device [IUD]). It usually affects women older than 25 years and may involve prostaglandins.

    c. Dysmenorrhea affects more than half of women of reproductive age at some point during their reproductive years and is a cause of recurrent disability in 10–15% of women during their early reproductive years.

    d. The incidence of primary dysmenorrhea peaks during the late teens and early 20s; the incidence of secondary dysmenorrhea increases with age.

  2. Clinical features

    a. Women with primary dysmenorrhea have cramping in the central lower abdomen or pelvis radiating to the back or thighs, beginning before or at the onset of menses, and lasting for 1–3 days. Physical examination is normal.

    b. Symptoms of secondary dysmenorrhea are similar but also may include bloating, menorrhagia, and dyspareunia. It is less related to the first day of flow.

    c. Adenomyosis (implantation of endometrial tissue in the myometrium) results in a tender, symmetrically enlarged, "boggy" uterus.

  3. Laboratory studies

    a. The diagnosis of primary dysmenorrhea is established on the basis of history and physical examination.

    b. Specific Tests for secondary dysmenorrhea target possible pelvic pathology.

  4. Treatment

    a. Primary dysmenorrhea

      (1) Start nonsteroidal anti-inflammatory drugs just before the expected menses and continue for 2–3 days.

      (2) Oral contraceptives, application of heat, and regular exercise also reduce pain.

      (3) Resistant cases may respond to tocolytic agents, calcium channel blockers, or progestogens.

    b. Secondary dysmenorrhea

      (1) Obvious underlying conditions should be treated and IUDs removed.

      (2) Symptomatic treatment may be sufficient.

      (3) Hysteroscopy, dilation and curettage (D&C), and laparoscopy allow both diagnosis and treatment.

C. Premenstrual syndrome (PMS)

  1. General characteristics

    a. PMS lacks agreed-on diagnostic criteria, pathophysiologic mechanisms, and optimal treatment.

    b. Hypothesized causes include abnormal levels of estrogen, progesterone, cortisone, prolactin, antidiuretic hormone, endogenous opiates, melatonin, serotonin, and/or prostaglandins; vitamin and mineral deficiencies; reactive hypoglycemia; menstrual toxins; and psychological, social, evolutionary, and genetic factors.

    c. The reported incidence is 10–90%, and it is debilitating in 10%. The prevalence is the greatest during the fourth and fifth decades. Seventy percent of women have some premenstrual symptoms.

    d. Fewer than 4% of women meet criteria for premenstrual dysphoric disorder. This diagnosis indicates premenstrual symptoms severe enough to cause dysfunction in daily living.

    e. An association exists among postpartum depression, perimenopausal depression, other affective disorders, and PMS.

  2. Clinical features

    a. Symptoms are associated with the menstrual cycle and begin 1–2 weeks before menses (i.e., during the luteal phase) and end 1–2 days after the onset of menses.

    b. A monthly symptom-free period during the follicular phase (i.e., from day 1 of menses to ovulation) must exist (Fig. 7-1).

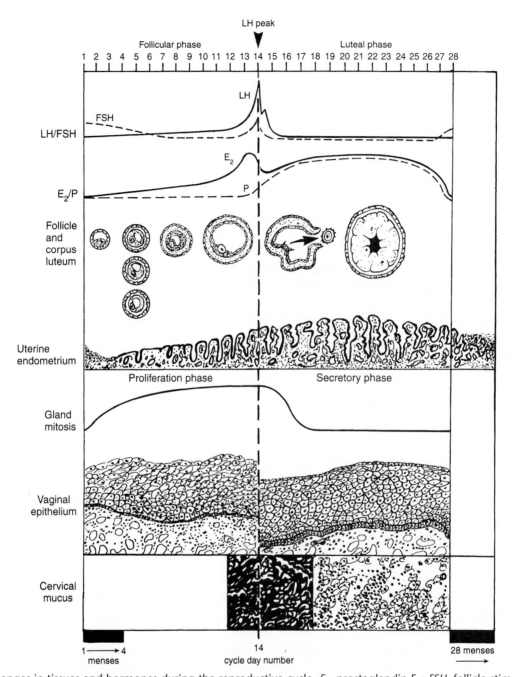

Composite changes in tissues and hormones during the reproductive cycle. E_2, prostaglandin E_2; *FSH*, follicle-stimulating hormone; *LH*, luteinizing hormone; *P*, progesterone.
(From Beckmann CB, Ling FW, Laube DW, et al., eds. Obstetrics and Gynecology. 3rd ed. Baltimore: Lippincott Williams & Wilkins, 1998:417.)

    c. The most common complaints are mood alteration and psychological effects (e.g., irritability, anxiety, depression, sleep and appetite changes, poor concentration, fatigue, insomnia).

    d. Symptoms related to fluid retention are edema, weight gain, and breast pain.

    e. Bloating, constipation, and backache also may occur.

  3. Tests include daily charting of symptoms; the specific constellation of symptoms is less important than their cyclical pattern of occurrence.

  4. Treatment

    a. Lifestyle modification includes caffeine reduction, salt restriction, low fat and high complex carbohydrate intake, emphasis on fresh foods, increased exercise, relaxation tapes, and stress reduction. Education of the patient and her family is essential.

b. Drug treatment

(1) Pyridoxine (vitamin B$_6$) and evening primrose oil show no benefit over placebo in clinical trials but relieve breast tenderness and depression in some women.

(2) Oral contraceptives may improve, worsen, or not change symptomatology; clinical studies have not shown progesterone to be useful.

(3) Diuretics (e.g., spironolactone) may be used for fluid-retention symptoms.

(4) Nonsteroidal anti-inflammatory drugs are useful for pain but also seem to relieve other symptoms.

(5) Selective serotonin reuptake inhibitors have proven to be beneficial in some patients; anxiolytics, including buspirone and cyclic alprazolam, may relieve anxiety.

D. Menopause

1. General characteristics

a. By definition, menopause is the last menses, and perimenopause (usually lasting 3–5 years) is the time surrounding it.

b. Mean age at natural menopause is 51.5 years; 95% of women stop menstruating between 44–55 years.

c. The subjective experience of menopause varies by individual and is influenced by cultural expectations and life circumstances.

d. Premature menopause is cessation of menses before age 40 and usually is termed "premature ovarian failure."

e. The ovaries continue to produce testosterone and androstenedione; estrone is the predominant post-menopausal circulating estrogen.

2. Clinical features

a. Vasomotor symptoms vary in intensity; when they occur frequently at night, they may cause insomnia, tiredness, and irritability. They resolve in 2–3 years (3–6 weeks with estrogen replacement therapy).

b. Urogenital atrophy may cause poor vaginal lubrication, dyspareunia, dysuria, and urge incontinence.

c. Accelerated bone loss may result in osteoporosis.

d. Estrogen-related cardiovascular protection declines.

e. One of the most disabling effects is changes in the sleep cycle.

f. The skin thins and becomes less elastic, and facial hair may increase. Hair loss increases, and nails become brittle.

g. Confusion, loss of memory, lethargy, inability to cope, depression, and loss of interest in sex have been associated with menopause. Causes are not clear, but symptoms may be relieved with hormone administration.

3. Laboratory studies. FSH of greater than 30 mIU/mL is diagnostic of menopause.

4. Treatment

a. Women should be treated based on individual risk factors and symptoms.

b. Lifestyle modifications may ameliorate symptoms and decrease risks.

c. Combined hormone replacement therapy appears to increase the risks for cardiovascular disease, breast cancer, and cognitive changes. Other possible risks include migraine and gallbladder disease.

d. Contraindications include undiagnosed vaginal bleeding, acute vascular thrombosis, and history of estrogen-dependent tumors.

e. Calcium and vitamin D supplementation, bisphosphonates, or calcitrol may be used in women at risk for osteoporosis.

f. Topical estrogens may improve urogenital symptoms, but any unopposed estrogen administration places a woman at increased risk for endometrial cancer.

II. UTERINE DISORDERS

A. Dysfunctional uterine bleeding (DUB)

1. General characteristics

a. DUB is abnormal uterine bleeding in the absence of an anatomic lesion, usually caused by a problem with the hypothalamic–pituitary–ovarian hormonal axis.

    b. DUB most commonly occurs shortly after menarche and during perimenopause because of increased anovulatory cycles. Other causes include polycystic ovarian syndrome, exogenous obesity, and adrenal hyperplasia.

2. Clinical features. Clinical features include an unremarkable physical examination in a very young or menopausal woman.

3. Laboratory studies

    a. CBC, possibly iron studies, prothrombin time and partial thromboplastin time, urinary human chorionic gonadotropin level, documentation of ovulation, thyroid function tests, serum progesterone level, liver function tests, and prolactin and serum FSH levels are needed.

    b. Pap smear, endometrial biopsy, pelvic ultrasonography, hysterosalpingography, hysteroscopy, and/or dilation and currettage may be indicated based on history and physical examination.

4. Treatment

    a. Treatment depends on severity of bleeding and may include observation, iron therapy, and volume replacement.

    b. Cyclic estrogens with progestins added to the last 10–15 days of the reproductive cycle for 3–6 months may establish a normal pattern.

    c. Oral contraceptives

        (1) Oral contraceptives should not be used in women who smoke or who have hypertension, diabetes, history of vascular disease, breast cancer, liver disease, or focal headaches.

        (2) Older women without risk factors can be prescribed oral contraceptives.

    d. Cyclic progestins alone may be used in younger patients.

    e. D&C may be both diagnostic and curative.

    f. Refractory cases may require endometrial ablation or vaginal hysterectomy.

B. Leiomyomata (uterine fibroids)

1. General characteristics

    a. Fibroids are more common in African-American women with a positive family history.

    b. Fibroids depend on estrogen and appear with increased frequency in women who have endometrial hyperplasia, anovulatory states, and estrogen-producing ovarian tumors.

    c. Women with fibroids have a fourfold increase in the risk of endometrial cancer.

2. Clinical features

    a. Most women have no symptoms but do have a firm, enlarged, irregular uterine mass. Some will have symptoms of pressure in the pelvis.

    b. Menorrhagia, intermenstrual bleeding, and dysmenorrhea are common. Bleeding is the most common presenting symptom.

3. Diagnostic procedures may include ultrasound, D&C, and hysteroscopy.

4. Treatment

    a. Observation is recommended in most cases of leiomyomata.

    b. Symptomatic patients may undergo myomectomy, hysterectomy, or D&C.

    c. GnRH agonists and mifepristone may reduce tumor size; in women with small leiomyomata, GnRH agonists may restore fertility.

    d. Use of arterial embolization is increasing.

C. Endometrial cancer

1. General characteristics

    a. Postmenopausal women make up 75% of patients; median age at presentation is 58 years.

    b. There are two types of endometrial cancer: estrogen-dependent, which generally is found in younger, perimenopausal women, and estrogen-independent, which is found in older, postmenopausal woman.

    c. Prognosis is influenced by histologic appearance, age (older women have poorer outcomes), and extent of spread.

    d. Endometrial cancer is the most common gynecologic malignancy and the fourth most common malignancy in women in the United States.

    e. Risk factors include obesity, nulliparity, late menopause, diabetes mellitus, unopposed estrogen stimulation, hypertension, gallbladder disease, and chronic tamoxifen use.

    f. Oral contraceptives seem to have a protective effect.

  2. Clinical features

    a. The cardinal symptom is inappropriate uterine bleeding (90% of patients).

    b. Obesity, hypertension, and diabetes mellitus may be present.

  3. Laboratory and diagnostic testing

    a. Women with postmenopausal bleeding should have a Pap smear, endocervical curettage, and endometrial biopsy. Endometrial biopsy has an accuracy rate of 90–95%.

    b. Other tests include fractional D&C and transvaginal ultrasonography.

  4. Treatment

    a. Total hysterectomy combined with bilateral salpingo-oophorectomy is the basis of treatment and staging.

    b. Radiotherapy may be indicated.

    c. Recurrence is treated with high-dose progestins or antiestrogens.

D. Endometriosis/adenomyosis

  1. General characteristics

    a. Endometriosis is a condition in which endometrial glands and stroma are found outside the endometrial cavity.

    (1) Most sites are found in the pelvis or on the ovary (60%), but it also may be distant (e.g., lung).

    (2) It most commonly occurs in nulliparous women in their late 20s or early 30s. First-degree relatives have a 7% chance of developing endometriosis.

    (3) Infertility is common.

    b. Adenomyosis is the extension of endometrial glands into the uterine musculature.

  2. Clinical features

    a. Endometriosis presents with dysmenorrhea, deep-thrust dyspareunia, dyschezia (difficulty passing bowel movement), intermittent spotting, and pelvic pain; signs include tender nodularity of the cul-de-sac and uterine ligaments.

    b. Adenomyosis presents with severe secondary dysmenorrhea and menorrhagia, but many patients are asymptomatic.

  3. Laboratory and diagnostic testing

    a. Diagnostic testing for endometriosis includes ultrasonography and laparoscopy or laparotomy.

    b. Endometrial biopsy, fractional D&C, or hysteroscopy in a patient with suspected adenomyosis will rule out endometrial cancer.

  4. Treatment

    a. Endometriosis treatment is based on severity of symptoms, location and severity of disease, and desire for childbearing.

    (1) Surgery may be conservative or definitive; large endometriomas must be resected.

    (2) Treatment with danazol or a GnRH agonist around surgery improves fertility.

    (3) Combined oral contraceptives or progestins may relieve symptoms.

    (4) Mifepristone also may be used.

    b. Adenomyosis may be treated with D&C, a GnRH agonist, mifepristone, or hysterectomy.

E. Prolapse

  1. General characteristics

    a. Prolapse of the uterus typically occurs after pregnancy, labor, and vaginal delivery but also may occur in nulliparas.

    b. Prolapse is less common in Asian and African-American women than in white women.

    c. Any condition that increases intra-abdominal pressure may predispose a woman to prolapse, including obesity, chronic cough, and repetitive heavy lifting.

    d. Iatrogenic causes include failure to correct pelvic support defects during surgery.

2. Clinical features

  a. Symptoms vary but usually are worse after prolonged standing or late in the day and are relieved by lying down.

  b. Uterine prolapse is graded as 0 (no descent) to 4 (through the hymen).

  c. With moderate prolapse, patients describe a falling-out sensation or a feeling of sitting on a ball.

3. Laboratory testing is not indicated.

4. Treatment

  a. Nonsurgical approaches include weight reduction, smoking cessation, pelvic muscle exercises, and use of a vaginal pessary.

  b. Surgical treatment relieves symptoms, restores normal anatomic relationships and visceral function, and allows coitus.

III. OVARIAN DISORDERS

A. Ovarian cysts

  1. General characteristics

    a. Cysts are the most common ovarian growth.

    b. Most cysts are functional; these include follicular, corpus luteum, and much less commonly, theca lutein cysts.

  2. Clinical features. Cysts may present as asymptomatic masses, with pain and menstrual delay or with hemorrhage because of rupture.

  3. Diagnostic studies. Cysts usually are confirmed by pelvic ultrasound.

  4. Treatment

    a. Follow for one or two cycles in premenopausal women with cysts smaller than 8 cm.

    b. Large or persistent cysts require laparoscopic evaluation.

    c. Cysts in postmenopausal women are presumed to be malignant until proved otherwise.

    d. Oral contraceptives have not been validated in treating functional cysts.

B. Polycystic ovarian syndrome (PCOS)

  1. General characteristics

    a. Formerly known as Stein-Leventhal syndrome, PCOS is the most common cause of androgen excess and hirsutism.

    b. Patients with PCOS have bilaterally enlarged polycystic ovaries, amenorrhea or oligomenorrhea, and infertility.

    c. Patients usually have a normal puberty and adolescence, followed by progressively longer episodes of amenorrhea.

    d. The underlying abnormality is thought to be hypothalamic pituitary dysfunction and insulin resistance, although the pathophysiology is not entirely clear. A genetic predisposition exists.

    e. Patients are at increased risk for endometrial hyperplasia and carcinoma because of unopposed estrogen stimulation.

  2. Clinical features

    a. Half of patients with PCOS are hirsute, and many show truncal obesity.

    b. Patients usually present for treatment of hirsutism or infertility. Others present with intractable acne or menstrual irregularities (oligomenorrhea or amenorrhea).

    c. Acanthosis nigricans sometimes is found.

    d. Impaired glucose tolerance is present in 30% of patients; frank diabetes mellitus (type 2) is present in 8%.

  3. Laboratory studies

    a. Ultrasound may demonstrate a characteristic "string of pearls" appearance within the ovaries.

    b. Laboratory testing reveals mildly elevated serum androgen levels, increased LH:FSH ratio, lipid abnormalities, and insulin resistance.

  4. Treatment

    a. Weight reduction improves hirsutism, lipid and glucose parameters, and fertility.

    b. Hirsutism is treated with androgen-lowering agents, including oral contraceptives.

    c. Infertility usually is treated with clomiphene citrate; in refractory cases, wedge resection of the ovary is used.

    d. Lipid abnormalities and insulin resistance should be managed medically.

C. Ovarian cancer

    1. General characteristics

        a. High-risk women are older, nulliparous, white, and have a positive family history of ovarian or endometrial cancer.

        b. Long-term oral contraceptive use may be protective because of the suppression of ovulation.

        c. A leading cause of death, ovarian cancer is the fifth most common cancer in U.S. women and the third most common gynecologic malignancy, with the highest mortality rate; 60% of patients die within 5 years.

    2. Clinical features

        a. Diagnosis often is delayed because of lack of specific symptoms. Women may present with ascites, abdominal distention, vague GI symptoms, or a fixed mass.

        b. Most patients are diagnosed between 40 and 60 years of age.

    3. Laboratory studies

        a. The *BRCA1* gene is associated in 5% of cases; cancer antigen 125 may be used to follow treatment, particularly in postmenopausal women.

        b. An association exists with mutations in the *P53* tumor-suppressor gene.

        c. Transvaginal or abdominal ultrasonography is useful in distinguishing benign from potentially malignant masses.

    4. Treatment. Treatment involves surgery plus chemotherapy and radiotherapy.

IV. CERVICAL DYSPLASIA AND NEOPLASIA

A. General characteristics

    1. Human papilloma virus (HPV) infection (especially types 16, 18, 31, 33, and 45) is strongly linked to cervical neoplasia; types 6 and 11 are linked with condylomata acuminata.

    2. Other risk factors include early age at first intercourse, early childbearing, multiple sexual partners or a high-risk sex partner, history of sexually transmitted disease, low socioeconomic status, African-American heritage, and cigarette smoking.

    3. Atypical changes at the transformation zone of the cervix initiate cervical intraepithelial neoplasia (CIN), the preinvasive phase of cervical cancer. The transformation zone is involved in 95% of cases.

        a. Mild dysplasia (CIN-1): may progress to moderate dysplasia (CIN-2), severe dysplasia (CIN-3), and carcinoma in situ (CIS); may stay the same; or may regress.

        b. About one-third of patients with CIN-3 develop microinvasive and frankly invasive carcinoma.

        c. CIN most commonly occurs in women in their 20s, CIS in those aged 25–35 years, and cervical cancer after age 40.

B. Clinical features

    1. Most women with abnormal Pap smears or other screening tests have no symptoms.

    2. Advanced or invasive cervical cancer may cause abnormal vaginal bleeding and vaginal discharge, and tumor may be seen on clinical examination.

    3. The mean age at diagnosis is 47 years overall but 39 years in lower socioeconomic status groups.

C. Laboratory studies

    1. Pap smear, liquid-based specimen, and other cytologic screening techniques are highly effective and should begin when a woman becomes sexually active or reaches age 18, whichever comes first. Annual Pap smear reduces the incidence of invasive cervical carcinoma by 95%.

    2. Abnormal cytologic screenings (Table 7-1) indicate a need for further diagnostic testing.

        a. Biopsy of suspicious lesions is mandatory.

        b. Colposcopy with biopsies is the most appropriate technique for histological evaluation.

        c. Conization is used when the results of colposcopy are unsatisfactory or endocervical curettage scrapings indicate severe disease.

    3. HPV DNA testing is now standard.

TABLE 7-1   The 2001 Bethesda System for Reporting Cervical and Vaginal Cytologic Diagnoses

Specimen type
  Conventional smear (Pap smear), liquid-based, or other type

Adequacy of the specimen
  Satisfactory for evaluation
  Unsatisfactory for evaluation (specify reason)

General categorization (optional)
  Negative for intraepithelial lesion or malignancy
  Epithelial cell abnormality (see *Interpretation/result*)
  Other (see *Interpretation/result*)

Automated review

Ancillary testing

Interpretation/result
  Negative for intraepithelial lesion or malignancy
    Organisms
      Trichomonas vaginalis
      Fungal organisms morphologically consistent with *Candida* spp.
      Shift in flora suggestive of bacterial vaginosis
      Bacteria morphologically consistent with *Actinomyces* spp.
      Cellular changes associated with herpes simplex virus
    Other nonneoplastic findings
      Reactive cellular changes associated with inflammation (includes typical repair)
      Radiation
      Intrauterine device
      Glandular cells status posthysterectomy
      Atrophy
    Other
      Endometrial cells (in a woman ≥40 years of age)

Epithelial cell abnormalities
  Squamous cell
    ASC-US; cannot exclude HSIL (ASC-H)
    LSIL, encompassing HPV, mild dysplasia, CIN
    HSIL, encompassing moderate and severe dysplasia, CIN-2 and -3, CIS
    Squamous cell carcinoma
  Glandular cells
    Atypical (AGC)
      Endocervical cells
      Endometrial cells
      Glandular cells NOS
    Atypical, favor neoplastic
      Endocervical cells
      Glandular cells NOS
  Endocervical AIS
  Adenocarcinoma
    Endocervical
    Endometrial
    Extrauterine
    NOS

Other malignant neoplasms (specify)

Educational notes and suggestions (optional)

AGC, atypical glandular cells; *AIS,* adenocarcinoma in situ; *ASC-H,* atypical squamous cells of high-grade lesion cannot be ruled out; *ASC-US,* atypical squamous cells of undetermined significance; *CIN,* cervical intraepithelial neoplasia; *CIS,* carcinoma in situ; *HPV,* human papilloma virus; *HSIL,* high-grade squamous intraepithelial lesion; *LSIL,* low-grade squamous intraepithelial lesion; *NOS,* not otherwise specified.

D. Treatment is based on the classification of disease.

  1. Mild lesions may resolve spontaneously.

  2. Preinvasive neoplasia may be treated with electrocautery or cryocautery, laser therapy, conization, large-loop excision of transitional zone, or loop electrodiathermy excision procedure.

  3. Hysterectomy and pelvic lymphadenectomy or radiation therapy are indicated for more severe abnormalities.

4. Gardasil is a vaccine against HPV associated with cervical cancer. The Centers for Disease Control and Prevention has recommended that all girls aged 11–12 years receive the series of three injections over 6 months; it is available to all women aged 9–26 years. It prevents four types of HPV in those not previously exposed, targeting HPV that causes 70% of all cervical cancers and 90% of genital warts. Boosters may be needed every 5 years, but final word is not know.

V. VAGINAL AND VULVAR DISORDERS

A. Pelvic organ prolapse

1. General characteristics

a. Pelvic organ prolapse refers to protrusion of the pelvic organs into or out of the vagina.

b. Organ prolapses may occur in isolation but usually are combined.

c. Prolapse may result from excessive stretching of pelvic fascia, ligaments, and muscles during pregnancy, labor, and delivery; from increased intra-abdominal pressure; or from iatrogenic factors.

d. Anterior vaginal prolapse includes cystocele or cystourethrocele.

e. Apical includes uterovaginal or vaginal vault prolapse.

f. Posterior includes enterocele and rectocele.

2. Clinical features

a. The amount of discomfort and other symptoms varies among patients. Most symptoms are worse after standing and late in the day and may be relieved by lying down.

b. Grading of prolapse: 0 = no descent, 1 = descent between normal position and ischial spines, 2 = descent between ischial spines and hymen, 3 = descent within hymen, and 4 = descent through hymen.

3. Laboratory studies are not indicated.

4. Treatment includes pelvic floor exercises, vaginal pessaries, and surgical treatment.

B. Neoplasm of the vulva and vagina

1. General characteristics

a. Neoplasia in this area is the rarest of the gynecologic neoplasms.

b. Most vulvar malignancies are squamous cell carcinomas and occur in postmenopausal women (mean age at diagnosis, 65 years).

c. Vaginal neoplasms are less common than cervical or vulvar neoplasms.

d. Women with in utero exposure to diethylstilbestrol (DES) are at increased risk for clear cell adenocarcinoma of the vagina.

e. Vaginal melanoma also occurs.

2. Clinical features

a. Vulvar cancer more often is found in women who are obese and who have hypertension, diabetes mellitus, and arteriosclerosis. A history of chronic vulvar itching is common.

b. Vulvar cancer in younger women is associated with HPV infection and smoking; 25% of patients have coexisting cervical carcinoma.

c. Most vaginal intraepithelial neoplasms occur in the upper one-third of the vagina and are asymptomatic.

d. Diethylstilbestrol-exposed women may have vaginal adenosis and structural changes of the cervix, vagina, and upper genital tract, leading to increased risk of miscarriage, premature delivery, and ectopic pregnancy.

3. Laboratory studies

a. Application of acetic acid or staining with toluidine blue may help to direct biopsies of suspicious vulvar lesions.

b. Vaginal biopsy for suspected vaginal invasive neoplasm should be directed by colposcopy or Lugol staining.

c. Clear cell adenocarcinoma is diagnosed by careful inspection and palpation of the vagina and cervix, followed by biopsies.

4. Treatment

a. Local excision, topical 5-fluorouracil, and laser therapy are used for early vulvar lesions.

b. Surgical excision is required for most vaginal neoplasms; primary vaginal cancer is treated with radiotherapy.

c. For clear cell lesions, radical hysterectomy and vaginectomy or radiation therapy is effective.

VI. BREAST DISORDERS

A. Benign breast disorders

    1. General characteristics

        a. Mastodynia (mastalgia), or breast tenderness, is common, often cyclical, and increases in women taking contraceptive pills or hormone replacement therapy.

        b. Mastitis, or breast infection, and breast abscesses most often are caused by *Staphylococcus aureus* and occur primarily, but rarely, in primigravid lactating women.

        c. Abscesses also may result from secondary infection of a galactocele.

        d. Fibrocystic changes (the most frequent benign condition of the breast) include cysts, papillomatosis, fibrosis, adenosis, and ductal epithelial hyperplasia.

        e. Fibroadenomas are the second most common benign breast disorder and occur in young women; they are more common in black women.

    2. Clinical features

        a. Persistent, noncyclic breast pain suggests underlying cancer; cyclic pain suggests luteal-phase tenderness.

        b. Mastitis and abscesses present with tenderness, heat, significant fever, chills, and other flu-like symptoms.

        c. Fibroadenomas typically are round, firm, smooth, discrete, mobile, and nontender.

        d. Fibrocystic changes are most common in women 30–50 years of age and may present as asymptomatic masses or as painful and tender masses. Pain, size fluctuation, and multiple lesions distinguish fibrocystic changes from carcinoma.

    3. Laboratory studies

        a. Mammography, ultrasonography, and biopsy may be indicated for breast complaints; however, young women's breasts usually are radiodense. Ultrasound differentiates between solid and cystic masses.

        b. Because *Staphylococcus aureus* is present in approximately 50% of patients with mastitis, culture of purulent material or milk usually is not done.

        c. In suspected cysts, fine-needle aspiration is both diagnostic and therapeutic; cysts usually contain straw-colored fluid.

        d. In a woman younger than 25 years, a fibroadenomatous mass should be biopsied.

    4. Treatment

        a. Treat mastodynia with reassurance, vitamin B_6, bromocriptine, tamoxifen, or danazol.

        b. Treat mastitis with a penicillinase-resistant antibiotic and hot compresses. Breast feeding may continue, because the source is likely to be the infant's oropharynx.

        c. Surgical treatment may be required for abscesses or duct ectasia.

        d. Many types of fibrocystic breast problems need no treatment other than a supportive bra. Aspirate cysts and excise fibroadenomas.

        e. The role of caffeine restriction in the treatment of fibrocystic changes is controversial; some patients respond to low-salt diet, vitamin E supplementation, or hydrochlorothiazide premenstrually.

B. Breast neoplasms

    1. General characteristics

        a. Most women with breast cancer have no identifiable risk factors other than female sex and increasing age (mean age at diagnosis, 60–61 years); *BRCA1* and *BRCA2* genes are associated with 5–10% of cases of breast cancer but appear in only 1% of the population.

        b. Associated factors include nulliparity, early menarche, late menopause, long-term estrogen or radiation exposure, and delayed childbearing.

        c. Ductal carcinomas account for 80–85% of breast cancers; the remainder are lobular carcinomas. Lobular CIS and atypical ductal hyperplasia predispose to cancer.

        d. Paget's disease is a ductal carcinoma presenting as an eczematous lesion of the nipple.

        e. All invasive lobular carcinomas and two-thirds of ductal carcinomas are estrogen-receptor positive.

        f. Breast cancer is the most common female malignancy and the second leading cause of death from cancer in women.

2. Clinical features

    a. Breast cancer most often presents as a single, nontender, firm, immobile mass: 45% occur in the upper outer quadrant and 25% under the nipple and areola.

    b. Rarer presentations include nipple discharge, dimpling, skin thickening, breast pain, and eczematous changes.

3. Diagnostic studies

    a. A combination of physical examination, mammography (the best screening tool), and fine-needle or sterotactic core-needle biopsy are highly accurate in establishing the diagnosis. Open biopsy may be required.

    b. Ultrasonography and excisional biopsy may be indicated. Biopsy specimen should undergo estrogen- and progesterone-receptor analysis as well as histologic analysis.

4. Treatment

    a. Staging should occur before treatment begins.

    b. Breast conservation therapy (lumpectomy), modified radical mastectomy, and partial mastectomy have equivalent survival rates when surgery is followed by radiation therapy.

    c. Adjuvant chemotherapy and/or hormonal manipulation benefit some women.

    d. Tamoxifen is used to treat women with estrogen receptor–positive disease and postmenopausal women.

VII. CONTRACEPTIVE METHODS

A. Traditional methods

    1. Coitus interruptus, postcoital douching, and use of household wraps are ineffective and unreliable.

    2. Lactational amenorrhea may be effective in delaying conception for 6 months after birth if the woman breast feeds exclusively and amenorrhea is maintained.

    3. Periodic abstinence methods rely on abstinence from just before the time of ovulation until 2–3 days thereafter; pregnancy rates for these methods average 5–25 per 100 woman-years.

        a. Calendar methods predict the day of ovulation based on average menstrual patterns, are based on the relatively constancy (14-day) of the luteal phase, and have a 35% failure rate.

        b. The basal body temperature method requires recording daily vaginal or rectal temperature before any activity is undertaken. A slight drop in temperature occurs 24–36 hours after ovulation, then rises 0.3–0.4°C, remaining at a plateau for the rest of the cycle.

        c. Combining the calendar and basal body temperature methods for contraception results in only 5 pregnancies per 100 couples per year.

        d. The cervical mucous method requires daily evaluation of the mucus; fertile mucus resembles egg white.

        e. The symptothermal method combines the cervical mucous and basal body temperature methods; it is probably the most reliable periodic abstinence method.

B. Oral hormonal contraceptives are the most effective reversible means of pregnancy prevention.

    1. All oral contraceptives contain synthetic steroids (similar to natural estrogens and progestins) used in doses and combinations that inhibit ovulation.

        a. The estrogen component is usually ethinyl estradiol or mestranol.

        b. The progestin component is one of the 19-nortestosterones, including norethindrone acetate, norethindrone, levonorgestrel, ethynodiol diacetate, desogestrel, norgestimate, DL-norgestrel, gestodene, and drospirenone.

    2. Use of combined estrogen–progestin pills begins with the onset of menses or the following Sunday; active pills are taken for 21 days, followed by 7 days of no pills or placebos. A newer method allows for 84 days of active pills; this results in limiting menses to four times per year.

    3. Withdrawal bleeding begins within 3–5 days of the last active pill.

    4. Minipills (progestin only) are half as effective as combination pills and may cause amenorrhea. They are most useful in lactating woman and in those older than 40 years.

    5. Noncontraceptive advantages

        a. Less benign breast disease, iron deficiency anemia, and pelvic inflammatory disease as well as fewer ovarian cysts.

        b. Protection against ectopic pregnancy; reduced risk of ovarian and endometrial cancer; reduced dysmenorrhea and menorrhagia; and improvements in hirsutism, acne, and symptoms of endometriosis. Oral contraceptives also may protect against rheumatoid arthritis.

6. Disadvantages
- **a.** Increased risk of thromboembolic disease, particularly in smokers, and abnormal lipids.
- **b.** Possible increased risk of breast cancer and, rarely, hypertension, cholelithiasis, and benign liver tumors.

7. Adverse effects
- **a.** Missed periods, intermenstrual bleeding, bloating, acne, nausea, headaches, and weight gain.
- **b.** Most of these problems resolve within the first few months of use and are rare with current low-dose formulations.

8. Theoretical failure rate for combination pills is less than 1%; actual rates are 4–6%.

C. Injected, implanted, and transdermal hormonal contraceptives

1. IM injection of a depot formulation of synthetic sex hormones may be pure progestin or a combination of progestin and estrogen; both inhibit anterior pituitary function.
- **a.** The most common is medroxyprogesterone acetate, 150 mg every 90 days.
- **b.** The failure rate is 0.3% in the first year.
- **c.** Fertility rates return to normal within 18 months of discontinuation.

2. The Norplant system relies on the implantation of six rods that release levonorgestrel. Efficacy is very good, but side effects are common, including menstrual irregularity, headache, and weight gain.

3. The transdermal patch is applied once a month. It is not effective in women who weigh more than 200 pounds.

4. A hormone-impregnated vaginal ring is inserted for 3 weeks and then removed for 1 week; withdrawal bleeding should occur.

D. IUDs

1. The mechanism of action is unknown, but leukocyte aggregation may produce an environment that is hostile to a fertilized ovum.

2. Two devices currently are available in the United States.
- **a.** Progestasert (usable for 1 year)
- **b.** Copper T (usable for 10 years)

3. Failure rates are less than 1% per year for copper T and 1–1.5% for Progestasert.

4. IUDs usually are inserted during menses.

5. Disadvantages and adverse effects include: uterine perforation; higher incidence of spontaneous abortion if pregnancy occurs; increased risk of ectopic pregnancy, cramping, or bleeding with menses; and risk of pelvic infection.

6. Absolute contraindications include current pregnancy, undiagnosed vaginal bleeding, acute infection, past salpingitis, and suspected gynecologic malignancy.

7. Relative contraindications include nulliparity, previous ectopic pregnancy or sexually transmitted disease, multiple sexual partners, severe dysmenorrhea, uterine abnormalities, anemia, valvular heart disease, and young age.

E. Barrier methods include the male and female condom, cervical caps, and diaphragms, which provide some additional protection against sexually transmitted infections. The common spermicides are nonoxynol-9 and octoxynol-3.

F. Emergency (postcoital) contraception is provided by high-dose estrogen–progestin or progestin-only tablets given within 72 hours of unprotected intercourse. It may be effective up to 5 days after unprotected intercourse. Nausea and vomiting is a frequent adverse effect of the former. Another method is postcoital insertion of an IUD.

G. Other methods of controlling fertility include induced abortion and sterilization.

VIII. INFERTILITY

A. General characteristics

1. Infertility generally is defined as a failure to conceive after 1 year of unprotected intercourse. Surveys estimate that up to 15% of reproductive-age couples in the United States are infertile.

2. Female factors include ovulatory (central, peripheral, metabolic), pelvic (infection, structural, endometriosis), and cervical (congenital, acquired) causes.

3. Male factors include endocrine and anatomic disorders, abnormal spermatogenesis or motility, and sexual dysfunction.

B. Clinical examination typically is normal.

C. Laboratory studies

    1. Semen analysis should precede any other testing.

    2. Basal body temperature, ovulation prediction tests, and progesterone levels confirm ovulation.

    3. Luteal-phase endometrial biopsy, FSH levels, prolactin, and thyroid-stimulating hormone tests may be helpful.

    4. Postcoital testing measures sperm survival.

    5. Hysterosalpingography determines tubal patency and uterine abnormalities.

    6. Other tests that may be useful include laparoscopy, sperm penetration assay, sperm antibody testing, ultrasonography, and hysteroscopy.

D. Treatments currently have an overall success rate of about 85%.

    1. Clomiphene citrate, 50–100 mg for 5 days beginning on day 3, 4, or 5 of the cycle, should be given to anovulatory women to promote ovulation.

    2. Artificial insemination is an alternative for couples with abnormal postcoital tests.

    3. Other treatments depend on the cause of the infertility, the couple's resources, and the age of the woman.

    4. Assisted reproductive technologies include in vitro fertilization, gamete intrafallopian transfer, zygote intrafallopian transfer, and surrogate options.

IX. PELVIC INFLAMMATORY DISEASE

A. General characteristics

    1. Pelvic inflammatory disease includes acute salpingitis (gonococcal or nongonococcal), IUD-related pelvic cellulitis, tubo-ovarian abscess, and pelvic abscess.

    2. It usually is polymicrobial (mixed aerobic and anaerobic). Most are bacterial, but viral, fungal, or parasitic causes are known.

    3. Complications include infertility and ectopic pregnancy.

B. Clinical features

    1. Lower abdominal and pelvic pain typically is bilateral. Nausea (with or without vomiting), headache, and lassitude are common. Fever may or may not be present.

    2. Examination reveals lower abdominal and pelvic pain and cervical motion tenderness. Purulent discharge and inflammation of Bartholin's or Skene's glands may be present.

    3. An adnexal mass may indicate a tubo-ovarian abscess.

C. Laboratory studies

    1. DNA probes for gonorrhea and chlamydia have largely replaced Gram staining and culture of any discharge.

    2. Ultrasound should be used to establish the diagnosis of adnexal masses.

    3. Diagnostic culdocentesis or laparoscopy may be required.

D. Treatment

    1. Women with mild disease should be treated as outpatients with antibiotics, antipyretics, analgesics, and bed rest.

    2. Women with severe disease should be hospitalized for IV antibiotic therapy and possible surgery.

    3. Sex partners should be evaluated and treated.

Obstetrics

Lori Parlin Palfreyman

I. ROUTINE PRENATAL CARE AND PRENATAL DIAGNOSTIC TESTING

A. Routine prenatal care

  1. General characteristics

    a. An initial obstetric history includes subjective symptoms (Table 8-1) of pregnancy as well as the patient's general medical, obstetric, and family history (Table 8-2).

    b. The due date or expected date of confinement (EDC) can be calculated using the Nägele's or McDonald's rule: EDC = first day of last menstrual period − 3 months + 7 days. This is based on a 28-day menstrual cycle and must be adjusted for shorter or longer cycles

    c. The patient's obstetric history can be expressed as gravida (G; number of total pregnancies) and parity (P; number of deliveries), denoted as a sequence of four digits (P_ _ _ _) signifying the number of term infants, premature deliveries (20–36 weeks of gestation), abortions (therapeutic and/or spontaneous occurring before 20 weeks of gestation), and living children.

    d. The initial visit should take place 6–8 weeks after the last menstrual period. Generally, a woman is examined every 4 weeks until the 28th week of gestation, every 2–3 weeks up to 36 weeks of gestation, and then weekly thereafter.

    e. After the initial visit, each subsequent prenatal visit includes a focused history and examination, including maternal weight gain, edema, fetal movement, blood pressure, check of fundal height, fetal heart tones, and a urinalysis for glucosuria and proteinuria. Vaginal examination to assess cervical dilation is added after 37 weeks or as indicated.

  2. Clinical features

    a. Uterine growth throughout pregnancy (Fig. 8-1)

      (1) At 20 weeks, the fundus is at the umbilicus.

      (2) From 21 weeks on, the height of the uterine fundus should correlate roughly (±2 cm) to the number of weeks of gestation.

    b. Fetal heart tones can be appreciated beginning at 10–12 weeks using handheld Doppler; normal fetal heart rate is 120–160 bpm.

    c. Quickening, or the first awareness of fetal movements, usually occurs at 18–20 weeks in a primigravida and as early as 14–18 weeks in a multigravida.

    d. Common complaints, such as backache, increasing varicosities, heartburn, hemorrhoids, and fatigue, can be associated with an otherwise healthy pregnancy.

B. Laboratory and prenatal diagnostic testing

  1. Table 8-3 lists the most common laboratory and prenatal testing by gestational age.

  2. Ultrasound

    a. Early pregnancy

      (1) Ultrasound can detect fetal heart activity as soon as 5–6 weeks after the last menstrual period.

      (2) Ultrasound is an accurate modality for detecting multiple gestations, establishing or confirming EDC, checking for fetal viability, correlating appropriate growth in relation to gestational age, checking for placental status and location, evaluating vaginal bleeding, and checking amniotic fluid level.

      (3) It also can be used to help detect lethal malformations and as a follow-up to abnormal α-fetoprotein testing.

    b. Late pregnancy

      (1) Ultrasound is used late in pregnancy to monitor fetal well-being in the form of a scored examination (biophysical profile [BPP]).

      (2) The biophysical profile examines five parameters, scaled on a 10-point system, including nonstress test (NST), amniotic fluid level, gross fetal movements, fetal tone, and fetal breathing.

TABLE 8-1 Manifestations of Pregnancy

Symptoms
  Amenorrhea
  Nausea/vomiting
  Breast tenderness
  Quickening (fetal movement)
    Nullipara: 18–20 weeks
    Multipara: 14–16 weeks
  Easy fatigability
  Urinary frequency, nocturia, infection

Signs
  Chadwick's sign (bluish discoloration of vagina and cervix)
  Increased basal body temperature
  Skin changes
    Melasma/chloasma (dark patches on face)
    Linea nigra
  Positive pregnancy test
  Hagar's sign (softening between fundus and cervix)
  Uterine growth
    12 weeks: at symphysis pubis
    16 weeks: midway between pubis and umbilicus
    20 weeks: at umbilicus
    After 20 weeks: 1 cm for every week of gestation
    Contractions after 28 weeks that are infrequent are benign
  Fetal heart tones
  Palpation of fetus
  Ultrasound of fetus
  Radiography of fetus

TABLE 8-2 Patient History on Initial Prenatal Office Visit

Menstrual history
  Last menstrual period

Present pregnancy
  See Table 8-1

Previous pregnancies
  Vaginal vs. cesarean section
  Complications

Medical history
  Cardiovascular
  Asthma
  Systemic lupus erythematosus
  Bleeding disorders
  Seizure disorders

Surgical history
  Abdominal surgery

Family history
  Chromosomal abnormalities
  Mental retardation
  Diabetes

Social history
  Alcohol
  Drugs
  Diet

Source: Adapted from DeCherney A. Current Obstetric and Gynecology Diagnosis and Treatment. 10th Ed. NY: McGraw-Hill Companies, 2007.

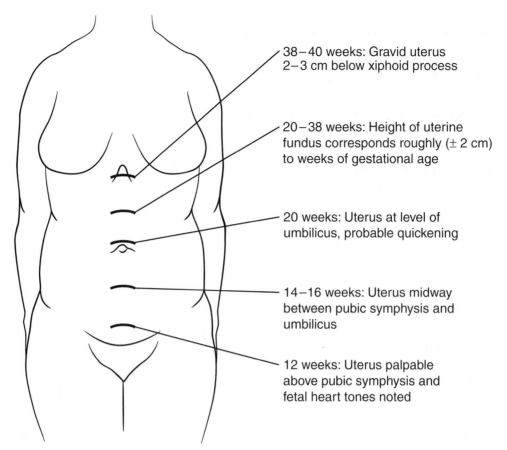

FIGURE 8-1 Uterine size and position throughout gestation.

TABLE 8-3	Prenatal Laboratories and Screening Tests

Early
  CBC
  Blood type and Rh
  Rubella titer
  Hepatitis B serum antigen
  Cultures for chlamydia and gonorrhea, as needed
  Offer all women HIV testing
  Offer all couples screening for cystic fibrosis, sickle cell, other conditions per maternal and
    paternal history
  Urinalysis
  Coombs' test (irregular antibody screen)
  Serologic testing for syphilis
  Pap smear

10–13 weeks
  Nuchal translucency screening, β-hcg, pregnancy-associated plasma protein A (PAPP-A)
  Chorionic villus sampling

15–18 weeks
  Quadruple screen (α-fetoprotein, human chorionic gonadotropin, unconjugated estriol inhibin)
  Amniocentesis

28 weeks
  In unsensitized Rh patients, repeat antibody titers (followed by Rh immunoglobulin)
  Screen for gestational diabetes
  Hemoglobin and hematocrit

35 weeks
  Vaginal–rectal culture for group B streptococci
  Hemoglobin and hematocrit

Source: Suggestions from the American College of Obstetricians and Gynecologists. ACOG Practice Bulletin, Clinical Management Guidelines for Obstetrician-Gynecologists. Obstetrics and Gynecology. Vol 109, No. 1, January 2007.

3. Triple screen
   a. The triple screen is a multiple-marker serum screening test offered to all women between 15 and 18 weeks of gestation.
   b. It can be performed up to 22 weeks of gestation but is less accurate during the later weeks.
   c. The triple screen checks levels of α-fetoprotein (a major circulating protein of the early fetus), human chorionic gonadotropin (hCG), and unconjugated estriol.
   d. It is useful in detecting up to 75–85% of open neural tube defects, such as spina bifida and anencephaly, and 70–90% of cases of trisomy 18 and trisomy 21.
   e. Abnormally high levels indicate increased risk for neural tube defects; abnormally low levels indicate increased risk for Down syndrome.
   f. If a triple screen is abnormal, follow-up tests may entail either a repeat α-fetoprotein, a comprehensive ultrasound with a thorough detailed examination of fetal anatomy, and/or amniocentesis.

4. Nuchal translucency screening test (also known as a nuchal fold scan)
   a. Ultrasound measurement of the nuchal space is performed at 10–13 weeks. It screens for trisomies 13, 18, and 21 as well as for Turner's syndrome.
   b. Indications are listed in Table 8-4.
   c. If an abnormally wide measurement for gestational age is detected, chorionic villus sampling or amniocentesis is offered.
   d. When combined c̄ pregnancy-associated plasma protein A (PAPP-A) and β-hcg, the detection rate is signifantly increased.

5. Chorionic villus sampling (CVS)
   a. CVS is performed between 10 and 13 weeks; a catheter or needle is used to biopsy placental cells.
   b. Indications for CVS are listed in Table 8-4.
   c. The advantage of CVS is its ability to be performed during the first trimester, allowing the option of a first-trimester termination if a major malformation is detected. Also, preliminary results are available within 48 hours after the procedure.
   d. The disadvantage of CVS is that unlike amniocentesis, CVS specimens cannot be used in α-fetoprotein testing for neural tube defects. Also, the risk of spontaneous abortion after CVS is slightly higher than that after amniocentesis (0.5–1% versus 0.25–0.5%)

6. Amniocentesis
   a. Amniocentesis involves the withdrawal of amniotic fluid via needle under ultrasound guidance for prenatal diagnosis.
   b. It is usually performed between 15 and 18 weeks of gestation.
   c. Indications for amniocentesis are listed in Table 8-4.
   d. There is a lower risk of spontaneous abortion following second-trimester amniocentesis than following first-trimester CVS (0.25–0.5% versus 0.5–1%). Also, amniocentesis can offer a wider array of genetic testing.
   e. The disadvantage of amniocentesis is that it is performed during the second trimester, so if termination of the pregnancy is chosen, a more complicated procedure is involved. Also, results from the test are not available for a minimum of 7 days.

TABLE 8-4 Indications for Nuchal Translucency Screening, Chorionic Villus Sampling, or Amniocentesis

Maternal age of 35 years or older

Previous child with chromosomal abnormality

Patient or father of baby with chromosomal anomaly

Family history of chromosomal anomaly

Neural tube defect risk (amniocentesis only)

Abnormal triple screen (amniocentesis only)

7. Fetal monitoring

a. Handheld Doppler ultrasound is used to assess fetal heart tones at each prenatal visit after 10 weeks of gestation

b. External Doppler monitor, along with an external stress gauge for uterine contractions (together called the NST), is used near term to monitor fetal well-being. It also is used to assess risks for those with preexisting maternal conditions and pregnancies with complications.

c. Baseline fetal heart rate is 120–160 bpm.

d. A normal (reactive) NST requires two accelerations of fetal heart rate in 20 minutes of up to 15 bpm from the baseline heart rate for a duration of 15 seconds and the absence of decelerations.

e. Contractions usually decrease the flow of blood to the placenta. This is poorly tolerated by the stressed fetus and leads to hypoxia and concomitant relative bradycardia.

f. Decelerations have been defined as a decline in fetal heart rate of 15 bpm or lasting more than 15 seconds or a slow return to baseline. Persistent late decelerations, which begin AFTER the peak of the contractions, are nonreassuring and warrant intervention.

II. COMPLICATIONS OF PREGNANCY

A. Ectopic pregnancy

1. General characteristics

a. Ectopic pregnancy is the implantation of a pregnancy anywhere but the endometrium.

b. More than 95% of ectopic pregnancies occur in the fallopian tube, and 55% of tubal pregnancies occur in the ampulla of the tube.

c. The most common cause of ectopic pregnancy is occlusion of the tube secondary to adhesions.

d. Risk factors for ectopic pregnancy include a history of a previous ectopic pregnancy, previous salpingitis (caused by pelvic inflammatory disease), previous abdominal or tubal surgery, use of an intrauterine device, assisted reproduction, exposure to diethylstilbestrol (DES), and progestin-only contraception.

2. Clinical features

a. The presentation of ectopic pregnancy is widely variable and may depend on the site of implantation.

b. The classic presentation includes unilateral adnexal pain, amenorrhea or spotting, and tenderness or mass on pelvic examination (Table 8-5). Other symptoms may include dizziness or syncope as well as GI symptoms.

c. Signs and symptoms associated with a ruptured ectopic pregnancy are severe abdominal or shoulder pain associated with peritonitis, tachycardia, syncope, and orthostatic hypotension.

3. Laboratory studies

a. Serum levels of hCG normally double every 48 hours. If serial increases of hCG are less than expected, ectopic gestation should be suspected until the diagnosis has been definitively excluded.

b. Transvaginal ultrasound is diagnostic in 90% of cases of ectopic gestation.

c. Women with an hCG titer of greater than 1,500 mU/mL should show evidence of a developing intrauterine gestation on a transvaginal ultrasound. If no such evidence is found, ectopic pregnancy is the clinical diagnosis.

TABLE 8-5 Signs and Symptoms Associated with Ectopic Pregnancy			
Sign/Symptom	**% of Cases**		
Pain	60–80%	Pelvic mass	20%
Abnormal menstruation	75%	Enlarged uterus	25%
Gastrointestinal symptoms	80%	Tachycardia, hypotension	75%
Dizziness or syncope	58%	Shock	25%

Source: Cunningham FG, et al. Williams Obstetrics NY: McGraw-Hill, 2005, Chapter 10

4. Treatment

    a. Medical treatment with methotrexate, a folic acid analog, can be used to treat up to 80% of ectopic gestations when diagnosed early. Criteria for methotrexate treatment include a serum hCG titer of less than 5,000 mU, ectopic mass less than 3.5 cm on ultrasound, a patient who is hemodynamically stable, and a patient who is deemed to be compliant for follow-up.

    b. Surgical treatment involves removal of the ectopic gestation using laparoscopy or laparotomy.

        (1) Laparoscopy is the preferred method.

        (2) Laparotomy usually is reserved for patients with known significant abdominal adhesions or those who are clinically unstable.

    c. Follow-up testing using serum hCG levels or pelvic examination is crucial to exclude any remaining evidence of pregnancy.

B. Spontaneous abortion

    1. General characteristics

        a. Abortion is the termination of pregnancy, by any means, before 20 weeks of gestation.

        b. Spontaneous abortion is the spontaneous, premature expulsion of the products of conception; it occurs in up to 15–20% of clinically recognized pregnancies.

        c. Eighty percent of spontaneous abortions occur during the first trimester of pregnancy; of these, up to 50% are associated with chromosomal abnormalities.

        d. Possible maternal factors that increase the risk of spontaneous abortion include smoking, infection, maternal systemic disease, immunologic factors, drug use, and environmental factors (e.g., lead, formaldehyde).

        e. Complications of an improperly treated spontaneous abortion are Rh sensitization, infection, hemorrhage requiring blood transfusion, potential blood coagulopathies (e.g., disseminated intravascular coagulation secondary to retained tissue), and sepsis.

    2. Clinical features

        a. Table 8-6 indicates the various classifications of spontaneous abortion.

        b. Bleeding is variable on examination.

        c. Uterine size often does not correlate appropriately to the last menstrual period, and the fundus of the uterus may be boggy or tender.

    3. Laboratory studies

        a. Serial hCG titers, serum progesterone, or serial ultrasounds may be required to confirm a viable pregnancy.

        b. Ultrasound findings in a nonviable pregnancy may include inappropriate development or interval growth, poorly formed or unformed fetal pole, and fetal demise.

        c. Blood type and Rh status are necessary tests to preclude Rh sensitization in the mother.

    4. Treatment

        a. If the pregnancy has been definitively determined to be no longer viable, the uterus must be emptied.

        b. If the pregnancy is early and the patient is managed expectantly, careful follow-up with pelvic examinations, serial hCG titers, and transvaginal ultrasound can be used to determine whether the abortion is complete.

        c. Dilation and curettage also may be necessary to ensure complete emptying of the uterus or as one form of induced abortion. Morbidity is caused by uterine perforation or cervical laceration.

TABLE 8-6 Classification of Spontaneous Abortions^a

Type	Vaginal Bleeding	Cervix Open	Products of Conception Passed
Threatened	Yes	No	No
Inevitable	Yes	Yes	Not yet, but no way to maintain pregnancy
Incomplete	Yes	Yes	Partial
Complete	Yes	Yes	Yes
Missed	No	No	No (fetal demise has occurred without symptoms)

^aThree or more consecutive abortions is classified as recurrent, and any abortion with associated sepsis is classified as septic.

d. Immunoglobulin should be administered to Rh-negative women in the event of either a threatened or spontaneous abortion.

e. Septic or infected abortion requires complete evacuation of the uterine contents, medical support, and antibiotics.

C. Gestational trophoblastic disease (GTD)

  1. General characteristics

   a. GTD is a spectrum of diseases arising from the placenta and includes complete and partial hydatidiform moles, placental site invasive moles, trophoblastic tumors, and choriocarcinomas.

   b. GTD is divided into benign and malignant forms. Hydatidiform moles (also called a molar pregnancy) is the benign form of GTD.

  2. Hydatidiform moles are divided into complete and incomplete molar pregnancies. Complete molar pregnancies are the most common form of GTD.

   a. Complete hydatidiform moles are characterized by an empty egg and the appearance of "grape-like vesicles" or a "snowstorm pattern" on ultrasound. Twenty percent progress to malignancy.

   b. Partial hydatidiform moles have a fetus present, but the fetus is nonviable. Ten percent progress to malignancy.

  3. Clinical features. A complete or partial molar pregnancy most commonly present with abnormal vaginal bleeding, uterine size greater than dates, hyperemesis gravidarum, or preeclampsia-like symptoms before 20 weeks of gestation.

  4. Laboratory studies

   a. With complete molar pregnancy, the hCG level often is greater than 100,000 mU/mL. Persistently elevated levels of hCG may indicate gestational trophoblastic tumor.

   b. Ultrasound of a complete hydatidiform mole shows a characteristic "sack of grapes" or "snowstorm" appearance consistent with the swelling of the chorionic villi. Ultrasound may aid in establishing the diagnosis of a partial molar pregnancy.

  5. Treatment

   a. Treatment depends on tumor classification. Benign tumors and low-risk metastatic tumors can be treated with chemotherapy. Metastatic high-risk tumors require a combination of chemotherapy with or without adjuvant radiation and surgery.

   b. Surgical treatment includes suction curettage (for those desiring to preserve fertility) and hysterectomy. These treatments all carry high cure rates of 80–100%.

   c. After evacuation, patients must be monitored with serial hCG to diagnose and manage sequelae properly. Contraception is recommended for 6–12 months after remission.

D. Multiple gestation

  1. General characteristics

   a. The overall incidence of multiple birth in the United States is 3% and has been increasing during the past 30 years, in part as a result of the use of assisted reproductive techniques and ovulation induction. Twins occur in 1 out of every 94 births.

   b. With multiple gestations, all the same symptoms of pregnancy generally occur, but they often are more severe. Prenatal visits should occur more frequently than with single gestations.

   c. Types

    (1) Two-thirds of twins are dizygotic, or fraternal (i.e., formed by the fertilization of two ova). The incidence of dizygotic twins is increased in those with a family history of twins, those taking fertility drugs, mothers with above-average weight and height, and African-American women.

    (2) Monozygotic twins (i.e., those formed from the fertilization of one ovum) occur randomly and are associated with fetal transfusion syndrome and discordant fetal growth.

   d. Maternal complications

    (1) The most common complications of multiple gestation are spontaneous abortion and preterm birth.

    (2) Other problems that occur with greater frequency are preeclampsia and anemia.

   e. Fetal complications include intrauterine growth restriction, cord accidents, death of one twin, congenital anomalies, abnormal or breech presentation, and placental abruption or previa.

E. Gestational diabetes

1. General characteristics

  a. Gestational diabetes mellitus is carbohydrate intolerance of variable severity that is only present during pregnancy.

  b. The lifetime risk of developing diabetes after pregnancy in women who have had gestational diabetes is increased to greater than 50% (versus 5% in the general population). If insulin is required during the pregnancy, there is a 50% risk of developing diabetes within 5 years from the pregnancy.

  c. Recurrence of gestational diabetes is common, occurring in 60–90% of subsequent pregnancies.

  d. Maternal complications associated with gestational diabetes mellitus include preeclampsia, hyperacceleration of general diabetic complications, and traumatic birth, including shoulder dystocia.

  e. Fetal complications associated with gestational diabetes mellitus include macrosomia, prematurity, fetal demise, and delayed fetal lung maturity.

2. Clinical features

  a. Patients with gestational diabetes usually are asymptomatic.

  b. Risk factors for the development of gestational diabetes include a history of a previous large-birth-weight infant, obesity, age older than 25 years, glucosuria, a previous poor obstetric outcome, family history of diabetes, or being a member of the following ethnic groups: African American, Asian, Hispanic or Indian.

3. Laboratory studies

  a. Screening recommendations

   (1) Screen high-risk women as soon as feasible, then conduct a repeat screening at 24–28 weeks.

   (2) All other women should be screened at 24–28 weeks.

   (3) Screening consists of administering a nonfasting, 50-g glucose challenge test, followed by a serum glucose level 1 hour later. If the 1-hour serum glucose value is greater than 130–140 mg/dL, a 3-hour glucose tolerance test is performed.

   (4) The 3-hour glucose tolerance test consists of a 100-g glucose load in the morning after an overnight fast. Serum glucose levels are taken at fasting and then at 1, 2, and 3 hours after the glucose load. If two or more of the values are abnormal, the patient is diagnosed as a gestational diabetic (Table 8-7).

  b. Antepartum testing using biophysical profiles and NSTs often is used in gestational diabetes beginning at 34 weeks of gestation.

  c. Women who have had gestational diabetes should be screened at 6 weeks postpartum for diabetes and at yearly intervals thereafter.

4. Treatment

  a. Careful management of gestational diabetes with diet and exercise is essential.

  b. Patients with gestational diabetes must check their blood glucose levels after fasting overnight and after each meal. In addition, fasting or 2-hour postprandial blood sugar measurements should be done at each office visit.

TABLE 8-7	**Diagnosis of Gestational Diabetes Mellitus with a 100-g Oral Glucose Load**[a]	
Test	**Results mg/dL**	**nmol/L**
Fasting	95	5.3
1 hr	180	10.0
2 hr	155	8.6
3 hr	140	7.8

Source: American Diabetic Association.
[a]Two or more of the venous plasma concentrations must be met or exceeded for a positive diagnosis. The test should be done in the morning after an overnight fast of between 8 and 14 hours and after at least 3 days of unrestricted diet and unlimited physical activity. The subject should remain seated and should not smoke throughout the test.

    c. Patients who have fasting blood sugar measurements of greater than 105 mg/dL or 2-hour postprandial blood sugar measurements of greater than 120 mg/dL may require insulin.

    d. To help avoid the development of diabetes later in life, the patient should be advised to obtain and maintain ideal body weight. Annual evaluations of fasting glucose concentrations are recommended.

F. Preterm labor and delivery

    1. General characteristics

      a. Preterm delivery is the delivery of a viable infant before 37 weeks of gestation and occurs in 8–10% of births.

      b. Preterm delivery is the most common cause of neonatal deaths not resulting from congenital malformations.

      c. Low-birth-weight infants born prematurely often have significant visual or hearing impairment, developmental delays, cerebral palsy, and lung disease.

      d. The cause of preterm labor is poorly understood. Risk factors include smoking, cocaine use, uterine malformations, cervical incompetence, infection (vaginal group B streptococci or urinary tract infection), and low prepregnancy weight

      e. Complications of maternal or fetal health, such as hypertension, diabetes mellitus, or abruptio placentae, are associated with preterm delivery.

    2. Clinical features

      a. Preterm labor is defined as regular uterine contractions between 20 and 36 weeks of gestation that are 5–8 min apart (or less) and the presence of one or more of the following signs:

        (1) Cervical dilatation of 2 cm or greater at presentation.

        (2) Cervical dilatation of 1 cm or greater on serial examinations.

        (3) Cervical effacement of greater than 80%.

      b. Late symptoms of preterm labor include painful or painless contractions, pressure, menstrual-like cramps, watery or bloody discharge, and low back pain.

    3. Laboratory studies

      a. Ultrasound sometimes is used to examine the length of the cervix.

      b. Examination of the cervicovaginal secretions for fetal fibronectin, a glycoprotein, has been used as a marker for preterm labor.

      c. Vaginal cultures and urinalysis with culture and sensitivity also should be obtained.

    4. Treatment

      a. Management techniques include bed rest, oral or IV hydration, antibiotics to treat subclincal infection, steroids administered to the mother to enhance fetal lung maturity, and tocolytics, if indicated.

      b. Tocolytics are used in an attempt to stop contractions.

        (1) Magnesium sulfate ($MgSO_4$) inhibits myometrial contractility mediated by calcium. Side effects include nausea, fatigue, and generalized muscle weakness.

          (a) $MgSO_4$ can lead to decreased reflexes, respiratory depression, and cardiac collapse.

          (b) In the case of $MgSO_4$ toxicity, calcium gluconate can be given.

        (2) β-Mimetic adrenergic agents, including ridodrine and terbutaline, stimulate β-receptors to relax smooth muscle to decrease uterine contractions. Side effects include maternal and fetal tachycardia, emesis, headaches, and pulmonary edema.

        (3) Calcium channel blockers inhibit smooth muscle contractility by decreasing intracellular Ca^{2+} ions, which therefore relax uterine muscle. Side effects include maternal hypotension and tachycardia.

      c. The goal in treatment of these patients is to identify those at risk and to diagnose the condition before labor is irreversibly established. Cervical cerclage (i.e., closure of cervix by mechanical means) is an option for women with known cervical incompetence or a history of preterm birth.

G. Premature rupture of membranes (PROM) and preterm premature rupture of membranes (PPROM)

    1. General characteristics

      a. PROM is rupture of the amniotic membranes before the onset of labor at or beyond 37 weeks of gestation, and it occurs in approximately 8% of all pregnancies. Most women (90%) will go into spontaneous labor within 24 hours after PROM.

      b. PPROM occurs before 37 weeks of gestation and precedes 30–40% of all preterm deliveries.

   c. The major risk associated with both PROM and PPROM is infection (chorioamnionitis and endometritis). This risk increases with time and hastens delivery.

   d. Cord prolapse also can occur with ruptured membranes if the head is not well engaged.

2. Clinical features

   a. Symptoms of ruptured membranes are a gush or persistent leakage of fluid from the vagina, vaginal discharge, and occasionally, simply pelvic pressure.

   b. Ruptured membranes can be confirmed with direct visualization of pooling using a sterile speculum, use of nitrazine paper, and the fern test. Ultrasound can be used to check the amniotic fluid index.

   c. Digital examination should be avoided unless delivery is imminent.

   d. Cord prolapse is identified as a rope-like, soft, elongated mass on speculum or bimanual examination.

3. Treatment

   a. PROM (after 37 weeks)

      (1) If expectant management is feasible, the patient should be hospitalized and the fetus carefully monitored.

      (2) Active management of PROM involves induction with prostaglandin cervical gel or misoprostol and/or oxytocin. The goal of this treatment is to expedite delivery to decrease rates of infection.

   b. PPROM (20–36 weeks)

      (1) If there is no sign of maternal or fetal infection or distress, expectant management is preferred. The patient should be put on strict bed rest.

      (2) If under 34 weeks of gestation, steroids (betamethasone) should be administered to enhance fetal lung maturity.

      (3) Antibiotics often are administered to prevent infection and to help prolong the pregnancy, because they have been shown to decrease infant mortality.

      (4) NST and BPP should be performed daily to assess fetal well-being.

      (5) Amniocentesis can be performed to check for lung maturity.

H. Hypertension in pregnancy

   1. Chronic hypertension is hypertension that presents before 20 weeks of gestation.

   2. Pregnancy-induced hypertension (PIH) is hypertension that presents after 20 weeks of gestation but has no other associated symptoms.

      a. Chronic hypertension and PIH are treated in the same manner: monthly ultrasound to check for intrauterine growth retardation, serial blood pressure and urine protein, and weekly NST during the third trimester.

      b. The basic underlying pathophysiology of PIH is thought to be vasospasm or arteriolar constriction.

      c. Medication for chronic hypertension and PIH is only given in severe cases. Methyldopa is the treatment of choice, with labetalol as an alternative.

   3. Preeclampsia/eclampsia

      a. General characteristics

         (1) To be diagnosed as preeclampsia/eclampsia, the symptoms must occur after 20 weeks of gestation. It most often occurs near term but can occur up to 2 weeks postpartum.

         (2) Preeclampsia is the triad of hypertension, edema, and proteinuria. Preeclampsia is categorized into mild or severe preeclampsia (Table 8-8).

         (3) HELLP syndrome is the presence of severe preeclampsia with the addition of **H**emolysis, **E**levated **L**iver enzymes, and **L**ow **P**latelets.

         (4) Eclampsia is severe preeclampsia with the addition of seizures.

         (5) The most common risk factor for preeclampsia is nulliparity. Other risk factors include extremes of age (<20 or >35 years), multiple gestation, diabetes, and chronic hypertension.

         (6) Maternal complications of preeclampsia include progression to eclampsia or HELLP syndrome, abruptio placentae, renal failure, cerebral hemorrhage, pulmonary edema, and disseminated intravascular coagulation.

         (7) Fetal complications include hypoxia, low birth weight, preterm delivery, and perinatal death.

TABLE 8-8	Classification of Mild Versus Severe Preeclampsia	
	Mild Preeclampsia[a]	**Severe Preeclampsia**
Blood pressure	140/90 mm Hg, **or** increase of 30 mm Hg systolic and 15 mm Hg diastolic from prepregnancy blood pressure	160–180/110 mm Hg
Proteinuria	300 mg/24 hr **or** trace to 1+ on dipstick	>2 g/24 hr, **or** 2+ or more on dipstick
Symptoms/signs	Nondependent edema	Elevated creatinine Liver enzyme elevation Headaches Visual disturbances Right upper quadrant pain

    b. Clinical features

        (1) Symptoms include edema of the face and hands, sudden weight gain, headache, visual disturbances, nausea, vomiting, right upper quadrant pain, and decreased urine output.

        (2) Signs include hypertension, proteinuria, and hyperreflexia.

    c. Laboratory studies

        (1) Sterile urine protein, 24-hour urine protein level, CBC, fibrinogen, and PT/PTT are followed.

        (2) Chemistry panel including liver function studies, creatinine, and uric acid levels aid in identifying risk for complications.

    d. Treatment

        (1) Delivery of the infant is the ultimate treatment for hypertensive disorders of pregnancy.

        (2) Mild preeclampsia

            (a) If the patient is reliable, she may be followed as an outpatient. Alternately, the patient may be hospitalized with expectant management. Whether or not the patient is followed as an in- or an outpatient, delivery through induction is indicated after 37 weeks of gestation.

            (b) $MgSO_4$, administered by IV drip, is the first-line medication for inpatient management to decrease chance of seizures. $MgSO_4$ should be continued for 24 hours after delivery.

            (c) Hydralazine or labetalol sometimes are given for acute management of blood pressure.

            (d) Betamethasone is given before 34 weeks of gestation to enhance fetal lung maturity.

        (3) Severe PIH or eclampsia are indications for prompt delivery regardless of gestational age.

I. Rh incompatibility

    1. General characteristics

        a. If the infant's blood type is not identical to the mother's blood type, the mother may develop antibodies against the infant's blood (i.e., Rh sensitization). For example, if mother is Rh-negative and fetus Rh-positive, the mother may develop antibodies against the infant's blood, and hemolysis can occur.

        b. The most common problem of mismatched blood involves the rhesus D factor (Rh factor). Approximately 15% of the population is Rh-negative. Although 98% of isoimmunizations are secondary to the Rh factor, 43 other antigens exist.

        c. Immunoglobulin (Rho-Gam) is administered routinely at 28–29 weeks of gestation to all Rh-negative mothers for prophylactic protection. After delivery, if the baby is found to be Rh-positive, the mother receives Rho-Gam again to protect subsequent pregnancies. When Rho-Gam is given, it helps to prevent development of these antibodies to the infant's blood in 99% of cases.

        d. The most common time of maternal/fetal blood mixing is at delivery. After any event that may allow fetal cells to enter maternal circulation, however, Rho-Gam should be given if incompatibility exists. Common events include ectopic pregnancy, spontaneous or therapeutic abortion, CVS, amniocentesis, or trauma.

        e. If antibodies develop, they will attack subsequent Rh-incompatible infants and can lead to severe fetal anemia and death (fetal hydrops).

    2. Laboratory studies

      a. Routine prenatal blood work should include blood type, Rh factor, and Coombs' test for antibodies.

      b. Antibody titers of less than 1:16 probably will not adversely affect the pregnancy.

      c. In a sensitized pregnancy, a combination of Coombs' test, amniocentesis, and ultrasound is used to follow the developing fetus for evidence of distress or fetal hydrops.

   3. Treatment

      a. Routinely give immunoglobulin (Rho-Gam), 300 mg, to Rh negative, nonimmunized women at 28 weeks of gestation and within 72 hours of delivering an Rh-positive infant.

      b. Rh immunoglobulin also is to be administered at amniocentesis and other instances of potential uterine bleeding, as noted previously.

      c. Massive fetal–maternal hemorrhage may require larger doses of immunoglobulin.

J. Abruptio placentae

   1. General characteristics

      a. Abruptio placentae is the premature separation of a normally implanted placenta after the 20th week of gestation but before birth.

      b. Abruptio placentae is the most common cause of third-trimester bleeding.

      c. Several risk factors are known for the development of abruptio placentae: trauma, smoking, hypertension, decreased folic acid, cocaine use, alcohol (>14 drinks/week), uterine anomalies, high parity, previous abruption (recurrence rate is 10–17%), and advanced maternal age.

      d. Types of abruption include external abruption (more common, less severe), when blood escapes from the uterus, and concealed abruption (less common, more severe), when blood is retained between the detached placenta and the uterus. Figure 8.2 depicts common types.

      e. Abruption can lead to liberation of tissue thromboplastin or consumption of fibrinogen, thereby activating the extrinsic clotting mechanism. This could eventually lead to disseminated intravascular coagulation.

   2. Clinical features

      a. Painful vaginal bleeding occurs in the majority of cases (85%).

      b. Uterine, abdominal, or back pain is a frequent symptom of abruptio placentae and, if bleeding is concealed, may be the only symptom.

      c. The uterus becomes hypertonic, irritable, or tender when the placenta has abrupted, and it may be enlarged.

      d. Evidence of fetal distress may or may not be present, depending on the degree of separation.

      e. Complications of abruptio placentae, in addition to the obvious compromise of placental blood flow to the fetus and hemorrhage, are renal failure, coagulation failure, and death.

   3. Laboratory studies

      a. Diagnosis is clinical.

      b. Ultrasonography is not reliable in establishing the diagnosis of this problem.

   4. Treatment

      a. Delivery of the fetus and placenta is the definitive treatment of abruptio placentae. However, management depends on the degree of separation and the age of the fetus.

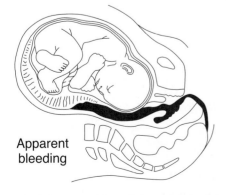
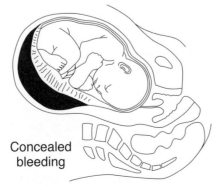
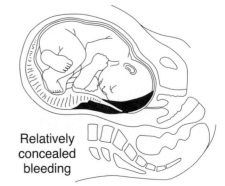

Apparent bleeding   Concealed bleeding   Relatively concealed bleeding

FIGURE 8-2 Types of abruptio placentae: external (apparent) and concealed.

  b. Blood type, cross-match, and coagulation studies are indicated in an unstable patient, as is placement of a large-bore IV line.

  c. Cesarean section most often is the preferred route for delivering the infant in cases of abruptio placentae.

K. Placenta previa

 1. General characteristics

  a. Placenta previa occurs when the placenta partially or completely covers the cervical os.

  b. Performing a digital examination in a patient with placenta previa is contraindicated, because it can incite severe bleeding.

  c. Placenta previa occurs in 0.3–0.5% of pregnancies and is associated with advanced age, smoking, high parity, and any process that could cause scarring of the lower uterine segment (e. g., cesarean delivery).

 2. Clinical features

  a. Painless vaginal bleeding is the hallmark of placenta previa.

  b. Bleeding may continue from the placenta's implantation site after delivery, because the lower uterus contracts poorly.

 3. Laboratory studies

  a. Ultrasonography is the test of choice for establishing the diagnosis of placenta previa.

  b. When the patient is hemodynamically unstable, studies for blood type, cross-match, and coagulation should be ordered; a large-bore IV line should be placed.

 4. Treatment

  a. Before term, watchful waiting is warranted if the patient is stable.

   (1) Blood transfusion may be necessary during the period of waiting for fetal maturity.

   (2) Placenta previa often is diagnosed before 20 weeks of gestation (on routine ultrasound). Up to 50% of affected placentas "migrate" up the uterine wall, however, because of growth, so they are not ultimately present at term.

   (3) Patients with previa should abstain from vaginal penetration.

  b. Cesarean section is the preferred method of delivering the infant in cases of placenta previa.

III. LABOR AND DELIVERY

A. Routine vaginal labor and delivery

 1. General characteristics

  a. Approximately 20% perinatal morbidity and mortality occur during the intrapartum period in otherwise healthy pregnancies.

  b. Most infants present with a vertex (head-down) presentation. However, other possibilities include breech, face, transverse, and compound (arm or leg).

 2. Clinical features

  a. Cervical examination to assess labor

   (1) Dilatation

    (a) Opening of the cervical os.

    (b) Expressed in centimeters (fully dilated is 10 cm).

   (2) Effacement

    (a) Cervical softening and thinning out.

    (b) Expressed as a percentage (up to 100%).

   (3) Station

    (a) Location of the presenting part (usually the head) in relation to the maternal ischial spines.

    (b) The level at the spines is denoted as "0" station. Stations above the spines are expressed in negative numbers (e.g., −1 cm, −2 cm) and stations below the spine in positive numbers (e.g., +1 cm, +2 cm).

  b. Stages of labor

   (1) The first stage of labor begins at the onset of true, regular contractions and ends at full dilatation. The length of the first stage of labor generally is 6–20 hours for nulliparous women and 2–14 hours for multiparous women (or 1–1.5 cm/hr).

(2) The second stage of labor begins at full dilatation and ends with the delivery of the infant. The length of the second stage of labor generally is 30 minutes to 3 hours (average, 50 minutes) for nulliparous women and 5–60 minutes (average, 20 minutes) for multiparous women.

(3) The third stage of labor begins after the delivery and entails separation and expulsion of the placenta. The length of the third stage of labor generally is 0–30 minutes but usually is about 5 minutes.

(4) The hour after delivery sometimes is called the fourth stage and is critical in assessing and treating tears, lacerations, and hemorrhage.

  c. Bloody show, which is the passage of a small amount of blood-tinged mucus that has been plugging the cervical os, often precedes true labor.

  d. Amniotic fluid rupture can occur before or during the first stage of labor.

3. Laboratory studies

  a. On admission, urinalysis for protein, glucose, and hematocrit should be obtained.

  b. Fetal monitoring is used in labor to assess the fetus' response to labor.

(1) An external fetal monitor is attached to maternal abdomen and assesses an estimated fetal heart rate via transmitted sound waves.

(2) An internal fetal monitor is an electrode attached to the infant's head and gives the most accurate fetal heart rate pattern because it transmits the true R wave (as with an electrocardiogram) of electroactivity. The cervix must be dilated at least 2 cm and membranes ruptured to attach an internal fetal monitor.

(a) Accelerations of an increase of 15 bpm for 15 seconds above the normal baseline heart rate (120–160 bpm) is reassuring and denotes fetal well-being.

(b) Early decelerations mirror the images of the contractions and denote fetal head compression. They often are present as a woman approaches the second stage of labor and are considered to be benign.

(c) Variable decelerations are rapid drops in fetal heart rate with a return to baseline with variable shape and no identifiable pattern. They often occur with cord compression and, if mild or infrequent, are benign.

(d) Late decelerations are fetal heart rate drops during the second half of the contractions. They denote uteroplacental insufficiency and always are worrisome.

(e) When a nonreassuring fetal heart rate is present, the following management is appropriate: stop oxytocin (if applicable), change maternal position, administer oxygen via face mask, and measure fetal scalp pH.

4. Treatment

  a. Regular cervical examinations for dilatation, station, and effacement are necessary to check the progress of labor.

  b. Continued blood pressure, temperature, and pulse readings are critical to exclude late PIH, toxemia, and infection.

  c. Analgesia is offered to provide comfort and to prevent fatigue.

  d. After crowning of the presenting part, pressure applied from the coccygeal region upward will extend the head at the proper time and help to protect the perineal musculature.

  e. When the head has been delivered, the baby can be suctioned with a rubber suction bulb.

  f. When the rest of the body passes, the cord is clamped and cut.

  g. Episiotomy (surgical incision to prevent traumatic tearing) sometimes is used to protect the perineum as the head crowns for such indications as a large baby or a short perineum.

  h. Signs of placental separation include umbilical cord lengthening, a fresh show of blood flow, fundus rising, and the uterus becoming firm and globular.

  i. The infant is suctioned, kept warm, and assessed for Apgar score at 1 and 5 minutes after delivery (Table 8-9).

  j. The placenta and umbilical cord should be examined to ensure that the entire placenta and membranes are passed and that the cord contains three vessels (two arteries and one vein).

  k. Oxytocin, ergonovine maleate, or methylergonovine maleate sometimes are used in the third stage of labor to reduce blood loss by stimulating contractions.

B. Abnormal labor and delivery

  1. General characteristics

    a. Abnormal labor, or dystocia, occurs when the cervix fails to dilate progressively over time and the fetus fails to descend.

Letter	Points Sign	0	1	2
A	Activity (muscle tone)	Absent	Arms and legs flexed	Active movement
P	Pulse	Absent	<100 bpm	>100 bpm
G	Grimace (reflex irritability)	No response	Grimace	Sneezes, coughs, pulls away
A	Appearance (skin color)	Blue-gray, pale all over	Pink, except extremities	Pink all over
R	Respiration	Absent	Slow, irregular	Good, crying

TABLE 8-9 Apgar Scoringᵃ

Source: Adapted with permission from Childbirth.org. Apgar scoring for newborns. Copyright © 1994–1998 by Childbirth.org. Available at: www.childbirth.org/articles/apgar.html; accessed on: June 9, 2003.
ᵃA score is determined for each sign at 1 min and at 5 min after birth; if there are problems with the neonate, a score is determined at 10 min as well. Scores are classified as follows: 7–10 = normal; 4–7 = may require some resuscitative measures; ≤3 = immediate resuscitation required.

   b. Common causes include abnormalities with the pelvis, powers, or passenger.

    (1) Pelvis refers to the passage through the pelvic structures. Sometimes, the pelvis is not large enough to allow the infant to pass through, which denotes cephalopelvic disproportion.

    (2) Powers refers to the contractions, which are needed to dilate the cervix and to expel the infant. If contractions are inadequate, oxytocin (Pitocin) can be given IV to enhance labor.

    (3) Passenger refers to the baby. The head usually is the biggest part. The bigger the baby is in relation to the pelvis, the larger the likelihood of cephalopelvic disproportion.

2. Clinical features

   a. Inability to deliver vaginally after full cervical dilatation is a good marker of true dystocia.

   b. Macrosomia, nonvertex presentation and the adequacy of the pelvis can be evaluated by clinical examination before the onset of labor.

3. Treatment

   a. Inadequate uterine contractions can be augmented with oxytocin after the maternal pelvis and fetus are assessed.

   b. If maternal pushing is inadequate, rest or assisted delivery with vacuum extraction or forceps may be used. Forceps or vacuum extractors are used to shorten the second stage of labor and may be indicated for fetal distress or maternal indications only if the head is engaged and the cervix is fully dilated.

   c. The diagnosis of dystocia is a leading indication for cesarean section.

   d. If the cord is prolapsed, manual elevation of the presenting part in the knee–chest position is necessary for temporary reduction of the cord while administering a tocolytic agent. Emergent delivery is required.

   e. If the baby is in a nonvertex presentation, external version with ultrasound guidance can be attempted after 37 weeks of gestation.

C. Cesarean delivery and vaginal birth after cesarean delivery (VBAC)

1. General characteristics

   a. Cesarean section is defined as the birth of the fetus through an incision in the abdominal and uterine walls and constitutes 21–25% of deliveries in the United States.

   b. The most frequent indications for cesarean section are repeat cesarean (one-third of cesareans), dystocia or failure to progress, breech presentation, and fetal distress.

   c. The success rate of VBAC depends on the indications for and the number of the previous cesarean sections.

    (1) When dystocia was the indicator for a previous cesarean delivery, the rate of successful VBAC is the lowest. Conversely, women who have a cesarean delivery for malpresentation (e.g., breech) have a higher rate of success with VBAC.

    (2) Although the incidence of uterine rupture in a VBAC after use of a low transverse incision is relatively low (0.2–1.5%), it can lead to death of the fetus and significantly increased morbidity and mortality of the mother.

   d. Risks of cesarean section include a greater likelihood of thromboembolic events, increased bleeding, and development of infection.

2. Treatment

   a. Prophylactic antibiotics often are used after a cesarean section to prevent infection.

TABLE 8-10	Induction of Labor	
Indications	**Relative Contraindications**	**Absolute Contraindications**
Prolonged pregnancy	Breech presentation	Cephalopelvic disproportion
Diabetes mellitus	Oligohydramnios	Placenta previa
Rh isoimmunization	Multiple gestation	Uterine scar from previous classical cesarean section
Preeclampsia	Prematurity	Transverse lie
Premature rupture of membranes	Grand multiparity	Myomectomy
Chronic hypertension	Previous cesarean section with transverse scar	
Placental insufficiency	Fetal macrosomia	
Suspected intrauterine growth retardation		

Source: Adapted from DeCherney A. Current Obstetric and Gynecology Diagnosis and Treatment. 10th Ed. NY: McGraw-Hill Companies, 2007.

    b. A low transverse uterine incision usually is made because of the decreased blood loss associated with its use, the ease of repair, and the lower likelihood of rupture compared with that of a classical incision (incidence with a classical incision is 4–9%). A classical incision is vertical through the entire length of the uterus.

D. Induction of labor

    1. General Characteristics

        a. Induction of labor can be done by medical or surgical means.

        b. Induction of labor is considered when prolongation of pregnancy might expose the mother or fetus to complications and when vaginal delivery is not contraindicated (Table 8-10).

    2. Methods

        a. Early induction of labor (when minimal dilatation or effacement has occurred) is initiated with prostaglandin gel put directly on the cervix; this may be repeated once in 12 hours. This helps to soften or "ripen" the cervix.

        b. Later induction (when the cervix is dilated >1 cm and some effacement has occurred) is initiated with oxytocin (Pitocin) given IV, with systematic increases in the oxytocin level until strong contractions are occurring approximately every 3 minutes.

        c. Amniotomy, or artificially rupturing the membranes with a small hook, also can induce labor

E. Postpartum hemorrhage

    1. General characteristics

        a. Postpartum hemorrhage is defined as blood loss requiring transfusion or a 10% decrease in hematocrit between admission and the postpartum period. It is the third leading cause of maternal mortality in advanced gestation.

        b. Early postpartum hemorrhage occurs less than 24 hours after delivery and is associated with abnormal involution of the placental site, cervical or vaginal lacerations, and retained portions of placenta.

        c. Late postpartum hemorrhage occurs more than 24 hours after delivery to 6 weeks postpartum and most commonly is caused by subinvolution of the uterus, retained products of conception, or endometritis.

    2. Clinical features

        a. Complaints of increased bleeding after delivery signal a need to evaluate for hemorrhage.

        b. A subinvoluted uterus will feel enlarged and soft on examination, and the patient may present with complaints of increased bleeding, pain, fever, and foul-smelling lochia.

    3. Laboratory studies

        a. Hemoglobin and hematocrit tests are necessary to quantify complaints of bleeding.

        b. Ultrasonography sometimes can detect obvious retained placental fragments.

    4. Treatment

        a. Initially, uterine massage and compression can be used.

        b. Establish IV access, and prepare blood components.

        c. Use of IV oxytocin, ergonovine, methylergonovine, or prostaglandins often is first-line treatment for early postpartum hemorrhage.

      d. Subinvolution of the uterus often responds to oral agents that increase uterine contraction (e.g., methyler-gonovine maleate, ergonovine maleate). Antibiotic treatment also may be necessary.

      e. Postpartum hemorrhage may require surgical intervention, depending on the cause and severity.

F. Endometritis

  1. General Characteristics

      a. Endometritis most commonly occurs after cesarean section or when membranes are ruptured more than 24 hours before delivery.

      b. Findings most commonly present 2–3 days postpartum. Fever higher than 30.0°C and uterine tenderness are highly suspicious for endometritis.

      c. Parametrid and adnexal tenderness, peritoneal irritation, and decreased bowel sounds may occur.

  2. Laboratory studies

      a. WBC count commonly is more than 20,000/mcL.

      b. Causative bacteria vary widely from hospital to hospital, but anaerobic streptococci are most common.

      c. Urinalysis also should be performed.

  3. Treatment

      a. Antibiotics are administered until afebrile for 24 hrs.

         (1) Clindamycin plus gentamicin is the first-line treatment.

         (2) Ampicillin is added if there is no response in 24–48 hours.

         (3) Metronidazole is added if sepsis is present.

      b. A single dose of antibiotic at the time of cord clamping reduces the incidence of endometritis.

IV. PUERPERIUM

A. Definition. The 6-week period after delivery is known as the puerperium or the postpartum period.

B. Normal puerperium

  1. General characteristics

      a. Immediately after delivery, the uterus is below the umbilicus.

         (1) After 2 days, the uterus shrinks, or involutes.

         (2) After 2 weeks, it descends into the pelvic cavity.

         (3) After about 4 weeks, it is back to its antenatal size.

      b. Lochia, or bleeding that occurs after delivery, represents the sloughing off of decidual tissue. It can last for 4–5 weeks postpartum.

      c. In a nonnursing mother, menses resume 6–8 weeks postpartum. In contrast, nursing mothers typically are anovulatory and may remain amenorrheic for the duration of lactation.

  2. Clinical features

      a. The first postpartum visit should be approximately 6 weeks after delivery. This should include a thorough history with attention to bleeding, breast or bottle feeding, pelvic pain, sexual and contraceptive history, bowel and bladder function, and emotional well being.

      b. On pelvic examination at 6 weeks, the perineum should be well healed and the uterus back to its pregravid size.

      c. Occasionally, a lactating mother will have atrophic vaginitis.

  3. Laboratory studies

      a. During the first postpartum visit, hemoglobin and hematocrit are performed as dictated by history.

      b. If the patient had developed gestational diabetes, a fasting blood sugar screen should be ordered.

  4. Treatment

      a. It is important to emphasize contraceptive counseling at the postpartum examination.

      b. Vitamin supplementation should be continued for the nursing mother.

      c. Atrophic vaginitis can be treated with vaginal estrogen as needed.

Rheumatology and Orthopaedics (Musculoskeletal System)

Petar A. Breitinger and Jennifer Roach

I. ARTHRITIS/RHEUMATOLOGIC CONDITIONS

A. Osteoarthritis (OA)

1. General characteristics

a. OA is the most common arthropathy among adults, particularly the elderly.

b. OA is characterized as progressive loss of articular cartilage with reactive changes in the bone, resulting in destruction and pain of the joint.

c. Among persons aged 65 years or older, 80% display radiographic signs of the disease.

2. Clinical features

a. Decreased range of motion, joint crepitus, and pain gradually worsening throughout the day are features of OA.

b. Common sites of involvement are the distal interphalangeal (DIP) joint (Heberden's nodes), proximal interphalangeal joint (Bouchard's nodules), wrist, hip, knee, and spine.

c. Joints can become unstable during the late stages of OA.

3. Laboratory studies and imaging

a. Laboratory tests are nonspecific.

b. Radiographs show asymmetric narrowing, subchondral sclerosis, cysts, and marginal osteophytes.

4. Treatment

a. Weight reduction, exercises, acetaminophen, salicylates, and intra-articular steroids are important in managing OA.

b. Surgical arthrodesis, osteotomy, and total joint arthroplasty are indicated in advanced cases.

B. Rheumatoid arthritis (RA)

1. General characteristics

a. RA is a chronic disease with synovitis affecting multiple joints and other systemic extra-articular manifestations.

b. Females are affected more often than males (3:2 ratio), with onset typically occurring between 40 and 60 years of age. The juvenile form occurs in patients younger than 16.

c. A cascade of events leads to joint destruction. Hyperplastic synovial tissue (pannus) may erode cartilage, subchondral bone, articular capsule, and ligaments.

2. Clinical features

a. Malaise, fatigue, and morning stiffness for more than 6 weeks are seen.

b. Arthritis affects the hands (i.e., ulnar deviation and subluxation of the metacarpal phalangeal joints, radial deviation of the wrists, swan-neck and boutonniere deformities) and the feet (i.e., claw toes, hallux valgus).

c. Knee, elbow, shoulder, ankle, and neck involvement is common.

d. Subcutaneous nodules are common and are associated with a positive rheumatoid factor.

e. Systemic involvement may manifest itself as rheumatoid vasculitis (causing ischemic ulcers and peripheral neuropathy), pericarditis, or pulmonary disease (e.g., pleural effusions, fibrosing alveolitis, nodules).

3. Laboratory studies and imaging

a. Aspiration and joint fluid analysis are the most useful laboratory tests to exclude the presence of gout or infectious arthritis (Table 9-1).

b. Erythrocyte sedimentation rate (ESR) and C-reactive protein are elevated.

c. Rheumatoid factor is sensitive in 80% of cases, with a specificity of 95%.

d. Periarticular erosion and osteopenia are seen on radiographs.

4. Treatment

a. Consultation with a rheumatologist is recommended for initiation of treatment and development of a long-term plan.

TABLE 9-1	**Differentiation of Joint Fluid Analysis**			
	Color	**WBCs (µL)**	**PMNs**	**Glucose**
Osteoarthritis	Yellow	200–300	<25%	Equal to serum
Rheumatoid arthritis (or other inflammatory conditions)	Yellow to opalescent	3,000–50,000	≥50%	>25 but less than serum
Septic	Yellow to green	>50,000	>75%	<25

Polymorphonucleocytes XXX; WBCs, white blood cells.

    b. Physical therapy should be implemented.

    c. Pharmacologic management should be early and aggressive to prevent or delay joint destruction.

        (1) Nonsteroidal anti-inflammatory drugs (NSAIDs) and aspirin may control symptoms.

        (2) Disease-modifying antirheumatic drugs (DMARDs) are begun early to delay progression of disease.

            (a) Methotrexate is the drug of choice.

            (b) Other DMARDs include tumor necrosis factor inhibitors (etanercept, infliximab, adalimumab), antimalarials corticosteroids, sulfasalazine, and leflunomide.

            (c) Combination therapy may be required.

    d. Reconstructive surgery is indicated for severe cases.

C. Juvenile RA

    1. General characteristics

        a. Characterized by chronic synovitis and a number of extra-articular manifestations.

        b. Females are affected more often than males (2:1 ratio) and have an earlier age of onset (females, 1–3 years of age; males, 8–12 years of age).

        c. The three types are systemic (20%), pauciarticular (50%), and polyarticular (30%).

    2. Clinical features

        a. Systemic

            (1) This type is characterized by spiking fevers (>102.7°F), myalgias, polyarthralgias, and a typical rash (maculopapular with central clearing) appearing in the evening.

            (2) The rash may be elicited by scratching the skin in susceptible areas (Koebner's phenomenon).

            (3) There are minimal articular findings, but splenomegaly, lymphadenopathy, pericarditis or myocarditis may occur.

        b. Pauciarticular. This type is characterized by involvement of larger joints, usually four or fewer for 6 consecutive weeks, and development of chronic uveitis (girls at higher risk) and spinal arthritis (boys at higher risk).

        c. Polyarticular

            (1) This type resembles adult RA with its symmetric involvement of the small joints of the hands and feet, involving five or more joints.

            (2) Markedly receding chin is caused by the closure of the ossification center of the mandible.

    3. Laboratory studies and imaging

        a. There are no specific diagnostic tests.

            (1) ESR is increased or normal with the systemic type.

            (2) The antinuclear antibody (ANA) test may be increased in the pauciarticular type and indicates a tendency for uveitis.

        b. Imaging studies may be similar to adults with soft-tissue swelling and osteoporosis findings. Joint destruction is less frequent.

    4. Treatment

        a. Anti-inflammatory medications (NSAIDs) and physical therapy are most beneficial. Methotrexate or hydroxychloroquine may be used as second-line agents, early on, if systemic signs are present.

        b. Monitor children with juvenile RA for any growth abnormalities, nutritional deficiencies, and school/social impairment.

D. Other types of arthritis

   1. Infectious (septic) arthritis

     a. Pathogenesis

       (1) The hematogenous spread of bacteremia, periarticular osteomyelitis, infection caused by diagnostic or therapeutic procedure (e.g., intra-articular injection), or infection elsewhere (e.g., cellulitis, bursitis) may lead to infectious arthritis. Bacterial septic arthritis usually involves a single joint (most commonly the knee, followed by hip, shoulder, ankle, and wrist) in 90% of cases.

       (2) Sexually active young adults are at risk for septic arthritis caused by infection with *Neisseria gonorrhoeae*.

       (3) *Staphylococcus aureus* is the most common pathogen in joint infections.

       (4) Patients usually present with acute swelling, fever, joint warmth and effusion, tenderness to palpation, and increased pain with minimal range of motion in the involved joint.

     b. Treatment

       (1) Aggressive treatment with IV antibiotics is required.

       (2) Arthrotomy (surgical opening into a joint to drain and debride the infection) and arthrocentesis (puncture of joint space with a needle for synovial fluid analysis and culture) often are required. Arthrotomy usually is not required when *Neisseria gonorrhoeae* is the infecting organism but is definitely required for infection involving the hip joint.

       (3) Oral antibiotics should follow the IV antibiotics.

   2. Psoriatic arthritis

     a. General characteristics

       (1) This is an inflammatory arthritis with onset in patients 30–50 years of age.

       (2) Skin involvement precedes joint disease by months to years.

     b. Clinical features

       (1) The course usually is mild and intermittent, affecting a few joints.

       (2) Symmetric involvement of the hands, feet, and cuticles and irregularity, pitting, and splitting of the nails are seen.

       (3) Sausage-finger appearance (caused by arthritis and tenosynovitis of the flexor tendon) is a common feature.

       (4) Asymmetric oligoarticular arthritis involving two to three joints at a time occurs.

       (5) Symmetric arthritis may occur and is similar to that of RA.

     c. Laboratory studies and imaging

       (1) ESR is elevated; normocytic normochromic anemia is seen.

       (2) Hyperuricemia may occur when skin involvement is severe.

       (3) Rheumatoid factor is normal.

       (4) "Cup and saucer" appearance of the proximal phalanx is demonstrated on radiography.

     d. Treatment

       (1) Drug treatment of psoriatic arthritis is similar to that of RA.

       (2) Methotrexate, an immunosuppressive drug, is beneficial for both the skin inflammation and the arthritis. Because of its potential toxicity, it should be avoided in patients with HIV.

       (3) Reconstructive surgery (arthrodesis or joint replacement) is indicated for painful end-stage arthropathy.

   3. Reiter's syndrome

     a. General characteristics

       (1) Reiter's syndrome is a seronegative arthritis, predominantly affecting men, with a triad of urethritis, conjunctivitis, and oligoarthritis.

       (2) It often is secondary to sexually transmitted disease (chlamydial urethritis or others) or gastroenteritis.

     b. Clinical features. Patients have dactylitis (sausage digits of either the toes or the fingers); painful oral ulcers; penile lesions (balanitis circinata); ulcers on the extremities, palms, and soles; and plantar heel pain.

     c. Laboratory studies and imaging

       (1) Laboratory analysis should include ESR, alkaline phosphatase, CBC, HLA-B27, and C-reactive protein.

       (2) Evidence of metatarsal head erosion appears on radiographs.

       (3) Calcaneal periostitis is present.

   d. Treatment
   (1) Physical therapy and NSAIDs are effective.
   (2) The underlying condition (e.g., sexually transmitted disease, gastroenteritis) must be treated.
E. Gout
   1. General characteristics
   a. Gout is a systemic disease of altered purine metabolism and subsequent sodium urate crystal precipitation into synovial fluid.
   b. It is more common in men than in women (9:1).
   2. Clinical features
   a. The most common feature is initial attack of the metatarsal phalangeal joint of the great toe (podagra).
   b. Other joints of the feet, ankles, and knees also commonly are affected.
   c. Pain, swelling, redness, and exquisite tenderness develop suddenly at and surrounding the joint. In chronic gout, tophi (chalky deposits of urate crystals) can form adjacent to the joint.
   3. Laboratory studies
   a. Joint fluid analysis is diagnostic if negatively birefringent urate crystals are seen. Positively birefingent crystals (calcium pyrophosphate) are suggestive of pseudogout. The diagnosis of gout also may be inferred by clinical examination.
   b. Serum uric acid level of greater than 8 mg/dL is diagnostic.
   4. Treatment
   a. Elevation and rest may alleviate symptoms. Dietary modifications stressing decreased ingestion of purines and alcohol can reduce elevated urate levels.
   b. Pharmacotherapy
   (1) NSAIDs generally are the initial drug of choice (i.e., indomethacin, 50 mg/day for 2 days, tapered off during the following week).
   (2) Colchicine (mechanism of action is unknown) reduces the inflammatory response to deposited crystals, diminishes phagocytosis, and terminates most acute attacks in 6–12 hours. Side effects, however, can be intolerable.
   (3)   Allopurinol may be used to decrease production of uric acid and to prevent further attacks.
   (4) Corticosteroids may be used if other medicines are not tolerated and for patients with chronic renal insufficiency.
F. Pseudogout
   1. General characteristics
   a. Pseudogout affects peripheral joints, usually in the lower extremity, and results from intra-articular deposition of calcium pyrophosphate.
   b. It shows marked similarity to gout, with recurrent and abrupt onset of attacks.
   2. Clinical features
   a. Painful inflammation results when crystals are shed into the joint.
   b. The joints most commonly involved are the knee, wrist, and elbow.
   3. Laboratory studies and imaging
   a. Calcium pyrophosphate crystals are found in joint aspiration.
   b. Radiographs show fine, linear calcifications in cartilage.
   4. Treatment
   a. NSAIDs and intra-articular steroid injections are beneficial.
   b. Treat joint destruction with surgical procedures similar to degenerative arthritis.
G. Systemic lupus erythematosus (SLE)
   1. General characteristics
   a. SLE is an autoimmune disorder characterized by ANAs and involvement of multiple organs.
   b. SLE commonly affects women of childbearing age. Prevalence also is found among certain familial and ethnic groups.

   2. Clinical features

   a. The diagnosis of SLE is based on the presence of certain criteria, including malar or discoid rash, photosensitivity, oral ulcers, arthritis, serositis, renal disorder, neurologic disorder, hematologic disorder, immunologic disorder, or ANA.

   b. Common musculoskeletal features

   (1) Arthralgias and symmetrical nonerosive arthritis are found.

   (2) SLE predominantly affects small joints of the hand, wrist, and knees.

   3. Laboratory studies

   a. Routine laboratory studies should include CBC, BUN, creatinine, urinalysis, ESR, and serum complement (C3 or C4).

   b. Antibodies to Smith antigen, double-stranded DNA, or depressed levels of serum complement may be used as markers for progression of the disease.

   c. ANA is present 100% of the time but is not specific for SLE.

   4. Treatment

   a. Mild or new cases

   (1) Salicylates or NSAIDs should be administered.

   (2) Hydroxychloroquine, 200 mg once or twice a day, also is effective.

   (3) Corticosteroids also are used at low doses.

   b. Acute illness with renal or central nervous system involvement

   (1) High-dose steroids may be used, tapering off as symptoms improve.

   (2) NSAIDs may serve as an adjunct therapy.

   (3) Antimalarial medications may be helpful, depending on the cause.

   (4) Pulsed high-dose steroids or immunosuppressive medications can be used in patients with glomerulonephritis or in those who are unresponsive to the above treatment.

H. Polymyositis

   1. General characteristics

   a. Polymyositis is an inflammatory disease of striated muscle affecting the proximal limbs, neck, and pharynx. The skin also can be affected (dermatomyositis).

   b. Other organ systems affected include joints, lungs, heart, and GI tract.

   c. Cause is unknown.

   d. Women are more commonly affected than men.

   2. Clinical features include insidious, painless, proximal muscle weakness; dysphagia; skin rash similar to the SLE-like butterfly distribution on the face; polyarthralgias; and muscle atrophy.

   3. Laboratory studies

   a. Muscle enzymes (creatine phosphokinase, aldolase, aspartate aminotransferase, alanine aminotransferase, lactate dehydrogenase), serum myoglobin, and electromyelography are sensitive but nonspecific for detecting muscle inflammation.

   b. Muscle biopsy should be performed to confirm the diagnosis of inflammatory myositis.

   4. Treatment. Polymyositis is treated with high-dose steroids, methotrexate, or azathioprine.

I. Polymyalgia rheumatica

   1. General characteristics

   a. Polymyalgia rheumatica is characterized by pain and stiffness in the neck, shoulder, and pelvic girdles and is accompanied by constitutional symptoms (e.g., fever, fatigue, weight loss, depression).

   b. Affects women twice as often as men.

   c. Cause is unknown.

   d. Age of onset is older than 50 years.

   2. Clinical features

   a. Stiffness usually is the predominant feature, being severe after rest and in the morning.

   b. Musculoskeletal symptoms usually are bilateral and symmetrical.

    3. Laboratory studies. ESRs are markedly elevated (>45 mm Hg).

    4. Treatment. Patients respond quickly to low-dose corticosteroid therapy, which usually is required for 2 years.

J. Polyarteritis nodosa

    1. General characteristics

        a. Small and medium artery inflammation involving the skin, kidney, peripheral nerves, muscle, and gut.

        b. The male to female ratio is 3:1.

        c. Onset generally is between 40 and 60 years old, although it occurs in every age group.

        d. Onset of disease has been associated with drugs, vaccines, bacterial infections, and viral infections (hepatitis B and C).

    2. Clinical features

        a. Fever, anorexia, weight loss, abdominal pain, peripheral neuropathy, arthralgias, and arthritis are commonly seen.

        b. Skin lesions, including palpable purpura and livedo reticularis, occur in some patients.

        c. Hypertension, edema, oliguria, and uremia may be present in the 75% of patients with renal involvement.

    3. Laboratory studies

        a. The diagnosis usually is established by vessel biopsy or angiography.

        b. Elevated ESR, RBC casts, proteinuria, and low serum albumin also may be present.

    4. Treatment

        a. Initial management is with high doses of prednisone.

        b. Cytotoxic drugs and immunotherapy also may be used.

K. Systemic sclerosis (scleroderma)

    1. General characteristics

        a. Scleroderma is of unknown cause and is characterized by deposition of collagen in the skin and, less commonly, in the kidney, heart, lungs, and stomach.

        b. The female to male ratio is 4:1.

        c. The peak age of onset is between 30 and 50 years.

    2. Clinical features

        a. Skin involvement occurs in 95% of patients. Changes most often begin with swelling in the fingers and hands and may spread to involve the trunk and the face.

        b. Shiny skin with tautness and atrophy occurs in later stages.

        c. Raynaud's phenomenon, vasospasm of the digital arteries, is the initial complaint in 70% of patients.

        d. Calcinosis, Raynaud's phenomenon, esophageal motility disorders, sclerodactyly, and telangiectasias (CREST syndrome) is seen in a subset of patients.

        e. The diffuse form of scleroderma may include involvement of the GI tract, lung, heart, or kidney.

        f. More than 50% of patients develop joint swelling and stiffness and pain in the finger, wrist, and knee joints.

    3. Laboratory studies

        a. ANA is present in 90% of patients with systemic sclerosis.

        b. There are no other reliable tests that can be used to follow disease activity and progression.

        c. Patients should be monitored for development of hypertension, heralding kidney involvement.

    4. Treatment

        a. There is no cure for scleroderma.

        b. Treatment is aimed at keeping joints mobilized, with supportive treatment for other organ systems involved.

L. Sjögren's syndrome

    1. General characteristics

        a. Sjögren's syndrome is an autoimmune disorder that destroys the salivary and lacrimal glands.

        b. It also may be a primary or secondary complication to a preexisting connective tissue disorder.

        c. The incidence peaks during the sixth decade, and it is seen in females more often than in males.

    2. Clinical features

        a. Dry mouth (xerostomia) and dry eyes (xerophthalmia or keratoconjunctivitis sicca) are characteristic features of primary Sjögren's syndrome.

b. The parotid gland also may be enlarged.

c. Secondary Sjögren's syndrome presents with evidence of associated conditions (RA, SLE, polymyositis, scleroderma).

3. Laboratory studies

a. Rheumatoid factor is present in 70% of cases, ANA in 60% of cases, and elevated ESR in 70% of cases.

b. A Schirmer's tear test evaluates tear secretions by the lacrimal glands. Wetting of less than 5 mm of filter paper placed in the lower eyelid for 5 min is positive for decreased secretions.

4. Treatment. Management is mainly symptomatic, with the goal of keeping mucosal surfaces moist.

M. Fibromyalgia

1. General characteristics

a. The cause and pathogenesis are poorly understood.

b. Fibromyalgia can occur with RA, SLE, and Sjögren's syndrome.

2. Clinical features

a. Patients have nonarticular musculoskeletal aches, pains, fatigue, sleep disturbance, and multiple tender points on examination.

b. Anxiety, depression, headaches, irritable bowel syndrome, dysmenorrhea, and paresthesias are associated with this condition.

3. Laboratory studies

a. Fibromyalgia is recognized by the typical pattern of pain and other symptoms as well as by exclusion of contributory or underlying diseases.

b. There are no routine laboratory markers; it often is a diagnosis of exclusion.

c. Abnormality of the T-cell subsets has been described.

4. Treatment

a. Tricyclic antidepressants often are helpful.

b. Aerobic exercises improve the functional status by encouraging physical activity rather than avoidance of activity.

c. Patient education, stress reduction, and treatment of psychological problems may alleviate symptoms.

II. BONE AND JOINT DISORDERS

A. Tendinitis and tenosynovitis

1. General characteristics

a. Tendinitis refers to inflammation of the lining of the tendon sheath.

b. Tenosynovitis is inflammation of the enclosed tendon sheath.

c. Common causes include overuse injuries and systemic disease (e.g., arthritides).

2. Clinical features

a. Tendinitis and tenosynovitis commonly appear in the following sites: rotator cuff, flexor carpi ulnaris, flexor carpi radialis, flexor digitorum, hip, hamstring, quadriceps, patella, Achilles tendon, semimembranous tendon.

b. Tendinitis and tenosynovitis generally occur together, causing pain with movement, swelling, and impaired function.

c. The conditions may resolve over several weeks, but recurrence is common.

3. Treatment

a. Ice, rest, and stretching help to relieve inflammation.

b. NSAIDs or injection with corticosteroids combined with anesthesia may be used. Intratendon injection should be avoided because of the risk of rupture.

c. Excision of scar tissue and necrotic debris should be performed. The scar tissue is caused by repetitive microtrauma to the tissue, and the most common site is the muscle–tendon unit.

B. Bursitis

1. General characteristics

a. Bursitis is an inflammatory, periarticular disorder of the bursa (a thin-walled sac lined with synovial tissue).

b. The inflammation is caused by repetitive friction, trauma, or systemic disease (e.g., RA, gout, infection).

2. Clinical features

    a. The common sites of presentation are subacromial, subdeltoid, trochanteric, olecranon, Achilles bursitis (pump bump), ischial bursitis (weaver's bottom), and prepatellar and suprapatellar (housemaid's knee).

    b. Pain and tenderness may persist for weeks.

3. Treatment of bursitis includes prevention of the precipitating factors, rest, NSAIDs, and steroid injections.

C. Osteomyelitis

  1. General characteristics

    a. Osteomyelitis is an inflammation of the bone caused by a pyogenic organism (most commonly *Staphylococcus aureus*) and is described by duration (acute, chronic), cause (hematogenous, exogenous, surgical, true contiguous spread), site (spine, hip), extent (size of defect), and type of patient (infant, child, adult, immunocompromised host).

    b. Types

      (1) Acute hematogenous osteomyelitis most commonly affects the long bones of children.

      (2) Patients with sickle-cell anemia are at risk for salmonella osteomyelitis.

      (3) Osteomyelitis is termed chronic hematogenous osteomyelitis when, after the original acute infection has completed appropriate treatment (antibiotics, surgery), viable colonies of bacteria harbored in necrotic and ischemic tissue cause a recurrence of infection.

      (4) Exogenous osteomyelitis results from open fracture or surgery.

  2. Clinical features

    a. Acute hematogenous osteomyelitis

      (1) Pain, loss of motion, and soft-tissue swelling occur.

      (2) Drainage is rare.

    b. Chronic hematogenous osteomyelitis

      (1) Recurrent acute flare-ups of tender, warm, sometimes swollen areas occur at indefinite intervals over months or years.

      (2) Bone necrosis, soft-tissue damage, and bone instability can occur.

    c. Exogenous osteomyelitis. Clinical findings are similar to chronic osteomyelitis.

  3. Laboratory studies and imaging

    a. WBC count increases in acute osteomyelitis. C-reactive protein and ESR can be mildly elevated in acute and chronic osteomyelitis. WBC count may be normal in chronic osteomyelitis.

    b. Causative organism is identified by blood culture or bone biopsy (best).

    c. Radiographic evidence of osteomyelitis lags behind symptoms and pathologic changes by 7–10 days.

    d. Late sequestra (i.e., dead bone surrounding granulation tissue) and involucrum (i.e., periosteal new bone) take several weeks to months to appear.

    e. MRI shows the changes before plain-film radiography.

    f. Bone scan shows increased uptake in the area of infection and decreased uptake in the area of sequestra.

  4. Treatment

    a. A 6-week course of IV antibiotic therapy is recommended, followed by 1–2 weeks of oral antibiotics.

    b. Immobilization and surgical drainage may be indicated.

    c. Intermittent long-term antibiotics suppress the clinical manifestations of chronic hematogenous osteomyelitis.

    d. Surgical treatment is required to remove sequestra, sinus tract (the abnormal channel permitting escape of exudate to the surface), infected bone, and scar tissue.

    e. Exogenous osteomyelitis is managed the same as chronic hematogenous osteomyelitis; if present, external or internal fixation devices need to be removed.

D. Neoplasms

  1. General characteristics

    a. Types

      (1) Common tumors are listed in Table 9-2.

      (2) Prostate, breast, lung, kidney, and thyroid are the primary carcinomas that most commonly metastasize to the bone. The spine is the most common site of bony metastases.

TABLE 9-2	Common Bone Tumors and Tumor-Like Conditions	
Tissue of Origin	**Benign**	**Malignant**
Cartilage	Osteochondroma	Chondrosarcoma
	Enchondroma	Variants of chondrosarcoma
	Chondroblastoma	Dedifferentiated
	Chondromyxoid fibroma	Clear cell
		Mesenchymal
Bone	Osteoid osteoma	Osteosarcoma
	Osteoblastoma	Variants of osteosarcoma
		Parosteal
		Periosteal
		Telangiectatic
		Postradiation
		Arising in Paget's disease
Marrow elements	Eosinophilic granuloma	Ewing sarcoma
		Plasmacytoma
		Multiple myeloma
		Lymphoma of bone
Fibrous tissue and tissue	Nonossifying fibroma	Fibrosarcoma
of uncertain origin	Aneurysmal bone cyst histiocytoma	Malignant fibrous histiocytoma
	Simple bone cyst	
	Giant cell tumor	
	Fibrous dysplasia	
	Desmoplastic fibroma	

Source: Reprinted with permission from Wilson F, Lins P. Gen Orthop 1997;12:302

b. Incidence

(1) Benign tumors of the bone and soft tissue are more common than primary malignant tumors.

(2) Ecchondroma (cartilaginous tumor) is the most common primary benign bone neoplasm of the hand and is asymptomatic unless complicated by pathologic fracture.

(3) Lipomas (soft, nontender, movable mass) and ganglions (soft, nontender, transilluminant mass, usually on the dorsum of the hand) are common benign soft-tissue masses.

(4) Mucous cysts are ganglia originating from the DIP joint and often are associated with Heberden's nodules.

(5) Soft-tissue sarcomas occur three times more often than primary bone malignancies.

(6) The most common types of primary sarcomas of bone are chondrosarcoma, Ewing's sarcoma, and osteosarcoma.

(7) Multiple myeloma is the most common primary malignant bone tumor.

c. Age groups

(1) Ewing's sarcoma is found in patients between 5 and 25 years of age, usually in the diaphyses of long bones, ribs, and flat bones. Osteosarcomas are most common in individuals 10–20 years of age, arising in the metaphyseal area of the long bones.

(2) In adults 60 years of age or older, metastatic carcinoma is the most common source of bone lesion. Chondosarcomas also increase in incidence in adults older than 60 years and can present within the central metaphyseal area.

2. Clinical features

a. Night pain often is associated with malignancy.

b. A painful mass attached to bone is likely to be malignant; however, some malignant tumors are nonpainful.

    c. Severe pain preceded by dull, aching pain may indicate pathologic fracture.

    d. Systemic symptoms, such as fever, weight loss, anorexia, or fatigue, should be noted.

    e. Rule out areas of metastases, such as the lungs, breasts, prostate, thyroid, and kidneys.

3. Laboratory studies

    a. Routine laboratory studies are noncontributory, but with suspected malignancy, routine labs can provide a baseline for patients who will need chemotherapy.

    b. Alkaline phosphatase is elevated when the bone is broken down and remodeled.

    c. Serum and urine electrophoretic studies can detect the specific abnormal globulin of multiple myeloma.

    d. Biopsy is essential to diagnose whether benign or malignant, the cell type, and the grade of lesion.

        (1) Open incisional biopsy is best.

        (2) The capsule is then closed tightly to prevent bleeding and local spread.

4. Imaging studies

    a. Radiology

        (1) Radiographic signs may help to distinguish benign from malignant tumors, because certain tumors have a characteristic appearance.

        (2) Radiography also may help to determine a tumor's location and may narrow the diagnostic possibilities.

    b. CT is the best imaging technique if a lesion involves the cortical bones.

    c. MRI is most helpful if marrow, soft tissue, or osseous tumors are suspected.

    d. Bone scans can evaluate distant osseous metastasis and periosteal involvement of soft-tissue masses.

5. Treatment

    a. The goals of treatment are to relieve pain and to maintain function.

    b. For benign tumors, simple excision is the treatment.

    c. Malignant neoplasms

        (1) Wide surgical resection is used when feasible.

        (2) The success of chemotherapy, either alone or in conjunction with radiation therapy, depends on the type of tumor, its location, and its metastases.

        (3) Limb salvage (using cadaver allograft or endoprosthetic devices) is part of definitive treatment.

        (4) Radiation therapy followed by local resection is the common treatment for soft-tissue sarcomas.

E. Osteoporosis

1. General characteristics

    a. Osteoporosis is a disease of abnormal bone remodeling.

        (1) It is characterized by a decrease in total bone volume, although the bone that is present is normal, just less dense.

        (2) This decrease in mass leads to an increased susceptibility to fractures.

    b. Osteoporosis is divided into two categories, either primary or secondary:

        (1) Primary osteoporosis is further divided.

            (a) Type I (postmenopausal) occurs primarily in women but can occur in men. It is the most prevalent form of primary osteoporosis.

            (b) Type II (age-related) occurs in both men and women.

        (2) Secondary osteoporosis is recognized by conditions in which bone is lost because of the presence of other diseases (malignancies, corticosteroid use, GI disorders or hormonal imbalances).

    c. Risk factors include modifiable (alcoholism, smoking, low body weight, sedentary lifestyle, low calcium and vitamin D intake, corticosteroid use, recurrent falls) and nonmodifiable (advanced age, Caucasian or Asian race, female gender).

2. Clinical features

    a. Type I commonly is associated with loss of estrogen in postmenopausal women and with testosterone deficiency in men.

        (1) The trabecular bone primarily is affected.

        (2) The vertebrae, hip, and distal radius are the most common fracture sites.

    b. Patients ≥75 years of age with poor calcium absorption are at high risk for type II.

        (1) Both trabecular and cortical bone are affected.

        (2) The hip and pelvis are the most common fracture sites.

3. Laboratory studies and imaging

    a. Calcium, hydroxyproline (index of bone dissolution), and serum alkaline phosphatase (index of bone deposition) levels are tested to rule out other abnormalities (e.g., hyperthyroidism, hyperparathyroidism, Cushing's syndrome, hematologic disorders, malignancy); they are normal in osteoporosis.

    b. Dual-energy x-ray absorptiometry is the most helpful way to measure bone density with the least amount of radiation. Screening bone density is recommended in the following groups:

        (1) All postmenopausal women younger than 65 years who have one or more additional risk factors.

        (2) All postmenopausal women older than 65 years.

        (3) Postmenopausal women who present with fractures.

        (4) All women considering therapy for other conditions in which the bone mineral density will affect that decision.

        (5) Women who have been on hormone replacement therapy (HRT) for prolonged periods.

        (6) Men who experience fractures after minimal trauma.

        (7) Patients with evidence of osteopenia on radiography or a disease known to increase risk for osteoporosis.

    c. Biopsy can be used to evaluate the severity.

    d. Radiographs show features of decreased bone density when 30% bone loss is present.

4. Treatment

    a. Preventative measures include physical activity, calcium and vitamin D supplementation, and estrogen therapy, either alone or with progesterone.

        (1) Conjugated estrogen (0.625 mg daily or the equivalent) and estradiol (0.5 mg) daily provides effective bone protection.

            (a) HRT does carry an increased risk of myocardial infarction, stroke, dementia, and breast cancer and needs to be weighed individually for the potential benefits of decreasing fractures.

            (b) To reduce the risks of HRT, low-dose estrogen regimens are preferred.

        (2) Selective estrogen-receptor modulators, such as raloxifene, may be helpful for women who cannot take estrogen.

    b. Vitamin D (400 U daily) should be taken by persons older than 75 years or those who lack sun exposure.

    c. IM injections of testosterone enanthate, 150–200 mg every 3–4 weeks, may be considered for men who have osteoporosis associated with low testosterone.

    d. Bisphosphonates (alendronate, ibandronate, pamidronate, risedronate, and zoledronic acid) decrease bone formation and resorption and decrease fracture risk by 50%.

    e. Calcitonin can be used for bone density gain with results similar to HRT, but it does not prevent hip fractures.

        (1) Calcitonin also has a modest analgesic effect after acute fracture.

        (2) It may be given subcutaneously, IM, or intranasally. The intranasal form, 200 U daily, has the fewest side effects.

    f. Intermittent low-dose parathyroid hormone has been shown to increase bone density in patients with glucocorticoid-induced osteoporosis.

III. FRACTURES, DISLOCATIONS, SPRAINS, AND STRAINS

  A. Classification of fractures

    1. Examples of location are proximal, middle, and distal third.

    2. Examples of direction are transverse (at a right angle to the axis of the bone), spiral (bone has a twisted appearance; also called torsion), oblique (fracture line between horizontal and vertical direction), comminuted (splintered or crushed), and segmental (double).

    3. Examples of alignment are angulation (deviation from straight line) and displacement (abnormal position of fracture fragments), such as dorsal displacement of the bone fragment in a Colles' fracture of the wrist and volar displacement of the bone fragment in a Smith's fracture of the wrist; both may be complicated by injury to the median nerve or radial artery.

4. Examples of associated factors are open fracture (disruption of the skin), closed fracture (skin is intact), and dislocation (displacement of bone from a joint).

B. Imaging studies

1. Plain-film radiographs are sufficient to visualize most fractures.
   a. Both anteroposterior (AP) and lateral films should be taken to ensure visualization of the boney structures 90° away from each other.
   b. Concurrent fractures also may be seen at the joints proximal and distal to the fracture (e.g., distal tibia, proximal fibula, dome of the talus, lateral malleolus).
2. Radionucleotide bone scanning shows increased uptake at the site of the occult fracture or stress fractures (common in athletes and associated with disuse osteopenia when weight bearing starts after long periods of immobilization).
3. CT is now a better diagnostic method than plain-film radiography or bone scans. It allows visualization of the bone's articular surface otherwise obscured by overlying structures (e.g., carpal bones, elbow, tibial plateau).
4. CT is helpful in establishing the diagnosis of pelvic, facial, or intra-articular fractures.
5. MRI is not required unless evaluating soft-tissue structures.

C. Treatment

1. The following types of fractures are initially treated with analgesics, immobilization, and emergent referral to an orthopaedist after adequate stabilization of the patient.
2. Open fractures
   a. Ideally, open fractures must be debrided and irrigated (in the operating room) within 4–8 hours of injury.
   b. IV antibiotics (first- and second-generation cephalosporins and aminoglycosides) should be administered for 48 hours after fracture and for 48 hours after surgical procedures. Always inquire about tetanus status.
   c. Immobilization and fixation should be performed to preserve function.
3. Intra-articular fractures (the fracture line enters a joint cavity)
   a. Open treatment may be indicated to restore and maintain articular congruity.
   b. When stable, consider active range of motion.
4. Femur fractures
   a. Treat neck fractures first with screws; then, treat shaft fractures with intramedullary rods or plates.
   b. There is significant potential for hemorrhage with fractures of the femur.
5. Fractures of the tibia and fibula in adults
   a. Fractures of the tibia and fibula are associated with ligamental, meniscal, and vascular injuries.
   b. For simple fractures, reduction can be closed (manipulation or traction); for more complicated fractures, open reduction combined with internal fixation (ORIF) is required.

D. Fractures in children

1. The physis, or growth plate, is more susceptible to fracture than to injury to attached ligaments.
   a. Swelling and tenderness over the physis are the common findings when fractured.
   b. Growth plate fractures are classified with the Salter-Harris classification system (Fig. 9-1).
   c. Comparison films may be helpful.
2. Incomplete fractures occur when the line of fracture does not include the whole bone.
   a. Torus fractures occur when one side of the cortex buckles as a result of a compression injury (e.g., falling on an outstretched hand). Treatment is 4–6 weeks in a cast.
   b. Greenstick fractures
      (1) These fractures occur in long bones when bowing causes a break in one side of the cortex.
      (2) When the angulation of the fracture is less than 15°, a long arm or leg cast can be applied for 4–6 weeks.
      (3) Fractures with angulation of greater than 15° need referral to an orthopaedic surgeon.
3. When radiographs of a young child show multiple fractures at various stages of healing, abuse should be suspected and the child referred to a protective agency.

1 **2** **3** **4** **5**

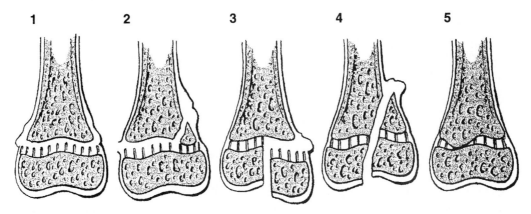

FIGURE 9-1 The Salter-Harris classification of fractures involving the physis. *1,* Fracture through epiphyseal plate. *2,* Epiphyseal fracture with associated metaphyseal fragment. *3,* Fracture through the epiphysis into the articular surface. *4,* Fracture through the distal metaphysis, epiphyseal plate, and epiphysis. *5,* Impaction of the epiphyseal plate.
(From Jarrell BE, Carabasi RA III. NMS Surgery. 3rd ed. Baltimore: Williams & Wilkins, 1996; redrawn with permission from Salter RB, Harris WR. Injuries involving the epiphyseal plate. J Bone Joint Surg Am 1963;45:587.)

E. Dislocations and subluxations

  1. General characteristics

    a. Dislocation is total loss of congruity that occurs between the articular surfaces of the joint.

    b. Subluxation is any less serious loss of congruity, such as that in nursemaid's elbow (subluxation of the head of the radius, occurring when a child, especially a 1- to 3-year-old, is suddenly lifted by the upper limb and the radial head slips anteriorly from the elbow joint out of the annular ligament).

  2. Sites of dislocation

    a. Common sites of dislocation are the anterior shoulder, anterior hip (abducted radiographs show the inferior margin of the acetabulum overlapped by the femoral head) and posterior hip (abducted radiographs show the femoral head posterior to the acetabular rim; a common complication of a posterior dislocation is osteonecrosis of the femoral head), and dislocations of the posterior elbow.

    b. Less common sites of dislocation are the navicular and subtalar joints, as part of a combination Lisfranc fracture (a dislocation of the tarsometatarsal joint complex), and the second metatarsal joint (often one metatarsal is fractured at the base and the others are dislocated).

  3. Treatment

    a. After assessment of the neurovascular status, most dislocations are treated with closed reduction.

    b. Dislocations that reduce spontaneously require immobilization for 2–4 weeks, followed by range-of-motion activity and return to normal activity.

    c. If associated fractures or interposed soft-tissues are present, the patient needs to undergo open reduction and internal fixation.

    d. It is imperative to assess the neurovascular status after reduction.

F. Strains and sprains

  1. A strain is an injury to the bone–tendon unit at the myotendinous junction or the muscle itself.

  2. A sprain involves collagenous tissue, such as ligaments or tendons.

  3. A strain or sprain injury often follows a sudden stretch.

    a. It can lead to avulsion of tendon (e.g., mallet finger avulsion or stretch of the terminal extensor tendon, which is treated with extensor splinting for 6 weeks).

    b. It also can lead to ligamentous sprain (e.g., stretch of the anterior talofibular ligament, which causes the common ankle sprain).

  4. Treatment. Both strains and sprains require supportive therapy: rest, ice, compression, and elevation (RICE).

IV. DISORDERS OF THE HEAD AND NECK

A. Temporomandibular joint (TMJ) disorder

1. General characteristics

a. TMJ disorder, which is the most common cause of facial pain, is pain that affects the TMJ and muscles of mastication.

b. Causes

(1) Neuropsychologic components, such as psychologic stress, may play a role.

(2) Joint capsulitis from bruxism, such as grinding of teeth, clenching of teeth, and posturing of the jaw, may cause TMJ disorder.

(3) Hypermobility syndrome and malocclusion may lead to pain in the jaw area.

2. Clinical features

a. Pain is aggravated by movement of the jaw.

b. There may be restricted range of motion; a click or pop may be felt or heard.

3. Imaging studies

a. Initial radiographic studies are normal.

b. Arthritis is a late finding.

c. Other systemic causes, such as OA, RA, growth abnormalities, and tumor, need to be ruled out.

4. Treatment

a. Most cases resolve without identification of the cause.

b. Referral to a specialist, such as an odontologist or oral and maxillofacial surgeon, is required if the symptoms warrant.

B. Neck pain

1. General characteristics

a. Spondylosis is the most common condition affecting the cervical spine.

(1) Degenerative changes occur in the disk, most frequently in C5-6, with the formation of osteophytes and disk narrowing.

(2) Later, facet joints and the joints of Luschka are affected.

(3) Paresthesias and numbness occur in the fingers. Pain increases with extension and decreases with flexion of the neck.

b. Compression by central disk protrusion or osteophytes causes long-tract signs (e.g., clonus, Babinski's sign) and gait disturbance.

2. Treatment

a. Conservative treatment involves the use of a cervical collar, traction, exercise, and analgesics.

b. In advanced disease, cervical fusion or diskectomy may be necessary.

C. Other conditions of the neck

1. Whiplash and extension injury are common causes of pain and can last 18 months or longer.

a. Injury occurs as a result of a rear impact, with rapid extension followed by flexion of the cervical spine.

b. Treatment includes a soft cervical collar (short term), application of ice or heat, analgesics, and gentle active range of motion.

2. Rheumatoid spondylitis is found in most of the patients with adult RA.

a. Ligamentous stretching causes progressive atlantoaxial and midcervical subluxation.

b. Surgical stabilization is used to treat RA of the cervical spine.

V. DISORDERS OF THE SHOULDER AND UPPER EXTREMITY

A. Shoulder pain

1. Shoulder pain can be referred pain caused by cervical spondylosis.

2. Pain, if localized to a particular area of the shoulder, may be the site of pathology; referred pain is diffuse and cannot be well localized.

B. Rotator cuff syndrome

1. General characteristics

    a. This syndrome occurs with eccentric overload (e.g., a throwing athlete), underlying glenohumeral instability, poor muscle strength, and training errors.

    b. A common cause in adults is impingement of the supraspinatus tendon as it passes beneath the subacromial arch.

2. Clinical features

    a. Dull aching in the shoulder is the main clinical feature.

    b. The pain is caused by inflammation, fibrosis, and tears.

    c. The pain may interfere with sleep and is exacerbated by abduction of the arm.

3. Laboratory studies and imaging

    a. Radiographs are helpful in ruling out calcific tendinitis, glenohumeral or acromioclavicular arthrosis, and bone tumors.

    b. Arthrography or MRI can be used to diagnose tears.

4. Treatment

    a. Aggravating factors, such as repetitive throwing, other overhead activities, and improper mechanics, must be avoided.

    b. NSAIDs may help to alleviate inflammation and pain.

    c. Local steroid injections may be considered.

    d. Physical therapy may provide relief. Begin nonoperative management of the cuff tears with a range of motion and strengthening program.

    e. Arthroscopic subacromial decompression should be considered for adults with persistent impingement.

    f. If the patient is still symptomatic after 1 month, surgical repair must be done to avoid progression of the tear.

C. Shoulder dislocations

1. General characteristics

    a. Fall on outstretched arm in abduction and extension is the most common cause of shoulder dislocation.

    b. Anterior shoulder dislocations are more common than posterior shoulder dislocations.

    c. As with all orthopaedic reductions, postreduction films should be obtained.

2. Clinical features

    a. Patient usually presents supporting the affected extremity with the other arm.

    b. Loss of shoulder contour is observed, with the elbow pointing outward.

    c. Careful neurovascular assessment must be performed to rule out axillary, musculocutaneous nerve, brachial plexus, or axillary artery injury before reduction attempts.

3. Diagnostic imaging should, at minimum, include an AP view of the shoulder as well as a transthoracic "Y" view. Humeral head deformities, Hill-Sachs lesions, may be noted in recurrent dislocations. Bankart lesion, a tear of the glenoid labrum, may be picked up on MRI.

4. Treatment options include first reduction using a number of methods.

    a. The Milch maneuver is accomplished in the prone position with weights to affect reduction.

    b. The Kocher maneuver can be used with slow external reduction and gentle downward traction on the affected arm.

    c. The Hippocratic maneuver has been used, but this entails using the practitioner's shoeless foot (in the axilla) to push the humeral head back into place along with longitudinal traction.

    d. Immobilization in a Velpeau sling is required after reduction for 6–8 weeks.

    e. Early mobilization of patients older than 55 years should be undertaken to avoid frozen shoulder.

D. Other conditions of the shoulder

1. Adhesive capsulitis (frozen shoulder) is an inflammatory process that may follow injury to the shoulder or arise on its own (common in diabetes).

    a. It is characterized by pain and restricted glenohumeral movement.

    b. Arthrography may demonstrate synovitis, capsular contraction, and fibrinous adhesions.

    c. Treatment includes NSAIDs, passive range of motion, and occasionally, manipulation under anesthesia.

2. OA of the humeral head usually is secondary to osteonecrosis.

    a. Pain, stiffness, and limited range of motion are features of the condition.

    b. Radiographs show osteophytes and joint space narrowing.

    c. Treatment includes NSAIDs, cortisone injections, activity modification, and débridement or total joint replacement in severe cases.

3. Rupture of the long head of the biceps tendons

    a. This rupture can occur as a result of spontaneous or forced overload.

    b. In the elderly, this rupture may be caused by degeneration or attritional changes.

    c. Treatment. Rupture is managed by surgical tenodesis to humerus if more than 5–10 days have elapsed since the injury.

E. Fractured clavicle

    1. General characteristics

        a. This is the most common fracture in children and adolescents.

        b. It can be found in up to 3% of live births.

        c. It is usually caused by a fall on an outstretched arm.

    2. Clinical features

        a. Visible deformity usually is present.

        b. The arm is supported by the contralateral extremity.

        c. Look for brachial plexus injuries (pain, weakness, reflex and sensory abnormalities).

        d. The proximal portion may be displaced superiorly because of the attachment of the sternocleidomastoid muscle.

    3. Imaging studies. An AP view generally will visualize the fracture.

    4. Treatment

        a. In children, the figure-of-eight bandage is sufficient. A sling may be added to prevent translocation of the distal segment but usually is not necessary.

        b. In adults, a sling generally is enough to treat the fracture.

F. Acromioclavicular separations

    1. General characteristics

        a. Also referred to as a "separated shoulder."

        b. It involves a "tearing" of the acromioclavicular and/or coracoclavicular ligaments.

        c. It is usually caused by a fall or impact on the tip of the shoulder.

    2. Clinical features. Patients may have a clinically apparent step off at the acromioclavicular joint.

    3. Imaging studies

        a. An AP view of both shoulders usually is necessary.

        b. Mild separations may require stress films that are obtained while the patient holds a weighted object to reveal the separation.

    4. Treatment

        a. Conservative management is possible for mild to moderate injuries, because they can be managed with a sling and analgesia.

        b. More severe injuries usually will require operative repair.

G. Humeral head fractures

    1. General characteristics

        a. Most fractures of the proximal humerus occur in older patients with osteoporosis.

        b. The female to male ratio is 2:1.

    2. Clinical features

        a. Pain, swelling, and tenderness, especially in the region of the greater tuberosity, are the most common findings.

        b. Ecchymosis typically does not appear until after 24–48 hours.

        c. The patient will hold the affected extremity against the chest wall.

        d. Look for injuries to the brachial plexus and/or axillary artery.

3. Imaging studies
   a. AP, lateral, and "Y" view typically are diagnostic.
   b. Humeral fractures are assessed most commonly by the Neer classification. Displaced fractures are two-part, three-part, or four-part based on whether or not the fracture parts (e.g., head, greater tuberosity, lesser tuberosity, shaft) are involved.
4. Treatment
   a. Closed reduction with the application of a Velpeau sling can treat most nondisplaced fractures. Early mobilization with pendulum exercises is indicated to prevent frozen shoulder.
   b. ORIF is reserved for the management of displaced fractures.
H. Humeral shaft fractures
   1. General characteristics
      a. The mechanism of injury includes motor-vehicle accidents, falls on an outstretched hand, and penetrating injuries, such as gunshot wounds.
      b. The degree of comminution and amount of soft-tissue injury relate directly to the amount of energy causing the fracture.
   2. Clinical features
      a. Pain, arm swelling, deformity, and shortening are all possible initial complaints.
      b. Radial nerve injury should be looked for carefully.
   3. Imaging studies. AP and lateral views that include the elbow and shoulder should be performed.
   4. Treatment
      a. Initial treatment usually is the application of a coaptation splint.
      b. The coaptation splint can be followed by a hanging cast, Sarmiento brace, or operative repair.
   5. Complications
      a. Fractures of the humeral shaft may be associated with radial nerve injury at the time of fracture.
      b. Radial nerve injuries also may develop during reduction and as a delayed complication because of incorporation of the nerve by a callus.
I. Supracondylar humerus fractures
   1. General characteristics. The usual mechanism of fracture is a hyperextension injury to the elbow.
   2. Clinical features
      a. Initially, patients may have pain with minimal swelling. Extension of swelling around the elbow is a delayed finding.
      b. Full neurovascular examination must be performed. Special attention to brachial artery injuries should be given. The brachial artery is the most spastic artery in the body and can lead to Volkmann's contractures.
   3. Imaging studies
      a. AP and lateral views generally are sufficient to make the diagnosis.
      b. In children, always obtain comparative views.
   4. Treatment
      a. Closed reduction in the operating room with posterior splint application for displaced fractures in children.
      b. Adults should have ORIF.
   5. Complications
      a. Besides Volkmann's ischemic contractures, injuries to all three nerves have been described.
      b. Varus (gunstock) or valgus deformities of the elbow also may result from arrest of the medial or the lateral growth plate, respectively.
J. Hand and wrist pain
   1. OA and RA are the most common painful conditions of the hand and wrist.
      a. OA commonly affects the carpometacarpal joint of the thumb and DIP joints.
      b. OA of the wrist can be posttraumatic or follow osteonecrosis of the lunate (Kienböck's disease).

2. Clinical features

    a. OA presents with Heberden's nodes and mucous cysts in DIP joints and Bouchard's nodes in proximal interphalangeal joints.

    b. RA causes rupture of extensor tendons, erosion subluxation, edema, or dislocation of joints.

    c. Dupuytren's disease affects the palmar aponeurosis, ring, little, and middle fingers, with painful nodules, pitting, and contractures.

3. Treatment

    a. There is no nonsurgical treatment for this condition.

    b. Surgical release is indicated for contractures of the metacarpal phalangeal joint that are greater than 30° and for proximal phalangeal contractures of any degree, pain (rare), or nerve compression (digital).

K. Carpal tunnel syndrome

1. General characteristics

    a. Carpal tunnel syndrome, the most common neuropathy, involves compression of the median nerve under the transverse carpal ligament.

    b. It can be precipitated by premenstrual fluid retention, early RA with thickening of the synovial tendon sheath, acromegaly, pregnancy, repetitive flexion or extension of the wrist (e.g., production line work, keyboard work), and alcohol abuse.

2. Clinical features

    a. Classic findings of night pain, numbness, paresthesias (sparing the little finger), clumsiness, and weakness are seen.

    b. Thenar atrophy may occur.

    c. Tinel's sign (tingling with percussion over the volar aspect of the wrist) may be noted.

    d. Phalen's test (symptoms with full flexion of the wrist for >1 min) may be positive.

3. Laboratory studies

    a. Helpful studies include glucose, thyroid panel, rheumatoid factor, ESR, and diagnostic steroid injections.

    b. Tests of nerve sensory conduction, if greater than 3.5 milliseconds, are helpful but not always diagnostic.

4. Treatment

    a. Activity modification, volar wrist splint, and NSAIDs (except in pregnancy) make up the initial recommended treatment.

    b. Steroid injections may be used.

    c. A daily vitamin B_6 supplement may be helpful.

    d. Surgical intervention may be needed to decompress the nerve.

L. Fractures and dislocations of the hand

1. A boxer's fracture is a fracture of the metacarpal neck of the fifth finger.

    a. Examination reveals loss of prominence of fifth knuckle with tenderness and pain.

    b. Inspect for a puncture wound over the metacarpal phalangeal joint. If the fracture was caused by a punch to another's mouth, it also may be necessary to treat with antibiotics (*Eikenella corrodens* is an organism specific to human mouth).

    c. Fractures with 25–30° of angulation should be reduced with the application of gutter splint or casting for at least 4 weeks.

2. A Colles' fracture is a distal radius fracture with dorsal angulation.

    a. The most common injury of the wrist, a Colles' fracture results from a fall onto the dorsiflexed hand and is described as a silver fork deformity.

    b. Cast immobilization is adequate after reduction.

3. Gamekeeper's thumb is a sprain or tear of the ulnar collateral ligament of the thumb.

    a. There usually is a history of a sprained thumb or a fall on the hand.

    b. Examination reveals ligamentous laxity of the ulnar collateral ligament, with instability and weakness of pinch.

    c. Surgical repair is indicated for a complete rupture; a partial rupture may be treated by immobilization with a thumb spica cast.

M. Lateral epicondylitis ("tennis elbow")

  1. General characteristics

  a. Most common overuse injury of the elbow.

  b. Most common during the fourth decade of life.

  c. Involvement of the tendinous insertion of the extensor carpi radialis brevis.

  2. Clinical features

  a. Pain on lifting objects, primarily when the arm is in the prone position.

  b. Duplicate pain by having patient extend their elbow, hold the forearm in the prone position, and then extend the fingers and wrist against resistance.

  3. Imaging studies

  a. AP and lateral views of the elbow may demonstrate osteophytes overlying the lateral epicondyle.

  b. MRI is useful in demonstrating tendon disruption.

  4. Treatment

  a. Cease the provocative activity for at least 6 weeks.

  b. Counterbalance braces (tennis elbow braces) are beneficial.

  c. Instruct the patient to pick up objects with the extremity in supination.

  d. Physical and occupational therapy are important adjuncts to care.

  e. A 3-mL injection of equal parts betamethasone sodium phosphate, 2% lidocaine, and 0.5% marcaine can be used.

    (1) Use of this injection is controversial, because tendon ruptures have been documented with this treatment.

    (2) It has been shown effective for the short term (6 weeks).

  f. NSAIDs frequently are used. Because anti-inflammatory agents are being used more for their analgesic effect, however, their use also is controversial.

  g. Surgery is reserved for those patients who fail at least 6 months of conservative management.

N. Medial epicondylitis ("golfer's elbow" or "baseball elbow")

  1. General characteristics. This affects the flexor–pronator muscles at their origin, anterior to the medial epicondyle.

  2. Clinical features

  a. A history of repetitive stress is obtained in most patients.

  b. Pain is reproduced by resisted pronation or flexion of the wrist.

  c. Patients may complain of paresthesias in the distribution of the ulnar nerve.

  3. Imaging studies. MRI typically is not indicated but is useful for assessing the ulnar nerve.

  4. Treatment

  a. Conservative management, including NSAIDs and physical and occupational therapy, most commonly is used.

  b. A medial counterforce brace frequently is applied.

  c. Surgical intervention to debride the epicondyle usually is not necessary but is an option.

O. Olecranon bursitis

  1. General characteristics

  a. Caused either by an acute injury or by repetitive trauma to the olecranon bursa.

  b. Less frequently, it can result from breaks in the skin, leading to a septic cause. The most common organism is *Staphylococcus aureus*.

  2. Clinical features

  a. Swelling overlying the olecranon process is the most common finding. This swelling may be mildly painful, but in chronic cases, it usually is painless.

  b. Range of motion usually is preserved.

  3. Imaging studies generally are not indicated unless there is a significant history of trauma or a fracture is suspected.

4. Treatment

  a. Aspiration with an 18-gauge needle using a Z tract is both diagnostic and therapeutic. Fluid should be sent for culture and sensitivity.

  b. NSAIDs and warm compresses are used for their analgesic properties.

  c. Surgical removal of the bursa is reserved for septic bursal sacs that are nonresponsive to conservative management.

P. Radial head injuries

  1. General characteristics

    a. Fractures of the radial head result from a fall on the outstretched hand.

    b. Subluxation of the radial head in children, or nursemaid's elbow, is caused by excessive longitudinal traction. It is most common before the age of 4.

  2. Clinical features

    a. Fractures of the radial head present with pain over the lateral aspect of the elbow that worsens with forearm rotation. It is the most common fracture of the elbow in adults.

    b. Children who have sustained a subluxation of the radial head (nursemaid's elbow) usually present with the extremity fully pronated, partially flexed, and held tightly to the side.

  3. Imaging studies

    a. AP and lateral films of the elbow usually are sufficient to establish the diagnosis. Displacement of the anterior fat pad implies the presence of a hemarthrosis. CT is useful in determining the degree of comminution.

    b. AP and lateral films usually are performed to rule out fracture in children who are suspected of having a subluxed radial head.

  4. Treatment

    a. Treatment of radial head fractures depends on the type of fracture.

    b. Radial head subluxations can be reduced by holding the affected arm just above the wrist and just below the elbow. The practitioner then places thumb of the proximal hand over the radial head while fully supinating the forearm and applying posteriorly directed pressure. The objective is to effect a "screwing" action and place the radial head back within the annular ligament.

Q. Scaphoid (navicular) fracture

  1. General characteristics

    a. This is the most commonly fractured carpal bone.

    b. Blood supply is from the radial artery by way of lateral and distal branches. The proximal pole of the scaphoid has a poor blood supply that is further compromised with fractures through the waist of the bone; this can lead to avascular necrosis or nonunion of the scaphoid.

  2. Clinical features

    a. Cardinal finding is pain over the anatomic snuffbox.

    b. Swelling over the region in association with ecchymosis implies a fracture–dislocation.

    c. Often confused with a "sprain" of the wrist, so clinical suspicion is key.

  3. Imaging studies

    a. AP, lateral, and scaphoid views should be ordered. If negative initially, films may be repeated after 2–3 weeks, at which time the fracture may become apparent.

    b. Bone scan, MRI, and even CT have been used to avoid a delay in diagnosis, because this can increase the likelihood of nonunion.

  4. Treatment

    a. A delay in diagnosis should be avoided. Suspicion of scaphoid fracture without radiologic evidence should be treated as a fracture in a long arm thumb spica cast until bone scan or MRI can be performed.

    b. The usual treatment of scaphoid fracture is long arm thumb spica cast for 4 weeks, followed by change to a short arm thumb spica cast if there is adequate healing.

    c. Displacement of 1 mm or greater requires ORIF.

  5. Complications include nonunion of the fracture or development of avascular necrosis. In avascular necrosis, radiography may reveal a ground-glass appearance of the proximal pole or an increased bone density.

R. DeQuervain's disease

1. Clinical characteristics

a. DeQuervain's disease is a stenosing tenosynovitis involving the abductor pollicis longus and extensor pollicis brevis.

b. It is more common in females older than 30 years and in diabetics.

2. Clinical features

a. Pain and tenderness occur at the wrist and base of the thumb. Radiation of pain may be up the forearm.

b. Swelling and thickening of the tendon sheath may be appreciated during examination.

c. The patient places the thumb within his or her fist, and the wrist is then ulnarly deviated, reproducing the pain (Finkelstein's test).

3. Imaging studies. Not usually required.

4. Treatment

a. Conservative treatment for at least a month using a thumb spica splint, NSAIDs, and physical/occupational therapy is required.

b. Injection of steroid into the tendon sheath can be employed if conservative measures fail. No more than three injections should be given.

c. Surgical decompression of the first dorsal compartment may be required in cases that are resistant to all conservative measures.

VI. DISORDERS OF THE BACK

A. Low back pain and sciatica

1. General characteristics

a. The most common causes of low back pain are prolapsed intervertebral disk and low back strain.

b. When back pain is unrelated to the mechanical use of the back, it can be referred from the intra-abdominal, pelvic, or retroperitoneal areas.

2. Clinical features

a. Pain originating in the back and radiating down the leg suggests nerve root irritation.

b. Pain from musculoskeletal causes may be localized to an area of point tenderness.

c. Sciatica (pain in the distribution of the sciatic nerve) is pain felt in the buttock, posterior thigh, and postero-lateral aspect of the leg around the lateral malleolus to the lateral dorsum of the foot and the entire sole.

d. Unilateral low back and buttock pain that gets worse with standing in one position may have sacroiliac joint involvement.

e. Pain in the elderly that is increased by walking and is relieved by leaning forward suggests spinal stenosis.

3. Laboratory studies and imaging

a. Radiographs of the spine in nontraumatic low back pain often are not required when pertinent directed history and physical examination reveal no sign of a serious condition.

b. CT is helpful in demonstrating bony stenosis and identifying lateral nerve root entrapment.

c. MRI can be useful in identifying cord pathology, neural tumors, herniated disks, and infections.

4. Treatment

a. Short-term bed rest (maximum of 2 days) with support under the knees and neck and administration of NSAIDs or analgesics are the first components of treatment.

b. Progressive ambulation to normal activities may follow if pain has subsided.

c. A fitness program, including postural exercises (e.g., McKenzie exercises for disk derangement) should be implemented for back rehabilitation.

d. If no improvement occurs in 6 weeks, perform further evaluation with bone scan, CT, MRI, or electromyelography and a medical workup to rule out spinal tumor or infection.

e. If studies are normal, continue back rehabilitation.

f. When conservative treatment fails, confirm candidates for surgical intervention (~5% of those who present with low back pain).

B. Scoliosis and kyphosis

1. Scoliosis

    a. General characteristics

        (1) Scoliosis is defined as lateral curvature of the spine.

        (2) Some curves are secondary to underlying causes (i.e., upper or lower motor neuron disease, myopathies).

        (3) Idiopathic adolescent scoliosis is the most common spinal deformity evaluated by a clinician.

        (4) Girls between onset of the puberty growth spurt and cessation of spinal growth are at the greatest risk for idiopathic scoliosis.

        (5) The vertebrae at the apex of the curve are used for its description. Right thoracic curves (T7 or T8) are the most common, followed by the double major (right thoracic, left lumbar), left lumbar, and right lumbar.

        (6) A thoracic curve to the left is rare; other spinal cord pathology needs to be ruled out before making a diagnosis of scoliosis.

    b. Clinical features

        (1) Physical examination reveals asymmetry in the shoulder and iliac height; asymmetric scapular prominence; and a flank crease with forward bending, showing right thoracic and left lumbar prominence.

        (2) Gait and neurologic examination are normal.

        (3) Curves of less than 20°, diagnosed less than 2 years postmenarche, and Risser stage 2–4 are less likely to progress than are other curves.

    c. Imaging

        (1) Single, standing AP radiographs should be obtained when a patient has scoliometer (a device used for measuring curves) readings of greater than 5°.

        (2) Vertebral levels are identified on radiographs.

            (a) The greatest anterior tilt is measured by the Cobb method (measurement is perpendicular to the end plate of the most tilted [end] vertebra).

            (b) Curves of greater than 15% are significant.

        (3) Accurate measurement is best performed by an orthopaedic specialist.

    d. Treatment

        (1) Curves of 10–15° are treated by 6-month follow-up of the forward-bending test and the scoliometer test.

        (2) Curves of 15–20° need serial AP radiograph follow-up every 3–4 months for larger curves and every 6–8 months for smaller curves or for patients near the end of growth.

        (3) Curves of 20° or greater need referral to an orthopaedist for continuous monitoring and management.

2. Kyphosis

    a. General characteristics

        (1) Kyphosis is defined as increased convex curvature of the thoracic spine.

        (2) Scoliosis also is present in one-third of patients with kyphosis.

        (3) Juvenile kyphosis (Scheuermann's disease) is idiopathic osteochondrosis of thoracic spine.

        (4) Tuberculosis of the spine (the most common extrapulmonary location of tuberculosis after the lymph nodes) causes progressive kyphosis (Pott's disease).

    b. Clinical features

        (1) When several vertebrae are involved, there is a round back appearance; when only one vertebra is involved, there is an angular curve.

        (2) If the curve is a result of faulty posture, it will disappear with spinal flexion.

        (3) Excessive lumbar lordosis is common.

    c. Imaging. Standing lateral films.

    d. Treatment

        (1) Curves of 45–60° should be observed every 3–4 months and exercises prescribed for lumbar lordosis and the thoracic spine.

        (2) Curves of greater than 60° or with persistent pain can be treated using a Milwaukee brace.

        (3) Surgery is indicated when curvature is unresponsive to conservative treatment.

C. Spinal stenosis

   1. General characteristics

   a. Spinal stenosis is nerve compression caused by narrowing of the spinal canal or neural foramina.

   b. Types

   (1) Central stenosis (compression of the thecal sac) can be idiopathic or developmental.

   (2) Lateral stenosis (impingement of the nerve root lateral to the thecal sac) often accompanies central stenosis or is an isolated entity in young adults and the middle-aged.

   c. Spinal stenosis usually is symptomatic in late middle age and is more common in men than in women.

   2. Clinical features

   a. Neural claudication and exacerbation of pain with walking is typical. The pain is relieved by leaning forward.

   b. Variable back and leg pain may occur.

   3. Imaging

   a. Radiographs show soft-tissue and thecal narrowing.

   b. Plain CT, postmyelographic CT, and MRI are standard imaging modalities.

   4. Treatment

   a. Conservative management includes rest, isometric abdominal exercises, pelvic tilt, Williams flexion exercises, NSAIDs, and weight reduction.

   b. Lumbar epidural corticosteroid injections provide symptomatic relief; 25% of patients will gain sustained relief of symptoms following steroid injection.

   c. Decompression and fusion are indicated when studies are positive for neural compressive pathology and quality of life is unacceptable to the patient.

D. Ankylosing spondylitis

   1. General characteristics

   a. Ankylosing spondylitis is inflammation and progressive fusion of the vertebrae.

   b. This condition involves onset of back pain, stiffness, and hip pain during the third and fourth decades of life and is seen more commonly in men than in women.

   c. This disorder affects the sacroiliac joint symmetrically and the spine in a progressively ascending manner.

   2. Clinical features

   a. Lumbar motion is restricted.

   b. Limited motion in the shoulders and hips, synovitis of the knees, plantar fasciitis, and Achilles tendinitis are seen.

   c. Patients also have hip contractures and fixed cervical, thoracic, and lumbar hyperkyphosis.

   d. Fracture of the fused osteopenic spine may occur (commonly cervical), as may sciatica.

   e. Extra-articular manifestations may occur, including uveitis, cardiac abnormalities, and interstitial lung disease.

   f. Noninvasive tests for spine and thoracic mobility include the Schober test, thoracolumbar rotation and flexion, finger-to-floor distance, cervical rotation, occiput–wall distance, and chest expansion.

   3. Laboratory studies and imaging

   a. Evaluation of ESR and HLA-B27 are indicated.

   b. The "bamboo appearance" on radiography occurs because of radiographic obliteration and marginal syndesmophyte ossification of the paraspinal ligaments.

   c. Generalized osteopenia of the spine may be seen.

   4. Treatment

   a. Underlying and complicating conditions must be treated.

   b. Spine fractures need intervention and stabilization.

E. Cauda equina syndrome

   1. General characteristics. This is a rare condition involving a large midline disk herniation that compresses several nerve roots, usually at L4 to L5 level.

    2. Clinical features

        a. Bowel and bladder function is severely impaired.

        b. Leg pain, numbness, and/or paralysis are noted.

    3. Treatment. This is a surgical emergency requiring immediate referral.

VII. DISORDERS OF THE HIP AND LOWER EXTREMITY

A. Aseptic necrosis of the hip

    1. General characteristics

        a. Aseptic necrosis (also known as osteonecrosis or avascular necrosis) of the hip results from loss of blood supply to the trabecular bone, which causes a collapse of the femoral head.

        b. It can occur at any age but is seen with greater frequency during the third to fifth decades of life and often is bilateral.

        c. In children, it is known as Legg-Calvé-Perthes disease; it may develop in children aged 2–11, with a peak incidence between 5 and 9 years of age.

        d. The cause generally is unknown, but it often is seen in patients with a history of trauma, steroid use, alcohol abuse, RA, radiation therapy, and SLE.

    2. Clinical features

        a. Dull ache or throbbing pain localized to the groin, lateral hip, or buttocks.

        b. Pain with weight bearing and activity that is relieved with rest.

        c. Loss of rotation (internal and external) or abduction and an antalgic limp.

        d. Adverse outcomes include secondary osteoarthritis, femoral head collapse, and disability.

    3. Imaging

        a. MRI is the study of choice for early detection.

        b. Radiographs may be normal early in the course of disease; later, progression of necrosis may reveal a crescent sign in lateral films.

        c. Bone scans are useful but are less sensitive than MRI.

    4. Treatment

        a. Protected weight bearing for early stage disease is considered to be a temporary treatment.

        b. Core decompression or a vascularized bone graft may be used for noncollapsed necrosis.

        c. With collapse or bilateral involvement, total hip arthroplasty is the procedure of choice.

B. Slipped capital femoral epiphysis (SCFE)

    1. General characteristics

        a. SCFE is a weakening of the epiphyseal plate of the femur, resulting in a displacement of the femoral neck. It may be bilateral.

        b. It typically presents in children between 10 and 16 years of age.

        c. Boys are affected more often than girls, and there is a higher incidence in African Americans, the athletically inclined, and obese children.

        d. Most cases of SCFE are idiopathic, but in the younger child, consider a metabolic cause (hypothyroidism or hypopituitarism).

    2. Clinical features include a history of insidious hip, thigh, or knee pain associated with a painful limp.

    3. Imaging. Lateral radiographs show posterior and medial displacement of the epiphysis.

    4. Treatment

        a. Definitive treatment for chronic SCFE is pinning in situ.

        b. Child should be placed on crutches and should avoid weight bearing before and after surgery.

        c. Traction may be considered for acute SCFE.

C. Meniscal injuries

    1. General characteristics

        a. Meniscal injury occurs with excessive rotational force of the femur on the tibia.

      b. The medial meniscus is injured more frequently than the other menisci.

      c. Injuries may be isolated or may occur with other ligamentous ruptures.

  2. Clinical features

      a. Patients report joint line pain on the side of the injury, which may be palpable during examination.

      b. Inability to fully extend the knee is described as locking.

      c. The patient may describe a feeling of the knee giving way.

      d. Swelling occurs gradually, over several hours.

      e. Walking up and down stairs or squatting is difficult and may be painful.

      f. The McMurray test (flexion of the knee and hip with internal and external rotation of the tibia) may be helpful in detecting a meniscal tear.

  3. Imaging

      a. Radiographs usually are negative.

      b. MRI has an accuracy rate of 95% in confirming meniscal tears.

  4. Treatment

      a. Initial treatment is conservative: activity modification, anti-inflammatories, quadriceps strengthening exercises, and time.

      b. Indications for arthroscopy include persistent symptoms unresponsive to conservative treatment or irreducible locking.

D. Osgood-Schlatter disease

  1. General characteristics

      a. Osgood-Schlatter disease is apophysitis of the tibial tubercle caused by trauma or overuse.

      b. The age of onset is between 8 and 15 years. Males are affected two to three times more often than females.

      c. A self-limited disease, it usually heals when the epiphysis closes.

  2. Clinical features

      a. Patients complain of anterior knee pain, with localized pain and swelling over the tibial tubercle.

      b. Pain typically is related to activity and is relieved with rest.

  3. Imaging. Lateral radiography usually is normal.

  4. Treatment

      a. The patient should abstain from physical activity for as long as several months.

      b. Stretching, ice, and anti-inflammatories after exercise are indicated.

E. Cruciate ligament injuries

  1. General characteristics

      a. Anterior cruciate ligament (ACL) is more commonly injured than the posterior cruciate ligament (PCL).

      b. ACL injury is commonly associated with a pivoting motion during running, jumping or cutting activities.

      c. Women are affected more often than men.

  2. Clinical features

      a. Patients usually report hearing a pop and complain of knee instability.

      b. Hemarthrosis develops quickly within 3 to 4 hours.

      c. Lachman test is the most sensitive for diagnosing an ACL tear.

  3. Imaging

      a. Radiographs are done to rule out associated fracture.

      b. MRI is useful as an adjunct to physical exam to diagnose an ACL tear.

  4. Treatment

      a. Non-operative treatment with physical therapy and bracing is appropriate in patients who do not participate in competitive activities or who do not report instability with desired activities.

      b. Surgical reconstruction with autograft or allograft is appropriate in patients who are younger than 40 years of age, those who participate in competitive activities or those who report instability with desired activities.

      c. Complications from surgery may include limited or loss of full range of motion (ROM) or anterior knee pain.

F. Ankle sprain/strain
  1. General characteristics
    a. Ankle sprains are one of the most common sports-related injuries; 85% result from an inversion injury.
    b. Ankle sprains most often involve the lateral ligaments, particularly the anterior talofibular ligament (ATL).
  2. Clinical features
    a. Patients will often report hearing a pop and will present with ecchymosis and tenderness of the lateral ankle.
    b. Stability of the ankle should be assessed using the "anterior drawer" sign.
  3. Imaging
    a. Radiographs should be used to rule out a fracture, especially if the patient is unable to weight bear or has tenderness to palpation over a bone.
  4. Treatment
    a. Treatment should be tailored to the severity of the sprain, but always should include "RICE" (rest, ice, compression, elevation).
    b. Patients should use crutches for the first 48 to 72 hours and a brace should be used for support.
    c. Referral to physical therapy may speed recovery. Length of recovery could be 3 to 4 months.
G. Achilles tendonitis
  1. General characteristics
    a. Pain is attributed to inflammation and degeneration of the Achilles tendon and its attachment to the calcaneus.
    b. It is common in runners and in patients who suddenly increase their activity level.
    c. It is considered an overuse injury and is usually the result of improper stretching and training.
    d. If untreated, it may result in rupture of the Achilles tendon.
  2. Clinical features
    a. Patients usually report a gradual onset of pain during activity or after activity is completed.
    b. The pain is located on the posterior calf, 2 to 6 cm above the insertion of the Achilles tendon.
    c. Patients will be tender over the posterior calf above the calcaneus and will report pain on passive dorsiflexion and resisted plantar flexion.
    d. Ankle ROM and strength should be normal.
    e. The Thompson test should be done to rule out Achilles tendon rupture.
  3. Imaging
    a. Radiographs may show a soft tissue shadow and calcifications along the tendon and its insertion.
    b. MRI may show hypertrophy of the Achilles tendon or help rule out a rupture.
  4. Treatment
    a. The patient should be started on a regimen of NSAIDs and physical therapy for stretching and strengthening exercises.
H. Bunions (hallux valgus)
  1. General characteristics
    a. The most common deformity of the metatarsophalangeal joint (MTP) is hallux valgus and is the result of a lateral deviation of the proximal phalanx.
    b. Bunions are more common in women than men (10:1). They are often caused by wearing tight, pointed shoes.
    c. Other causes include congenital deformity and systemic diseases such as rheumatoid arthritis.
  2. Clinical features
    a. Patients will often complain of medial eminence pain, metatarsal head pain, deformities of the toes and the inability to find shoes that fit.
    b. Exam may show a hallux valgus deformity, MTP enlargement and pain and crepitation on movement of the MTP joint.
    c. Patients may also have limited ROM and pain on extreme ROM of the MTP joint.

3. Imaging

    a. Weight-bearing radiographs of the foot will show the valgus deformity of the proximal phalanx; an angle of greater than 15 degrees is considered abnormal.

4. Treatment

    a. Encourage patients to buy shoes with a wide toe box and to use pads on the medial eminence of the bunion deformity or between the first and second toes if they are rubbing together.

    b. Surgical treatment is for severe deformity or pain that is not relieved with conservative measures.

I. Morton's neuroma

  1. General characteristics

    a. Result of traction of the interdigital nerve against the transverse metatarsal ligament causing degeneration of the nerve and chronic inflammation.

    b. It usually affects the third web space and is more common in women than men (10:1).

  2. Clinical features

    a. Patients complain of pain and localized numbness when walking and standing that is relieved with rest.

    b. Pain is usually localized to the web space and, often, a mass is palpable.

    c. Squeezing the forefoot will often reproduce the symptoms.

  3. Imaging

    a. Plain radiographs are normal.

    b. MRI is sensitive but not usually needed as the diagnosis is made clinically.

  4. Treatment

    a. Conservative treatment using a soft metatarsal pad and shoes with a wide toe box are helpful.

    b. Steroid injections into the web space can be helpful.

    c. Surgical removal of the neuroma is possible in cases that are not resolved with conservative treatment, but the patient should be aware that both toes will be chronically numb.

J. Plantar fasciitis

  1. General characteristics

    a. Plantar fasciitis is very common in runners and overweight patients.

    b. It is caused by microscopic tears in the plantar fascia at the calcaneal origin.

  2. Clinical features

    a. Patients will complain of pain with the first few steps in the morning and heel pain at night.

    b. Exam will show pain at the calcaneal origin and an inflexible Achilles tendon.

  3. Imaging

    a. Plain radiographs are typically normal, but may reveal a calcaneal fracture or bone spur.

    b. MRI may reveal calcifications of the plantar fascia.

  4. Treatment

    a. Conservative treatment is recommended for 6 to 12 months, including physical therapy for stretching of the plantar fascia and the Achilles tendon, heel pads, arch supports and massage of the area with a tennis ball.

    b. Steroid injections should be used with caution due to the risk of rupture of the plantar fascia. Surgery is reserved for extreme cases.

10

Endocrinology

Rebecca Lovell Scott

I. THYROID DISORDERS

A. Hyperthyroidism (thyrotoxicosis)

1. General characteristics

    a. Hyperthyroidism involves elevated thyroid hormone concentrations and may be caused by excess production, leakage, or exogenous hormone administration.

    b. The most common cause (90% of cases) is Graves' disease.

        (1) Graves' disease is an autoimmune disorder in which autoantibodies attach to thyroid-stimulating hormone (TSH) receptors and stimulate thyroid hyperfunctioning. It most often occurs in women who are 20–40 years of age.

        (2) A familial tendency exists, as does an association with HLA-B8 and HLA-DR3.

        (3) Graves' disease also may be found in individuals with other autoimmune disorders (e.g., pernicious anemia, myasthenia gravis, diabetes mellitus).

        (4) Persons with Graves' disease are at increased risk of Addison's disease, alopecia areata, celiac disease, cardiomyopathy, and hypokalemic periodic paralysis.

    c. Other causes include toxic adenomas; subacute and postpartum thyroiditis; exogenous thyroid hormone ingestion; trophoblastic tumors and, rarely, pituitary tumors; and administration of amiodarone, which causes either active elaboration of excessive thyroid hormone (type I) or destructive thyroiditis (type II).

    d. Thyroid storm is the abrupt onset of more florid symptoms of thyrotoxicosis.

2. Clinical features

    a. Symptoms include heat intolerance, sweating, weight loss (or gain), increased appetite, nervousness, loose stools, frequent urination, muscle cramps, irritability, fatigue, weakness, dyspnea on exertion, and menstrual abnormalities (typically excess bleeding).

    b. Patients also may have sinus tachycardia or atrial fibrillation, premature atrial contractions, palpitations, precordial chest pain, warm moist skin, fine hair, stare, onycholysis, fine resting finger tremor, lid lag, hyperreflexia, and muscle weakness.

    c. Hyperthyroidism caused by Graves' disease

        (1) Patients will have a goiter, frequently with a bruit.

        (2) Between 20 and 40% of patients will have mild ophthalmopathy (chemosis, conjunctivitis, proptosis); between 5 and 10% will have severe ophthalmopathy (exophthalmos, possibly diplopia, corneal drying). Changes may be asymmetric.

        (3) Pretibial myxedema occurs in 3% of patients.

    d. Findings may be limited to one organ system and may include isolated atrial fibrillation, psychosis, or myopathies.

    e. Complications include atrial fibrillation, hypercalcemia, osteoporosis, impotence, nephrocalcinosis, decreased libido, gynecomastia, and decreased sperm count.

    f. Chronic thyrotoxicosis may cause osteoporosis, clubbing, and finger swelling.

    g. Asian or Native-American men with thyrotoxicosis may develop hypokalemic periodic paralysis lasting 7–72 hours, often after IV dextrose, oral carbohydrate, or vigorous exercise.

    h. Thyroid storm

        (1) Thyroid storm follows stressful illness, thyroid surgery, or radioactive iodine administration.

        (2) It presents with high fever, tachycardia, vomiting, diarrhea, dehydration, marked weakness, and muscle wasting; extreme restlessness, confusion, and emotional lability may also occur.

        (3) Although rare, its mortality rate is high.

3. Laboratory studies
   a. Laboratory studies are based on levels of thyroid hormones; TSH is secreted by the pituitary gland and stimulates thyroid hormone production. Thyroid hormone levels are affected by severe illness, cirrhosis, nephrotic syndrome, a variety of drugs, high estrogen states, and acute psychiatric illness.
   b. In primary hyperthyroidism, TSH (the most sensitive indicator) is low.
   c. Serum thyroxine (T_4), triiodothyronine (T_3), free T_4, free T_4 index, and thyroid resin uptake usually will be elevated.
   d. TSH-receptor antibody and antithyroglobulin or antithyroperoxidase antibody levels usually are high in Graves' disease; serum antinuclear antibody and anti–double stranded DNA antibodies usually are elevated.
   e. In subacute thyroiditis, erythrocyte sedimentation rate may be elevated.
   f. Thyroid radioactive iodine uptake and scan reveal high uptake in Graves' disease and toxic multinodular goiter.
   g. MRI of the orbits is preferred for evaluation of ophthalmopathy.
4. Treatment
   a. β-Blockers control symptoms (tachycardia, tremor, diaphoresis, anxiety, palpitations) in any hyperthyroid episode and are the initial treatment of choice for thyroid storm and periodic paralysis.
   b. Thiourea drugs (methimazole or propylthiouracil)
      (1) These drugs control hyperthyroidism within several weeks and are taken for 12–24 months.
      (2) They are useful in preparing patients for surgery or radioactive iodide treatment.
      (3) Propylthiouracil is the drug of choice for pregnant and breast-feeding women.
      (4) Thiourea drugs are associated with lower risk of posttreatment hypothyroidism compared to other medical or surgical treatments.
      (5) Agranulocytosis is a rare complication.
   c. Radioactive iodine (^{131}I) ablation is preferred to surgery for permanent control, particularly in the elderly. Surgery is preferred for pregnant women, patients with large goiters, and when malignancy is likely.
   d. Iodinated contrast agents provide temporary treatment and may be helpful in highly symptomatic patients.
   e. Ophthalmopathy may respond to high-dose, tapered prednisone treatment, particularly in nonsmokers.
   f. Atrial fibrillation is not likely to convert electrically while the patient is hyperthyroid.
      (1) Digoxin may be used in large doses and β-blockers with caution.
      (2) Anticoagulation with warfarin is used to prevent thromboembolism.
      (3) Congestive heart failure must be treated as usual, along with aggressive treatment for hyperthyroidism.
   g. Thyroid storm is a life-threatening emergency requiring prompt and specific treatment. The treatment for thyroid storm includes administration of β-blockers, hydrocortisone, supportive therapy, and attempts to control hyperthyroidism.

B. Hypothyroidism and myxedema
   1. General characteristics
      a. Hypothyroidism almost always results from autoimmune thyroiditis, previous thyroid surgery, or radiation therapy.
      b. Hashimoto's thyroiditis (autoimmune thyroiditis, chronic lymphocytic thyroiditis) frequently leads to hypothyroidism.
   2. Clinical features
      a. Signs and symptoms tend to be vague and nonspecific.
      b. Common complaints include fatigue, lethargy, anorexia, constipation, depression, menstrual abnormalities muscle stiffness, memory impairment, cold intolerance, and dry skin.
      c. Signs include edema, weight gain, weakness, bradycardia, hyporeflexia, dementia, and psychosis.
   3. Laboratory studies
      a. TSH will be elevated in primary disease.
      b. Low total T_4 and free T_4 are likely; T_3 may be normal.
      c. Presence of antithyroid peroxidase and antithyroglobulin antibodies in the serum confirm autoimmune disease.
   4. Treatment with synthetic T_4 is best monitored by serial TSH levels.

C. Thyroiditis

   1. General characteristics

      a. Hashimoto's (chronic lymphocytic) thyroiditis is the most common thyroid disorder in the United States and may be associated with other autoimmune or polyglandular syndromes. It often is associated with other autoimmune disorders.

         (1) It tends to be familial and is more common in women.

         (2) Frequency is increased with dietary iodine supplementation, certain drugs, and exposure to head and neck radiation during childhood.

      b. Subacute (granulomatous, de Quervain's, giant cell) thyroiditis may present either with acute symptoms or silently.

         (1) It is most common in young or middle-aged women.

         (2) A viral cause is suspected; the incidence peaks in summer.

      c. Postpartum thyroiditis occurs soon after parturition and usually resolves completely.

      d. Suppurative (infectious) and Reidel's (invasive fibrous, woody) thyroiditis are rare.

   2. Clinical features

      a. In Hashimoto's thyroiditis, the thyroid is diffusely enlarged, firm, and finely nodular; changes may be asymmetric.

         (1) Signs and symptoms usually are of hypothyroidism (more likely in smokers), but transient thyrotoxicosis may occur.

            (a) It usually is not painful, although neck tightness occurs.

            (b) Depression and chronic fatigue are common and may persist after treatment.

            (c) Autoimmune xerostomia and keratoconjunctivitis may occur, as may mild myasthenia gravis.

         (2) In elderly women (10% of cases), the gland is atrophic and fibrotic.

      b. Subacute thyroiditis presents as an acute, painful glandular enlargement with dysphagia.

         (1) Patients may have thyrotoxicosis and malaise followed by hypothyroidism.

         (2) Manifestations last from weeks to months and usually resolve within 12 months.

      c. Postpartum thyroiditis manifests with hyperthyroidism 1–6 months after delivery and lasts for 1–2 months. Some evidence suggests a link to postpartum depression.

      d. Fever, pain, redness, and a fluctuant neck mass are common in suppurative thyroiditis.

   3. Laboratory studies

      a. Testing for Hashimoto's disease involves screening for serum antithyroid peroxidase and antithyroglobulin antibodies, which will confirm autoimmune disease.

      b. In subacute disease, erythrocyte sedimentation rate is high, and antithyroid antibodies are low.

      c. T_4 and T_3 resin uptake are markedly elevated in acute and subacute disease. Radioactive iodine uptake initially is very low.

   4. Treatment is based on specific manifestations.

      a. Hashimoto's thyroiditis requires lifelong replacement with thyroid hormone for hypothyroidism or large goiter, with watchful waiting in others.

      b. Subacute thyroiditis is treated with aspirin; other treatment is directed at symptoms.

D. Thyroid cancer

   1. General characteristics

      a. The most common form (76% of cases) is papillary carcinoma; other forms are follicular (16%), medullary (4%), anaplastic (1%), and lymphoma/metastatic disease (3%).

      b. Women are affected two to three times more often than men; the incidence increases with age.

      c. Cancer usually presents as a single nodule; however, only 5% of all palpable thyroid nodules are malignant.

      d. Cancer risk is associated with childhood neck or head irradiation or exposure to radioactive isotopes of iodine, with peak occurrence 20–25 years later.

      e. Papillary, follicular, medullary, and anaplastic cancers are all associated with genetic mutations and translocations.

      f. One-third of medullary carcinoma is sporadic, one-third familial, and one-third associated with multiple endocrine neoplasia type 2. Families of patients with medullary disease should have genetic testing.

      g. Papillary carcinoma is the least aggressive and anaplastic the most aggressive.

2. Clinical features

    a. Patients most often present with painless neck swelling and have a single, palpable, firm nodule. Pain, hoarseness, and hemoptysis also may occur.

    b. The nodule may enlarge over a short period.

    c. Patients may have evidence of metastatic disease, including thyrotoxicosis.

    d. The gland often is stony and hard.

    e. Medullary carcinoma causes flushing, diarrhea, fatigue, and Cushing's syndrome; anaplastic carcinoma has signs of pressure or invasion, such as recurrent laryngeal nerve palsy (hoarseness).

3. Laboratory studies

    a. Thyroid function tests often are normal.

    b. TSH should be measured to exclude primary thyroid disease.

    c. Fine-needle biopsy is essential.

    d. Hot nodules on radionuclide scanning usually are benign.

    e. Metastatic and follicular tumors have high serum thyroglobulin; medullary tumors have high serum calcitonin and carcinoembryonic antigen.

    f. Ultrasound of the neck is useful in determining size and location; other possible tests include radioisotope scanning, chest radiography, MRI, CT, and positron-emission tomography.

4. Treatment

    a. Surgical resection and near-total thyroidectomy are indicated.

    b. T_4 therapy prevents hypothyroidism and reduces the risk of recurrence.

    c. Radioactive iodine ablation is used for residual disease.

    d. Metastatic bone disease is treated with external radiation and brain metastasis with gamma-knife radiation therapy.

II. PARATHYROID DISORDERS

A. Hypoparathyroidism and pseudohypoparathyroidism

1. General characteristics

    a. Hypoparathyroidism most commonly is found after thyroidectomy, but it also may be caused by heavy metal toxicity, granulomas, Reidel's thyroiditis, tumors, infection, autoimmune problems, or neck irradiation.

    b. Functional disease may occur in the presence of magnesium deficiency.

    c. Pseudohypoparathyroidism results from a group of diseases characterized by hypocalcemia caused by renal resistance to parathyroid hormone.

    d. Di George's syndrome includes hypoparathyroidism plus congenital facial and cardiac anomalies.

    e. Hypoparathyroidism is a possible manifestation of polyglandular autoimmunity type 1.

2. Clinical features

    a. Acute disease causes tetany, carpopedal spasm, cramping, convulsions, circumoral and distal extremity tingling, and irritability.

    b. Positive Chvostek's sign* and Trousseau's phenomenon** cataracts, and teeth and nail defects indicate associated hypocalcemia.

    c. Findings in patients with chronic disease include lethargy, anxiety, parkinsonism, mental retardation, personality changes, and blurred vision caused by cataracts.

    d. Dry skin, loss of eyebrow hair, brittle nails, and hyperreflexia may be present.

3. Laboratory and diagnostic studies

    a. Corrected serum calcium, urinary calcium, and parathyroid hormone levels are low.

    b. Serum magnesium may be low.

    c. Serum phosphate will be high; alkaline phosphatase will be normal.

    d. CT or radiography of the skull may show dense bones and basal ganglia calcifications.

---

* (Facial muscle contraction after tapping the facial nerve)
** (Carpal spasm with blood pressure cuff inflation)

   e. Electrocardiographic findings include prolonged QT intervals and T-wave abnormalities.

   f. Slit-lamp examination may show early posterior lenticular changes.

   g. Radiography may demonstrate chronic increased bone mineral density, especially in the lumbar spine.

4. Treatment

   a. Emergency treatment for tetany includes airway maintenance and slow administration of IV calcium gluconate.

   b. Maintenance therapy includes oral calcium and vitamin D preparations to keep serum calcium at 8–8.6 mg/dL.

   c. Magnesium supplementation may be required.

   d. Transplantation of cryopreserved parathyroid tissue may restore normocalcemia.

   e. Monitoring of treatment includes measurement of serum and urine calcium levels.

   f. Phenothiazines and furosemide should be avoided.

B. Hyperparathyroidism

1. General characteristics

   a. This condition is more common in women compared to men and in those older than 50 years of age.

   b. Causes include parathyroid adenoma and, less commonly, hyperplasia or carcinoma. Multiglandular disease and carcinoma are more common in persons younger than 30 years.

   c. Many malignancies also cause hypercalcemia and have clinical findings similar to those of hyperparathyroidism.

2. Clinical features

   a. Hypercalcemia most commonly is identified on routine chemistry panels in asymptomatic patients; abnormal screening studies should be repeated.

   b. Patients may have polydipsia and polyuria caused by nephrogenic diabetes insipidus.

   c. Excessive calcium and phosphate excretion may lead to renal stones, and nephrocalcinosis and renal failure may occur.

   d. Bone pain and arthralgias are common; cortical bone or diffuse bone demineralization, trabecular bone increase, pathologic fractures, and cystic bone lesions may occur (jaw is most common).

   e. Mild hypercalcemia is likely to be asymptomatic; if the hypercalcemia is more severe, it causes thirst, anorexia, nausea, vomiting, constipation, anemia, weight loss, peptic ulcer disease, pancreatitis, hypertension, and depressed deep tendon reflexes.

   f. Depression, muscle weakness, fatigability, paresthesias, pruritus, psychosis, and coma occur in severe disease.

   g. Symptoms can be summarized as "bones, stones, abdominal groans, psychic moans, with fatigue overtones."

   h. Secondary hypercalcemia is caused by many malignant tumors (e.g., breast, lung, pancreas, uterus) and, in older persons, by multiple myeloma.

   i. Other secondary causes of hypercalcemia include granulomatous disorders, calcium or vitamin D ingestion, familial hypocalciuric hypercalcemia, adrenal insufficiency, hyperthyroidism, certain medications, prolonged bed rest, and acute renal failure.

3. Laboratory studies

   a. Hypercalcemia (Ca >10.5 mg/dL) is the hallmark; serum phosphate often is less than 2.5 mg/dL.

   b. Urine calcium excretion generally is low for the degree of hypercalcemia. Excess loss of phosphate in the urine occurs, and serum phosphate is low to normal.

   c. Elevated parathyroid hormone levels confirm the diagnosis.

   d. The immunoradiometric assay (the best immunoassay) is both sensitive and specific in distinguishing primary hyperparathyroidism from other causes of hypercalcemia.

   e. All patients should be screened for familial benign hypocalciuric hypercalcemia with a 24-hour urine for calcium and creatinine before treating for hyperparathyroidism.

4. Treatment

   a. Surgical treatment is recommended for symptomatic and certain asymptomatic patients. Hypocalcemia is a common complication, as is transient hyperthyroidism.

   b. Medical treatment includes intensive hydration, inhibitors of bone resorption (i.e., bisphosphonates), calcium-receptor agonists, and avoidance of immobility; postmenopausal estrogen supplementation and propranolol may be helpful.

   c. Patients should avoid thiazide diuretics, large doses of vitamins A and D, and calcium-containing antacids and supplements.

III. DIABETES MELLITUS (DM)

A. General characteristics

   1. Most patients with diabetes have type I (1,000,000 patients in the United States) or type II (17.2 million patients in the United States).

   2. Rare types include maturity-onset diabetes of the young, diabetes caused by mutant insulins or insulin receptors, diseases of the exocrine pancreas, endocrinopathies, drug- and chemical-induced, and other genetic syndromes.

   3. Insulin-resistance syndrome (metabolic syndrome, syndrome X) is a constellation of hyperglycemia, hyperinsulinemia, dyslipidemia, and hypertension; it predisposes patients to coronary artery disease (CAD) and stroke. Patients also may have hyperuricemia, abdominal obesity, as well as prothrombotic and proinflammatory states.

   4. Diabetic retinopathy is the leading cause of blindness among people in the United States who are older than 60 years. Other ocular problems include premature cataracts and glaucoma.

   5. Diabetic nephropathy causes approximately one-third of end-stage renal disease in the United States. Patients with type I have a 30–40% chance, whereas those with type II have a 15–20% chance of serious renal disease.

   6. Patients with diabetes have accelerated large-vessel atherosclerosis, putting them at increased risk for stroke and CAD. Large vessel atherosclerosis in diabetic patients also is the cause of at least half the nontraumatic lower extremity amputations in the United States.

   7. Neuropathy is the most common complication of DM.

   a. It causes a characteristic peripheral symmetric polyneuropathy and may cause a peripheral mononeuropathy or mononeuropathy multiplex.

   b. Painful foot neuropathy may be physically and emotionally disabling.

   c. Nerve damage also causes autonomic dysfunction, leading to erectile dysfunction, atonic bladder, and delayed gastric emptying.

   8. Skin changes associated with DM include slow wound healing, necrobiosis lipoidica diabeticorum, and acanthosis nigricans.

B. Type I DM

   1. General characteristics

   a. Type I occurs most often in young people (10–14 years of age) of normal or low weight, particularly among individuals of Scandinavian ancestry; nonautoimmune type I disease occurs primarily in those of Asian or African origin.

   b. There is little or no endogenous insulin secretion.

      (1) Plasma glucagon is elevated.

      (2) Pancreatic B cells fail to respond to stimuli and undergo destruction. If untreated, this is a catabolic state with ketosis.

   c. Most type I DM is an autoimmune disease (90%), with 95% of patients having HLA-DR3 or HLA-DR4 antigens. HLA-DQ genes are even more specific, and 85% of patients have islet cell antibodies.

   d. Extrinsic factors affecting pancreatic B-cell function include mumps and coxsackie B4 virus infection, toxic chemicals, and destructive cytokines and antibodies.

   2. Clinical features

   a. The most common findings include polydipsia, polyuria, and rapid weight loss despite normal or increased appetite, associated with a random plasma glucose of 200 mg/dL or greater.

   b. Blurred vision is common; weakness, postural hypotension, and paresthesias may occur.

   c. Untreated type I DM results in diabetic ketoacidosis, leading to anorexia, nausea, vomiting, dehydration, stupor, and ultimately, coma. Fruity breath suggests ketoacidosis.

   3. Laboratory studies

   a. A random plasma glucose of more than 200 mg/dL with classic symptoms or fasting levels of 126 mg/dL or greater on more than one occasion is diagnostic.

   b. Most patients with new-onset type I DM will have a severely elevated glucose, warranting no further diagnostic study.

    c. Patients are likely to have glycosuria; they also may have ketonemia and/or ketonuria.

    d. Glycosylated hemoglobin (HbAI) reflects glycemic control over the preceding 8–12 weeks.

       (1) Levels of HbAIc (the major form) are highly specific and so are used to follow treatment.

       (2) Serum fructosamine reflects control over the preceding 2 weeks.

    e. Patients should use a portable glucometer to monitor control.

    f. Well-controlled type I DM results in normal lipid values.

4. Treatment

    a. Diet is central to management.

       (1) Diet must be individualized according to the patient's activity level, food preferences, and need to attain and maintain ideal weight.

       (2) Patients with type I DM should limit their intake of carbohydrates and administer 1 U of regular or lispro insulin for each 10–15 g ingested. They should limit their cholesterol to 300 mg daily; protein should make up 10–20% of total daily calories, saturated fat 8–9%, and other fats 8–9%.

       (3) A diet high in soluble fiber improves glucose through slowed absorption and improves cholesterol levels; insoluble fiber improves colonic transit.

       (4) Patients should eat meals and snacks at regular intervals.

       (5) Artificial sweeteners appropriate for patients with diabetes include aspartame, saccharin, sucralose, and acesulfame potassium.

    b. Insulin may be delivered by subcutaneous injection or by insulin pump.

       (1) Glycemic response depends on depth of injection, injection site, proximity of site to muscles being exercised, and temperature.

       (2) Regular insulin is absorbed most rapidly from the abdomen, but any site with loose skin may be used. Analog insulins are less affected by site of injection.

       (3) Human insulin causes markedly less antibody response than animal insulin and is available in regular, neutral protamine hagedorn, lente, and ultralente formulations.

       (4) Analog insulins include rapid-acting (lispro, aspart, glulisine) and very-long-acting (glargine) forms.

       (5) Rapid-acting insulins (lispro, aspart, glulisine) reach peak serum values in 1 hour and have a 4-hour duration of action; they may be taken 20 minutes before a meal.

       (6) Regular insulin is short-acting and is used before meals; the effect appears in 30 minutes and lasts for 5–7 hours. IV administration is useful in diabetic ketoacidosis and in perioperative management of patients with diabetes.

       (7) Neutral protamine hagedorn insulin and lente insulin are intermediate-acting forms; their peak effect is in 8–12 hours.

         (a) These forms often are used in combination with regular or lispro insulin for improved control.

         (b) Because of the 18- to 24-hour duration of action, most patients require at least two doses per day.

       (8) Ultralente insulin is long-acting but must be given twice daily; glargine may be given once a day but cannot be mixed with other human insulins. Both are used to provide basal coverage.

    c. Daily aspirin (81–325 mg) reduces the risk of diabetic atherothrombosis.

    d. Careful foot care, moderate exercise, meticulous personal hygiene, and prompt treatment of infection are imperative.

    e. Pancreas transplant at the time of renal transplant is becoming more common.

C. Type II DM

  1. General characteristics

    a. Type II DM, a heterogeneous group of diseases, occurs most often in middle-aged or older people; however, it is increasingly found in younger persons.

    b. Overweight and obesity are the strongest contributing factors. Distribution of fat to the upper body is associated with the highest risk, and exercise and weight loss decrease the risk.

    c. Type II DM has a strong genetic component.

    d. In the United States, type II DM accounts for 90% of diabetes cases and is found most often in African Americans, Hispanics, and Pima Indians.

      e. In type II DM, insulin levels are high enough to prevent ketoacidosis, but tissues are resistant. Impaired pancreatic B-cell response to glucose also often is present. Resistance is increased with aging, sedentary lifestyle, and abdominovisceral obesity.

      f. Untreated type II DM can lead to hyperosmolar nonketotic states.

2. Clinical features

      a. Many patients have polyuria and polydipsia; ketonuria and weight loss are rare.

      b. Patients also may present with fatigue, pruritus, recurrent candidal vaginitis, blurred vision, or poor wound healing.

      c. Many patients, particularly those who are obese, have few symptoms; DM is discovered during routine laboratory testing. Distribution of fat to the upper body is associated with increased risk.

      d. Women who have delivered large babies or had polyhydramnios, preeclampsia, or unexplained fetal loss are at increased risk.

3. Laboratory studies

      a. The diagnostic criteria for type II DM are the same as those for type I DM: random glucose >200 mg/dL or fasting glucose ≥ 126 mg/dL on more than one occasion.

      b. An oral glucose tolerance test may be needed in symptomatic patients with fasting glucose levels of less than 126 mg/dL.

      c. HbAIc and fructosamine are used to monitor chronic control.

      d. Diabetic dyslipidemia includes high triglycerides, low high-density lipoprotein (HDL), and alteration of low-density lipoprotein (LDL) to smaller, denser particles. It is very common in type II DM.

4. Treatment

      a. Diet must be individualized, as for type I DM. In obese patients, the goal should be weight loss, which may restore insulin responsiveness.

      b. Cholesterol, protein, fat, fiber, and artificial sweetener recommendations are the same as in type I DM.

      c. Regular exercise also is correlated with better glucose control.

      d. Oral hypoglycemic agents potentiate insulin secretion.

          (1) The most common are the sulfonylureas; of these, glyburide, glipizide, and glimepiride are second-generation agents with few drug interactions.

          (2) Other, newer insulin-stimulating drugs are repaglinide and nateglinide.

      e. Metformin, which reduces hepatic glucose production, may be added as a second agent.

      f. Thiazolidinediones (rosiglitazone, pioglitazone) sensitize peripheral tissues to insulin and may be used either alone or in combination with a sulfonylurea, metformin, or insulin.

      g. α-Glucosidase inhibitors (acarbose, miglitol) delay absorption of carbohydrate from the intestine.

      h. Approximately one-third of patients with type II DM require insulin.

      i. Exenatide stimulates the insulin response in response to glucose and prevents glucagon release after meals.

      j. Acceptable glucose levels are 90–130 mg/dL before meals and after an overnight fast and 180 mg/dL or less at 1 hour and less than 150 mg/dL at 2 hours postprandially. Patients should monitor glucose levels regularly.

      k. Careful foot care, moderate exercise, meticulous personal hygiene, and prompt treatment of infection are imperative.

      l. Daily aspirin (81–325 mg) reduces the risk of diabetic atherothrombosis.

D. Hypoglycemia

1. General characteristics

      a. Fasting hypoglycemia occurs secondary to some endocrine disorders, liver malfunction, and renal failure; primary hypoglycemia is caused by either hyperinsulinism (e.g., exogenous administration, insulinoma) or extrapancreatic tumors.

      b. Postprandial or reactive hypoglycemia is classified as early (2–3 hours after eating) or late (3–5 hours after eating).

      c. Other causes include postgastrectomy, functional, β-cell dysfunction, alcohol related, factitious, immunopathologic, and pentamidine induced.

2. Clinical features

      a. Symptoms begin at plasma glucose levels of 60 mg/dL; cognitive impairment begins at 50 mg/dL.

      b. Fasting hypoglycemia often is subacute or chronic and presents with neuroglycopenia.

c. Postprandial hypoglycemia usually is acute and presents with sweating, palpitations, anxiety, and tremulousness.

d. The Whipple's triad consists of a history of hypoglycemic symptoms, a fasting blood glucose of 40 mg/dL or less, and immediate recovery on administration of glucose.

3. Laboratory studies depend on the suspected cause.

4. Treatment is directed at the underlying cause.

IV. ADRENAL DISORDERS

A. Chronic adrenocortical insufficiency (Addison's disease)

1. General characteristics

a. The most common cause is autoimmune destruction of the adrenal cortex (80% of cases).

b. It may occur alone or as part of polyglandular autoimmune syndrome or other genetic disorders.

c. Pituitary failure causes secondary adrenocortical insufficiency.

d. Adrenal crises may be precipitated by infection, trauma, surgery, stress, or cessation of corticosteroid medication.

2. Clinical features

a. Addison's disease begins insidiously with nonspecific problems, such as fatigue and weakness. Anorexia and weight loss usually are present, as is irritability.

b. Most patients have myalgias and arthritis; many have GI symptoms.

c. Many patients develop sensory hypersensitivities.

d. Some patients crave salt.

e. Orthostatic hypotension is common.

f. Delayed deep tendon reflexes are found.

g. Hyperpigmentation is found only in primary disease (i.e., when adrenocorticotropic hormone [ACTH] is elevated).

h. Other findings include small heart, hyperplasia of lymphoid tissues, and scant axillary and pubic hair.

i. Addisonian crisis is heralded by acute pain (abdomen, low back), vomiting, diarrhea, dehydration, hypotension, and altered mental status. If untreated, it can be fatal.

3. Laboratory studies

a. Laboratory findings include hyperkalemia (only in primary disease), hyponatremia, hypoglycemia, hypercalcemia, and low urea nitrogen.

b. Neutropenia, mild anemia, relative lymphocytosis, and eosinophilia may occur.

c. Low (<3 μg/dL) 8:00 AM plasma cortisol accompanied by elevation of the plasma ACTH (>200 mg/dL) is diagnostic. Low levels of ACTH indicate secondary disease.

d. The cosyntropin stimulation test also is diagnostic. A serum cortisol rise of more than 20 μg/dL after administration of cosyntropin is normal; anything less is suspicious.

e. Antiadrenal antibodies will be present in 50% of patients; antithyroid antibodies are found in 45% of patients.

4. Treatment

a. Primary disease is treated with oral hydrocortisone or prednisone; many patients also require fludrocortisone acetate for its sodium-retaining effect.

b. Dehydroepiandrosterone may be given to some women who have adrenal insufficiency.

c. Addisonian crisis requires aggressive IV saline, glucose, and glucocorticoids.

B. Cushing's disease and syndrome (hypercortisolism)

1. General characteristics

a. Cushing's syndrome may be exogenous or endogenous. The exogenous form is caused by chronic excess glucocorticoid, most commonly from corticosteroid drugs used to treat other diseases.

b. Cushing's disease is caused by excess secretion of ACTH by the pituitary, often resulting from a small, benign pituitary adenoma.

(1) Cushing's disease is the major cause of endogenous Cushing's syndrome.

(2) It is most common in premenopausal women.

c. Adrenocortical tumors and nonpituitary ACTH-producing tumors (most often small cell lung carcinoma) also may cause Cushing's syndrome.

2. Clinical features

    a. Hypercortisolism may present as obesity, hypertension, and DM.

        (1) Obesity is centripetal, and extremities may appear wasted.

        (2) Fat deposition also causes the characteristic buffalo hump, moon facies, and supraclavicular pads.

    b. The most specific signs are proximal muscle weakness and pigmented striae more than 1 cm wide; patients may present with backache and headache.

    c. Oligomenorrhea or amenorrhea and erectile dysfunction are common.

    d. Disorders of calcium metabolism may cause osteoporosis, vertebral fractures, hypercalciuria, and kidney stones. Avascular necrosis may occur.

    e. Wound healing, acne, easy bruisability, and superficial skin infections occur.

    f. Psychiatric symptoms range from emotional lability to psychosis.

3. Laboratory studies

    a. Excretion of free cortisol in the urine of greater than 125 mg/dL in 24 hours is diagnostic.

    b. In Cushing's disease, the overnight dexamethasone suppression test will result in a plasma cortisol of greater than 10 mg/dL (<5 mg/dL is normal).

    c. The cortisol excretion test and plasma cortisol test should be confirmed with a low-dose dexamethasone suppression test. False positives are caused by rifampin, phenytoin, primidone, phenobarbital, carbamazepine, estrogens, and pregnancy.

    d. Plasma ACTH of less than 20 pg/mL suggests adrenal tumor; higher levels suggest pituitary or ectopic production.

    e. CT may show adrenocortical or other tumors. MRI is better to identify pituitary tumors.

    f. Hyperglycemia and hypokalemia are not unusual.

4. Treatment

    a. Treatment of Cushing's disease is transsphenoidal resection of the pituitary adenoma and hydrocortisol replacement; an alternative is gamma-knife radiosurgery.

    b. Surgical removal of tumors is the treatment of choice for Cushing's syndrome.

    c. Radiation and chemotherapy may be used for nonresectable tumors.

    d. Adrenal inhibitors also can be used.

        (1) Metyrapone and/or ketoconazole may suppress hypercortisolism.

        (2) Parenteral octreotide suppresses ACTH in one-third of cases.

V. PITUITARY DISORDERS

A. Acromegaly or gigantism

1. General characteristics

    a. Acromegaly almost always is caused by a pituitary adenoma and involves excessive growth hormone.

    b. It usually is sporadic but may be familial; it also may be part of multiple endocrine neoplasia type 1.

2. Clinical features

    a. Excessive growth of hands, feet, jaw, and internal organs occurs in acromegaly.

    b. Gigantism occurs if disease ensues before closure of the epiphyses.

    c. Other features include doughy, moist handshake; carpal tunnel syndrome; deep, coarse voice; obstructive sleep apnea; goiter; hypertension and cardiomegaly; weight gain and insulin resistance; arthralgias and arthritis; colon polyps; hyperhydrosis; cystic acne; acanthosis nigricans; headaches; decreased libido; erectile dysfunction; and menstrual abnormalities.

3. Laboratory studies

    a. Serum prolactin, insulin-like growth factor I, glucose, liver enzymes, BUN, TSH, free T_4, inorganic phosphorus, and calcium are measured after an overnight fast.

    b. Serum growth hormone is measured 1 hour after glucose syrup ingestion.

    c. Radiology

      (1) MRI is superior to CT for pituitary adenomas, which are present in 90% of patients with acromegaly.

      (2) Radiography may show enlarged sella turcica, thickened skull, tufting of the terminal phalanges, and thickening of the heel pad.

   4. Treatment

     a. Treatment generally is endoscopic transnasal, transsphenoidal pituitary microsurgery to remove the adenoma.

     b. Dopamine agonists are used in patients who fail surgery.

     c. Somatostatin analogs are beneficial for persistent disease.

     d. Pegvisomant, a growth hormone–receptor antagonist, provides symptomatic relief and normalizes insulin-like growth factor I in about 90% of patients.

     e. Stereotactic radiosurgery is used for treatment failures.

B. Dwarfism

   1. General characteristics. The prototype chondroplasia is achondroplasia, the most common nonlethal type.

   2. Clinical features

     a. Achondroplastic dwarfs

       (1) These dwarfs have short limbs, long and narrow trunks, large heads with midface hypoplasia, and prominent brows.

       (2) They have delayed motor milestones and fall below normal height standards.

       (3) Intelligence is normal.

       (4) Neurologic complications, bowing of the legs, obesity, dental problems, and frequent otitis media are common.

     b. A substantial reduction in height may occur in children who have type I DM.

     c. Although not usually apparent at birth, pituitary dwarfism may present in male infants with hypoglycemia and micropenis.

     d. Children with constitutional growth delay are small but otherwise of normal appearance.

   3. Laboratory studies. The achondroplasia group of disorders are all caused by mutations in the *FGFR3* gene.

   4. Treatment

     a. Surgical correction of orthopaedic problems is indicated in achondroplasia.

     b. Use of human growth hormone is controversial.

C. Diabetes insipidus (DI)

   1. General characteristics

     a. DI is uncommon and caused by deficiency of or resistance to vasopressin.

     b. Primary DI may be familial or sporadic.

     c. Secondary DI is caused by hypothalamic or pituitary pathology caused by tumor, anoxic encephalopathy, surgery, accidental trauma, infection, sarcoidosis, multifocal Langerhans cell granulomatosis, or metastatic disease.

     d. Vasopressinase-induced DI may be seen during late pregnancy and the puerperium.

     e. Nephrogenic DI occurs in the presence of normal secretion of vasopressin with inappropriate response by the kidney.

   2. Clinical features

     a. Intense thirst, craving for ice water, and large-volume polyuria are most common; other possible presentations are hypernatremia and dehydration.

     b. Unremitting enuresis may be present in partial disease.

   3. No single laboratory study can diagnose DI.

     a. Serum tests include glucose, BUN, calcium, uric acid, potassium, and sodium.

     b. Urine collection for 24 hours is needed for volume, glucose, and creatinine; dipstick testing shows a low specific gravity, usually less than 1.006.

     c. Central DI may be confirmed with a vasopressin challenge test.

   4. Treatment

     a. Desmopressin acetate is the treatment of choice for central DI and for DI associated with pregnancy and the puerperium.

b. Mild cases may require no treatment except adequate hydration.

c. Central and nephrogenic DI respond partially to hydrochlorothiazide.

d. Nephrogenic DI may respond to indomethacin, either alone or in combination with hydrochlorothiazide, desmopressin, or ameloride.

VI. OTHER ENDOCRINE DISORDERS

A. Metabolic bone disease

1. Osteoporosis (see Chapter 9)

2. Osteomalacia and rickets

a. General characteristics

(1) Osteomalacia and rickets are diseases of defective mineralization.

(2) Osteomalacia is found in adults; rickets is found in children.

(3) Both most often are caused by a deficiency of vitamin D; they also may be caused by calcium or phosphate deficiency or by aluminum toxicity. Other causes include disorders of bone matrix and inhibitors of mineralization.

(4) Phenytoin may induce osteomalacia.

b. Clinical features

(1) Patients with osteomalacia present with diffuse muscle weakness (especially in the pelvic girdle) and bone pain.

(2) Children develop permanent skeletal deformities.

c. Laboratory studies

(1) In osteomalacia, radiography shows generalized decrease in bone density; Milkman lines or Looser zones (pseudofractures) are diagnostic.

(2) Both osteomalacia and rickets may be diagnosed by bone biopsy, although biopsy is not necessary.

(3) Hypocalcemia, hypocalciuria, hypophosphatemia, secondary hyperparathyroidism, increased alkaline phosphatase, and decreased 25-hydroxyvitamin D may be present.

d. Treatment

(1) Ergocalciferol (50,000 U by mouth twice per week for 6–12 months, followed by 1,000 U daily) treats vitamin D deficiency.

(2) Phosphate supplementation and vitamin D are required for renal phosphate wasting.

(3) Oral calcium should be given with meals to treat nutritional calcium deficiency.

(4) Aluminum-containing antacids should be discontinued.

(5) Patients on phenytoin should be treated prophylactically.

3. Paget's disease of bone (osteitis deformans)

a. General characteristics

(1) Paget's disease of bone involves localized dysplastic bone formation.

(2) It affects 3% of adults and 5–11% of those in their 80s. Prevalence is highest among the elderly in the northeastern United States.

(3) Patients may have a family history of Paget's disease.

(4) Long-standing lesions in 1–3% of patients transform into osteosarcoma.

b. Clinical features

(1) Most patients (three-quarters) are asymptomatic.

(2) Bone and joint pain often is the first symptom.

(a) Common sites of involvement are spine, pelvis, femur, humerus, and skull.

(b) Patients may present with pathologic fractures or other symptoms related to the site (e.g., headache, increased hat size, warmth).

(3) Patients also may have bowed tibias and kyphosis.

(4) Deafness is the most common neurologic finding.

(5) Cardiac output may increase and progress to failure.

    c. Laboratory studies

      (1) Serum calcium and phosphate are normal; alkaline phosphatase is high.

      (2) Hypercalciuria is common, and urinary hydroxyproline is elevated in active disease.

      (3) Hypercalcemia occurs in patients on bed rest.

      (4) The extent of the disease should be determined by skeletal radiography (dense, expanded bone; fissures in long bone) and bone scans.

    d. Treatment

      (1) Prompt cyclic administration of bisphosphonates (alendronate, etidronate, tiludronate, risedronate, zoledronic acid, or pamidronate) is the treatment of choice.

      (2) Nasal calcitonin-salmon is an alternative treatment.

B. Dyslipidemia

  1. General characteristics

    a. Dyslipidemias are highly associated with atherosclerosis, especially CAD.

    b. Reducing total cholesterol in patients with known cardiovascular disease reduces total mortality in both men and women and in middle-aged and older patients; in patients without cardiovascular disease, results are less conclusive.

    c. LDL cholesterol is associated with increased risk of atherosclerotic heart disease, and HDL cholesterol is associated with decreased risk.

    d. Hypertriglyceridemia is a risk factor for CAD, especially in women and diabetics. Severe elevations can cause pancreatitis.

    e. Genetic forms of dyslipidemia are rare, but patients with a history of familial hypercholesterolemia, familial combined hyperlipidemia, familial hyperchylomicronemia, or dysbetalipoproteinemia must be screened.

    f. Secondary hyperlipidemia has many possible causes, including diabetes, alcohol use, hypothyroidism, hypercortisolism, acromegaly, obesity, sedentary lifestyle, renal and liver problems, estrogens, thiazide diuretics, and β-blockers.

  2. Clinical features

    a. Most patients have no symptoms or signs.

    b. Eruptive and tendinous xanthomas are pathognomonic for hyperlipidemia.

    c. Nearly two-thirds of all people with xanthelasmas (the commonest form of xanthomas, affecting the eyelids) have normal lipid profiles.

    d. Patients with severe hypercholesterolemia may develop premature arcus senilis; lipemia retinalis is seen with triglyceride levels of greater than 2,000 mg/dL.

  3. Laboratory studies

    a. Patients with any evidence of cardiovascular disease should be screened with a fasting complete lipid profile; those with cardiac risk factors should be screened with at least a total cholesterol.

    b. Screening for patients with no evidence of cardiovascular disease and no other risk factors should begin at 35 years of age for men and 45 years of age for women.

    c. Risk factors for cardiovascular disease include family history, hypertension, cigarette smoking, diabetes mellitus, low HDL cholesterol, older age, and male gender.

    d. Screening may include total cholesterol alone, total and HDL cholesterol, or LDL and HDL cholesterol levels only.

  4. Treatment

    a. Nonpharmacologic therapy

      (1) Initial dietary changes should include reducing total dietary fat to 25–30% and saturated fat to less than 7% of calories; some diets reduce fat even further. The Mediterranean diet reduces LDL cholesterol without reducing HDLs. Dietary cholesterol should not exceed 200 mg daily.

      (2) Soluble fiber, garlic, soy, pecans, plant sterols and vitamin C also may help to reduce LDL cholesterol.

      (3) The diet should be high in antioxidant-containing fruits and vegetables.

      (4) Patients should be encouraged to increase aerobic exercise to increase levels of HDL.

b. Pharmacologic treatment

    (1) Patients with high LDL cholesterol and a significant risk of CAD should take aspirin, 81–325 mg daily, unless contraindicated. This will reduce the risk of thromboembolism.

    (2) Postmenopausal estrogen replacement increases HDL and reduces LDL cholesterol.

    (3) Niacin is associated with reduced long-term mortality and has an optimal effect on lipids, but it is poorly tolerated at full doses because of flushing of the skin.

    (4) Resins that bind bile acids in the intestine include cholestyramine, cholesevelam, and colestipol. These resins reduce the incidence of coronary events in middle-aged men, but they have no effect on mortality.

    (5) 3-Hydroxy-3-methylglutaryl–coenzyme A reductase inhibitors (e.g., lovastatin, pravastatin, simvastatin, fluvastatin, rosuvastatin, and atorvastatin)

        (a) These inhibit the rate-limiting enzyme in formation of cholesterol.

        (b) They also reduce CAD and total mortality in secondary prevention.

        (c) Myositis is a common side effect, especially in patients also taking niacin or a fibrate.

    (6) Fibric acid derivatives include gemfibrozil, clofibrate, and fenofibrate.

        (a) They reduce synthesis and increase breakdown of very-low-density lipoproteins.

        (b) Their side effects include cholelithiasis, hepatitis, and myositis.

        (c) Clofibrate is associated with a statistically significant increase in cancer mortality.

    (7) Ezetimibe blocks intestinal absorption of dietary and biliary cholesterol and may be used as monotherapy or in combination with a statin.

11

Neurology

William H. Marquardt

I. CEREBROVASCULAR DISEASE

A. Stroke

   1. General characteristics

   a. Stroke is the third most common cause of death in the United States and the most disabling neurologic disorder.

   b. The overall incidence of stroke has decreased over the past three decades, likely secondary to increased awareness and a more aggressive focus on prevention.

   c. The incidence of stroke increases with age, is higher in men than in women, and is higher in blacks than in whites.

   d. The major risk factors for stroke include hypertension, hypercholesterolemia, diabetes, oral contraceptives, cigarette smoking, heavy alcohol use, AIDS, and elevated blood homocysteine levels.

   e. Ischemic strokes account for 80% of all strokes. Two-thirds of ischemic strokes are thrombotic, and one-third are embolic. Emboli commonly arise from the heart, aortic arch, or large cerebral arteries.

   f. Hemorrhagic strokes, which usually are secondary to hypertension, account for 20% of strokes.

   2. Clinical features

   a. Signs and symptoms of stroke begin abruptly and, by definition, last longer than 24 hours. They correlate with the area of the brain that is supplied by the affected vessel, especially with ischemic events.

   b. In most cases, hemiparesis or hemisensory deficit is revealed on history and physical examination. One can localize the lesion to one side, contralateral to these deficits.

   c. Strokes involving the anterior circulation (anterior choroidal, anterior cerebral, middle cerebral arteries), which supplies the cortex, subcortical white matter, basal ganglia, and the internal capsule, commonly are associated with hemispheric signs and symptoms (aphasia, apraxia, hemiparesis, hemisensory losses, visual field defects).

   d. Strokes involving the posterior circulation (vertebral and basilar arteries), which supplies the brainstem, cerebellum, thalamus, and portions of the temporal and occipital lobes, commonly are associated with evidence of brainstem dysfunction (coma, drop attacks, vertigo, nausea, vomiting, ataxia).

   e. Thrombotic strokes evolve in a step-wise fashion and often are preceded by transient ischemic attacks. Embolic strokes occur abruptly and without warning. Hemorrhagic strokes are less predictable because of complications of blood dispersion, cerebral edema, and increased intracranial pressure.

   3. Laboratory studies

   a. Routine blood tests include CBC, erythrocyte sedimentation rate, platelet count, prothrombin time, partial thromboplastin time, cholesterol and lipids, and blood glucose level.

   b. Additional blood tests may include Venereal Disease Research Laboratory (VDRL) for syphilis, antinuclear antibodies, and serum lipids depending on patient risk factors.

   c. CT is recommended during the acute phase and is the best modality for differentiating ischemic versus hemorrhagic stroke.

   d. Additional imaging tests to evaluate stroke patients include MRI, carotid ultrasound, echocardiography, and angiography.

   e. Electrocardiography may reveal arrhythmia or a recent myocardial infarction as the possible source of embolus.

   f. Lumbar puncture and angiography should be reserved for patients with suspected hemorrhage or vascular malformations.

   4. Treatment

   a. Acute treatment is aimed at reversing the ischemia and salvaging tissue in the core and surrounding penumbra.

   b. Thrombolytic therapy (recombinant tissue plasminogen activator) is given to reduce the extent of deficit; it is most effective within 3 hours of symptoms but can be tried up to 12 hours.

      (1) The major complication is bleeding.

      (2) Contraindications include recent bleeds, chronic anticoagulant therapy, arterial puncture, or blood pressure above 185/110 mm Hg.

   c. Antiplatelet therapy is initiated for ischemic stroke and transient ischemic attack, whereas anticoagulant therapy is indicated in the setting of cardiac embolus.

   d. Endarterectomy may be indicated if 70–99% stenosis of the common or internal carotid artery is present.

   e. Hemorrhagic stroke is treated with conservative and supportive measures, including management of hypertension and antiedema therapy (mannitol and corticosteroids).

   f. Supportive therapy, follow-up physical therapy, and social supports are important.

B. Transient ischemic attack (TIA)

   1. General characteristics

   a. TIAs are noted most frequently in older patients and in those at risk for vascular disease.

   b. Sudden onset of focal neurologic deficits is secondary to disturbance of cerebral circulation.

   c. TIAs typically relate directly to either the carotid or the vertebral vascular distribution.

   d. Most TIAs only last for a few minutes, but symptoms may persist for more than 1 hour. By definition, symptoms resolve completely within 24 hours.

   e. Although TIAs are brief and transient, one-third of these patients will have a stroke within 5 years.

   2. Clinical features

   a. If the TIA is related to a disturbance in carotid circulation, patients may demonstrate hand–arm weakness with sensory loss, ipsilateral visual symptoms or aphasia, or amaurosis fugax. Carotid bruit may be present, but with a high-grade stenosis (>95%), bruit may be absent.

   b. Those experiencing vertebrovascular TIA may demonstrate diplopia, ataxia, vertigo, dysarthria, cranial nerve palsies, lower extremity weakness, perioral numbness, or drop attacks.

   c. The differential diagnosis of TIA includes generalized seizure, migraine, syncope, and mass lesions.

   3. Diagnostic studies

   a. Arteriography is the definitive study, but magnetic resonance angiography also is used and is less invasive.

   b. Cardiac workup should be done to exclude arrhythmia and new murmurs. The heart is a very common source of emboli.

   c. A hematologic workup must be done to identify coagulopathies.

   (1) An erythrocyte sedimentation rate will effectively rule out temporal arteritis.

   (2) Other studies include CBC with differential, cholesterol, prothrombin time, partial thromboplastin time, and antiphospholipids.

   d. Other studies to evaluate possible cardiogenic or carotid emboli are two-dimensional echocardiography, electrocardiography, and carotid Doppler imaging.

   4. Treatment

   a. Because a TIA may indicate an impending stroke, prophylactic antiplatelet therapy is initiated when the TIA is not cardiogenic. This therapy might include aspirin, ticlopidine, clopidogrel, sulfinpyrazone, or dipyridamole.

   b. Cardiogenic TIA requires anticoagulation, initially with IV heparin for those who are admitted to the hospital and with warfarin for long-term therapy.

   c. Carotid endarterectomy may be indicated in patients with anterior circulation TIAs and moderate- to high-grade carotid stenosis on the side appropriate to account for the symptoms.

   d. Vital adjunct therapies include control of blood pressure, serum cholesterol, and atrial fibrillation. Patients also must be urged to discontinue cigarette smoking and to avoid excessive use of alcohol.

C. Cerebral aneurysm

   1. General characteristics

   a. A ruptured cerebral arterial aneurysm or, less commonly, an arteriovenous malformation causes bleeding into the subarachnoid space.

   b. Ruptured saccular (berry) aneurysm accounts for approximately 75% of nontraumatic cases of subarachnoid hemorrhage (SAH) and has a mortality rate of 50%. It most often occurs during the fifth and sixth decades of life, with an approximately equal gender distribution.

   c. Intracranial arteriovenous malformation counts for less than 10% of SAHs. It occurs twice as often in men and typically during the second to fourth decades.

2. Clinical features

a. The classic SAH presents as sudden onset of an unusually severe, generalized headache, which patients may describe as "the worst headache I've had in my life." The headache may be followed by nausea and vomiting and an altered state of consciousness.

b. The headache may remain unchanged for several days and subside only slowly over 1–2 weeks.

c. Frequently, blood pressure rises precipitously as a result of the hemorrhage.

d. Patients with SAH may develop a temperature of up to 102°F (38.9°C) and frequently display confusion, stupor, coma, and nuchal rigidity or other signs of meningeal irritation.

e. A herald bleed, or aneurysmal leak, occurs in up to 40% of patients, producing a less severe but atypical headache and accompanied by focal neurologic signs resulting from pressure on the brain or cranial nerves.

3. Laboratory studies

a. CT is the initial investigational modality for suspected SAH; more than 90% of patients with aneurysmal rupture will be identified in this way.

b. Evaluation of cerebrospinal fluid (CSF) reveals markedly elevated opening pressures and grossly bloody fluid.

c. Cerebral angiography should be done to evaluate the entire vasculature when convenient, because as many as 20% of individuals will have multiple aneurysms.

d. Electroencephalography (EEG) may indicate the side or site of hemorrhage or may show only diffuse, non-specific changes.

4. Treatment

a. Supportive medical treatment involves prevention of elevated arterial or intracranial pressures that might lead to rerupture of the affected vessel. It also may include strict bed rest, mild sedation, or administration of stool softeners to prevent straining.

b. Management of hypertension is important, but care must be taken to prevent hypotension and inadequate cerebral perfusion.

c. Surgical management includes the clipping or wrapping of aneurysms, depending on the clinical state of the patient, and removal or embolization of an arteriovenous malformation by intra-arterial catheter.

II. SEIZURE DISORDERS

A. General characteristics

1. Idiopathic seizures usually begin between 5–20 years of age and have no specific cause.

2. Secondary seizures may result from congenital abnormalities and perinatal injury, metabolic disorders, trauma, tumors, vascular disease, infectious diseases, or degenerative diseases, such as Alzheimer's disease.

3. Seizures are transient disturbances of cerebral function caused by abnormal paroxysmal neuronal discharges in the brain.

4. Seizures are characterized as either generalized or partial, depending on whether the disturbance affects the entire brain or only a portion.

5. Status epilepticus, either convulsive or nonconvulsive, is diagnosed when seizures fail to cease spontaneously or recur so frequently that full consciousness is not restored between successive episodes.

B. Clinical features

1. Generalized seizures are characterized by a sudden loss of consciousness and are either convulsive (grand mal or tonic-clonic) seizures or nonconvulsive (absence) seizures.

a. Generalized convulsive seizures are associated with a postictal obtundation and confusion lasting from minutes to hours.

b. Generalized nonconvulsive seizures are associated with only minor motor activity, such as blinking.

2. Partial seizures

a. Simple partial seizures are not accompanied by an impairment of consciousness. There may be isolated tonic or clonic activity of a limb or transient altered sensory perception, which may spread to include the entire side of the body in a "jacksonian march."

b. Complex partial (temporal lobe) seizures often are characterized by an aura (transient abnormalities in sensation, perception, emotion, or memory), followed by impaired consciousness lasting for seconds to minutes. Nausea or vomiting, focal sensory perceptions, and focal tonic or clonic activity may accompany a complex seizure.

C. Laboratory studies

1. In generalized absence seizures, EEG typically shows generalized spikes and associated slow waves.

2. In simple partial seizures, EEG may show a focal rhythmic discharge at the onset of the seizure, but occasionally, no ictal activity will be seen.

3. EEG in complex partial seizures often reveals interictal spikes or spikes associated with slow waves in the temporal or frontotemporal areas.

4. Other laboratory studies, such as CBC, blood glucose, liver and renal functions, and serologic test for syphilis, are indicated to evaluate potential metabolic or toxic causes.

D. Treatment

1. Correction of hyponatremia, hypoglycemia, or drug intoxication may be all that is necessary to control seizures.

2. Anticonvulsant therapy typically is not indicated in the setting of a single, unprovoked seizure in a patient with a normal neurologic examination and normal brain imaging and EEG.

3. The goal of medical therapy is to prevent seizures by using a single agent in progressive doses until seizures are controlled or toxicity occurs.

   [handwritten: Tegretol]
   [handwritten: Dilantin]

   a. Generalized convulsive, simple partial, and complex partial seizures typically are treated with carbamazepine, phenytoin, and valproic acid; phenobarbital and primidone are less effective. Newer anticonvulsants, such as gabapentin, topirimate, lamotrigine, oxcarbazine, levetiracetam, and zonisamide, also are effective.

   [handwritten: Topamax] *[handwritten: Keppra]*

   b. Felbamate typically is reserved for patients who are unresponsive to other medications or combinations because of serious potential side effects.

   [handwritten: Depakene]

   c. Valproic acid or ethosuximide is used for generalized, nonconvulsive (absence) seizures.

   [handwritten: Zarontin]

4. Because of the possibility of permanent brain damage secondary to hyperthermia, circulatory collapse, or excito-toxic neuronal damage, status epilepticus is a medical emergency.

   a. Immediate management must ensure a patent airway, including positioning the patient to prevent aspiration of stomach contents.

   b. Management of hyperthermia, related to increased motor activity and high levels of circulating catecholamines, may include a cooling blanket or induction of motor paralysis with a neuromuscular blocking agent.

   c. Diazepam or lorazepam is administered IV until the seizures stop; a loading dose of phenytoin or fosphenytoin also is given.

III. MULTIPLE SCLEROSIS (MS)

A. General characteristics

1. MS is characterized by inflammation associated with multiple foci of demyelination in the central nervous system (CNS) white matter.

2. Patients with MS typically follow either a relapsing–remitting pattern of episodes or a chronic progressive course. A secondary progressive form also is seen, in which the relapsing–remitting pattern changes to one of progressive degeneration.

3. MS is thought to be an immunologic disorder associated with CNS immunoglobulin production and alteration of T lymphocytes. A viral infection may act as a precipitant.

4. Based on numerous studies of twins, familial cases, and the association with specific HLA antigens (HLA-DR2), a genetic relationship is considered to be likely.

5. MS typically begins between 18 and 45 years of age; women are affected more often than men.

B. Clinical features

1. Patients initially may present with any of an array of symptoms, including focal weakness, numbness or tingling, optic neuritis, diplopia, focal neuralgias, balance problems, or urinary symptoms.

2. Symptoms last for days to weeks and affect different areas over different events.

3. Patients often develop cognitive and psychological deficits.

4. The diagnosis must be questioned if signs and symptoms are not related to multiple areas of the CNS over time.

C. Laboratory studies

1. The diagnosis cannot be based exclusively on laboratory findings.

2. MRI with gadolinium is very effective for visualizing white matter lesions in the CNS.

3. CSF can reveal a sterile inflammation with a mild protein elevation, elevated immunoglobulin G index, oligo-clonal bands, and increased myelin basic protein.

4. Visual, auditory, and somatosensory-evoked potentials are helpful for assessing nerve transmission.

D. Treatment

1. Corticosteroids may hasten maximal recovery from acute exacerbations. High-dose IV corticosteroids often are used in the setting of optic neuritis.

2. Interferon-β decreases the frequency of relapses, especially moderate and severe attacks.

3. Daily subcutaneous injections of glatiramer acetate also decrease the frequency of relapses, especially in mild disease.

4. Otherwise, therapy is symptomatic.

   a. Amantadine and pemoline can improve fatigue.

   b. Baclofen and diazepam improve spasticity.

   c. Several agents may relieve urologic dysfunction.

IV. DEMENTIA

A. General characteristics

1. Dementia is characterized by a progressive impairment of intellectual functioning, with compromise in at least two of the following spheres of mental activity: language, memory, visuospatial skills, emotional behavior, personality, and cognition.

2. Alzheimer's disease is the most common form of dementia; other forms are referred to as senile dementia.

B. Alzheimer's disease

1. General characteristics

   a. Alzheimer's is the most common cause of chronic dementia, constituting 60–80% of patients with dementia.

   b. The disease is characterized by steadily progressive memory loss and other cognitive deficits and typically begins during the sixth or seventh decade of life.

   c. Genetic factors have been identified, and familial cases have been mapped to chromosomes 1, 14, 19, and 21.

   d. Alzheimer's disease has a characteristic pathology, consisting of intracellular neurofibrillary tangles and extra-cellular neuritic plaques.

2. Clinical features

   a. The diagnosis can be established when an otherwise alert patient exhibits progressive memory loss and other cognitive deficits, such as disorientation, language difficulties, inability to perform complex motor activities, inattention, visual misperception, poor problem-solving abilities, inappropriate social behavior, or hallucinations.

   b. Intellectual decline should be present in two or more areas of cognition and documented by a mental status examination or similar scale.

   c. Formal neuropsychological testing can confirm the diagnosis and document the progression of disease.

3. Laboratory studies

   a. Laboratory tests include CBC, heavy metal screens, serum electrolytes, calcium, glucose, thyroid-stimulating hormone, vitamin B_{12}, renal and liver function tests, and drug and alcohol levels

   b. MRI or CT is helpful only in ruling out other treatable causes of dementia.

4. Treatment

   a. Standard medical therapy, initially in low doses, is useful in treating insomnia, agitation, and depression.

   b. A trial of acetylcholinesterase inhibitors, such as tacrine, donepezil, galantamine, or rivastigmine, may improve memory function. Memantine is a N-methyl-D-aspartic acid (NMDA) receptor antagonist that is thought to regulate glutamate and has been approved for use in severe Alzheimer's disease

   c. The patient will require vigilant family supervision. Day care centers and respite care are adjuncts to family supervision.

C. Senile dementia

1. General characteristics

   a. Between 15 and 20% of patients with a chronic dementia have a vascular dementia, usually referred to as multi-infarct dementia, which includes lacunar and multiple cortical infarcts.

(1) Multi-infarct dementia is more common in men than in women.

(2) It is associated with hypertension, with or without a history of TIA or stroke.

b. A similar percentage of patients (15–20%) has evidence of both vascular and Alzheimer-type dementia; the correct diagnosis for the large majority of these patients is Alzheimer's disease.

2. Clinical features

a. Senile dementia usually manifests as forgetfulness in the absence of depression and inattentiveness. Symptoms typically occur in a step-wise fashion.

b. Social graces may be well maintained, so mental status testing is important to establish the diagnosis.

c. Progression of the disease leads to loss of computational ability, problems with word-finding and concentration, difficulty with routine daily activities, and ultimately, complete disorientation and social withdrawal.

3. Laboratory studies. Laboratory testing and imaging are useful only in establishing other, treatable causes of dementia.

4. Treatment

a. Control of hypertension and metabolic disorders may help to slow the progression of symptoms.

b. As in Alzheimer's disease, standard medical regimens can be used to treat insomnia, agitation, or depression.

c. Caregivers should identify and reduce home hazards and arrange, as necessary, community services or preparation of an advance directive.

V. HEADACHE

A. Tension headache

1. General characteristics

a. Tension headaches were once thought to be caused by muscle contraction. Current theory relates tension headaches to abnormal neuronal sensitivity.

b. There may be an associated history of significant stress or minor trauma to the head or neck.

c. Tension headache is the most frequent type of headache and is very costly (because of loss of productivity).

2. Clinical features

a. Tension headaches are typified by a band-like pain around the head or generalized head pain. Discomfort usually is reported as steady or aching (nonpulsatile) and is not associated with focal neurologic symptoms. It typically is bilateral and without photophobia, phonophobia, nausea, or vomiting.

b. Pain may be episodic or chronic. Stress, sleep deprivation, hunger, and eyestrain are typical precipitants.

c. Posterior cervical and occipital muscles, or the scalp, may be tender, but the physical examination generally is normal.

3. Laboratory studies

a. Routine laboratory tests are helpful only in ruling out concurrent illness or an underlying rheumatologic condition.

b. Imaging studies, lumbar puncture, or EEG are done only if there is a high index of suspicion for structural lesion.

4. Treatment

a. Medical treatment generally is with simple analgesics, such as aspirin, acetaminophen, or nonsteroidal anti-inflammatory drugs (NSAIDs).

b. When appropriate, local heat and muscle relaxants may be employed for muscle-tension discomfort. Physical therapy and stress reduction techniques also are helpful.

c. In the setting of depression or significant stress or chronic recalcitrant tension headaches, antidepressants or psychotherapy may be indicated.

B. Migraine headache

1. General characteristics

a. Migraine headaches more typically present unilaterally, with throbbing or pulsating discomfort. Patients often identify migraine triggers, including chocolate, red wine, hard cheeses, monosodium glutamate, hormonal changes, exertion, fatigue, and stress.

    b. Patients often relate a family history of migraine disease. Women are affected more commonly than men; migraines often follow the menstrual cycle pattern.

    c. The pathophysiology of migraines classically has been attributed to intracranial vasospasm followed by extracranial vasodilatation. More current theories relate to dysfunction of the trigeminovascular system, resulting in the perivascular release of substance P.

    d. Migraine often is associated with other diseases, such as seizure disorders, essential tremor, Tourette's syndrome, depression, anxiety, and stroke.

2. Clinical features

    a. As the name indicates, migraine with aura (formerly called classic migraine) presents with an aura, commonly involving visual changes, field cuts, or flashing lights affecting one visual hemifield.

        (1) The throbbing pain often is contralateral to the aura and associated with the other symptoms that are seen in migraine without aura.

        (2) Migraine with aura also can be associated with transient neurologic deficits and hemisensory loss.

    b. Migraine without aura (formerly called common migraine) frequently is accompanied by nausea, vomiting, photophobia, phonophobia, and anorexia.

    c. Patients also exhibit irritability and fatigue.

    d. Migraine patients often retreat to quiet, dark rooms and prefer to lie quietly.

3. Laboratory studies

    a. Routine laboratory tests are done only to help rule out other concurrent disorders.

    b. Imaging studies or lumbar puncture is done only in select clinical settings and then only to rule out causes of acute secondary headache.

4. Treatment

    a. Mild to moderate migraine headache

        (1) Abortive therapy may include aspirin, acetaminophen, NSAIDs, or isometheptene.

        (2) Subsequent measures for migraine might include serotonin-receptor agonists, such as various forms of the triptans (e.g., sumatriptan, zolmitriptan, rizatriptan, naratriptan, almotriptan, frovatriptan, eletriptan). Various forms of the ergotamines also are useful.

    b. In the setting of frequent migraine headache, prophylactic measures may be employed.

        (1) Medical prophylaxis for migraine might include β-blockers, tricyclic antidepressants, calcium channel blockers, NSAIDs, valproic acid, or topiramate.

        (2) Biofeedback therapy often is employed in migraine patients in the hope of reducing the number of headaches by helping patients deal more effectively with stress.

        (3) Botox injections may be helpful in patients with severe, intractable migraine.

    c. Patients with triggers should avoid exposure.

    d. Psychotherapy and stress reduction may be needed.

C. Cluster headache

1. General characteristics

    a. Cluster headaches are severe, unilateral, periorbital headaches that last for 30–90 minutes and occur several times a day over a period of weeks to months.

    b. The typical patient with cluster headaches is a middle-aged man.

2. Clinical features

    a. The unilateral pain of cluster headache often is accompanied by ipsilateral lacrimation, conjunctival injection, nasal congestion, and myosis and ptosis.

    b. Patients with cluster headache often pace incessantly around the room, because the pain is severe and is not relieved by rest.

3. Laboratory studies

    a. As in other headache syndromes, laboratory studies only help to identify other concurrent conditions and to rule out other causes of acute head and facial pain.

    b. Imaging studies or lumbar puncture is indicated only in specific clinical settings and to rule out other causes of acute cephalgia.

4. Treatment

    a. Abortive and symptomatic therapy for cluster headaches includes administration of 100% oxygen, injectable forms of ergotamines or sumatriptan, and analgesics (e.g., intranasal butorphanol) as indicated.

    b. Prophylactic therapy for cluster headaches includes lithium, calcium channel blockers, and oral corticosteroids.

VI. MOVEMENT DISORDERS

A. Benign essential (familial) tremor

    1. General characteristics

        a. The cause of benign essential tremor is unknown. It often is inherited in an autosomal dominant manner and may thus be called familial tremor.

        b. Tremor may begin at any age.

        c. It is enhanced by emotional stress; small quantities of alcohol commonly provide dramatic, temporary relief from the tremor.

        d. Although the tremor may interfere with manual skills, it causes only minimal disability.

    2. Clinical features

        a. Patients with benign essential tremor display a rhythmic, 6- to 8-Hz, to-and-fro movement, usually of the upper extremities but sometimes of the head (titubation).

        b. Speech also may be affected if the laryngeal muscles are involved.

    3. Laboratory studies. No laboratory testing is needed or warranted.

    4. Treatment

        a. Low doses of β-blockers, usually propranolol, may be useful in controlling tremor but, unless tremor is associated only with certain circumstances and intermittent dosing is adequate, will have to be used indefinitely.

        b. Primidone may be useful in controlling tremor if propranolol fails.

B. Parkinson's disease

    1. General characteristics

        a. Idiopathic Parkinson's occurs in all ethnic groups, with an approximately equal sex distribution, and most often begins between 45 and 65 years of age.

        b. Parkinson's disease is characterized by degeneration of cells in the substantia nigra, causing a deficiency of the neurotransmitter dopamine and an imbalance of dopamine and acetylcholine.

        c. Patients generally complain of problems related to their slowed movements, difficulty arising from a seated position, difficulty ascending and descending stairs, trouble with getting dressed, and difficulty with handwriting (micrographia).

    2. Clinical features

        a. The essential features that establish a diagnosis of Parkinson's disease are resting tremor, bradykinesia, rigidity, and postural instability.

        b. The tremor is most noticeable at rest, at 4–6 cycles/sec, and may be only very slight with voluntary effort. It typically is described as "pill-rolling."

        c. Initially, the tremor is confined to one limb or the limbs on one side, but eventually, it may be present in all limbs and the lips and mouth.

        d. Bradykinesia, or a generalized slowness of voluntary movements, is evident in the slow, shuffling gait; reduced arm swing; slowed rapid alternating movements; infrequent blinking; and mask-like facies.

        e. Rigidity is found on passive range of motion testing, and cogwheel rigidity may be noted.

        f. Postural instability is seen, including difficulty in standing from a seated position, unsteadiness on turning, difficulty in stopping, and a tendency to fall.

        g. Depression and cognitive impairment develop in more than 50% of patients over time.

    3. Laboratory studies

        a. Generally, no laboratory testing is needed or warranted.

        b. Blood tests and imaging studies can be done to rule out other causes.

4. Treatment

    a. Treatment is designed to best restore the balance between dopamine and acetylcholine by blocking the effect of acetylcholine with anticholinergic drugs, administering levodopa (the precursor of dopamine), or a combination of both.

    b. Amantadine, a mild anticholinergic, often is helpful for patients with mild symptoms but no disability.

    c. Benztropine and other anticholinergic drugs are particularly helpful in treating the tremor of Parkinson's disease and less helpful for bradykinesia.

    d. Levodopa is converted to dopamine in the body and improves all symptoms of Parkinson's disease. Carbidopa, when added to levodopa in various combinations, allows lower doses of levodopa and reduced side effects.

    e. Dopamine agonists, such as bromocriptine, act directly on dopamine receptors and often are reserved for patients who become refractory to levodopa therapy.

    f. Selegiline, a monoamine oxidase B inhibitor, inhibits breakdown of dopamine, and studies indicate it may arrest progression of the disease.

    g. Catecholamine-O-methyl-transferase (COMT) inhibitors reduce the metabolism of levodopa to 3-O-methyldopa and result in more stable plasma levels and more constant dopaminergic stimulation of the brain. Two COMT agents, tolapone and entacapone, are available as adjuncts to levodopa/carbidopa therapy.

    h. Physical therapy may help some patients, and quality of life may be improved with household modifications or the availability of special utensils.

    i. Psychological support for both the patient and the family are helpful.

C. Huntington's disease

    1. General characteristics

        a. Huntington's disease is an inherited, autosomal dominant disorder that occurs throughout the world in all ethnic groups, with a prevalence of less than 5 per 100,000.

        b. The gene responsible for Huntington's disease is on chromosome 4.

        c. Symptoms of the disease usually do not develop until after 30 years of age. By this time, those who are affected often have already had children who may be similarly affected.

    2. Clinical features

        a. The disease is characterized by progressive chorea and dementia; it is usually fatal within 15–20 years.

        b. The earliest mental changes often are behavioral, with irritability, moodiness, and antisocial behavior that generally progress to an obvious dementia.

        c. The earliest physical signs may be a mere restlessness or fidgetiness, but eventually, severe choreiform movements and dystonic posturing occur.

    3. Laboratory studies. CT demonstrates cerebral atrophy as well as atrophy of the caudate nucleus.

    4. Treatment

        a. Huntington's disease has no cure, and progression of the disease cannot be halted.

        b. Symptomatic treatment for the disease may include phenothiazines to control dyskinesia, and haloperidol or clozapine to control any behavioral disturbances.

        c. Children of Huntington's patients should receive genetic counseling in conjunction with genetic testing, which now is available for making a definitive diagnosis even in the presymptomatic state.

D. Cerebral palsy

    1. Cerebral palsy is a chronic impairment of muscle tone, strength, coordination, or movements. It is believed to result from cerebral injury before birth, during delivery, or in the perinatal period.

    2. Clinical features are widely varied and include spasticity (75% of patients), ataxia, seizure disorders, and mental retardation as well as disorders of speech, hearing, vision, and sensory perception.

    3. Physical examination may reveal hyperreflexia, microcephaly, limb-length discrepancies, cataracts, retinopathy, and congenital heart defects.

    4. Diagnostic testing is done to rule out other neurologic disorders. Depending on the presentation, MRI, immunoglobulin G, immunoglobulin M, urine acid tests, blood amino acids, lactate, pyruvate, and ammonia concentrations may aid in the diagnostic quest.

    5. Treatment is supportive, with the goals of attaining maximum function and potential physical, occupational, and speech ability. Pharmacologic treatment of spasticity and seizures often is required.

VII. DISEASES OF PERIPHERAL NERVES

A. Bell's palsy

1. General considerations

a. Unilateral facial muscle weakness is noted without evidence of other neurologic disease and without apparent cause. More than 60% of cases occur on the right side.

b. Although the cause of the weakness is unknown, it is seen more frequently in pregnant women and in people with diabetes. It often is associated with trauma, infection, neoplasia, or toxins.

c. There can be a paralysis of all muscles supplied by the cranial nerve VII (complete palsy) or variable weakness in different muscles (incomplete palsy).

2. Clinical features

a. Facial muscle weakness typically begins abruptly but may progress over a matter of hours to 2 days. Paralysis involves the forehead and lower face; patients cannot close the eye, raise the brow, or smile on the affected side.

b. Pain about the ipsilateral ear often precedes the facial weakness or is noted concurrently with the weakness.

c. Depending on the site of the nerve lesion, patients may demonstrate impairment of taste, lacrimation, or hyperacusis.

d. Clinical evaluation reveals no abnormality beyond the motor function of cranial nerve VII.

3. Diagnostic studies

a. Bell's palsy is a clinical diagnosis. Specific diagnostic confirmation with nerve conduction studies or EMG are only done in patients with atypical or prolonged Bell's palsy.

b. Appropriate diagnostic procedures may be done to identify other conditions that may produce facial palsy, including tumors, Lyme disease, AIDS, and sarcoidosis.

4. Treatment

a. Approximately 60% of cases resolve spontaneously and require no treatment, although the course is varied and may extend from a few days to a few months.

b. A poorer prognosis, with possible incomplete recovery, is associated with patients presenting with severe pain and complete palsy, hyperacusis, or advanced age.

c. A course of oral prednisone, with or without acyclovir, if begun soon after the onset of symptoms, has been shown to increase the percentage of patients who completely recover and should be considered in those at risk of a poor prognosis.

B. Diabetic peripheral neuropathy

1. General considerations

a. Peripheral nerve abnormalities in patients with diabetes are common and present as a mixed polyneuropathy (motor, sensory, and autonomic) in 70% of cases. The remainder of cases involves largely sensory neuropathies.

b. Less commonly, patients may develop mononeuropathies involving specific peripheral or cranial nerves.

c. Neuropathy generally is related to the duration and severity of hyperglycemia, but it may be the presenting symptom in occult diabetes. Neuropathy is the result of vascular insufficiency or nerve infarction.

2. Clinical features

a. Symptoms are more common in the lower extremities than in the arms and consist of numbness, pain, dysesthesias (burning), or paresthesias.

b. A distal polyneuropathy also can be diagnosed before the development of any symptoms, in the form of reduced deep tendon reflexes or impaired vibratory sensation.

c. Autonomic complications related to diabetes include postural hypotension, cardiac arrhythmias, impaired thermoregulatory sweating, and disturbances of bowel, bladder, gastric, and sexual function.

3. Diagnostic studies

a. Serial nerve conduction studies can be completed to document the presence, severity, and course of the neuropathy.

b. Additional diagnostic workup may be appropriate to rule out other causes of polyneuropathy, including uremia, alcoholic or nutritional deficiencies, connective tissue disease, vasculitis, vitamin B_{12} deficiency, hypothyroidism, or amyloidosis.

4. Treatment
   a. Tight control of hyperglycemia is vital, but there are no specific treatments for diabetic peripheral nerve complications, with the exception of an entrapment neuropathy that may respond to a decompression procedure.
   b. Phenytoin, mexiletine, or carbamazepine may be helpful in controlling the shooting or stabbing neuropathic pain.
   c. Amitriptyline, gabapentin, or fluphenazine may be useful in controlling deep, constant, aching pain.
   d. Postural hypotension may respond to salt supplementation, lower extremity pressure stockings, or medications, such as fludrocortisone or midodrine.

C. Guillain-Barré syndrome (acute idiopathic polyneuropathy)
   1. General considerations
      a. Guillain-Barré syndrome is an idiopathic polyneuropathy often following minor infections, immunizations, or surgical procedures, but in many cases, no cause is identified.
      b. Recent clinical and epidemiologic evidence seems to indicate a relationship with a preceding infection with *Campylobacter jejuni.*
   2. Clinical features
      a. Patients generally present with symmetrical extremity weakness that begins distally and ascends; proximal muscles tend to be affected more often than distal muscles. Deep tendon reflexes may be decreased or absent. Cranial nerves are affected in 45–75% of patients.
      b. Sensory abnormalities are common but generally less marked than the motor symptoms.
      c. Pain is present in more than 85% of cases and can be severe in a subset of patients.
      d. Significant autonomic dysfunction may be noted, including tachycardia, cardiac irregularities, labile blood pressure, disturbed sweating, impaired pulmonary function, sphincter disturbances, or paralytic ileus.
      e. Guillain-Barré syndrome can be life-threatening if the muscles of respiration or swallowing are involved.
   3. Diagnostic studies
      a. Electrophysiologic studies may reveal marked slowing of nerve conduction velocities, both motor and sensory. These studies also may document denervation or axonal loss.
      b. CSF evaluation typically yields an elevated protein, but the cell counts are normal.
   4. Treatment
      a. Patients should be hospitalized with close monitoring of respiratory status, because autonomic involvement may rapidly result in complications and death from orthostatic hypotension or arrhythmias.
      b. Plasmapheresis, instituted as early as possible, is very effective in reducing the time required for recovery and may reduce the likelihood of residual neurologic deficits. In patients who are severely affected, plasmapheresis also may shorten the time on a respirator as well as the length of time it may take to walk independently.
      c. IV immunoglobulin also is very effective and is used in preference to plasmapheresis in adults with cardiovascular instability and in children.
      d. Patients will benefit from physical, occupational, and speech therapy during rehabilitation.

D. Myasthenia gravis
   1. General characteristics
      a. Myasthenia gravis involves muscle weakness and fatigability, which improve with rest.
      b. The onset of myasthenia gravis usually is insidious, but the disorder sometimes is made evident by a coincidental infection that exacerbates the symptoms.
      c. The disorder may occur at any age but is more common in young women and older men.
      d. Antibodies directed against the acetylcholine receptor on the muscle surface cause an increased rate of receptor destruction leading to weakness.
   2. Clinical features
      a. Typical presenting problems include ptosis, diplopia, difficulty in chewing or swallowing, respiratory difficulties, limb weakness, or a combination of any of these.
      b. Symptoms may fluctuate in intensity during the day, and there is a tendency to have longer-term spontaneous relapses and remissions that may last for weeks.

    c. Clinical examination confirms the weakness and fatigability of affected muscles, which improve after a short rest.

    d. Sensation is normal, and there usually are no reflex changes.

    e. The diagnosis may be confirmed if marked clinical improvement is achieved by administering a short-acting anticholinesterase, edrophonium.

3. Laboratory studies

    a. Lateral and anteroposterior chest radiographs should be obtained to rule out a coexisting thymoma.

    b. Electrophysiologic studies may show a decrementing muscle response.

    c. Assay of serum for elevated levels of circulating acetylcholine-receptor antibodies is another way of establishing the diagnosis; this assay is positive in 80–90% of patients.

4. Treatment

    a. The mainstay of therapy is administration of a cholinesterase inhibitor, such as pyridostigmine, which produces a transient improvement in strength.

    b. Thymectomy often leads to improvement of symptoms.

    c. Corticosteroids, immunosuppressive agents, IV immunoglobulin, and plasmapheresis are effective in patients with refractory disease.

VIII. CNS INFECTION

A. Bacterial meningitis

    1. General characteristics

        a. Typical symptoms of meningitis are based on three processes: inflammation, increased intracranial pressure, or tissue necrosis.

        b. Causes of bacterial meningitis have changed over the past decades.

            (1) The primary causes today are *Streptococcus pneumoniae*, *Neisseria meningitidis*, and group B streptococci (especially in infants).

            (2) The rate of *Haemophilus influenzae* type b (Hib) meningitis has dramatically decreased since the widespread use of the Hib vaccine.

    2. Clinical features

        a. Fever, headache, vomiting, and a stiff neck are the typical signs and symptoms of meningitis, although all may not be present. A petechial rash is characteristic of *Neisseria meningitidis*.

        b. Symptoms typically are acute, with patients presenting within hours or 1–2 days of infection.

        c. Careful initial examination may reveal evidence of soft-tissue abscess, otitis, or other parameningeal infection.

        d. Meningeal signs may be absent or very subtle at the age extremes or be difficult to assess with impaired consciousness.

    3. Laboratory studies

        a. Prompt lumbar puncture and CSF analysis are essential. CT is performed before lumbar puncture to rule out evidence of a space-occupying lesion.

            (1) The CSF may be slightly turbid to grossly purulent.

            (2) CSF pressure is elevated in more than 90% of cases.

            (3) CSF WBC count is elevated, ranging from 1,000 to as high as 10,000 μL with increased neutrophils.

            (4) CSF protein concentrations of 100–500 mg/dL are most common.

            (5) CSF glucose levels often are decreased and may be less than 40 mg/dL.

        b. Gram stain and cultures of the CSF are diagnostic in more than 80% of cases.

    4. Treatment

        a. Antibiotic treatment is begun immediately if the CSF is not clear and colorless. The initial choice of antibiotic is based empirically on the patient's age.

            (1) Neonates receive ampicillin and gentamicin.

            (2) Infants up to 3 months of age receive the same combination, with higher doses of gentamicin.

(3) All children and adolescents up to 18 years of age generally receive chloramphenicol plus either a third-generation cephalosporin or ampicillin.

(4) Adults generally receive IV penicillin G or ampicillin.

(5) The elderly generally are treated with ampicillin plus a third-generation cephalosporin.

(6) If the meningitis is postsurgical or posttraumatic, the patient generally receives a third-generation cephalosporin with or without nafcillin to cover *Staphylococcus aureus* and Gram-negative bacilli.

b. Repeat lumbar puncture and CSF analysis are crucial to assess response to treatment.

(1) The CSF should be sterile after 24 hours.

(2) A decrease in pleocytosis and the proportion of neutrophils should be seen within 3 days.

B. Viral (aseptic) meningitis and encephalitis

1. General considerations

a. Viral meningitis most frequently is associated with enteric viruses during the summer and fall months: 50% are coxsackievirus A or B, 30% echoviruses, and 10–15% mumps virus.

b. Aseptic meningitis also may reflect an inflammatory process in the parameningeal area (i.e., sinusitis, otitis, abscess).

c. Viral encephalitis may not have an identifiable cause in many cases but frequently is associated with childhood exanthems, arthropod borne agents, and herpes simplex virus type 1.

2. Clinical features

a. Viral meningitis and encephalitis often present as an acute confusional state, especially in children and young adults.

b. Signs and symptoms generally are not as acute as in meningitis and may have persisted for several days.

c. Examination may reveal a number of systemic manifestations, suggesting a particular causal agent (e.g., rash, pharyngitis, adenopathy, pleuritis, carditis, jaundice, organomegaly, diarrhea).

d. In encephalitis, because it involves the brain directly, there may be markedly altered consciousness, seizures, personality changes, or other focal neurologic signs.

3. Laboratory studies

a. As with bacterial meningitis, prompt lumbar puncture and CSF analysis are crucial after assessing for evidence of increased intracranial pressure.

b. The CSF opening pressure generally is normal.

c. Cells present in the CSF are more likely to be lymphocytes or monocytes, and the WBC count generally is less than 1,000/μl.

d. The CSF protein, glucose, and serum blood counts are more likely to be normal.

4. Treatment

a. With the exception of infection with herpes simplex virus, the course of aseptic meningitis generally is benign and self-limited, and no specific therapy is required. Suspected herpes virus infection is treated with acyclovir.

b. Mild headaches can be treated with acetaminophen.

c. Seizures can be suppressed with anticonvulsants.

d. Breathing should be supported, if necessary.

C. Brain abscess

1. General characteristics

a. Brain abscess typically results from direct spread of infection from sinus, ear, or soft tissue; hematogenous spread to the brain is rare.

b. Abscesses may be localized to the extradural (epidural) space, subdural spaces, or in the brain parenchyma.

2. Clinical features

a. Brain abscess presents as a space-occupying lesion; symptoms may include vomiting, fever, altered mental status, and focal neurologic signs.

b. These signs and symptoms may have been preceded by previous evidence of otitis, sinusitis, or pharyngitis.

3. Laboratory studies

a. A lumbar puncture and CSF analysis should be performed, following CT.

b. CT or MRI is helpful in establishing the diagnosis, especially if performed using a contrast medium.

c. The bacteriology of brain abscess usually is polymicrobial and may include both Gram-positive and Gram-negative organisms.

4. Treatment

a. Acute treatment may involve respiratory and circulatory support, airway management, and monitoring of other vital functions.

b. Brain abscesses are treated with appropriate antibiotics that penetrate brain tissues well, including IV penicillin, chloramphenicol, and metronidazole.

c. Surgical excision or decompression may be required in cases of very large lesions or a delayed response to therapy.

IX. CNS TRAUMA

A. Brain injury

1. General characteristics

a. Head injury accounts for nearly half of the trauma-related deaths in young people.

b. Prognosis is directly related to the site and severity of brain damage.

c. Loss of consciousness for more than 2 minutes implies a worse prognosis.

d. The degree of retrograde and posttraumatic amnesia also is directly related to the severity of brain injury.

2. Clinical features

a. During the physical examination, special attention must be given to the level of consciousness and to the extent of any brainstem dysfunction.

b. In concussion, there may be a brief loss of consciousness with bradycardia, hypotension, and respiratory arrest for a few seconds.

c. In the setting of acute epidural hemorrhage, signs and symptoms may include headache, confusion, somnolence, seizures, and focal deficits occurring several hours after the injury.

d. Bruising may be on the side of the injury (coup injury) or on the contralateral side (contracoup injury).

3. Laboratory studies

a. Skull radiography or CT may detect skull fractures; further studies of the cervical spine should be done to look for related injuries.

b. CT also is important to demonstrate intracranial hemorrhage, to show evidence of cerebral edema, and to identify displacement of midline structures.

4. Treatment

a. Surgical evacuation may be necessary after acute epidural, acute subdural, and cerebral hemorrhage.

b. Increased intracranial pressures may be relieved by induced hyperventilation, IV mannitol infusion, and IV furosemide.

B. Spinal cord injury

1. General characteristics

a. Whiplash injury may cause spinal cord damage, but severe injury typically relates to fracture or dislocation causing compression or angular deformity of the cord.

b. Sites of injury may extend from the cervical to the upper lumbar region.

c. Extreme hypotension after acute injury may result in cord infarction.

2. Clinical features

a. Total cord transection

(1) Total cord transection results in immediate, flaccid paralysis and loss of sensation below the level of the lesion.

(2) Reflex activity is lost for a variable time, and there is urinary and fecal retention.

(3) With the slow return of reflex function, spastic paraplegia or quadriplegia develops, with hyperreflexia and extensor plantar responses.

b. Lesser cord injury

(1) Patients may be left with mild limb weakness or distal sensory disturbance.

(2) Sphincter function impairment may lead to urinary urgency and incontinence.

      c. A unilateral cord lesion produces an ipsilateral motor disturbance with accompanying impairment of proprioception and contralateral loss of pain and temperature below the lesion (Brown-Séquard syndrome).

      d. A central cord syndrome may lead to a lower motor neuron deficit and loss of pain and temperature, with sparing of posterior column functions.

      e. A radicular deficit may occur at the level of the injury; if the cauda equina is involved, there may be dysfunction in several lumbosacral roots.

   3. Laboratory studies

      a. No laboratory testing is needed or warranted.

      b. Imaging studies (plain-film radiography, CT, MRI) are indicated based on signs and symptoms.

   4. Treatment

      a. Treatment of spinal cord injury involves immobilization as well as decompressive laminectomy and fusion if there is cord compression.

      b. Early treatment with high-dose corticosteroids has been shown to improve neurologic recovery if started within 8 hours of the injury.

      c. Anatomic realignment of the spinal cord by traction and other orthopaedic procedures is important.

      d. Subsequent care of residual neurologic deficit requires therapy for spasticity and care of the skin, bowel, and bladder.

X. PRIMARY CNS NEOPLASMS

  A. General characteristics

   1. Approximately half of all primary intracranial neoplasms are gliomas, and the remainders are meningiomas, pituitary adenomas, neurofibromas, and others.

   2. Approximately 10% of spinal tumors are intramedullary; ependymoma is the most common.

   3. Certain tumors, especially neurofibromas, hemangioblastomas, and retinoblastomas, may have a familial basis.

   4. The most common source of intracranial metastasis is carcinoma of the lung, breast, kidney, and the GI tract.

  B. Clinical features

   1. Spinal tumors may lead to spinal cord dysfunction by direct compression, by ischemia secondary to arterial or venous obstruction, or by invasive infiltration.

   2. Intracranial tumors may produce a generalized disturbance of cerebral function and lead to evidence of increased intracranial pressure (i.e., personality changes, intellectual decline, emotional lability, seizures, headaches, nausea, malaise).

   3. Intracranial tumors also may produce focal deficits, depending on their location.

      a. Frontal lobe lesions often produce progressive intellectual decline, slowing of mental activity, personality changes, contralateral grasp reflexes, and possibly, expressive aphasia.

      b. Temporal lobe lesions may lead to seizures, olfactory or gustatory hallucinations, licking or smacking of the lips, depersonalization, emotional and behavioral changes, visual field defects, and auditory illusions.

      c. Parietal lobe lesions typically cause contralateral disturbances of sensation and may cause sensory seizures, a cortical sensory loss (impaired stereognosis) or inattention, or some combination of these.

      d. Occipital lobe lesions characteristically produce crossed homonymous hemianopia or a partial field defect, visual agnosia for objects and colors, or unformed visual hallucinations.

      e. Brainstem and cerebellar lesions produce cranial nerve palsies, ataxia, incoordination, nystagmus, and pyramidal and sensory deficits in the limbs on one or both sides.

   4. Symptoms of spinal tumors usually develop insidiously, with pain characteristically aggravated by coughing or straining and either localized to the back or felt diffusely in an extremity as motor defects, paresthesias, or numbness, especially in the legs.

   5. Physical examination of patients with spinal tumors may reveal localized spinal tenderness.

  C. Laboratory studies

   1. CT or MRI performed with contrast medium may detect the lesion, define its location and size, evaluate the extent to which the normal anatomy is distorted, and the degree of any associated cerebral edema or mass effect.

2. Arteriography may demonstrate stretching or displacement of normal cerebral vessels as well as the presence of tumor vascularity.

3. EEG may demonstrate a focal disturbance resulting from the neoplasm or a more diffuse change reflecting altered mental status.

4. CT myelography or MRI may be needed to identify and localize the site of spinal cord compression.

5. CSF removed at myelography often is xanthochromic and contains greatly increased protein concentration, normal cell content, and normal glucose concentration.

D. Treatment

1. Complete surgical removal of the tumor may be possible if it is extra-axial or is not in a critical or inaccessible region of the brain.

2. Surgical shunting of an obstructive hydrocephalus may dramatically reduce clinical deficits.

3. Radiation, chemotherapy, or both increases median survival rates, regardless of any preceding surgery.

4. Corticosteroids help to reduce cerebral edema and usually are started before surgery.

5. Anticonvulsants commonly are administered in standard doses.

6. Intramedullary cord lesions are treated by decompression and surgical excision and by irradiation.

7. Treatment of epidural spinal metastases consists of irradiation, irrespective of cell type.

XI. **SLEEP DISORDERS**

A. General characteristics

1. Dyssomnia (insomnia) complaints include difficulty getting to sleep or staying asleep, intermittent wakefulness during the night, early morning awakenings, or some combination of all these. Psychiatric disorders, including depression and manic disorders, often are associated with persistent insomnia.

2. Hypersomnia (excessive daytime sleepiness) generally is a more severe problem and may manifest in patients with sleep apnea, narcolepsy, or those who demonstrate nocturnal myoclonus.

3. Parasomnias (abnormal behaviors during sleep) include sleep terrors, nightmares, sleepwalking, and enuresis.

B. Clinical features

1. Taking a careful history of those with insomnia may reveal depression, abuse of alcohol, heavy smoking (>1 pack/day), inappropriate use of sedatives/hypnotics, or a medical history of uremia, asthma, or hypothyroidism.

2. Sleep apnea often is seen in obese, middle-aged and older men with hypertension and associated congestive heart failure.

3. Patients with narcolepsy experience sudden, brief sleep attacks; cataplexy; sleep paralysis; and hypnagogic hallucinations, which may precede sleep.

C. Laboratory studies

1. Polysomnography (sleep studies) assesses EEG activity, heart rate, respiratory movement, and oxygen saturation.

2. Thyroid studies may be helpful if hypothyroidism is suggested.

D. Treatment

1. Insomnia

a. In transient insomnia, de-emphasis and reassurance are sufficient treatment.

b. A variety of sleep hygiene rules should be discussed to remove numerous barriers to effective sleep. Sleep hygiene rules include avoidance of caffeine, nicotine or exercise prior to bedtime, establishment of regular sleep hours, relaxation techniques, etc.

c. Medications should be avoided if possible. Antihistamines may be effective for milder problems, however, and rapidly acting hypnotics may be used for short periods if necessary.

2. Treatment of sleep apnea includes weight reduction if appropriate and administration of air under continuous pressure through the nasopharynx during sleep (continuous positive airway pressure).

3. Narcolepsy is managed by administration of stimulants.

4. Nocturnal myoclonus typically is treated with clonazepam.

5. Sleep terror and sleep walking can be treated with benzodiazepines.

12 | Psychiatry

Melanie Trecartin

I. DIAGNOSIS OF PSYCHIATRIC DISORDERS

A. Background

1. Psychiatric diagnoses conform to the *Diagnostic and Statistical Manual of Mental Disorders* (DSM) published and periodically updated by the American Psychiatric Association.

2. The DSM is widely accepted because professionals from a number of specialties outside of psychiatry were involved in its conception and development.

3. The *International Statistical Classification of Diseases and Related Health Problems* (ICD) is published by the World Health Organization. It is similar to the DSM and is used in most countries of the world, except the United States and Japan.

B. The DSM endorses a criteria-based diagnostic approach that requires the following three conditions be met.

1. The condition is not caused by the direct effects of any drug.

2. The psychiatric disorder is not caused by the effects of a medical condition.

3. There is significant impairment of social functioning, occupational functioning, or both.

C. If a patient's signs and symptoms result from a medical condition or from substance abuse, the diagnosis should reflect this situation; in this case, the psychiatric symptoms take a secondary role. This relationship holds regardless of the behavior manifested by the patient.

D. The DSM contains a catchall category for each group, labeled "not otherwise specified" (NOS), which allows a diagnosis for patients with atypical symptoms.

1. NOS includes a mixed presentation, symptoms below the diagnostic threshold, or a presentation that does not meet the criteria for a specific disorder.

2. It allows a patient to be assigned to a diagnostic group while avoiding a forced classification based on incomplete or contradictory symptomatology.

E. The DSM employs a multiaxial system.

1. Axis I: All mental disorders, including substance abuse and developmental disorders.

2. Axis II: Personality disorders and mental retardation.

3. Axis III: Any general medical condition or physical disorder.

4. Axis IV: Psychosocial and environmental situations that contribute to the disorder (e.g., homelessness, economic difficulties).

5. Axis V: The global assessment of function (GAF), a rating system designed to assess the level of daily functioning based on social, occupational, and psychological assessment.

II. SCHIZOPHRENIA AND OTHER PSYCHOTIC DISORDERS

A. Definition

1. Brief psychotic disorder, schizophreniform disorder, and schizophrenia present with common symptoms, which are differentiated by severity and duration.

2. Psychotic disorders

a. Patients exhibit disordered thought content and thought processes as well as perceptual disturbances, such as illusions or hallucinations, delusions, and impaired reality orientation.

b. Patients' social and occupational functions are disrupted by problems with affect, motivation, perception, and communication or disorganized speech; memory and consciousness are not impaired.

c. Symptoms are categorized as positive (hallucinations, bizarre behavior, delusions) or negative (flat affect, apathy, poor grooming, social withdrawal, anhedonia, poor eye contact, poverty of speech).

3. Subtypes of schizophrenia

    a. Paranoid schizophrenia. The most common form; characterized by persecutory or grandiose delusions or auditory hallucinations.

    b. Disorganized schizophrenia. Characterized by disorganized speech or behavior and flat or inappropriate affect.

    c. Catatonic schizophrenia. A rare subtype; manifested by at least two of the following: motor immobility, excess motor activity that is without purpose, extreme negativism or mutism, peculiarly voluntary movement (bizarre postures, stereotyped movements, grimacing), and echolalia (mimicking sound) or echopraxia (mimicking behavior).

    d. Undifferentiated schizophrenia. Delusions and hallucinations are prominent, paranoid, disorganized, and catatonic symptoms are absent.

    e. Residual schizophrenia. Negative symptoms predominate, and there are only minimal positive symptoms.

B. Clinical features

    1. Schizophrenia usually runs a chronic and debilitating course. Prognosis is more favorable with late onset, acute (vs insidious) onset, obvious precipitating factor, and the presence of positive symptoms.

        a. An estimated 1–2% of the population is affected; it most commonly manifests in early adulthood. Onset before age 10 or after age 60 is rare.

        b. The prodromal phase, which precedes the first psychotic break, is manifested by functional decline, social withdrawal, and irritability. Onset of disease tends to be earlier for men (ages 10–25) than for women (ages 25–35).

        c. The psychotic phase consists of delusions, disorganized thought process and content, and perceptual disturbances.

        d. The residual phase generally occurs between psychotic episodes. It is characterized by blunted affect, odd thinking or behavior, and other negative symptoms.

    2. At least two of the following symptoms must be present during a 1-month period (or less if successfully treated), and continuous signs of the disorder must persist for at least 6 months. The presence of hallucinations or delusions is not necessary for a diagnosis.

        a. Delusions. Erroneous beliefs based on a misinterpretation of reality, such as paranoia, ideas of reference, thought broadcasting, delusions of grandeur, or delusions of guilt.

        b. Hallucinations. False perceptions in any of the sensory modalities, such as auditory (most common), tactile, olfactory, and visual. To qualify for the diagnosis, the hallucination must not occur as an isolated experience, in a clouded sensorium, or as part of a religious or cultural experience.

        c. Disorganized speech. Used as a marker for disorganized thought processes.

            (1) The patient is unable to stay on a topic (loose associations), unable to provide an answer related to questions (tangential response), or both.

            (2) The symptoms need to be severe enough to impair an individual's ability to communicate effectively.

        d. Grossly disorganized behavior. May be exhibited as unpredictable agitation, inappropriate sexual behavior, child-like silliness, catatonic motor behavior, or a reduced level of self-care and hygiene.

        e. Negative symptoms. Manifested as blunted affect, poor posture, or lack of goal-directed activities or initiative.

    3. Social functioning, occupational functioning, or both must be affected.

        a. This impairment may be manifested as an inability to hold a job for an extended period, inability to maintain relationships, or withdrawal from established friends and social relationships.

        b. The patient's educational progress may be disrupted or not completed.

C. Cause

    1. The cause is unknown.

    2. Theories consider neurotransmitter abnormalities, such as excess dopamine activity, elevated serotonin and norepinephrine, and decreased γ-aminobutyric acid (GABA). A dysfunctional limbic system is another potential site of pathology.

    3. Enlarged ventricles and cortical atrophy on CT are common in chronic disease.

D. Treatment

    1. Hospitalization is recommended for patients exhibiting suicidal ideation or an inability to care for themselves or who pose a threat to self or others.

    2. Pharmacotherapy

      a. No therapeutic intervention is totally effective in ameliorating all symptoms.

        (1) Patients with diagnostic subtypes react differently to the various neuroleptics available.

        (2) Combined use of antipsychotic drugs and psychosocial treatment is better than either treatment alone.

      b. Neuroleptic and antipsychotic medications

        (1) Typical neuroleptic and antipsychotic medications with dopamine-antagonist activity (haloperidol, chlorpromazine, thioridazine, loxapine, fluphenazine) are best for decreasing positive symptoms (i.e., delusions).

        (2) Atypical neuroleptics with serotonin- and dopamine-antagonist (SDA) activity (risperidone, olanzapine, sertindole, ziprasidone, clozapine, quetiapine) generally are preferred for the management of negative symptoms (i.e., withdrawal) and have fewer side effects. The SDAs are now the drugs of first choice to treat schizophrenia.

      c. Side effects, such as extrapyramidal symptoms, parkinsonian-like symptoms, neuroleptic malignant syndrome, and tardive dyskinesia, are more likely to be encountered with the typical neuroleptics. Clozapine may cause agranulocytosis; weekly blood counts are required.

      d. A 4- to 6-week medication trial is optimal before concluding nonresponse.

    3. Resistant cases may be treated with an antipsychotic medication combined with another drug, such as carbamazepine, valproate, or lithium.

    4. Behavior-oriented therapy targeted toward social skills training (as an adjunct along with group and/or family therapy) may be helpful. ·

  E. Other forms of psychoses

    1. Schizoaffective disorder

      a. This disorder meets the criteria for major depressive episode, manic episode, or mixed episode, during which criteria for schizophrenia also are met.

      b. Delusions or hallucinations lasting for 2 weeks without mood disorder symptoms help to differentiate schizoaffective disorder from mood disorder with psychotic features.

      c. It carries a better prognosis than schizophrenia but worse prognosis than a mood disorder.

    2. Delusional disorder

      a. This disorder is characterized by the presence of nonbizarre delusions (i.e., situations that occur in real life) for at least 1 month.

      b. The behavior is not obviously odd, and functioning is not significantly impaired.

      c. Subtypes include erotomanic (belief that another person is in love with the patient), somatic (delusions of a physical defect or medical condition), jealous (delusions of sexual partner's infidelity), and persecutory (delusion of mistreatment or persecution).

    3. Psychotic disorders may be caused by alcohol, illicit drug use, or medications (anticholinergics, antidepressants, hallucinogens, psychostimulants).

    4. Psychotic disorders can be caused by general medical conditions (central nervous system disease, endocrinopathies, vitamin deficiency states, HIV/AIDS, systemic lupus erythematosus).

    5. In brief psychotic disorder, symptoms are present for at least 1 day but for less than 1 month, and the patient returns to premorbid levels of functioning after the symptoms abate. This commonly is encountered after a catastrophic event.

    6. Schizophreniform disorder presents with the same symptoms as seen in schizophrenia; symptoms last between 1 and 6 months.

III. SOMATOFORM DISORDERS

  A. Somatization disorder

    1. General characteristics

      a. Patients present with vague physical complaints involving many organ systems that cannot be explained by general medical condition or substance use. Visits to health care providers are numerous, although no medical disorder is found.

    b. Patients commonly complain of symptoms related to the GI tract or to the reproductive or neurologic systems; they also may complain of pain. Periods of increased stress are associated with worsening of the somatic symptoms.

    c. This disorder occurs in females more often than in males and more often in low socioeconomic groups. Onset is before 30 years of age, most commonly during adolescence, and 50% of patients have a comorbid mental disorder. Lifetime prevalence is 0.2–2.0%. The course of illness is often chronic and debilitating.

  2. Treatment

    a. Treatment is regularly (i.e., monthly) scheduled visits with a health care provider.

    b. Patients often are very resistant to seeing a mental health care provider. Group and individual psychotherapy is beneficial to develop coping strategies.

    c. Secondary gain should be minimized and medications avoided.

B. Body dysmorphic disorder

  1. General characteristics

    a. This disorder is characterized by a preoccupation with an imagined defect in physical appearance or an exaggerated distortion of a minor flaw. The most likely concern is facial flaws.

    b. Patients feel self-conscious and fear humiliation; they go to great lengths to hide or correct their perceived anomaly.

    c. Visits to a dermatologist and/or plastic surgeon are common, although the patient usually is still not satisfied with his or her appearance.

    d. Age of onset is 15–30 years; females are affected more often than males.

  2. Treatment

    a. Serotonin-modulating drugs (fluoxetine, clomipramine) can be efficacious.

    b. Coexistent psychiatric disorders should be treated appropriately. The most common coexisting disorder is a major depressive episode, followed by anxiety disorder.

C. Conversion disorder

  1. General characteristics

    a. This disorder is characterized by one or more neurologic complaints that cannot be explained clinically.

    b. Symptoms are not intentionally produced and may be motor (involuntary movements, tics, blepharospasm, weakness), sensory (paresthesia and/or anesthesia, tunnel vision, deafness), seizure activity, or mixed (psychogenic vomiting, syncope, globus hystericus). The most common symptoms are shifting paralysis, blindness, and mutism.

    c. Patients display an unexpected lack of concern and indifference to their symptoms (la belle indifference).

    d. Symptoms tend to be episodic, lasting for days to a month, and may remit for a period of time only to recur during times of stress.

  2. Conversion disorder is common.

    a. There is a 20–25% incidence in general medical practice.

    b. It most commonly is diagnosed during adolescence and young adulthood and is two to five times more common in females than in males. With men, there often is an associated occupational or military accident.

  3. Treatment

    a. Psychotherapy, such as insight-oriented or behavioral therapy, can be of benefit.

    b. Hypnosis, anxiolytics, and relaxation therapy may help.

    c. Some patients have responded to amobarbital interviews to uncover underlying psychological factors. Lorazepam, especially if a patient has experienced a traumatic event, may be beneficial.

D. Factitious disorder

  1. General characteristics

    a. Patients with this disorder intentionally fake signs and symptoms of medical or psychiatric symptoms, with the primary motivation being to assume the sick role.

    b. It usually begins in early adulthood and carries a poor prognosis.

    c. Often, patients will seek hospital admission under different names and by feigning different illnesses. When (or if) confronted with their ruse, they usually become angry and abruptly sign out.

d. Obtaining a reliable past medical history is unlikely. Patients usually are familiar with the disease process that they are feigning; however, true disease processes must be ruled out.

e. Related disorders include Munchausen syndrome and Munchausen-by-proxy syndrome, which is a form of child abuse. Munchausen syndrome is a factitious disorder with predominantly physical complaints.

2. Treatment

a. Early recognition is paramount in the management of this disorder so as to avoid unnecessary and/or potentially dangerous procedures.

b. No specific psychiatric intervention has been notably effective, but psychotherapy (individual, family) is suggested.

c. Selective serotonin reuptake inhibitors (SSRIs) may be useful to reduce impulsive tendencies seen in acting-out factitious behavior.

E. Malingering

1. Malingering involves the deliberate production of physical or psychological symptoms, motivated by external gain. Some of these obvious, definable goals are avoiding responsibility, police or legal action, punishment, or dangerous or difficult situations; receiving monetary compensation (e.g., in a lawsuit) or free hospital room and board; and obtaining drugs.

2. Patients tend to express vague, poorly defined complaints and claim that these symptoms cause great distress and impaired functioning. Injuries often are found to be self-inflicted, and history reveals multiple, undiagnosed illnesses or previous injuries and even tampering with laboratory results.

a. Patients are uncooperative and refuse to accept a clean bill of health.

b. Their symptoms typically improve when the objective has been met or the ruse has been exposed.

F. Hypochondriasis

1. General characteristics

a. Hypochondriasis is a preoccupation with the belief of having or the fear of contracting a serious illness. This belief is not of delusional intensity; normal bodily sensations are misinterpreted as manifestation of disease.

b. This condition commonly is coexistent with symptoms of anxiety and depression.

c. The patient's fear persists even though medical investigation reveals no cause.

d. The course, although generally chronic, is episodic and may be exacerbated after a major stressor.

2. Treatment

a. Group and insight-oriented psychotherapy can be helpful, but patients usually are resistant to psychiatric care. Discussing mechanisms for coping with stress without reinforcing their perceived illness behavior is important.

b. Regularly scheduled appointments with a practitioner are recommended to provide reassurance.

c. Pharmacotherapy can be used if the patient has a concurrent or underlying anxiety or major depressive disorder.

G. Pain disorder

1. General characteristics

a. Pain is reported in one or more areas without any identifiable cause and results in significant distress and impairment in functioning.

b. These patients may describe atypical facial pain, low back pain, headache, pelvic pain, and other types of chronic pain syndromes.

(1) When a medical condition does coexist, the pain cannot be fully explained as a result of the condition.

(2) Patients tend to view the pain as a cause of all their problems.

c. Usually, there is an abrupt onset, and pain may increase in intensity over weeks or months.

(1) A long history of medical and surgical attention is common, because this tends to be a chronic (and sometimes disabling) disorder.

(2) Psychological factors are deemed to have an important role in the pathogenesis.

(3) Peak onset is 30–50 years of age; it is twice as common in women as in men.

2. Treatment

a. Psychotherapy, behavioral therapy (e.g., biofeedback and hypnosis), and pain control programs may be helpful. Pain reduction may not be feasible, so the treatment focus should be on rehabilitation.

b. Analgesics and sedatives generally are not beneficial and may lead to abuse or dependence.

(1) SSRIs and tricyclics have been used with some positive results and currently are the most effective drug therapy.

(2) Some patients benefit from amphetamines as an adjunct to SSRIs.

IV. MOOD DISORDERS

A. Definition

1. Mood disorders (affective disorders) are a group of clinically distinct entities identified by patterns of mood episodes, which are periods of time (weeks to months) in which some mood impairment is present. The defining feature is a change in mood from a premorbid state. Normally, people feel more or less in control of their moods; however this sense of control is lost in mood disorders, resulting in a feeling of great turmoil.

2. Mood episodes include major depressive episodes, manic episodes, hypomanic episodes, and mixed episodes.

3. Mood disorders include major depressive disorder, bipolar I, bipolar II, dysthymia, and cyclothymia.

4. Cause. The cause is largely unknown; however, neurochemical (serotonin, norepinephrine, dopamine, growth hormone, cortisol), genetic, and psychosocial factors (life events) have been implicated.

B. Mood episodes

1. Major depressive episode

a. Depressive signs and symptoms must be present for the better part of a 2-week period (Table 12-1).

b. At least one of the symptoms must include depressed mood or anhedonia (loss of interest or pleasure in all activities).

c. Patients should not exhibit manic signs or symptoms (Table 12-1).

d. The mood episode is not the result of bereavement.

2. Manic episode

a. Manic episode is characterized by an abnormally and persistently elevated, expansive, or irritable mood that lasts for at least 1 week.

b. At least three manic symptoms (four if mood is irritable) are present (Table 12-1).

c. Patients may exhibit psychotic features or require hospitalization to prevent harm to self or others.

d. Mania results in severe social and/or occupational dysfunction.

TABLE 12-1 Symptoms of a Mood Episode

Depression
  Depressed mood (either reported by the patient or observed by others)
  Anhedonia
  Excessive feelings of guilt
  Indecisiveness
  Lack of self-worth
  Sleep problems, such as insomnia or hypersomnia
  Cognitive problems (difficulty with memory and concentration)
  Psychomotor retardation or agitation
  Either decreased or increased appetite or a 5% or greater unintentional change
    in body weight over a 1-month period
  Decreased interest in sex
  Either suicidal ideation or thoughts of death without suicidal ideation
  Chronic fatigue or decreased energy

Mania
  Inflated self-esteem or grandiosity
  Irritability
  Decreased need for sleep
  Pressured speech
  Flight of ideas
  Distractibility
  Impaired judgment, resulting in pursuit of pleasurable activities with a high probability
    of adverse outcomes
  Psychomotor agitation

3. Hypomanic episode

a. Hypomanic episode is characterized by at least four continuous days of an abnormally and persistently elevated, expansive, or irritable mood.

b. At least three manic symptoms (four if the mood is irritable) must be present.

c. Although the patient's mood and functioning are changed from premorbid functioning, social and occupational functioning are not significantly affected, and there are no psychotic features.

d. Hypomanic episode does not require hospitalization.

4. Mixed episode

a. Mixed episode is characterized by rapidly alternating moods, with symptoms of both a manic episode and a depressive episode, which lasts for at least 1 week.

b. Symptoms typically are severe enough that there is marked impairment in occupational or social functioning.

C. Mood disorders

1. Major depressive disorder (MDD)

a. General characteristics

(1) MDD has a chronic course with relapses.

(a) Premorbid functioning may return between episodes.

(b) Between 5% and 10% of patients subsequently develop a manic episode.

(c) MDD is two to three times more common in females than in males. The lifetime prevalence of depressive syndromes is 13–20%.

(2) The suicide rates is estimated at 15%.

(a) Patients may be at highest risk after initiating treatment; therapy may bring out the energy that the patient previously lacked to undertake a suicide attempt.

(b) Higher suicide rates are associated with a previous attempt, white males older than 45 years, a detailed plan, a self-destructive pattern, a recent severe loss, poor support system, poor health, concurrent substance abuse, psychotic symptoms, and an inability to accept help.

b. Subtypes

(1) Seasonal affective disorder

(a) Seasonal affective disorder is characterized by the predominance of fall or winter onset and likely is caused by the lessening daylight hours; it typically remits in the spring.

(b) It is more common in colder climates and in young females; the average age at presentation is 40 years.

(c) Light therapy and SSRIs have been used successfully.

(2) Melancholia

(a) Melancholia is characterized by anhedonia, psychomotor retardation or agitation, anorexia, weight loss, depressed mood (especially in the morning), feelings of guilt, and sleep disturbance (most often early morning awakening). Suicidal ideation may be present.

(b) Melancholia characterizes about 50% of hospitalized patients with major depression.

(c) Patients respond better to pharmacotherapy than nonmelancholic patients do.

(3) Atypical depression

(a) Atypical depression is characterized by overeating and weight gain, oversleeping, reactive mood, leaden paralysis, and oversensitivity to interpersonal rejection.

(b) Monoamine oxidase inhibitors (MAOIs) often are useful.

(4) Catatonic depression

(a) Catatonic depression is characterized by motor immobility or stupor, blurred affect, purposeless motor activity, extreme withdrawal, negativism, bizarre mannerisms or posturing, echolalia, or echopraxia.

(b) It often is treated with antidepressants and antipsychotics simultaneously.

(5) Psychotic depression is characterized by the presence of delusions or hallucinations.

(6) Postpartum depression is characterized by the onset of symptoms within 4 weeks of delivery.

c. Pharmacotherapy

(1) If well tolerated, antidepressants should be continued for a minimum of 3–6 weeks to determine efficacy. Maintenance therapy should be continued long term (>6 months), both because of the high relapse rate and because future episodes may be more severe.

(2) SSRIs (fluoxetine, paroxetine, sertraline) are considered to be first-line therapy, because they have minimal adverse effects and are safer than other antidepressant classes.

(a) Selection of a particular SSRI should be based on side-effect profiles and the presenting problems.

(b) Side effects include GI upset, headache, and sexual dysfunction.

(3) Bupropion, venlafaxine, nefazodone, and mirtazaprine also are very effective and have a safer side-effect profile than tricyclic antidepressants (TCAs) or MAOIs. Nefazodone and mirtazapine have not been associated with decreased libido, erectile dysfunction, or anorgasmia.

(4) TCAs and tetracyclics cause side effects such as weight gain, orthostatic hypotension, anticholinergic effects, and somnolence. Overdosage with these agents is more lethal than with other antidepressants.

(5) MAOIs require a tyramine-free diet (no wine, beer, nearly all cheeses, aged foods, smoked meats) to avoid side effects, such as hypertensive crisis.

(6) Precautions

(a) Use of MAOIs with SSRIs can result in serotonin syndrome, which causes acute mental status changes, restlessness, diaphoresis, tremor, hyperthermia, seizures, and occasionally, coma and death.

(b) TCAs and MAOIs used concurrently can cause delirium and hypertension.

(c) The serious risks associated with MAOIs make this class of drugs the least likely to be used.

d. Electroconvulsive therapy (ECT)

(1) ECT is effective in all types of MDD. Usually, however, it is reserved for severely depressed patients or patients who are unresponsive or intolerant of psychiatric medications or when the clinical picture is so debilitating that rapid improvement is warranted.

(2) ECT can safely be used in pregnant and elderly patients, produces a rapid response, and has very few relative contraindications.

(3) Common adverse effects include postictal confusion and somatic complaints, such as headache, nausea, and muscle soreness.

(4) The greatest concern is memory loss, which often returns to baseline by 6 months after treatment.

e. Psychotherapy treatment for mood disorders. Most studies indicate that cognitive, interpersonal, and behavioral therapy are effective, especially in combination with pharmacotherapy.

2. Bipolar I disorder

a. General characteristics

(1) Bipolar I disorder is characterized by the occurrence of one or more manic or mixed episodes, which often cycle with depressive episodes, but the latter is not required for diagnosis. It commonly is known as manic depression.

(2) Manic episodes

(a) Episodes are characterized by a sudden escalation of mood, which is abnormally and persistently euphoric, expansive, or irritable.

(b) Patients may go for days without sleep; become excessively talkative or loud, socially outgoing, overly self-confident, hypersexual, or disinhibited; and display a flamboyant clothing style.

(3) Thought processes are difficult to follow because of racing thoughts, flights of ideas, and easy distraction. Judgment is quite impaired, resulting in spending sprees, promiscuity, or foolish business investments.

(4) Psychotic symptoms (e.g., hallucinations, paranoia, delusions) may be present.

(5) The course usually is chronic with relapses. In general, it carries a worse prognosis than MDD and has a high suicide rate.

(6) Epidemiology

(a) The lifetime prevalence is about 1%.

(b) The average age of onset is 30 years, and early onset is correlated with a higher incidence of psychotic symptoms and a poorer prognosis.

(c) First-degree relatives have an increased incidence of developing the disorder. Monozygotic twin concordance rates are about 75%.

b. Treatment

(1) Lithium, valproic acid, olanzapine, or carbamazepine typically are effective. Gabapentin, topiramate, and lamotrigine also show beneficial effects.

    (a) Lithium has a narrow therapeutic window, and plasma levels need to be monitored every 4–8 weeks.

    (b) Although usually well tolerated, lithium has side effects, including weight gain, tremor, nausea, increased thirst and urination, drowsiness, hypothyroidism, arrhythmias, and seizures.

(2) Antipsychotics (i.e., haloperidol or risperidone) or benzodiazepines (i.e., lorazepam or clonazepam) may be added if agitation or psychotic symptoms are present, especially at the initiation of treatment when acute manic episodes are likely.

(3) Acute depressive episodes can be treated with SSRIs or bupropion. Caution: antidepressant medication may precipitate mania.

(4) Secondary treatment measures include ECT, MAOIs, and TCAs (caution must be exercised, because these drugs can result in rapid cycling between mood states).

(5) Family, group, supportive, interpersonal, and/or cognitive therapy may help.

3. Bipolar II disorder

  a. General characteristics

    (1) Bipolar II disorder is characterized by at least one or more major depressive episodes and at least one hypomanic episode. The patient has never experienced a manic episode or a mixed episode.

    (2) Hypomanic symptoms are similar to manic symptoms but are less severe and cause less social impairment. Hypomania also usually does not present with psychotic symptoms, racing thoughts, or excess psychomotor agitation.

    (3) Prevalence is estimated at 0.5%; it appears to be slightly more common in females than in males.

  b. Treatment. Same as for bipolar I disorder.

4. Dysthymic disorder

  a. General characteristics

    (1) Dysthymic disorder is a chronic, persistent mild depression that is manifested by pessimism, brooding, generalized loss of interest, decreased productivity, feelings of inadequacy, and social withdrawal.

    (2) There are no psychotic or manic/hypomanic features.

    (3) MDD eventually will develop in 10–20% of patients. Bipolar disorder may develop in others, and 25% of patients will have lifelong dysthymic symptoms.

    (4) It is two to three times more common in women than in men; onset is during young adulthood.

  b. Diagnosis

    (1) Depressed mood for most of the day, for more days than not, for at least 2 years (at least 1 year in children and adolescents).

    (2) During the 2-year period, the person has not been without the symptoms for more than 2 months at a time, and no major depressive episode occurred during the first 2 years of symptoms.

    (3) At least two of the following conditions are noted: poor concentration or indecisiveness, hopelessness, poor appetite or overeating, insomnia or hypersomnia, low energy or fatigue, and lack of self-esteem.

  c. Treatment

    (1) Antidepressants (SSRIs, bupropion, TCAs, or occasionally, MAOIs) are effective.

    (2) Insight-oriented behavior and cognitive therapies are beneficial, especially when combined with pharmacotherapy.

5. Cyclothymic disorder

  a. General characteristics

    (1) Patients are described as moody, erratic, impulsive, and somewhat volatile.

    (2) This disorder (similar to bipolar II but less severe) is characterized by recurring periods of relatively less severe depressive episodes and hypomania over a 2-year period, with symptom-free periods lasting for no more than 2 months at any one time. The depressive episodes are not severe enough to be classified as a major depressive episode, and manic or mixed episodes have not occurred.

    (3) It has a chronic course, and there is a 15%–20% risk of bipolar disorder.

  b. Treatment. Similar to bipolar I disorder (mood stabilizers and antimanic drugs are first-line therapy).

6. Adjustment disorder

   a. General characteristics

   (1) This disorder is characterized by maladaptive behavioral or emotional symptoms that develop within 3 months after a stressful life event and end within 6 months of the event.

   (2) Among adolescents, precipitants include parental rejection and divorce, problems at school, and leaving home.

   (3) Among adults, stressors include marital discord, financial difficulties or loss of a job, marriage, or parenthood. Also included are natural disasters and racial/religious persecution.

   (4) The symptoms cause significant impairment in functioning.

   (5) Symptoms are not caused by bereavement.

   b. Treatment.

   (1) Adjustment disorder is treated with supportive psychotherapy or group therapy.

   (2) Short-term pharmacotherapy for associated insomnia, anxiety, or depression may be used but is not first-line treatment.

V. PERSONALITY DISORDERS

A. Definition

   1. Personality disorders are deeply ingrained, inflexible patterns of relating to others that are maladaptive and cause significant impairment in social or occupational functions.

   2. Patients are ego-syntonic and lack insight regarding their problems. Personality disorders are Axis II and are divided into three clusters.

   a. Cluster A (mad)

   (1) This cluster includes schizoid, schizotypal, and paranoid personality disorders.

   (2) Patients are viewed as weird or peculiar.

   (3) It is associated with psychotic disorders.

   b. Cluster B (bad)

   (1) This cluster includes antisocial, borderline, histrionic, and narcissistic personality disorders.

   (2) Patients are viewed as emotional and inconsistent.

   (3) It is associated with mood disorders.

   c. Cluster C (sad)

   (1) This cluster includes avoidant, dependent and obsessive-compulsive personality disorders.

   (2) Patients are viewed as fearful or anxious.

   (3) It is associated with anxiety disorders.

B. Cluster A personality disorders

   1. Paranoid personality disorder

   a. General characteristics

   (1) Paranoid personality disorder is characterized by a pervasive distrust and suspicion of others, beginning by early adulthood. Patients blame their own problems on others and seem hostile and angry.

   (2) Males more commonly are affected than females.

   b. Clinical features

   (1) Suspicion (without evidence) that others are exploiting or deceiving him or her.

   (2) Preoccupation with doubts regarding the loyalty or trustworthiness of acquaintances; doubts regarding fidelity.

   (3) Reluctance to confide in others.

   (4) Interpretation of benign remarks as threatening or demeaning.

   (5) Persistence of grudges; quick to counterattack.

   c. Treatment

   (1) Individual psychotherapy is the key.

   (2) Antianxiety medications or a short course of antipsychotics for transient psychosis may be needed.

2. Schizoid personality disorder

   a. General characteristics

      (1) This disorder is characterized by a lifelong pattern of voluntary social withdrawal, often perceived as eccentric and reclusive.

      (2) Patients are quiet and unsociable and have constricted affect. They have no desire for close relationships and prefer to be alone.

      (3) Males are affected twice as often as females.

   b. Clinical features

      (1) Patients neither enjoy nor desire close relationships (including family).

      (2) They generally choose solitary activities.

      (3) They show little (if any) interest in sexual activity with another person.

      (4) They are indifferent to praise or criticism.

      (5) An emotional coldness, detachment, or flattened affect is seen.

   c. Treatment

      (1) Group therapy and psychotherapy are recommended.

      (2) Low-dose, short-term antipsychotics or antidepressants can be given if indicated for comorbidity.

3. Schizotypal personality disorder

   a. General characteristics

      (1) This disorder is characterized by a pervasive pattern of eccentric behavior and peculiar thought patterns beginning in early adulthood.

      (2) The patient often is perceived as strange and eccentric.

   b. Clinical features

      (1) Patients have ideas of reference but not delusions of reference, which are beliefs or perceptions that irrelevant, unrelated, or innocuous things in the world are referring to them directly or have special personal significance.

      (2) Patients display odd behaviors, thoughts, speech, beliefs, or magical thinking inconsistent with cultural norms; these may include belief in clairvoyance or telepathy, bizarre fantasies or preoccupations, and belief in superstitions.

      (3) Unusual perceptual experiences (e.g., bodily illusions) may be noted.

      (4) Patients show suspiciousness and excessive social anxiety.

      (5) Inappropriate or restricted affect is seen.

   c. Treatment

      (1) Psychotherapy is the treatment of choice.

      (2) A short course of low-dose antipsychotics, antidepressants, or benzodiazepines to decrease anxiety can be used if necessary.

C. Cluster B personality disorders

   1. Antisocial personality disorder

      a. General characteristics

         (1) This disorder is characterized by an inability to conform to social norms.

         (2) A pervasive pattern of disregard for and violation of the rights and feelings of others is seen.

         (3) Patients are described as extremely manipulative, deceitful, impulsive, and totally lacking empathy or remorse. On interview, however, they can act exceedingly charming and seem normal.

         (4) It may begin in childhood as a conduct disorder.

            (a) These children may have a history of physical and/or sexual abuse.

            (b) Symptoms may decrease with age.

         (5) Multiple physical complaints, substance abuse, and depression are common.

         (6) An abnormal electroencephalogram may be seen.

         (7) Males are affected three times more often than females. There is a familial pattern, and it is more common in urban areas and prison populations.

   b. Clinical features

   (1) Patients show deceitfulness, lying, and conning others for personal gain.

   (2) Irritability and aggressiveness, manifested by repeated physical assaults, are noted, and patients have a reckless disregard for the safety of self or others.

   (3) Patients are irresponsible and are unable to sustain work.

   c. Treatment

   (1) Treatment is psychotherapy with socially based intervention.

   (2) Pharmacotherapy with SSRIs, lithium, valproate, carbamazepine, and possibly propranolol may help to reduce anxiety, impulsivity, and aggression. Caution must be exercised, however, because of the high potential for abuse.

2. Borderline personality disorder

   a. General characteristics

   (1) This disorder is characterized by an unstable and unpredictable mood, affect, and behavior as well as a poorly established self-image. Mood swings and impulsivity are common, and the patient always appears to be in a state of crisis.

   (2) Short and transient psychotic episodes, paranoid ideation, or dissociative symptoms may occur, especially during times of increased stress.

   (3) Self-mutilation and manipulative suicide attempts are common.

   (4) The patient desperately attempts to avoid abandonment.

   (5) Patients cannot tolerate being alone yet can exhibit intense anger toward their friends.

   (a) Splitting (i.e., seeing people as either all good or all bad) is common.

   (b) Patients have unstable and intense relationships.

   (c) Inappropriate anger or difficulty controlling anger is seen.

   (6) There is a high incidence of MDD; suicide rates peak during early adulthood.

   (7) Females are affected twice as often as males.

   b. Treatment

   (1) Treatment includes psychotherapy with social skills training, behavioral therapy, and individual and group therapy.

   (2) Pharmacotherapy in addition to psychotherapy yields better results.

   (a) Antipsychotics are used to control hostility and brief psychotic episodes.

   (b) Antidepressants are used to improve mood.

   (c) Benzodiazepines are used to help decrease anxiety.

   (d) Anticonvulsants have been beneficial to improve global functioning.

3. Histrionic personality disorder

   a. General characteristics

   (1) Individuals with this disorder are overly emotional, dramatic, and seductive; they are excitable, with a high degree of attention-seeking behavior and a tendency to exaggerate their thoughts and feelings.

   (a) Patients are flamboyant and extroverted, but their rapidly shifting emotions and superficiality renders them unable to maintain a deep, long-lasting relationship.

   (b) They are easily influenced by others.

   (c) Patients need to be the center of attention and may throw a temper tantrum if the attention shifts. They have a pattern of excessive emotionality and attention-seeking behavior and often are inappropriately seductive or provocative, with exaggerated expression and emotion.

   (2) Somatization and substance use disorders are common.

   (3) Speech can be excessively impressionistic and lacking in detail.

   b. Treatment

   (1) Treatment includes psychotherapy, either group or individual.

   (2) Antidepressants and/or anxiolytics may be useful for specific symptoms.

4. Narcissistic personality disorder

      a. General characteristics

        (1) Patients have an inflated self-image, pattern of grandiosity, need for admiration, and lack of empathy. They consider themselves to be special and expect to be treated as such, and they may have an arrogant, haughty attitude.

        (2) Although they have a sense of entitlement and grandiosity, their self-esteem is quite fragile. They have a need for excessive admiration, and they are prone to depression if criticized.

        (3) They have a preoccupation with fantasies of unlimited success, beauty, brilliance, and so forth. Aging is difficult and makes them prone to midlife crisis.

        (4) They may be exploitative and take advantage of others to meet their own needs.

      b. Treatment

        (1) This disorder is difficult to treat.

        (2) Psychotherapy is key.

        (3) Lithium has been used if mood swings are present. Antidepressants (especially SSRIs) are a useful adjunct.

  D. Cluster C personality disorders

    1. Avoidant personality disorder

      a. General characteristics

        (1) These individuals have an extreme sensitivity to rejection (inferiority complex).

        (2) Patients see themselves as unappealing.

        (3) They have intense social anxiety and feelings of inadequacy, which may lead to interpersonal withdrawal and total avoidance of any situation in which they may be criticized.

        (4) Although shy, they display a great desire for companionship, but with strong guarantees of unconditional acceptance. They may avoid occupational activities that involve interpersonal contact because of fear of rejection.

        (5) They show great restraint with intimate relationships because of fear of rejection.

        (6) Social phobia (fear of embarrassment or rejection in a particular setting) is common in this group.

      b. Treatment

        (1) Psychotherapy, social skills training, group therapy, and assertiveness training may be beneficial.

        (2) β-Blockers and SSRIs are useful for managing anxiety and depression and may help to reduce the patient's sensitivity to rejection.

    2. Dependent personality disorder

      a. General characteristics

        (1) These individuals have an enduring pattern of dependent, clinging, and submissive behavior; they cannot make their own decision without help from others.

        (2) Patients have difficulty disagreeing with others for fear of loss of support or approval.

        (3) They lack self-confidence, avoid positions of responsibility, and have a dislike of being alone. They are passive, self-doubtful, and reliant on others to take care of them.

        (4) Depression may ensue, especially if they experience loss of the person on whom they depend.

        (5) They go to extreme lengths to seek another relationship.

        (6) Social and occupational functioning are impaired; risk for depression is high. Some suffer physical or mental abuse because they fail to assert themselves.

        (7) They feel uncomfortable when alone for fear of being unable to care for self.

      b. Treatment

        (1) Psychotherapy, especially insight-oriented, behavioral, group, family therapy, and assertiveness training, may help.

        (2) Anxiolytics and antidepressants may be useful to target symptoms; benzodiazepines and SSRIs are used.

    3. Obsessive-compulsive personality disorder

      a. General characteristics

        (1) Obsessive-compulsive personality disorder is characterized by a pervasive pattern of orderliness (rules, lists, details), perfectionism, and inflexibility. Unlike personality disorders, these patients often have an awareness of their disorder and seek treatment on their own.

(2) Patients tend to be rigid, stubborn, and emotionally constricted, and they insist that others submit to their ways, causing difficulty with interpersonal and occupational relationships.

(3) Perfectionism interferes with the ability to complete tasks or form relationships.

(4) A change in routine threatens to upset their perceived stability and can lead to extreme anxiety.

(5) The course of this disorder is variable. The disorder may remit, or obsessions and compulsions may develop. Schizophrenia and MDD may develop.

(6) Obsessive-compulsive personality disorder is ego-syntonic (not distressing to the patient), whereas obsessive-compulsive disorder is ego-dystonic (distressing to the patient).

(7) Patients display excessive devotion to work and productivity to the exclusion of leisure activities; they have a reluctance to delegate tasks unless those tasks will be done the way that he or she wants.

(8) Miserly spending or hoarding of money is seen.

b. Treatment

(1) Psychotherapy and group or behavioral therapy are recommended.

(2) Clomipramine, clonazepam, and SSRIs may help if obsessive-compulsive symptoms occur.

E. Personality disorder NOS

1. This category contains disorders that do not fit into any of the true personality disorders.

2. Passive–aggressive

a. Characterized by procrastination, irritability, stubbornness, negativistic attitudes, and passive resistance to demands for adequate performance. These patients are sullen, argumentative, and envious/resentful toward those who seem to be more fortunate.

b. Patients lack self-confidence, make excuses for delays, find fault with others, and are intentionally inefficient. They complain of being misunderstood and unappreciated.

c. Treatment is psychotherapy. Antidepressants and benzodiazepines can be used only when clinically indicated for depressive symptoms.

3. Depressive

a. Manifested by chronic unhappiness; very similar to dysthymic disorder.

b. Patients tend to be gloomy and pessimistic, have low self-esteem, and may be overly conscientious with work performance and critical of self and others.

c. Treatment includes psychotherapy (insight-oriented, group or self-help) along with antidepressants (SSRIs).

4. Sadomasochistic

a. Sadism is the desire to cause pain to others by being sexually, physically, or mentally abusive; masochism generally is the seeking of humiliation rather than of physically inflicted pain.

b. Patients may exhibit sadism, masochism, or both.

5. Sadistic

a. Characterized by a pervasive pattern of demeaning, humiliating, and cruel behavior toward others.

b. Patients may be fascinated with violence, torture, or weapons and are aggressive without gain (e.g., sexual, monetary).

c. Treatment is insight-oriented psychotherapy.

VI. ANXIETY DISORDERS

A. Definition

1. Anxiety disorders are characterized by excessive amounts of anxiety that impede performance.

2. These disorders can result in physiologic symptoms, such as dizziness, palpitations, perspiration, loss of appetite, nausea, trembling, and other symptoms that cause the patient distress.

B. Generalized anxiety disorder

1. General characteristics

a. Generalized anxiety disorder is characterized by persistent, excessive anxiety regarding general life events that lasts for 6 months or more.

b. The patient has difficulty coping with the anxiety, which usually is expressed as worry or apprehension.

    c. There is a high (50–90%) comorbidity with other psychiatric disorders, such as MDD, specific and social phobias, and panic disorder.

    d. Diagnostic criteria include at least three of the following: restlessness or hypervigilance, easy fatigability, irritability, sleep disturbance, muscle tension, and difficulty concentrating. Medical disorders, such as thyroid dysfunction, stimulant abuse, alcohol withdrawal, caffeine intoxication, and cardiac arrhythmias, must be ruled out.

    e. Generalized anxiety disorder is very common, with lifetime prevalence estimated at 45%. It affects women twice as often as men. Age of onset is around age 20, although patients typically report feeling anxious for as long as they can remember.

  2. Treatment

    a. SSRIs and buspirone are effective; TCAs also may help.

    b. Benzodiazepines can be used as an adjunct for short-term management of severe symptoms but are not recommended for monotherapy because of the risk of dependence or abuse.

    c. Behavioral and insight-oriented therapy also should be initiated.

C. Panic attacks and panic disorder

  1. Panic attacks

    a. Panic attack is defined as a period of extreme anxiety that peaks within 10 minutes, typically declines within 30 minutes, and rarely lasts for longer than 1 hour.

    b. Panic attacks may have a definable trigger or be totally unexpected.

    c. Patients may experience palpitations or tachycardia, sweating, trembling, dyspnea, sensation of choking, chest discomfort, nausea, depersonalization (feel estranged from self and/or the external world), derealization (people, events, and surroundings appear to be changed or unreal), fear of losing control, fear of dying, lightheadedness, numbness or tingling, chills, or hot flashes.

  2. Panic disorder

    a. Panic disorder is characterized by recurrent, unexpected panic attacks that abruptly occur and are accompanied by debilitating fear of having additional attacks.

    b. The intense fear and physical symptoms may be accompanied by feelings of impending harm or death, fear of a heart attack or stroke, and/or fears of "going crazy."

    c. Panic disorder occurs in 1–5% of the population. It is two to three times more common in females than in males.

    d. Average age at onset is in the mid-20s, but it can occur at any age, including childhood.

  3. Diagnosis should specify panic disorder with or without agoraphobia (extensive avoidance of settings in which panic attacks have occurred).

  4. Cause

    a. Evidence points toward a biologic cause though genetics, and psychosocial factors most likely contribute.

    b. Nervous system dysregulation and abnormal activity of norepinephrine, serotonin, and GABA have been implicated.

    c. Some substances (e.g., IV sodium lactate or inhalation of carbon dioxide) have panic-inducing effects on patients with panic disorder yet rarely have any effect on those without panic disorder.

  5. Treatment

    a. For acute management of anxiety, a short course of benzodiazepines (alprazolam or lorazepam) is beneficial.

    b. For maintenance, SSRIs should be instituted as benzodiazepines are tapered. Paroxetine is especially beneficial; alternatives include fluvoxamine and sertraline. TCAs (especially clomipramine and imipramine) also have been used successfully. In general, doses should be started low and titrated slowly.

    c. Treatment should continue for 8–12 months, because relapse rates are high after medication is discontinued.

    d. Mild cases may be managed with psychotherapy alone. Cognitive, insight-oriented, relaxation training, and behavioral therapies have been shown to be effective.

D. Obsessive-compulsive disorder

  1. General characteristics

    a. Obsessions refer to persistent and recurrent thoughts, images, or impulses that are intrusive and inappropriate and cause significant anxiety.

b. Compulsions are the ritualistic or repetitive behaviors or thoughts that patients feel compelled to engage in to relieve the anxiety caused by the obsessions and to reduce distress. The behaviors or mental acts are excessive and have no realistic connection between the events the patient is trying to avoid.

c. Patients typically have insight and realize that their thoughts and behaviors are irrational and causing distress.

d. This disorder is ego-dystonic as opposed to obsessive-compulsive personality disorder, which is ego-syntonic (not distressing to the patient).

e. Two-thirds of patients are diagnosed before age 25 and one-third during adolescence.

f. Evidence indicates that neurotransmitter dysregulation, genetic, and psychosocial factors contribute to the disorder.

g. Common types of obsessive-compulsions, in order of frequency
   (1) Contamination. Patients wash their hands excessively or compulsively avoid objects presumed to be contaminated.
   (2) Pathologic doubt. Patients worry about such things as forgetting to lock the door or turn off the stove; these doubts result in repetitive checking.
   (3) Intrusive thoughts. Patients have obsessive thoughts without a compulsion; these thoughts may be of a sexual or aggressive nature.
   (4) Need for symmetry. Patients must order and arrange objects, leading to extreme precision and slowness.
   (5) Other. Religious obsessions, compulsive hoarding, nail biting, and trichotillomania (compulsively pulling out hair).

2. Treatment
   a. SSRIs, in doses often higher than normally prescribed, are considered to be first-line therapy; TCAs such as clomipramine also have shown efficacy.
   b. Patients who show only a partial remission of symptoms may undergo a trial of lithium, venlafaxine, buspirone, or clonazepam.
   c. Behavioral therapies should be initiated. Relaxation therapy may be beneficial.

E. Posttraumatic stress disorder (PTSD)

1. General characteristics
   a. PTSD results from exposure to or witnessing a physiologically or psychologically traumatic event that is out of the range of normal human experience. Symptoms can develop in as little as 1 week or many years after the event and can fluctuate over time, becoming worse during stressful times.
   b. PTSD is manifested by overwhelming sensations of helplessness, fear, and horror that impair occupational or social functioning.
   c. A patient may have a sense of repeatedly reliving the event, have intrusive memories or disturbing dreams of the event, or experience distress when exposed to stimuli that trigger event review.
   d. PTSD must be differentiated from brief psychotic, acute stress, adjustment, and borderline personality disorders. There is a high comorbidity with substance abuse and depression.
   e. PTSD is most common in young adults because of the nature of the precipitating event. In men, it most often results from combat experience; in women, it most often results from assault or rape.

2. For diagnosis, three or more of the following should be present for more than 1 month.
   a. Inability to recall an important aspect of the event.
   b. Avoidance of activities, places, or people that remind him or her of the event.
   c. Attempts to avoid thinking or talking about the event.
   d. Feelings of detachment or estrangement from others.
   e. Markedly decreased interest or anhedonia.
   f. Restricted range of affect.
   g. Belief that one's future has been foreshortened because of the event.
   h. An increased state of arousal characterized by at least two of the following: insomnia, irritability or angry outbursts, poor concentration, hypervigilance, or exaggerated startle response.

3. Treatment

    a. SSRIs (sertraline, paroxetine) are considered to be first-line treatment; TCAs (imipramine, doxepin, amitriptyline) may be effective. Buspirone, MAOIs, and anticonvulsants, such as carbamazepine and valproate, also may be effective.

    b. Crisis counseling should be initiated as a preventive measure when feasible. Support groups, family therapy, and cognitive or behavioral therapies are recommended. Hypnosis, coping mechanisms, and relaxation techniques can be beneficial as well.

F. Acute stress disorder

  1. General characteristics

    a. Symptoms of acute stress disorder occur within 1 month of the traumatic event and last from 2 days to 4 weeks, whereas symptoms of PTSD may develop any time after the event and last for more than 1 month.

    b. Common comorbidities include depression, anxiety, substance abuse, and cognitive difficulties (e.g., impaired concentration).

    c. It is most prevalent in younger ages.

  2. Clinical features

    a. Either during or after the event, the person has three or more of the following: sense of numbing or detachment, reduced awareness of surroundings (in a daze), derealization, depersonalization, or dissociative amnesia (inability to recall an important component of the trauma).

    b. Patients experience excessive anxiety or arousal (e.g., insomnia, irritability, poor concentration, hypervigilance, exaggerated startle response).

    c. The distressing event is reexperienced in at least one of the following ways: recurrent dreams, images, or thoughts; flashback; sensation of reliving the event; or exposure to reminders of the trauma, causing distress.

    d. Patients avoid stimuli that remind them of the trauma (e.g., activities, places, people).

    e. Distress results in marked impairment in important areas of functioning.

  3. Treatment

    a. Treatment includes cognitive and behavioral therapy and supportive counseling.

    b. Anxiolytics can be used to decrease insomnia and irritability.

    c. Similar measures to treat PTSD also can be employed to treat acute stress disorder, including support groups, family therapy, SSRIs, TCAs, and anticonvulsants.

G. Phobias (specific and social)

  1. General characteristics

    a. Phobias are considered to be the most common mental disorder in the United States.

    b. They are characterized by an irrational fear and persistent excessive anxiety when presented with an object or a situational event.

    c. Exposure results in an immediate increase in anxiety and can precipitate a panic attack.

    d. Because of the discomfort caused by the increased anxiety, the panic attack, or both, the situation or object is either feared and avoided or endured with considerable apprehension.

    e. Except for children, patients with this disorder know that their fear is excessive and unreasonable.

    f. Diagnosis of a phobia is made if the response to phobic stimuli interferes with the patient's daily routine, social, or occupational functioning.

    g. Common comorbidities are MDD, substance abuse, other anxiety disorders, and personality disorders.

  2. Specific phobia

    a. Specific phobias are more common than social phobias.

    b. Specific phobia and agoraphobia are two to three times more common in women than in men; social phobia affects men and women equally.

    c. Many phobias can begin in childhood, and the majority are in place by early adulthood.

    d. Specific phobia refers to the fear of a specific object or situation. There are five types.

      (1) Animal. The fear is of animals or insects; onset generally is during childhood.

      (2) Natural environment. The fear is of natural phenomena (e.g., storms, heights, water, lightning).

      (3) Blood-injection injury. The fear of invasive procedures is paramount; the phobic trigger may be the possibility of injury, the sight of blood, or fear of contamination by exposure to bodily fluids.

(4) Situational. The fear of bridges, tall buildings, flying, driving, and confined spaces are examples of this type.

(5) Other. This type includes fear of situations that may lead to choking, vomiting, or getting an illness; in children, the fear may be of loud noises or costumed characters.

3. Social phobia

a. Social phobia is the fear of social situations in which embarrassment or humiliation in front of other people may occur.

b. Common inciting events are public speaking, using public restrooms, and eating in public.

4. Agoraphobia

a. Agoraphobia is an intense anxiety about placing oneself into a situation in which an incapacitating problem could occur and no help would be available. The event usually is viewed by the patient as extremely embarrassing or humiliating.

b. Often, there is fear of being in public places where escape may be difficult in the event of a subsequent attack. Anxiety-producing situations may include riding on a train or bus; being in any crowded area, mall, supermarket, or theater; or just being alone outside the home.

c. Agoraphobia may occur with or without a history of panic disorder, although 50–70% of patients with agoraphobia have coexisting panic disorder. If the feared incapacitating event is a panic attack, then agoraphobia is diagnosed as secondary to the panic disorder.

d. Diagnostic criteria

(1) Any of the symptoms that are characteristic of a panic attack may be present. In addition, the patient may have a potentially incapacitating or embarrassing medical condition, such as a heart condition or a lack of bowel or bladder control.

(2) In extreme cases, symptoms may render the patient either unwilling or unable to leave home.

5. Treatment

a. For social phobias and agoraphobia, SSRIs (particularly paroxetine) are considered to be first-line therapy. If SSRIs are not successful, benzodiazepines, venlafaxine, buspirone, and lastly, TCAs (imipramine) may be initiated.

b. β-Blockers, such as propranolol, have been used successfully to reduce autonomic hyperarousal symptoms and tremor associated with performance situations.

c. Insight-oriented therapy should be initiated, and hypnosis may be helpful.

d. Specific phobias can be treated with short-term benzodiazepines and β-blockers; however, systemic desensitization/exposure therapy, hypnosis, supportive, and insight-oriented psychotherapy probably are more useful.

VII. EATING DISORDERS

A. Anorexia nervosa

1. General characteristics

a. Patients have a distorted body image and an intense fear of becoming fat, even though they are underweight.

b. This results in a self-imposed starvation, despite normal appetite and craving for food. Patients generally are less than 85% of expected weight for height.

c. Patients often feel that losing weight is a desired achievement of self-control, whereas gaining weight is thought of as an unacceptable lack of discipline. Patients deny the seriousness of their low body weight.

d. Patients may exercise excessively, and they commonly have food-related obsessions (e.g., hoarding food, collecting recipes).

e. There are two types of anorexia.

(1) Restricting. The patient eats very little and does not regularly engage in binge eating or purging behavior, such as induced vomiting, abusing laxatives or diuretics, or using enemas.

(2) Binge eating and purging. The patient eats in binges followed by purging behavior.

f. Physical signs include emaciation, orthostatic hypotension, bradycardia, hypothermia, dry skin, lanugo, peripheral edema, amenorrhea, salivary gland hypertrophy, dental erosion, calluses or abrasions on the back of the hand from induced vomiting, leukopenia, electrolyte abnormalities (hypochloremia, hypokalemia, elevated blood urea nitrogen, metabolic alkalosis), arrhythmias, and amenorrhea.

  g. Approximately 90% of patients are female. Anorexia nervosa is more common in developed countries and in professions that require thinness (e.g., modeling, ballet). Peak onset is during early adolescence.

  h. Causes

   (1) Biological, genetic, social, and psychological factors have been implicated.

   (2) The increased incidence of this disorder during the latter half of the 20th century may be the result of cultural and societal pressure on women to attain exceedingly thin physiques.

 2. Treatment

  a. Patients rarely seek treatment; family members usually are first to bring it to attention. A multidisciplinary approach to treatment is essential.

  b. Hospitalization often is indicated, especially if the patient is more than 20% below the expected body weight. There is a high (>10%) mortality rate. Fluid and electrolyte abnormalities must be corrected, and weight restoration is crucial.

  c. Outpatient management consists of behavioral therapy, family therapy, and supervised weight-gain programs.

  d. Certain antidepressants (amitriptyline, paroxetine, mirtazapine) can be used, especially when depression is present.

  e. An appetite stimulant may be of use, as might a drug that has weight gain as a side effect. Overall, medications do not play a major role in the treatment of this disorder.

B. Bulimia nervosa

 1. General characteristics

  a. Patients with bulimia employ binge eating as well as vomiting, use of laxatives and/or diuretics, excessive exercise, or other measures to avoid gaining weight.

  b. The binge eating causes emotional distress and a feeling of loss of control.

  c. Unlike patients with anorexia, those with bulimia commonly maintain a normal body weight, or they may even be overweight.

  d. There are two types of bulimia.

   (1) Purging. This involves self-induced vomiting as well as disuse of laxatives, diuretics, or enemas.

   (2) Nonpurging. The patient uses other compensatory behaviors, such as excessive exercise or fasting.

  e. Medical complications are seen more often in the purging type.

  f. Physical findings include dental erosion, esophagitis, calloused or abraded knuckles, hypochloremic hypokalemic alkalosis, hypomagnesemia, and salivary gland hypertrophy.

  g. Bulimia is significantly more common in females than in males. It is more prevalent than anorexia.

  h. The behavior is quite common, affecting about 36% of young females; the disorder is present in 1–3% of these young women.

  i. Patients with bulimia tend to be high achievers and respond to societal pressure to be thin.

  j. There is an increased rate of anxiety and mood disorders, bipolar I disorders, impulse control disorders, and history of sexual abuse.

 2. Treatment

  a. The prognosis for patients with bulimia is better than that for patients with anorexia. They also are more likely to seek treatment, both because their uncontrolled eating is ego-dystonic and because there is less denial.

  b. Antidepressants, such as SSRIs (fluoxetine), are useful, as are TCAs and MAOIs.

  c. Behavioral psychotherapies should be used in conjunction with family therapy. Group therapy with others suffering from bulimia also should be considered.

  d. Hospitalization usually is not necessary; exceptions are the presence of suicidal ideation or severe purging, resulting in significant metabolic or electrolyte disturbances.

C. Obesity (binge-eating disorder)

 1. General characteristics

  a. Obesity is defined as 20% or more over ideal body weight or a body mass index (BMI) of greater than 30. The BMI is calculated by weight divided by height (kg/m^2).

  b. Obesity affects more than half of the U.S. population and is more common in lower socioeconomic groups. Women are more likely than men to be obese.

c. Overeating; lack of exercise; and developmental, psychological, endocrine, and genetic reasons all contribute to the development of this disorder.

d. Obese patients often suffer emotional distress over their eating binges but do not purge or restrict eating in an attempt to control their weight. They admit to a loss of control over their eating behavior.

e. Diagnostic criteria

(1) Recurrent episodes of binge eating at least 2 days/week for 6 months, characterized by eating a larger amount of food in a 2-hour period than most average people would consume.

(2) The binge-eating episodes are associated with three or more of the following: eating faster than normal; eating until feeling uncomfortably full; eating to excess, even though not hungry; eating alone out of embarrassment; and feeling disgusted, guilty, or depressed after the episode.

(3) Episodes are not associated with any inappropriate compensatory weight loss behaviors (vomiting, fasting, excess exercise, laxatives), and patients are not fixated on body image

2. Treatment

a. Behavior modification therapy, food diaries, and development of new eating patterns (eating slowly, not eating between meals or when not seated) are beneficial. Implementation of a low-calorie, balanced diet and establishment of an exercise regimen are important. Group therapy helps to provide education and motivation.

b. Pharmacotherapy

(1) The use of sympathomimetics, such as amphetamine, dextroamphetamine, phentermine, phendimetrazine, and diethylpropion, can be used.

(2) Orlistat (Xenical), a lipase inhibitor, and sibutramine (Meridia), a mixed neurotransmitter reuptake inhibitor, also can be useful adjuncts.

c. Surgical methods (gastric bypass and gastroplasty) have been used for patients who are markedly obese.

VIII. SUBSTANCE ABUSE DISORDERS

A. General characteristics

1. The most commonly abused drugs are alcohol, nicotine, and caffeine; others include opiates, barbiturates, benzodiazepines, and over-the-counter medications.

2. Activation of the dopaminergic system has been implicated.

B. Types of abuse

1. Addiction is a nonscientific, nonmedical term denoting psychological and/or physical dependence that results in substance-seeking behavior that may or may not pose risks to the individual.

2. Physical dependence is the physiologic changes that occur with drug use and result in withdrawal symptoms on termination of use.

3. Psychological dependence refers to the craving or desire for the substance independent of the physiologic withdrawal symptoms.

4. Because both physiologic and psychological dependence occur together, a more appropriate term is substance dependence. This occurs when substance use results in impairment as manifested by three of the following within a 12-month period.

a. Tolerance. There is either a decreased effect over time when the same amount of substance is used or a need for an increased amount of a substance over time to achieve a baseline.

b. Withdrawal. There is a need to use the substance to relieve or avoid physical symptoms associated with deprivation of it.

c. There is a use of increasingly larger amounts of a substance over a longer period than desired.

d. There are unsuccessful efforts to stop or decrease the amount of a substance used.

e. There are significantly larger amounts of time spent in attempts to acquire or use the substance or to recover from its effects.

f. There is social, occupational, or recreational impairment.

g. There is continued use of a substance despite the awareness that doing so has adverse consequence.

5. Substance abuse is substance use that has not met the criteria for dependence but has resulted in impairment as manifested by at least one of the following within a 12-month period.

   a. Patient fails to meet home, school, or work obligations.

   b. Patient repeatedly uses the substance in hazardous situations (e.g., driving a car).

   c. Patient has recurrent substance-related legal problems.

   d. Patient continues to use the substance, even though he or she is experiencing interpersonal or social problems as a result.

   6. Substance intoxication refers to maladaptive behavioral or psychological changes attributed to recent ingestion of a substance. Intoxication is reversible and is not caused by a mental disorder or medical condition.

C. Epidemiology

   1. Lifetime prevalence of substance abuse or dependence is about 17%.

   2. The most likely age group is 18- to 34-year-olds. Men are more commonly affected than women.

   3. Substance abusers have a threefold risk in the United States of having a mental disorder (excluding those who use nicotine and caffeine).

D. Treatment

   1. Substance dependence is viewed as a chronic relapsing disease by the Substance Abuse and Mental Health Services Administration (SAMHSA). Relapses are not considered to be a failure in treatment but, rather, a step toward what will, it is hoped, be a complete remission of all symptoms.

   2. Risk factors can be assessed in an office setting through use of the CAGE screening test for alcohol abuse or drug use (Table 12-2).

   3. Nonpharmacologic modalities include education, coping skills, relaxation therapy, family therapy, various kinds of psychotherapy (insight-oriented, group), health and nutritional counseling, lifestyle changes, and aftercare programs.

   4. The 12-step program is a popular form of therapy for those with a number of different types of substance abuse (e.g., Alcoholics Anonymous, Narcotics Anonymous) as well as for family members (e.g., Al-Anon, Alateen).

   5. Pharmacologic therapy

   a. Some forms of dependence require intensive detoxification, rehabilitation, and/or ongoing medication to keep the patient free of drugs (e.g., daily methadone as therapy for a patient with a dependence on opiates).

   b. Withdrawal symptoms may ensue on discontinuation of substance abuse, especially if the use was prolonged or heavy.

   (1) Withdrawal typically begins with tremulousness/shakes/jitters that start 6–8 hours after cessation of alcohol.

   (2) Additional manifestations include psychomotor and perception symptoms (8–12 hours after cessation), seizures, and delirium tremens (generally within 72 hours of cessation but can occur after 1 week).

   c. Alcohol withdrawal commonly requires the use of benzodiazepines, such as diazepam (Valium) or chlordiazepoxide (Librium), as well as thiamine, folic acid, and multivitamin administration.

   d. Disulfiram (Antabuse) is an alcohol-deterrent medication that causes nausea when alcohol is consumed.

   e. Withdrawal from other central nervous system depressants can be managed with phenobarbital. Anxiolytics or neuroleptics can be used for acute agitation seen in stimulant withdrawal.

   f. Naloxone is used to reverse the effects of any opioid. Opioid abuse and withdrawal also can be managed in several ways, including a slow taper of methadone or clonidine along with adjuncts, such as ibuprofen for muscle cramps, loperamide for diarrhea, and promethazine for nausea.

   g. Nicotine and tobacco cravings can be treated with nicotine transdermal patches; nasal spray, gum, or inhaler; antidepressants, such as bupropion (Zyban); or clonidine.

   h. Marijuana, PCP, and hallucinogen withdrawal usually does not require medication; however, anxiolytics can be used. In the latter two, neuroleptics, such as haloperidol, can be used if acute psychotic symptoms are present.

TABLE 12-2	CAGE Screening Test for Alcohol Abuse or Drug Use
C (cut down)	Have you ever felt you should cut down on your drinking (or drug use)?
A (annoyed)	Have people annoyed you by criticizing your drinking (or drug use)?
G (guilty)	Have you felt bad or guilty about your drinking (or drug use)?
E (eye opener)	Have you ever had a drink (or used drugs) first thing in the morning to steady your nerves or to get rid of a hangover (eye opener)?

IX. CHILDHOOD DISORDERS

A. Attention-deficit disorder (ADD) or attention-deficit hyperactivity disorder (ADHD)

1. General characteristics

a. ADD and ADHD can manifest as hyperactivity and impulsivity or as inattentiveness. Most children manifest symptoms that result in a diagnosis emphasizing both attention deficits and hyperactivity.

b. Secondary symptoms include emotional immaturity and lability, poor social skills, and sometimes, motor incoordination. Disruptive behavior may result in peer rejection and deflated self-image. At home, these children often do not comply with parents' requests and can become explosive and irritable.

c. Between 2 and 20% of school-age children may be affected. It is two to five times more frequent in boys than in girls and is most common in the firstborn son.

d. Approximately 50% of affected children continue to have dysfunctional symptoms into adulthood.

e. A multifactorial cause is likely, including prenatal exposure to infections and toxins, prenatal complications, familial or genetic factors, psychosocial factors, and neurochemical dysregulation.

f. Diagnosis

(1) The diagnosis generally is established through parental and teacher rating scales, such as the Connors' scales.

(2) Diagnostic criteria

(a) Symptoms of hyperactivity, impulsivity, or inattentiveness resulting in impairment must have been manifest before 7 years of age.

(b) Symptoms must occur in at least two settings (e.g., home, school).

(3) At least six symptoms of inattention, hyperactivity/impulsivity, or both, as listed in Table 12-3, are developmentally inappropriate and present for at least 6 months.

2. Treatment

a. Treatment involves central nervous system stimulants in combination with behavioral therapies; a multimodal approach is crucial for success. Remissions may occur, most often between 12 and 20 years of age.

b. Pharmacotherapeutic agents, such as methylphenidate (Ritalin, Concerta, Metadate), dexmethylphenidate (Focalin), and amphetamine/dextroamphetamine (Adderall, Dexedrine), have been used successfully and are considered to be first-line treatment.

c. Atomoxetine (Strattera) is a selective norepinephrine reuptake inhibitor (nonstimulant) recently approved for treatment of ADD and ADHD. Efficacy is equal to that of the stimulants, and side effects are similar but less frequent. It is NOT a controlled substance and, therefore, will add convenience to therapy.

TABLE 12-3	**Symptoms of Attention-Deficit Disorder and Attention-Deficit Hyperactivity Disorder Used for Diagnostic Criteria**

Inattention symptoms
    Makes careless mistakes and has trouble attending to details
    Problems in sustaining attention; does not appear attentive when directly addressed
    Does not follow through or complete assigned work
    Forgetful
    Easily distracted from activities by other things going on at the same time
    Loses items critical to accomplishing assigned activities
    Avoids activities requiring sustained mental effort
    Has difficulty in organizing tasks

Hyperactivity and impulsivity symptoms
    Fidgets or squirms
    Leaves seat often
    Restlessness
    Difficulty playing quietly
    Talking excessively
    Blurting out
    Difficulty awaiting turn
    Interrupts or intrudes on others

        d. Antidepressants, including bupropion, venlafaxin, and guanfacine, and clonidine, can be used as adjuncts.

        e. Therapy should include behavior modification, educational and classroom management, and family therapy. Group therapy can improve social skills and self-esteem.

  B. Disruptive behavioral disorders

    1. Conduct disorder

      a. General characteristics

        (1) This disorder affects boys more often than girls.

        (2) There is a 40% risk of antisocial personality disorder in adulthood.

        (3) There is a high comorbidity with ADD and ADHD, learning disability, mood disorders, and substance abuse disorder.

        (4) Diagnostic criteria. The diagnosis is established based on a pattern of behavior that involves violation of the basic rights of others or of social norms, with at least three acts of the following types: aggression toward people and animals, destruction of property, deceitfulness, and serious violations of rules.

      b. Treatment

        (1) A multimodal approach is used, involving environmental and behavioral modifications and psychotherapy, with the use of pharmacotherapy for specific behaviors.

        (2) Haloperidol, risperidone, and olanzapine can be used to treat aggressive/assaultive behaviors.

        (3) The SSRIs may aid to reduce impulsivity and mood lability/irritability.

    2. Oppositional defiant disorder

      a. General characteristics

        (1) This disorder affects 16–22% of children. It will remit in 25%, but it also may progress to conduct disorder.

        (2) There is a high comorbidity with substance abuse disorders, mood disorders, and ADD and ADHD.

        (3) Diagnostic criteria. The diagnosis includes at least 6 months of negativistic, hostile, and defiant behavior, including at least four of the following: frequent loss of temper, arguments with adults, defying adults' rules, deliberately annoying others, easily annoyed, anger and resentment, spiteful, and blaming others for mistakes or misbehaviors.

      b. Treatment

        (1) Family intervention using training skills in child management for the parents/caregivers is crucial.

        (2) Individual psychotherapy, focusing on behavioral modification and problem-solving skills, is recommended.

  C. Pervasive developmental disorders

    1. Autistic disorder is characterized by impaired social interaction, impaired communications, and repetitive stereotyped patterns of behavior and activities.

    2. Asperger's disorder is characterized by impaired social interaction and restricted or stereotyped behavior, interests, or activities.

    3. Rett's disorder is characterized by decreasing head circumference per height and weight advances as well as loss of previously learned behaviors, social interactions, and motor and language development.

    4. Treatment. These disorders require supportive treatment.

X. ABUSE AND NEGLECT

  A. Child abuse

    1. Definition

      a. In most states, health care providers are required to alert the appropriate authorities if abuse or neglect of a child is suspected.

      b. When a young patient presents with any condition that appears questionable for physical, emotional, or sexual abuse or neglect, it is best to consult with a mental health professional or family social services.

      c. The child must be protected from further abuse as well as treated for current injuries.

2. Physical signs of abuse

    a. Any injury that cannot be adequately explained or is not consistent with the history given has the potential of being abuse.

    b. Bruises, lacerations, soft-tissue swelling, dislocations, or fractures and spiral fractures are common.

    c. Burns that are doughnut-shaped, in a stocking-gloved distribution, or symmetrically round (e.g., caused by a lit cigarette) are other signs.

    d. Bruises or injuries that form regular patterns on the face, back, buttocks, or thighs may be the result of abuse.

    e. Other physical signs are internal hemorrhages, abdominal injuries, bite marks, and injuries that have the shape of the instrument used to make them (e.g., belt, cord, hand).

3. General characteristics

    a. Psychiatric disturbances as a result of abuse are common and include anxiety, aggressive or violent behavior, PTSD, depression, suicide, substance abuse, poor self-esteem, dissociative disorders, and paranoid ideation.

    b. Abuse or neglect also can be manifested in subtle ways, such as failure to thrive.

    c. Munchausen-by-proxy syndrome

        (1) This is a form of abuse usually perpetrated by the mother. Symptoms are fabricated or clinical signs are induced in a child, resulting in repeated visits to a health care provider for relief.

        (2) The perpetrator induces the various signs and symptoms to receive attention as being either an attentive or a suffering parent.

    d. Corporal punishment within reason is not normally considered to be abuse; it becomes abuse if the parent indicates receiving gratification while administering the punishment.

    e. Neglect also can be considered when a client allows a minor to engage in potentially harmful behavior (e.g., alcohol consumption) or remain unattended. In some states, leaving a child younger than 13 years of age at home alone is considered to be neglect.

B. Sexual abuse

  1. General characteristics

    a. Approximately 25% of women and 12% of men report histories of being sexually abused as children.

    b. Common ages of abuse are between 9 and 12 years. Such abuse often involves a male who is known by the child.

  2. Any of the following should raise the suspicion of sexual abuse in a child.

    a. Evidence of a sexually transmitted disease.

    b. Bruises, pain, itching, or any trauma of the anal or genital area.

    c. Detailed knowledge about sexual acts that are inappropriate for age.

    d. Child initiates sexual acts with others, especially peers.

    e. Child exhibits sexual knowledge through play.

C. Spousal abuse

  1. General information

    a. When confronted with a patient who may be a victim of spousal abuse, the following actions are needed.

        (1) Immediate medical attention to address the physical sequelae.

        (2) Recognition of suspected abuse and engagement of the patient in nonthreatening questioning to confirm whether abuse has occurred. If abuse has occurred, it must be emphasized to the abused patient that someone does care and that there are alternatives.

    b. Provision of contact numbers for referral agencies (e.g., legal recourse, local emergency shelters, support groups). The decision to accept a referral ultimately is the patient's, but if help is offered and accepted, one must ensure that a referral can be made immediately.

  2. Precautions

    a. Caution is required in dealing with cases of spousal abuse.

        (1) The patient should be presented with options and allowed to decide which path to take.

        (2) The abused may close ranks with the abuser and confront the clinician for attempting to break up the family.

        (3) It is estimated that a woman who leaves an abusive partner has a 70% greater risk of being killed by the batterer than a woman who stays.

    b. Battered victims have suffered a blow to their ego defenses and may not be assertive enough to believe that their rights have been violated.

    c. It is not uncommon to find battered women who believe that they either deserved the beating or must accept the beatings as the price for a roof over their head and food on the table.

D. Elder abuse

  1. General characteristics

    a. Elder abuse affects 10% of the population older than 65 years. Most victims are very old, frail, and vulnerable.

    b. It can be physical, sexual, psychological, emotional, or financial, or it can be in the form of neglect.

  2. Forms of abuse

    a. Physical or sexual abuse is suspected in the presence of bruises, puncture wounds, fractures, cuts, burns, poor hygiene, soiled clothing, hair loss in clumps, weight loss or poor nutrition, dehydration, lack of eyeglass or hearing aids, injuries from use of restraints, genital or rectal injuries or bleeding, evidence of excessive drugging, or a lack of or delay in seeking medical attention.

    b. Psychological abuse can be manifested by threats, insults or verbal abuse, or refusal to allow travel, church attendance, or family visits.

    c. Financial abuse may come in the form of misuse of the patient's funds.

    d. Neglect includes the withholding of food, medicine, clothing, routine health care, or other basic necessities.

  3. Clinicians should be aware of the following.

    a. Previous history of abuse by the caregiver.

    b. Conflicting accounts of accidents by caregiver.

    c. Unwillingness of a caregiver to agree to implementation of treatment plans.

    d. Inappropriate defensiveness by the caregiver.

    e. A caregiver who will not allow, or who limits, the patient's responses to questions.

    f. Some states have the same reporting requirements for suspected elder abuse as for child abuse.

XI. RAPE CRISIS

A. Definition

  1. Rape is an act of aggression that may be perpetrated on a spouse, a known partner, or a stranger.

  2. Forced acts of fellatio and anal penetration are considered to be sodomy.

  3. Forced participation in any sexual acts can result in psychological sequelae.

  4. A patient who has been raped or sodomized may experience depression; lack of appetite; sleep disturbances; rage and anger; feelings of worthlessness; enduring patterns of sexual dysfunction; agoraphobia; fear of future violence, death, or contracting a sexually transmitted disease; feelings of being used or dirty; and anxiety attacks.

B. Approach to the patient

  1. History and physical examination, including genital and rectal examinations.

    a. Rape constitutes both a psychiatric emergency and a legal situation; all procedures should be documented, clothing saved, and samples taken.

    b. A rape kit, which has instructions on questions to include in the history, on how specimen samples are to be collected and under what conditions, and on how samples should be handled after collection, is valuable and ensures that the proper evidence is secured.

    c. Explain to the patient the purpose of all procedures, and inform the patient of what is being done before doing it. This provides the patient with a feeling of some control.

  2. Prevention of sexually transmitted diseases and pregnancy. Prophylactic antibiotic therapy should be initiated; the patient should be given the option of emergency contraception.

  3. Counseling. As soon as possible after the event, and preferably before leaving the emergency department, the patient should talk to a mental health professional, and follow-up counseling should be scheduled.

XII. UNCOMPLICATED BEREAVEMENT

A. Definition

1. Uncomplicated bereavement is defined as a normal response to a major loss.

2. Duration of the reaction depends on the suddenness of the loss, the relationship of the survivor to the deceased, and the age or physical condition of the person who has died.

3. Normal grief symptoms resolve within 1 year; the most severe symptoms occur within the first 2 months.

4. Some patients do develop major depressive disorder. This diagnosis is not made until grief symptoms fail to resolve.

B. General characteristics

1. The mourner experiences shock, confusion, sadness, numbness, or guilt. Symptoms of depression may be seen.

2. Mourners sometimes report illusions, such as briefly seeing or hearing the deceased, or they may deny certain aspects of the death. These are considered to be normal reactions; however, hallucinations that are persistent and/or intrusive, or the belief that the deceased is still alive, are not.

3. Treatment

a. Treatment consists of social contact and reassurances.

b. Patients probably are not helped by antidepressant medications. Benzodiazepines, in short courses only, may alleviate insomnia.

13 Dermatology

Edward D. Huechtker

I. DIAGNOSIS

A. History and physical examination

1. History

    a. A thorough history is the first step in accurate diagnosis of skin diseases.

    b. Past medical history, medication history, family history, psychosocial factors, recreational and employment risk, and diet and environmental exposures should be investigated.

2. Physical examination

    a. A general physical examination, paying particular attention to the skin, hair, nails, and mucocutaneous surfaces, should be carried out under natural or bright light.

    b. A magnifying glass may be useful.

3. Special signs and tests

    a. Darier's sign. Rubbing a lesion causes urticarial flare.

    b. Auspitz's sign. Pinpoint bleeding after scale is removed.

    c. Nikolsky's sign. Pushing a blister causes further separation of the dermis.

    d. Photopatch test. Documents photoallergy.

    e. Patch test. Demonstrates hypersensitivity reaction.

    f. Koebner's phenomenon. Minor trauma leads to more lesions.

4. Diagnostic techniques

    a. Diascopy

        (1) A glass slide or diascope is pressed against the skin to reveal changes produced in the underlying skin when pressure is applied.

        (2) Blanching indicates intact capillaries; extravasated blood (purpura) does not blanch.

    b. Potassium hydroxide preparation (KOH prep)

        (1) Microscopic examination of skin scrapings mounted in KOH, which dissolves keratin and cellular material but does not affect fungi.

        (2) This method readily identifies dermatophytes.

    c. Scrapings and smears

        (1) Blunt and sharp instruments facilitate specimen collections.

        (2) Various staining techniques and visualization methods (e.g., Tzanck smear, dark-field microscopy) bring out certain characteristics of the lesion or responsible pathogen.

    d. Wood's light examination is used to assess changes in pigment or to fluoresce infectious lesions.

    e. Acetowhitening, using acetic acid, facilitates examination of penile or vulvar warts.

    f. Biopsy (excisional, incisional, shave, punch) is indicated if pathologic confirmation is necessary.

B. Common dermatologic terminology

1. Common skin lesions are defined in Table 13-1.

2. The following descriptive terms also are useful.

    a. Telangiectasia. Dilated, superficial blood vessel.

    b. Lichenification. Thickened skin with distinct borders.

    c. Macerated. Swollen and softened by an increase in water content; the appearance skin gets when left in water too long.

    d. Verrucous. Irregular, rough, and convoluted surfaces.

TABLE 13-1	Common Skin Lesions
Papule	Solid, palpable lesion <10 mm in diameter
Nodule	Solid, palpable lesion >10 mm in diameter
Macule	Flat, nonpalpable lesion <10 mm in diameter
Patch	Flat, nonpalpable lesion >10 mm in diameter
Plaque	Plateau-like lesion >10 mm in diameter, may be a group of confluent papules
Vesicle	Circumscribed, elevated lesion containing serous fluid <5 mm in diameter
Bulla	Circumscribed, elevated lesion containing serous fluid >5 mm in diameter
Wheal	Transient, elevated lesion caused by local edema
Petechiae	Minute hemorrhagic spots that cannot be blanched by diascopy
Crust	Hard, rough surface formed by dried sebum, exudate, blood, or necrotic skin
Scale	Heaped-up piles of horny epithelium with a dry appearance

II. MACULOPAPULAR AND PLAQUE DISORDERS

A. Eczematous disorders

1. The terms eczema and dermatitis are used interchangeably. Eczema more commonly denotes endogenous disorders, and dermatitis denotes exogenous disorders.

2. There are many eczematous disorders, encompassing a wide range of polymorphic inflammatory reaction patterns.

3. Contact dermatitis

  a. General characteristics

    (1) Irritant contact dermatitis is caused by a chemical irritant in contact with the skin.

    (2) Allergic contact dermatitis denotes an allergic type IV cell-mediated hypersensitivity reaction. Occupational or personal contact with irritants, such as cleaning supplies, solvents, oils, abrasives, oxidizing or reducing agents, dust, nickel, enzymes, and plants, are common.

  b. Clinical features

    (1) Patients complain of itching and burning in the affected areas.

    (2) Acute lesions typically are well-demarcated areas of erythema and plaques; vesicles, erosions, and crusts may develop.

    (3) Chronic lesions show plaques and scaling with lichenification. Satellite papules and excoriations are common.

  c. Laboratory studies

    (1) Patch tests that result in similar reactions support the diagnosis.

    (2) Gram stains or cultures should be done if secondary infection is suspected.

  d. Treatment

    (1) Avoid or remove the offending agent. Wet dressings with Burow's solution and topical corticosteroids are sufficient in most cases.

    (2) Severe cases may necessitate systemic steroids.

    (3) Chronic lesions can be treated with topical steroids.

    (4) Supportive measures include cleaning with mild soaps or oatmeal preparations and antihistamines to help alleviate itching.

4. Atopic dermatitis

  a. General characteristics

    (1) This is a chronic relapsing skin disorder that begins in childhood.

    (2) It is a type I immunoglobulin E–mediated hypersensitivity reaction.

    (3) Many patients also have asthma or allergic rhinitis (atopy).

b. Clinical features

(1) Papules and plaques, with or without scales, are noted and may be associated with edema, erosion, and crusts.

(2) Patients complain of pruritus and dry, scaly skin. Scratching leads to lichenification, fissures, and worsening rash; secondary infections most commonly are caused by *Staphylococcus aureus*.

(3) The rash is most common on the flexural surfaces, neck, eyelids, forehead, face, and dorsum of the hands and feet.

(4) Dermatographism is characteristic.

c. Laboratory studies. Not routinely done, although cultures for suspected secondary infection may help to guide treatment.

d. Treatment

(1) Antihistamines help to reduce itching.

(2) Topical corticosteroids are the mainstay of treatment; avoid systemic corticosteroids.

(3) Hydration and topical emollients are key to management. Soaps should be avoided.

(4) Ultraviolet B (UVB) phototherapy is effective.

(5) Severe systemic cases may necessitate cyclosporine.

5. Nummular dermatitis

a. General characteristics

(1) This is a pruritic inflammatory disorder that typically affects young adults and the elderly.

(2) It typically occurs during the winter.

b. Clinical features

(1) Small, grouped vesicles coalesce to form coin-shaped plaques with an erythematous base.

(2) Crusting and excoriations occur.

c. Treatment

(1) This is a chronic disorder that responds to moisturizers or topical steroids.

(2) Tar baths or UVB phototherapy is helpful for refractory cases.

6. Seborrheic dermatitis

a. General characteristics

(1) Seborrheic dermatitis is common during infancy and puberty and in young to middle-aged adults.

(2) It occurs where sebaceous glands are most active (body folds, face, scalp, genitalia).

b. Clinical features

(1) Scattered yellowish or gray, scaly macules and papules with a greasy look are noted.

(2) Sticky crusts and fissures are found behind the ears, especially in infants. On the scalp, it manifests as cradle cap in infants and dandruff in adults.

c. Treatment

(1) Ultraviolet radiation is helpful; lesions resolve during the summer and flare during the fall and winter.

(2) Cradle cap. Treat with olive oil compresses and baby shampoo or ketoconazole shampoo or cream or with hydrocortisone.

(3) Dandruff. Use shampoos containing selenium or zinc and ketoconazole shampoo for acute flare-ups; tar shampoos or topical steroids can be used for severe cases.

(4) Other areas. Use ketoconazole shampoo or topical steroids; blepharitis is treated with gentle scrubs using baby shampoo, followed by a suspension of sulfa and/or steroid preparation or ketoconazole cream if needed.

7. Perioral dermatitis

a. General characteristics. Typically occurs in young women.

b. Clinical features. Papulopustules are on erythematous bases; may become confluent with plaques and scales; satellite lesions are common.

c. Laboratory studies. Culture to rule out staphylococcal infection.

d. Treatment

(1) Avoid topical steroids, because they will aggravate the lesions.

(2) Use topical metronidazole or erythromycin or oral minocycline, doxycycline, or tetracycline.

(3) Untreated lesions will fluctuate over time, similar to rosacea.

8. Stasis dermatitis

   a. General characteristics

      (1) Chronic venous insufficiency leads to edema, stasis dermatitis, hyperpigmentation, fibrosis, and ulceration.

      (2) Varicose veins, superficial phlebitis, and venous thrombosis commonly occur before skin changes.

      (3) Women are affected three times more often than men. Pregnancy will exacerbate both venous insufficiency and stasis dermatitis.

   b. Clinical features

      (1) Patients complain of heaviness or aching in the legs that is aggravated by standing and relieved with walking.

      (2) Dermatitis of the lower legs and feet manifests with inflammatory papules, scales, and crusts. Stippled pigmentation develops, and excoriations are common.

      (3) Ulcerations will occur in 30% of patients.

   c. Laboratory studies

      (1) Doppler studies, sonography, or venography exhibit chronic insufficiency.

      (2) Biopsy of lesions shows dilated vessels, tortuous veins, edema, and fibrin deposition.

   d. Treatment

      (1) Chronic venous insufficiency is treated with compression stockings. Sclerosis of varicose veins helps to prevent further dermatitis, but recurrence is common.

      (2) Vascular bypass or angioplasty may benefit severely compromised areas, but results are only fair.

      (3) Ulcers demand chronic treatment.

B. Lichen simplex chronicus

   1. General characteristics

      a. This is a long-term manifestation of atopic dermatitis.

      b. The skin of patients with atopic dermatitis is sensitive to minor trauma, including touch, rubbing, or scratching.

      c. Lichenification develops as well-circumscribed plaques that are highly pruritic. This sets up a cycle of itch–scratch lesions.

   2. Clinical features

      a. Solid, firm, thick plaques with little to no scaling are seen.

      b. Light touch precipitates a strong desire to scratch.

      c. Lesions can be single or multiple. Common areas include nuchal area, scalp, ankles, lower legs, upper thighs, exterior forearms, or genital areas.

      d. Black skin more typically shows a follicular pattern of smaller papules rather than larger plaques.

   3. Laboratory studies.

      a. A KOH prep is done to rule out fungal infection.

      b. Biopsy shows hyperplasia and hyperkeratosis.

   4. Treatment

      a. Topical steroids or tar preparations with occlusive dressing can be used

      b. Antihistamines will reduce itching.

C. Pityriasis rosea

   1. General characteristics

      a. Pityriasis rosea is characterized by a herald patch, which precedes a widespread symmetrical papular eruption.

      b. The cause is unknown but is thought to be viral (human herpes virus 7).

   2. Clinical features

      a. There may be a mild upper respiratory tract infection–like prodrome before the onset of the rash.

      b. The herald patch is a solitary round or oval pink plaque with a raised border and fine adherent scales in the margin. It typically precedes the rash by a week or so.

  c. The rash begins to appear on the trunk as round or oval, salmon-colored, slightly raised papular and macular lesions usually 1 cm in diameter.

  d. The long axis of each lesion usually follows the natural skin folds, giving a Christmas tree–like distribution. It is usually confined to the trunk.

  e. In the beginning, the lesions are covered with a fine scale that desquamates, leaving an inverse collarette scale around each lesion.

  f. Pityriasis rosea usually lasts for 3–8 weeks and disappears spontaneously.

 3. Treatment

  a. No treatment is indicated other than lotions or emollients for the scales.

  b. UVB phototherapy may be helpful if started during the first week of eruption.

  c. Lotions, antipruritics, or oral antihistamines may help if itching is bothersome.

D. Molluscum contagiosum

 1. General characteristics

  a. This is a common viral disease of the skin and mucous membranes caused by a poxvirus. It is common in children but can affect adults.

  b. In adults, the lesions are commonly in the groin areas and on the lower abdomen.

  c. The virus can be transmitted during sexual activity.

  d. In immunocompromised patients (such as HIV), lesions can be larger and be more widespread, including predominance on the head and neck.

 2. Clinical features

  a. Lesions manifest as discrete, flesh-colored, waxy, dome-shaped, umbilicated papules over the face, trunk, and extremities.

  b. They range in size from 3 to 6 mm and appear in groups.

  c. A white, curd-like material can be expressed from under the depression of the lesion.

 3. Laboratory studies. Biopsy may be needed in immunocompromised patients to rule out fungal dissemination.

 4. Treatment

  a. Treatment usually is not necessary, because the disease is self-limited.

  b. If therapy is indicated, it consists of local destruction of individual lesions either by curettage, cryotherapy, electrodessication, or an acid or exfoliative peel (e.g., tretinoin, imiquod [Aldara]). These treatments can be painful.

E. Lichen planus

 1. General characteristics

  a. This is an acute or chronic inflammatory dermatitis that occurs in adults. Females are more commonly affected than males.

  b. Lichen planus–like eruptions may occur in graft-versus-host disease, malignant lymphoma, and drug reactions.

 2. Clinical features

  a. Lichen planus is designated as the 4 P's—purple, polygonal, pruritic papule.

  b. Lesions are flat-topped, shiny, violaceous papules with surface white lines (Wickham's striae). They typically are grouped and most commonly occur on the flexor aspect of the wrists, lumbar area, eyelids, shins, and scalp.

  c. Mucosal lesions occur on the glans and penis and in the mouth. They usually are very painful, and they often ulcerate.

  d. Variants include follicular, vesicular, actinic, and ulcerative lesions.

  e. Lesions may affect hair (scarring alopecia) or nails (destruction of nail fold and bed with longitudinal splintering).

 3. Laboratory studies. Biopsy and immunofluorescence confirm the diagnosis.

 4. Treatment

  a. Topical steroids with occlusive dressings are used.

  b. Intralesional steroids or topical tretinoin is used for severe lesions.

  c. Cyclosporine mouthwash is used for oral lesions.

  d. Systemic therapy (cyclosporine, corticosteroids, or retinoids) may be needed in severe, painful cases.

  e. Psoralens plus ultraviolet A (PUVA) radiation therapy is helpful in generalized eruptions.

F. Dyshidrosis

1. General characteristics

 a. This dermatitis generally develops in people younger than 40 years. Half of those affected have an atopic background.

 b. Eruptions follow stress or occur in hot, humid weather.

2. Clinical features

 a. Early disease

  (1) Pruritus is common; pain develops if secondarily infected.

  (2) Small vesicles in clusters (tapioca appearance) are seen, and occasionally, bullae form.

 b. Late disease

  (1) Papules, scaling, lichenification, and erosions from ruptured vesicles are seen.

  (2) Painful fissures may develop.

 c. There is a predilection for the hands and feet.

3. Laboratory studies

 a. Culture is done to rule out secondary infection.

 b. KOH prep will rule out dermatophytosis.

4. Treatment

 a. Wet dressings with Burow's solution. Large bullae should be drained but kept intact.

 b. Fissures are treated with topical collodion.

 c. Topical steroids are used for localized lesions and systemic steroids for severe cases.

 d. Treat secondary infection with systemic antimicrobials.

G. Psoriasis

1. General characteristics

 a. Psoriasis affects 2% of the population (3–5 million people).

 b. Most patients have localized psoriasis, but more severe forms exist.

 c. A genetic predisposition exists, although only about one-third of the patients have family members with the condition.

 d. Psoriasis is a chronic, inflammatory, scaling condition of the skin that also may involve the mucous membranes. It seems that the earlier the onset of the disease, the more severe it will be. Psoriasis in HIV-positive patients can be very severe and resistant to treatment.

 e. The basic pathology is a greatly enhanced epidermal cell turnover (to a rate 28 times normal).

2. Clinical features

 a. Psoriasis patches usually are raised, pink to red papules and plaques with distinct margins and loosely adherent silvery scales. Peeling away a scale produces specks of bleeding from the capillaries (Auspitz's sign).

 b. Patches most often are found on the elbows, knees, and scalp but can be found anywhere on the body.

 c. Pruritus is common. Scratching leads to more lesions (Koebner's phenomenon).

 d. Patients with extensive disease also have nail involvement. The nails have tiny pits and ridges, are separated from the nail bed (onycholysis), and have oil spots.

 e. Psoriatic arthritis occurs in 5–10% of patients. It involves the distal joints of the hands and feet, typically is asymmetric, and may be present without lesions.

 f. Diagnosis is made by history and appearance. The symptoms usually are mild, but the lesions are unsightly and interfere with business and social activities.

 g. Variants

  (1) Psoriatic vulgaris is the most common type and involves chronic recurring scaling papules and plaques.

  (2) In psoriatic erythroderma, lesions involve the entire skin surface; this variant is exfoliative and serious.

  (3) Guttate psoriasis is characterized by acute eruption of typical and atypical lesions in a disseminated pattern; it spares the palms and soles and often appears after streptococcal pharyngitis.

  (4) Pustular psoriasis (von Zumbusch's syndrome) is an abrupt, life-threatening condition characterized by widespread pustules that coalesce to form lakes of pus; fever, malaise, and leukocytosis are seen.

3. Treatment

    a. In mild cases, treatment consists of topical corticosteroids and topical vitamin D preparations (calcipotriene).

    b. Systemic steroids help, but the disease often will flare after withdrawal.

    c. Coal tar or salicylic acid preparations and occlusive dressings are effective in controlling or removing scales.

    d. Moderate psoriasis may respond to tazarotene gel (topical retinoid).

    e. For more serious cases, UVB phototherapy, PUVA, and methotrexate have been effective but carry risks of skin cancer, cataracts, and hepatotoxicity.

    f. Pustular psoriasis may respond to acitretin, a synthetic retinoid, with or without ultraviolet treatment. This also is helpful in erythroderma and psoriatic arthritis but is teratogenic.

    g. Cyclosporine may be effective in severe recalcitrant disease, but recurrence after cessation is common.

III. VESICULOBULLOUS DISORDERS

A. Pemphigus vulgaris

    1. General characteristics

        a. This is a serious bullous autoimmune disease; immunoglobulin G antibodies induce acantholysis, resulting in a loss of cell-to-cell adhesion.

        b. The disorder occurs in middle-aged adults.

    2. Clinical features

        a. Lesions begin in the oral mucosa; skin lesions occur 6–12 months later. There may be pain or burning but not pruritus. Weakness and malaise are common.

        b. Lesions are round vesicles or bullae that contain clear liquid and easily rupture. They are discrete and randomly scattered. Erosions and crust occur because of the fragility of the blisters (Nikolsky's sign).

        c. Secondary infection as well as fluid and electrolyte imbalance are common causes of morbidity and mortality.

        d. Variants include pemphigus vegetans, pemphigus foliaceous, Brazilian pemphigus (fogo selvagem), pemphigus erythematosus, drug-induced pemphigus, and paraneoplastic pemphigus.

    3. Laboratory studies

        a. Immunofluorescence of serum or blister material highlights immunoglobulin G.

        b. Biopsy proves acantholysis.

    4. Treatment

        a. Systemic therapy is required. Start with prednisone, then add immunosuppressive agents, azathioprine, and/or methotrexate.

        b. Dapsone, gold, or cyclophosphamide may help in refractory cases.

        c. Supportive therapies include fluid and electrolyte replacement, cleansing baths, wet dressings, topical steroids, and antibiotics as needed.

B. Bullous pemphigoid

    1. General characteristics

        a. This autoimmune disorder occurs typically in patients in their sixth decade of life.

        b. Autoantibodies, complement fixation, neutrophil, and eosinophils cause bullous formation.

    2. Clinical features

        a. There may be a prodrome of urticarial or papular lesions.

        b. Bullae are large, tense, oval or round, and contain serous or hemorrhagic fluid. They rupture less easily than in pemphigus.

        c. Typically, bullae collapse and crust; at times, bleeding erosions occur.

        d. Axillae, thighs, groin, and abdomen commonly are affected. Mucous membrane lesions are less severe and less painful than in pemphigus vulgaris.

    3. Laboratory studies. Biopsy and immunofluorescence will confirm the diagnosis.

    4. Treatment

        a. Systemic prednisone at high doses until remission, then at a lower dose for maintenance.

        b. Azathioprine may be added.

        c. Mild cases or localized recurrences are treated with topical steroids.

IV. PAPULOPUSTULAR INFLAMMATORY DISORDERS

A. Acne vulgaris

1. General characteristics

a. Acne affects all age groups, from neonates to older adults. It is most prevalent in adolescents and more severe in males.

b. Pathology includes plugged follicles, retained sebum, bacterial overgrowth, and release of fatty acids. Androgens stimulate sebum production.

2. Clinical features

a. Acne is an inflammatory follicular, papular, and pustular eruption involving the pilosebaceous apparatus.

b. Acne lesions can be open comedones or closed, noninflammatory comedones.

(1) Open comedones often are referred to as "blackheads" because of melanin depositions on a keratin plug.

(2) Closed comedones, often called "whiteheads," are flesh-colored, 1-mm papules.

(3) Open or closed comedones can become erythematous papules, pustules, nodules, or cysts, ranging in size from 1–5 mm.

c. Sinus tracts occur with nodular acne. Inflammatory lesions can lead to hyperpigmentation and scarring.

3. Laboratory studies. Testosterone, follicle-stimulating hormone, luteinizing hormone, or dehydroepiandrosterone 5 levels can be measured if an endocrine disorder is suggested; however, the majority of acne is not endocrine based.

4. Treatment

a. Treatment for mild acne can be accomplished by keeping the affected areas clean and applying topical preparations, such as retinoids, azelaic acid, and salicylic acid.

b. If inflammatory lesions are present, topical benzoyl peroxide, tretinoin, erythromycin, clindamycin, or sodium sulfacetamide can be used.

c. In more serious or cystic acne, oral antibiotics should be used in conjunction with the topical preparations.

(1) Tetracyclines were the drug of choice early on and are still effective. Erythromycin, doxycycline, minocycline, trimethoprim/sulfamethoxazole, and clindamycin also frequently are used.

(2) The bacterium that is involved in acne is becoming resistant to some medications. It is best to treat as conservatively as possible and only for as long as necessary.

(3) Recurrence after cessation is common.

d. Accutane (oral isotretinoin)

(1) This medication can be prescribed only by a dermatologic provider approved by Roche.

(2) Side effects can be very serious, ranging from dry eyes, nose, and lips to epistaxis, joint pains, mood swings, and suicidal thoughts.

(3) Premature closure of the long bones, visual changes, hepatic enzyme elevation, leukopenia, triglyceridemia, and teratogenicity also occur.

B. Acne rosacea

1. General characteristics

a. Acne rosacea is a chronic acneiform disorder mainly affecting females between 30 and 50 years of age.

b. It is a disease of the pilosebaceous units associated with increased activity of capillaries, which leads to flushing and telangiectasias.

c. The outbreaks are episodic and typically occur in response to heat, alcohol, or hot, spicy foods. Coffee and tea stimulate outbreaks because of the heat, not the caffeine.

2. Clinical features

a. It is characterized by the insidious onset of scattered, small papulopustules and sometimes nodules; comedones do not occur. The face appears red or flushed.

b. There is a symmetric distribution on the face (cheeks, chin, forehead, glabella, nose). Sometimes, lesions appear on the neck, chest, back or scalp.

c. Later telangiectasia, hyperplasia, and lymphedema develop.

d. Patients often complain of disfiguring appearance.

e. When describing effects, the suffix -phyma, meaning "enlarged," is used: rhinophyma (nose), blepharophyma (eyelid), metophyma (forehead), otophyma (ear), or gnathophyma (mouth).

3. Treatment

  a. Reduce triggers, such as alcohol or hot beverages.

  b. Topical metronidazole, sodium sulfacetamide, or antibiotics often are sufficient.

  c. If topical treatment fails, systemic antibiotics, such as tetracycline, minocycline, or doxycycline, are tried until remission and then continued at lower doses for maintenance.

  d. Very severe cases may need oral isotretinoin under the care of a dermatologic specialist.

C. Folliculitis

  1. General characteristics

  a. Folliculitis is an inflammation of the hair follicles.

  b. It most commonly is caused by *Staphylococcus aureus* but can be caused by other organisms. Pseudomonal folliculitis has been reported in hot tub users.

  c. Noninfectious folliculitis is common among people working in hot, oily environments, such as engine workers on ships, machinists, or anyone working in a hot, dirty environment.

  d. Occlusion, perspiration, and rubbing from tight clothes also may cause folliculitis.

  e. Pseudofolliculitis is defined as ingrown hairs occurring in the beard area.

  2. Clinical features

  a. The lesions are erythematous papules or pustules. They usually are not painful but may burn.

  b. Sycosis is severe, deep-seated, recalcitrant folliculitis with surrounding eczema and crusting.

  c. Abscesses may form at the site of folliculitis.

  3. Treatment

  a. Gentle cleansing and mild compresses help. Protection from offending substances and use of drying agents also helps.

  b. Topical application of clindamycin or erythromycin works well on mild cases. Mupirocin (Bactroban) ointment also may be used.

  c. In more extensive cases, oral antibiotics may be necessary.

  d. Hot tub folliculitis usually resolves without treatment but may be treated with a fluoroquinolone.

D. Erythema multiforme (EM)

  1. General characteristics

  a. EM can be induced by drugs (sulfonamides, phenytoin, barbiturates, penicillin, allopurinol), following infections (herpes simplex virus, *Mycoplasma* sp.), or be idiopathic (50% of cases).

  b. Half of all cases occur in patients younger than 20 years.

  c. Previous history of EM is a strong risk factor for subsequent cases.

  2. Clinical features

  a. Lesions begin as macules and become papular, then vesicles and bullae form in the center of the papules.

  b. Lesions can be localized to the hands and feet or become generalized.

  c. Mucosal lesions (hallmark of EM major) are painful and erode.

  d. Patients complain of fever, weakness, and malaise. Lungs and eyes may be affected.

  3. Treatment

  a. Avoid target substances, and control herpes outbreaks with acyclovir.

  b. Severely ill patients are treated with systemic steroids.

E. Stevens-Johnson syndrome (SJS) and toxic erythema nodosa (TEN)

  1. General characteristics

  a. These are mucocutaneous blistering reactions most often caused by a drug reaction. Drugs associated with SJS or TEN include sulfonamides, aminopenicillins, quinolones, cephalosporins, tetracyclines, phenobarbital, carbamazepine, phenytoin, valproic acid, oxicam, allopurinol, and corticosteroids.

  b. SJS is thought to be a severe variant of EM, and TEN is thought to be a severe variant of SJS.

  c. SJS or TEN may occur in patients of any age or gender.

  d. The pathogenesis is unknown, but it is thought to be an immunologic response.

  e. The dangers are secondary infection, fluid loss, and electrolyte imbalance.

2. Clinical features

　a. Patients present with fever, photophobia, sore throat, mucosal inflammation, and sore mouth. The cutaneous lesions tend to be concentrated more on the trunk at first. The lesions may be painful or may sting.

　b. Progression occurs over 4 days: diffuse erythema, morbilliform lesions, necrotic epidermis, wrinkled surfaces, sheet-like loss of epidermis, and raised, flaccid blisters (Nikolsky's sign).

　c. TEN exhibits higher fever and more severe epidermal separation and loss compared with SJS.

　d. Regrowth of skin takes 3 weeks; it is delayed in pressure-point areas.

　e. About 90% of patients have mucosal lesions that are painful and eroding.

　f. Other complications include acute tubular necrosis, erosion in the lungs and gut, and bronchitis.

3. Laboratory studies

　a. Patients have anemia and lymphopenia.

　b. Biopsy is diagnostic.

4. Treatment

　a. Prompt withdrawal of offending or causative agent.

　b. Patients with extensive necrolysis should be transferred to a burn unit for care.

　c. Treat patients for fluid and electrolyte imbalance and any complications or infections.

　d. Treatment debate

　　(1) Corticosteroid treatment is being debated. Some feel massive doses are appropriate; others feel steroids may exacerbate the disease.

　　(2) The same controversy applies to antibiotic therapy, because antibiotics may be the causative agent.

F. Hidradenitis suppurativa

1. General characteristics

　a. Hidradenitis suppurativa is a disease of the apocrine gland areas (axilla, anogenital, scalp).

　b. It affects females between puberty and menopause (axillary disease) more often than it affects males (anogenital disease).

　c. Predisposing factors include obesity, history of acne, apocrine duct obstruction, and bacterial infection. There appears to be a genetic tendency.

2. Clinical features

　a. Tender inflammatory nodule or abscess. Lesions are not related to hair follicles.

　b. Open comedones and sinus tracts form and may drain purulent material.

　c. Fibrosis, scarring, and contractures may occur. Severity is variable.

3. Laboratory studies include culture for secondary bacterial infection.

4. Treatment

　a. Lesions are treated with intralesional triamcinolone, incision and drainage of abscesses, and excision of sinus tracts.

　b. Oral antibiotics are given until lesions resolve; prednisone is added if lesions are severe and should be tapered over 2 weeks.

　c. Severe cases, especially in the anogenital area, may benefit from psychological support.

V. LOCALIZED SKIN INFECTIONS

A. Furuncles and carbuncles

1. General characteristics

　a. Furuncles sometimes are referred to as "boils" or "risens." These lesions are deep-seated infections of the hair follicles; *Staphylococcus aureus* is the most common pathogen.

　b. A furuncle is an infection of a single follicle; a carbuncle includes more than one infected follicle as a conglomerate mass.

2. Clinical features

　a. These lesions present as red, hard, tender lesions in hair-bearing areas of the head, neck, or body.

　b. Lesions progress to become fluctuant and rupture spontaneously, draining pus and necrotic tissue.

   3. Treatment
      a. Treatment should be started with warm, moist compresses.
      b. Antibiotic therapy as well as incision and drainage are added as appropriate once the lesion is mature.
      c. Cloths used for warm compresses and/or towels used to clean or dry these lesions should be handled with care to prevent additional infection.

B. Cellulitis
   1. General characteristics
      a. Cellulitis is an acute, spreading inflammation of the dermis and subcutaneous tissue.
      b. Although the causative organism can be identified by culturing any drainage or discharge or by needle aspiration, it probably is best to begin treatment with antibiotics that will cover *Haemophilus influenza, Streptococcus* sp., and *Staphylococcus* sp.
   2. Clinical features
      a. The area involved is swollen, red, hot, and tender.
      b. The patient may have lymphadenopathy, fever, chills and malaise.
   3. Treatment
      a. Mild or early infections may be treated with an oral penicillinase-resistant penicillin, such as dicloxacillin or a cephalosporin. For patients who are allergic to penicillin, erythromycin is appropriate.
      b. In severe infections, first-generation cephalosporins are given IV. Patients started on parenteral therapy may be switched to oral therapy when the fever, chills, and malaise subside.
      c. It may be appropriate to mark the margins of involvement before treatment to follow the progression or regression of the area.
      d. If there is poor response to antimicrobial therapy or a necrotizing, soft-tissue infection is suspected, surgical intervention is mandatory.

C. Abscess
   1. General characteristics
      a. An abscess is a localized infection characterized by a collection of purulent material in a cavity formed by necrosis or disintegration of tissue.
      b. A sterile abscess is one formed without bacterial pathogen.
   2. Clinical features
      a. Abscess presents as a tender, erythematous, and often fluctuant area, indicating the formation of pus.
      b. The most common locations are axillary, buttocks, perirectal, and the head and neck.
      c. Discharge or drainage can be cultured, but usually, there is more than one causative organism.
      d. An abscess may develop at the site of therapeutic or drug-use injection.
   3. Treatment
      a. Early abscess should be treated with hot soaks for 20 minutes four times daily to bring it to a head. Once the lesion is fluctuant, it can be incised and drained and an iodoform gauze wick placed in the wound to facilitate drainage.
      b. Alternatively, hot soaks can be followed by a dressing saturated with a drawing salve.
      c. Oral antibiotics, such as dicloxacillin, a cephalosporin, or erythromycin, should be started if the patient has a fever or cellulitis surrounding the abscess.

VI. DERMATOPHYTOSIS

A. General characteristics
   1. Dermatophytosis is a superficial fungal infection that can affect the hair, nails, and skin.
   2. The three most common dermatophytes affecting humans are *Trichophyton, Microsporum,* and *Epidermophyton* sp.; *T. rubrum* is the most common dermatophyte in the industrialized world.
   3. When describing the area of infection, the word tinea (meaning "fungal infection") is followed by the affected part of the body: tinea pedis (foot), tinea cruris (groin), tinea corporis (trunk, legs, arms, or neck), tinea barbae (beard area), tinea unguium (nails), tinea manuum (hand), tinea facialis (face), and tinea capitis (head).

B. Clinical features

    1. Generally, dermatophytosis presents as an erythematous, annular patch with distinct borders and a central clearing. A fine scale usually covers the patch.

    2. Symptoms include itching, stinging, and/or burning. Maceration or peeling fissures are common between the digits.

    3. The nails present with a thickening discoloration and onychomycosis of the nail bed and plate.

    4. In tinea capitis, broken hair shafts are seen as black dots.

    5. A kerion (indurated, boggy, inflammatory plaque studded with pustules) can appear with any of these infections but most commonly is found with tinea capitis. It represents an intense inflammatory reaction to superficial dermatophytes.

C. Laboratory studies. A KOH prep should be done to confirm the presence of fungus.

D. Treatment

    1. There is a wide selection of topical creams, ointments, lotions, powders, and sprays to treat dermatophytosis. They should be used twice daily for 4 weeks or more. If vesicles are present, powders help to dry the area and to prevent maceration.

    2. Chronic or resistant infections or nail infection may require oral griseofulvin, itraconazole, terbinafine, or keto-conazole. Treatment may take 3 months.

    3. Kerions are treated with fluconazole or griseofulvin.

    4. Compliance and monitoring are very important in treating these infections.

        a. It is important to advise patients taking griseofulvin not to use alcohol in any form, because it may cause a reaction similar to that with disulfiram (Antabuse), including flushing, headache, nausea, vomiting, sweating, weakness, vertigo, chest pain, dyspnea, and confusion.

        b. Patients with hepatic disorders should be monitored closely when using oral medications.

        c. If the patient will be on these medications for a long period, such as when treating tinea unguium for several months, they should have liver enzymes monitored, starting with a baseline.

    5. Steroids should be avoided. Long-term use will exacerbate the condition and increase the risk of side effects.

    6. Local measures include keeping the skin clean and dry and wearing cotton socks and loose-fitting underclothes.

E. Tinea versicolor (Pityriasis versicolor)

    1. Tinea versicolor is caused by *Malassezia furfur,* a yeast found on the skin of humans. It is not understood why this yeast manifests in the spore and hyphal form in some patients, causing disease.

    2. Clinical features

        a. Tinea versicolor consists of hypo- or hyperpigmented macules that do not tan. Most patients are asymptomatic and notice the infection only during the summer, when their tan is spotted. The disease does not appear to be contagious.

        b. KOH prep of scrapings will show hyphae and spores (spaghetti and meatballs).

    3. Treatment

        a. Treatment consists of daily applications of selenium sulfide shampoo from the neck to the waist; the shampoo is left on for up to 15 min for 7 consecutive days. This can be repeated monthly for maintenance therapy as necessary.

        b. There are other, less popular topical methods of treatment as well as oral treatment with ketoconazole. Patients should not shower for 18 hours after taking oral ketoconazole, because it works by being delivered to the skin surface through the patient's sweat.

        c. Newer imidazole creams, lotions, and solutions are effective, but the expense is prohibitive.

VII. PARASITIC INFESTATIONS

A. Scabies

    1. General characteristics

        a. Scabies is infestation with *Sarcoptes scabiei,* an eight-legged mite.

        b. Scabies can be found in patients of any age but rarely in infants younger than 3 months.

2. Clinical features

a. Distribution is most common on the hands, genitalia, and axillary areas. Lesions often are seen in the web spaces between the fingers and toes, around the belt line, or at the edges of socks.

b. The lesions are pruritic burrows, vesicles, or nodules with excoriations and crusting.

c. Secondary infections typically are caused by group A streptococci.

3. Laboratory studies

a. Look for mites, eggs, or feces in a scraping. A drop of mineral oil before scraping facilitates yield.

b. Positive microscopy is confirmative but not always successful.

4. Treatment

a. Use 1% lindane or 5% permethrin in lotion or cream. It is applied to the skin from the chin to the bottom of the feet and is left on overnight (8 hours), then washed off in the morning. The treatment should be repeated in 7 days.

b. Antihistamines or topical steroids may help with the itching.

c. Lindane is more toxic and should be avoided in children younger than 2 years, people with extensive dermatitis, and those who are pregnant or lactating.

d. All bedclothes and clothing of infected patients and household contacts should be washed.

B. Spider bites

1. General characteristics

a. Although all spiders in the United States are venomous, only a few can puncture the human skin. The most important is the brown recluse (*Loxosceles reclusa*).

b. Most spider bites occur while the patient is sleeping or dressing in the morning after the spider crawled into the clothing during the night.

2. Clinical features

a. Generally, the patient will begin to feel pain 3 hours after a bite; systemic symptoms begin 4–6 hours after the bite.

b. An acute necrotic injury to the skin lasts 10–15 days.

c. Black widows can cause a neurologic overstimulation (e.g., muscle aches, spasms, rigidity). These spiders are not prevalent today.

d. The brown recluse can cause a significant reaction.

(1) The single bite is accompanied by an infarct of skin caused by rapid blood coagulation within the vessels.

(2) The lesion is a sinking macule, pale gray in color, slightly eroded in the center, and has a halo of very tender inflammation and hemorrhage.

(3) The lesion can extend to the muscle and be as large as the palm of the hand.

3. Treatment

a. Most spider bites can be managed with local care and analgesics.

b. Neurologic manifestations of black widow bites are treated with diazepam and calcium gluconate.

c. Brown recluse bites may be treated locally with wound cleansing and analgesia. Extensive débridement has not proven to be beneficial. Usually, the wound decreases significantly in 5–10 days.

d. Antivenin rarely is indicated and is not readily available.

C. Pediculosis

1. General characteristics

a. Lice are 1- to 3-mm, flat creatures with three pairs of legs. Females lay 300 nits during a lifetime. Nits are opalescent, found on hair shafts, and hatch in about 1 week.

b. *Pediculus humanus* var. *capitis* infects the scalp (head lice), and *P. humanus* var. *corporis* infects the body. *Phthirus pubis* infects the pubic area (crabs).

c. Transmission is person to person.

2. Clinical features

a. Pruritus is variable in severity. Excoriations may become secondarily infected.

b. Lice are visible but often difficult to find. Nits are more readily seen on the hair shafts.

3. Laboratory studies. Specimens can be viewed under the microscope to confirm the diagnosis.

4. Treatment
   a. Prevention is key; avoid sharing contact items, such as hats, brushes, and so forth. All contacts should be examined.
   b. Topical insecticides are effective. Permethrin, pyrethrins, and malathion are considered to be first-line treatments; lindane or ivermectin is an alternative.
   c. Special combs help to remove nits; petroleum jelly or other occlusive materials may help to suffocate the lice.
   d. Reapplication in 7–10 days is recommended to kill any newly hatched lice.

VIII. WARTS

A. General characteristics
   1. Warts are caused by the human papilloma virus (HPV). There are 77 known serotypes.
   2. HPV replicates in cutaneous and mucosal epithelium. Growths remain local and regress spontaneously.
   3. Common warts can arise on any skin surface. Genital warts (condylomata) are spread through sexual contact.

B. Clinical features
   1. Skin warts can be flat or superficial. Plantar warts are deeper. The surface is rough, resembling tiny heads of cauliflower.
   2. Warts of the oral cavity or larynx can be life-threatening if they block the airway. They commonly recur after excision.
   3. Anogenital warts occur almost exclusively on the squamous epithelial of the external genitalia and perianal area.
   4. Cervical warts are a risk factor for dysplasia, which may progress to cervical cancer.

C. Laboratory studies
   1. Microscopic study shows characteristic hyperplasia and hyperkeratosis. Koilocytotic squamous cells are present.
   2. The presence of HPV is confirmed by immunofluorescence. Molecular probes can detect HPV in cervical tissue.

D. Treatment
   1. Spontaneous regression is typical over time.
   2. Type, location, and age of patient dictate treatment. The extent of the lesions, the patient's motivation, and the patient's immunologic status also affect treatment choice.
   3. Salicylic acid plasters can be effective for common warts. Cryosurgery or electrodessication can be effective but risks scarring.
   4. Imiquod (Aldara) is a topical therapy patients can apply at home, but compliance is a problem.
   5. Intralesional interferon also may be effective if other treatments fail.
   6. Anogenital warts can be treated with trichloroacetic acid or topical podophyllin, but this may require many applications.
   7. Surgical excision is successful, but recurrence is common.
   8. A vaccine that is effective against four of the strains associated with cervical cancer and warts has been developed and is effective for at least 4–5 years. It is approved for females aged 9–26 years.

IX. TUMORS

A. Benign neoplasm
   1. A keratoderma is a generalized thickening of the horny layer of the epidermis.
      a. Types of keratoderma
         (1) Punctate keratodermas (found on the palms of the hands and the soles of the feet) and keratodermas on the digits are more prevalent in African-American patients. The lesions develop central plugs.
         (2) Solar keratoderma (actinic keratosis) is a premalignant condition brought on by cumulative exposure to the sun and is more prevalent in fair-skinned people. The thickened lesions progress very slowly to squamous cell carcinomas; they also can progress to a cutaneous horn.
         (3) Actinic cheilitis is actinic dermatosis of the lip.
         (4) Seborrheic keratosis is a benign plaque, beige to brown or black, with a velvety, warty surface that appears "stuck on."
      b. Treatment
         (1) Liquid nitrogen can be used successfully to treat keratodermas.
         (2) Electrodessication and curettage also are effective.

(3) Mild acid treatments and the application of Monsel's solution have been used.

(4) 5-Fluorouracil (applied topically twice daily for 2–4 weeks) is effective, but patients must be warned that their lesions will look worse before they look better.

2. Lipomas (adipose tumors) are benign neoplasms of mature fat cells that pose no harm to the patient. Surgical excision may be appropriate for cosmetic reasons or if the lipoma is located where it is constantly irritated.

3. Pyogenic granulomas (capillary hemangiomas). This term is a misnomer, because the lesion does not have an infectious cause.

    a. Clinical features

        (1) These bright red, raspberry-like nodules usually present on exposed parts of the body, such as the arms, hands, fingers, or legs.

        (2) They often appear after an injury or surgery but also can appear spontaneously.

    b. Treatment. Electrodesiccation and curettage or excision are used. Cauterization with silver nitrate and cryosurgery has not proved to be curative.

B. Malignant neoplasms

    1. Melanoma

        a. General characteristics

            (1) Although only approximately 3% of skin cancers are melanomas, they cause 66% of deaths from skin cancers.

            (2) Melanomas frequently metastasize widely to regional lymph nodes, skin, liver, lungs, or the brain.

        b. Clinical features

            (1) Melanomas usually are black or dark brown but can be flesh colored. They sometimes have blue, pink, or red components.

            (2) The lesions are irregular in outline, with an outward spreading of pigment. If the lesion changes in size over a relatively short period, malignant degeneration should be considered.

            (3) Although most commonly seen on the skin, a melanoma can occur anywhere on the body, including the eye and mucous membranes of the genitalia, anus, or oral cavity.

            (4) Lesions can be macular to nodular, and four types exist: lentigo maligna melanoma, superficial spreading malignant melanoma (most common), nodular malignant melanoma, and acral-lentiginous melanomas (palms, soles, nail beds).

        c. Prognosis can be estimated by the thickness of the lesion.

            (1) A melanoma entirely within the epidermis carries a very good prognosis.

            (2) As the thickness progresses beyond the epidermis, the prognosis diminishes.

            (3) The likelihood of survival is further diminished if the melanoma is on the upper back, upper arm, neck, or scalp.

        d. Treatment

            (1) Early detection is the key to successful treatment.

            (2) Since the 1970s, the 5-year survival rate has increased from 25–40% to more than 80%. However, the incidence of melanoma is on the rise and is occurring in younger individuals.

            (3) Patients with melanoma need to be referred to a dermatologist or surgeon for complete excision and follow-up.

    2. Squamous and basal cell carcinomas are the most common neoplasms of the skin. Metastasis is rare.

        a. Clinical features

            (1) The lesions are asymptomatic but may itch or bleed. The patient seeks treatment because the nodules do not heal.

            (2) Lesions most commonly present on areas that usually are exposed to the sun (face, head, neck).

            (3) There are several types of basal cell lesions.

                (a) Nodular. Translucent or pearly papule or nodule.

                (b) Ulcerating. Ulcer with a rolled border; often covered with a crust.

                (c) Sclerosing. Infiltrating carcinoma; white sclerotic patch with ill-defined borders.

                (d) Superficial. Erythematous, slightly scaly, thin plaques, often with a fine rolled or pearly border.

                (e) Pigmented. Thick, hard area of variegated pigmentation.

(4) Squamous cell lesions typically appear as sharply demarcated, scaling, or hyperkeratotic macule, papule, or plaque. Erythema, scaling, erosions, and crusts may occur.

b. Treatment

(1) Complete eradication of the lesions is recommended.

(2) Options include excision with clear margins, electrodessication with curettage, 5-fluorouracil, cryosurgery, radiation therapy, Mohs' micrographic surgery, and laser vaporization.

X. ULCERS, BURNS, AND WOUNDS

A. Ulcers

1. General characteristics

a. Diabetic ulcers, stasis ulcers, and arterial leg ulcers are common in the lower limbs.

b. Decubitus ulcers occur in areas of pressure in patients with limited mobility.

2. Clinical features

a. Diabetic ulcers tend to be deep, punched-out lesions over the malleoli, the plantar surfaces of the feet, or the toes. They usually are painless because of associated neuropathies.

b. Stasis ulcers are a result of chronic venous stasis. Stasis dermatitis develops initially, then ulcers that are wide but not deep develop, with irregular, undulating edges and a clean base. Elevation of the affected limb eases any pain.

c. Arterial ulcers usually do not become as large as venous ulcers and are not preceded by dermatitis. Arterial ulcers are painful, pulses are diminished or absent, and the distal area is cold.

d. Decubitus ulcers are a result of impaired blood supply caused by pressure. The sacrum and hip areas most commonly are affected. Complications include osteomyelitis, bacteremia, and sepsis.

e. There are four stages of decubiti.

(1) Stage I. Nonblanching erythema of intact skin.

(2) Stage II. Necrosis, superficial, or partial-thickness involving the epidermis and/or dermis; shallow ulcer.

(3) Stage III. Deep necrosis; crater ulcers with full-thickness skin loss; damage or necrosis can extend down to, but not through, fascia.

(4) Stage IV. Full-thickness ulceration with extensive damage and necrosis to muscle, bone, or supporting structures.

3. Treatment

a. All limb ulcers can be difficult to treat.

b. Diabetic and arterial ulcers are treated similarly.

(1) Lifestyle changes include smoking cessation and moderate exercise to enhance blood flow.

(2) Débridement is necessary if the wound is necrotic.

(3) Wet-to-dry dressings or hydrogels are standard treatment, because wounds heal better in a moist environment. Hydrocolloids (DuoDERM) and enzymatic preparations maintain moisture, enhance granulation, promote débridement, and improve rates of epithelialization.

c. Stasis ulcers are treated with elevation and compression to enhance venous return.

(1) The affected limb should be whirlpooled, the lesion painted with gentian violet, and an Unna's boot applied weekly.

(2) Wraps or support hose also may be used for compression; they should be applied while the leg is elevated and before the veins fill again.

d. Prevention is the key to managing decubitus ulcers.

(1) Repositioning, massaging prone areas, and frequent monitoring are essential.

(2) Efforts to minimize friction, use of an air mattress to reduce compression, meticulous hygiene, and good nutrition help.

(3) If an ulcer develops, moist sterile gauze (Gelfoam), DuoDERM, and/or surgical débridement may be necessary.

e. Topical and/or systemic antibiotics are indicated for any signs of infections.

B. Burns (see Chapter 15)

C. Open wounds

    1. Tetanus status should be assessed with any open wound.

        a. If the last tetanus booster was more than 10 years ago, an update is needed; if the wound is particularly dirty, a tetanus booster may be given sooner.

        b. If the tetanus status is unknown, the patient should receive tetanus immunoglobulin as well as the vaccine.

    2. Wounds should be cleansed well, irrigated, and closed unless they are more than 8 hours old or signs of infection exist. Dirty wounds may need antibiotic coverage.

XI. HAIR AND NAILS

A. Alopecia (loss of hair)

    1. Androgenetic alopecia (male pattern baldness)

        a. Male pattern baldness has a genetic component.

        b. Its extent is variable and unpredictable.

        c. Minoxidil solutions are most effective in persons with recent onset and smaller areas of hair loss.

    2. Alopecia areata is of unknown cause.

        a. It may be seen in thyroiditis, pernicious anemia, or Addison's disease.

        b. Tiny hairs typically are found. Loss can be patchy, involve only the scalp (alopecia totalis), or include the entire body (alopecia universalis).

        c. It may respond to systemic steroids, but relapse is common.

    3. Drug-induced alopecia may occur with thallium, vitamin A, retinoids, antimitotic agents, anticoagulants, oral contraceptives, and others.

B. Nails

    1. Onycholysis is distal separation of the nail plate from the nail bed.

        a. Common causes include excessive exposure to water, soaps, detergents, or alkalis; psoriasis; drugs; or thyroid disease.

        b. Onychomycosis indicates infection with fungi or yeast.

    2. Discolorations and crumbly nails are seen in dermatophytosis and psoriasis.

    3. Paronychia is an inflammation of the nail fold. Erythema, swelling, and throbbing pain may extend into the proximal nail fold and eponychium.

    4. Felon is a subcutaneous infection of the pulp space. This is a closed infection that may rupture or cause osteitis or osteomyelitis; the abscess should be drained.

    5. Congenital nail disorders include nail atrophy and clubbed fingers.

    6. Systemic disease may cause Beau's lines (transverse furrows), atrophy, clubbed fingers, spoon nails, stippling or pitting, and hyperpigmentation.

XII. PIGMENTATION DISORDERS

A. Acanthosis nigricans

    1. General characteristics

        a. This hyperpigmentation disorder can be hereditary or acquired.

        b. It commonly is associated with obesity, endocrine disorders, and paraneoplastic syndromes, or it may be drug induced.

    2. Clinical features. This develops insidiously. Initially, the skin darkens and appears dirty; later the skin is thick and velvety, with accentuated skin lines.

    3. Laboratory studies. If the disorder is thought to be associated with an underlying disorder, further investigation is needed.

    4. Treatment. There is no treatment except for that of any underlying disorder.

B. Melasma

    1. Melasma means "a black spot"; it is an acquired hyperpigmentation disorder of sun-exposed areas and may be associated with pregnancy or with oral contraceptives or other medications.

2. Clinical features

    a. Young adults are more commonly affected.

    b. Hyperpigmented macular areas evolve rapidly over weeks. The color usually is uniform.

3. Laboratory studies. Wood's lamp examination accentuates the hyperpigmented macules.

4. Treatment

    a. Treatment includes 3% hydroquinone solution in combination with 0.025% tretinoin gel. Alternatively, 4% hydroquinone and glycolic acid in a cream base may be used.

    b. Sun block is essential.

C. Vitiligo

    1. General characteristics

        a. Destruction of melanocytes can be associated with thyroid disease, pernicious anemia, diabetes mellitus, and Addison's disease, or it may be idiopathic.

        b. It occurs at any age, in every race, and in males and females equally. About 30% of patients report a family history.

        c. Macules of hypopigmentation may occur focally, segmentally, or in a generalized pattern.

    2. Treatment. Sunscreens, cosmetic cover-up products, or repigmentation therapies under the direction of an experienced dermatologist may be used.

    3. Vitiligo can be very psychologically distressing, especially in dark-skinned patients.

XIII. ANGIOEDEMA AND URTICARIA

A. General characteristics

    1. Urticaria is a group of disorders that can have many causes, most commonly food or drug allergies, heat or cold, and stress or infection.

    2. Urticaria affects 15–20% of the population.

    3. Hives or wheals are raised red areas on the skin or mucous membranes caused by the release of histamines, bradykinin, kallikrein, and other vasoactive substances from mast cells and basophils in the skin, causing small blood vessels to leak and resulting in intradermal edema.

    4. The wheals may be the size of a pencil eraser up to the size of a dinner plate, and they may coalesce into even larger areas.

    5. The lesions most commonly are pruritic but may sting or burn.

B. Acute urticaria may be self-limiting, lasting from a few minutes to hours.

    1. Most often, acute urticaria is an allergic reaction to food or drugs. Immunoglobulin E attaches itself to a receptor on the mast cell and causes a chemical release.

    2. Common causes of acute urticaria are things that are ingested, such as drugs like penicillin or other antibiotics, sulfa drugs and other medications, shellfish, peanuts, food preservatives in hot dogs, and canned foodstuffs.

    3. Other less common causes include things the skin may contact (e.g., laundry detergents, shampoos, perfumes and cleaning solvents) or things the patient may breathe (e.g., fabric softeners).

C. Chronic urticaria lasts more than six weeks. Typically, the lesions wax and wane.

    1. Chronic urticaria is idiopathic; exacerbations can be precipitated by stress.

    2. Females are affected twice as often as males.

D. Physical urticaria can be caused by reaction to heat or cold, water, infection, exercise, or sun exposure. Dermatographism is caused by pressure and can be bothersome.

E. Treatment

    1. Any known causes should be eliminating, but it is estimated that the cause is not found in up to 80% of cases.

    2. For acute or idiopathic urticaria, an H_1 antihistamine, such as diphenhydramine (Benadryl), hydroxizine (Vistaril), fexofenadine (Allegra), or cetirizine (Zyrtec), may be used orally.

    3. In chronic urticaria or in acute urticaria that does not respond initially, an H_2 antihistamine, such as famotidine (Pepcid) or ranitidine (Zantac), may be added to the H_1 regimen.

    4. Recurring urticaria or chronic urticaria may require steroids.

    5. If there is a concern that urticaria may progress to anaphylaxis, a prescription for an Epipen should be given to the patient along with education regarding how to use it.

14

Infectious Disease

Claire Babcock O'Connell

I. FEVER

A. General information

  1. The normal range of body temperature is 97–99.5°F (36.0–37.4°C), averaging 98.6°F (36.7°C). There is a normal diurnal variation of 1.25–2.5°F (0.5–1.0°C).

   a. Stimulation of monocyte–macrophage cells elaborates pyogenic cytokines, which cause an elevation of the set point of the body temperature (i.e., fever). Increased heat production causes shivering; reduction causes peripheral vasoconstriction.

   b. A body temperature of greater than 106°F (41.1°C) risks irreversible brain damage.

  2. Elevated temperature and the symptoms caused by change in body temperature are fairly well correlated with illness, particularly infection.

   a. The degree of elevation does not correlate with severity of illness.

   b. Children typically mount high fevers; the elderly and people on chronic medications (e.g., nonsteroidal anti-inflammatory drugs, steroids) may not mount a fever at all.

B. Fever of unknown origin (FUO) is defined as a temperature of greater than 101°F (38.3°C) for 3 weeks with no discernible cause despite at least 1 week of diagnostic workup.

  1. The most common causes of FUO are infections and multisystem disease (e.g., autoimmune disorders, neoplasms).

  2. No diagnosis is found in 25% of FUO cases.

C. Treatment of fevers is mainly for patient comfort. Reduction in temperature is not part of the therapy for the underlying cause.

  1. Fevers can be reduced by supportive measures, such as alcohol or cold sponge baths, ice bags, or ice-water enemas, or through administration of antipyretics, such as aspirin or acetaminophen. Avoid aspirin products in children because of the risk of Reye's syndrome.

  2. Empiric broad-spectrum antibiotics often are begun when infection is suspected.

II. BACTERIAL INFECTIONS

A. *Streptococcus* sp.

  1. General characteristics

   a. Streptococci are a group of Gram-positive, catalase-producing cocci that appear in chains. They can be aerobic, anaerobic, or facultative and are cultured on blood agar media: Complete hemolysis is identified as β-hemolytic, incomplete hemolysis as α-hemolytic, and no hemolysis as γ-hemolytic streptococci.

   b. The β-hemolytic streptococci are the most common pathogenic type.

    (1) Lancefield classified the β-hemolytic streptococci into groups, labeled A through O.

    (2) The group A β-hemolytic streptococci are the most common of all pathogenic streptococci.

   c. Humans are the only reservoir of group A β-hemolytic streptococci.

    (1) Asymptomatic carriers are frequent. The highest incidence of infection with group A β-hemolytic streptococci is in patients younger than 10 years.

    (2) Crowded conditions and person-to-person transmission is responsible for its perpetuity.

  2. Clinical manifestations

   a. Pharyngitis

    (1) An abrupt onset of sore throat and painful swallowing with fever and chills heralds infection.

    (2) There is enlargement of the cervical lymph nodes, edema and hypertrophy of pharyngeal mucosa, and erythema and exudates that may be punctate or confluent.

    (3) The disease usually is self-limited and typically resolves in 3–4 days, even without specific treatment. Untreated infections may lead to nonsuppurative complications.

b. Scarlet fever is characterized as strep throat with a rash.

    (1) The rash is a diffuse erythema that blanches; superimposed fine red papules may be appreciated only by touch (sandpaper rash). It is described as a sunburn with goose bumps.

    (2) The face typically is flushed, with circumoral pallor and a strawberry tongue.

    (3) The rash fades in 2–5 days, with fine desquamation.

c. Erysipelas is a painful macular rash with well-defined margins; it is characterized by an abrupt onset and rapid progression.

    (1) The rash typically is confined to the face, which becomes fiery red, but it may progress to the extremities. Flaccid bullae may develop.

    (2) The rash desquamates in 5–10 days.

d. Impetigo (*Streptococcus pyoderma*) is characterized by thick, crusted, golden "honey" yellow lesions.

    (1) There is a higher prevalence with poor hygiene and malnutrition.

    (2) The bacteria colonize unbroken skin and, with abrasions or bites, inoculate the intradermal space, where lesions develop.

    (3) Impetigo also can be caused by staphylococci (bullous impetigo).

e. Cellulitis manifests with local swelling, erythema, and pain.

    (1) The skin is pinkish and indurated.

    (2) Group A streptococci is the most common cause of cellulitis in the United States; it is common in patients with lymphedema, chronic stasis, or venous grafts.

    (3) Surgical débridement may be necessary if there is poor response to medical treatment.

f. Necrotizing fasciitis (flesh-eating bacteria) is a deep subcutaneous infection that results in destruction of fascia and fat.

    (1) Swelling, heat, erythema, and pain spread proximally and distally.

    (2) The skin darkens, and blisters and bullae with clear yellow fluid form.

    (3) Development of gangrene and necrosis is associated with mental status changes and delirium; mortality is high.

g. Toxic shock syndrome is a bacteremia with susceptible strains of streptococci following deep soft-tissue infection.

    (1) A viral-like prodrome and history of minor trauma, surgery, or varicella may be found.

    (2) Onset is abrupt with severe pain, typically in an extremity; abdominal infection may mimic peritonitis, pelvic inflammatory disease, myocardial infarction, or pericarditis.

    (3) Fever or hypothermia, confusion, combativeness, and coma develop. Patients develop shock and multiorgan failure. A violaceous or blue vesicular or bullous rash is an ominous sign. Mortality is 30% despite treatment.

    (4) Complications include endophthalmitis, myositis, peritonitis, septic arthritis, myocarditis, perihepatitis, meningitis, and sepsis.

    (5) Common laboratory findings include hemoglobinuria, elevated serum creatinine, low albumin, low calcium, mild leukocytosis and a severe left shift, and low platelets.

    (6) Management includes IV fluids (colloids and crystalloids) and antibiotics as well as pressors, mechanical ventilation, and surgical intervention as needed.

h. Nonsuppurative complications of group A β-hemolytic streptococcal infections

    (1) Acute glomerulonephritis (see Chapter 6)

    (2) Acute rheumatic fever (ARF) is a systemic immune process occurring 15 weeks after exposure to streptococcal pharyngitis.

        (a) Once rare, it has become more prevalent since the 1980s. Peak age is 5–15 years, and mortality is 1–2% despite treatment.

        (b) Jones' criteria for ARF diagnosis. The presence of two major criteria (carditis, erythema marginatum, subcutaneous nodules, Sydenham's chorea, arthritis) or one major and two minor criteria (fever, polyarthralgias, reversible prolongation of the PR interval, rapid sedimentation rate, history of rheumatic fever) plus evidence of recent β-hemolytic streptococci (culture or ASO titer) makes the diagnosis.

(c) Complications of ARF

(i) Congestive heart failure, rheumatic pneumonitis, and rheumatic heart disease (RHD) are possible complications. RHD most commonly results in valvular defects but also may cause arrhythmias, pericarditis, or effusions.

(ii) Patients with valvular defects must receive prophylactic antibiotics before any invasive procedures to prevent endocarditis.

(iii) Current recommendation is 2 g of amoxicillin orally 1 hour before dental or respiratory procedures; combination therapy (e.g., ampicillin plus gentamicin, vancomycin plus gentamicin) is recommended for GI or genitourinary procedures.

(d) Early treatment of streptococcal infection is imperative to reduce risk of ARF and RHD. Recurrence is common; those at high risk are given prophylactic antibiotics (penicillin, sulfadiazine, or erythromycin) during outbreaks of streptococcal pharyngitis.

(e) Patients with carditis have the poorest prognosis: 30% of patients will die within 10 years, two-thirds will develop detectable valvular abnormalities, and 10% will have permanent significant heart disease or cardiomyopathy.

3. Laboratory findings

a. The diagnosis of streptococcal infection is established by a combination of clinical manifestations, rapid reagent tests, and identification of the bacteria through Gram staining or culture.

b. An elevated WBC count, erythrocyte sedimentation rate, and other markers of infection may be found in severe infections or sepsis.

4. Treatment

a. For the most part, group A streptococci remains susceptible to penicillins; cephalosporins are also effective.

b. For patients who are allergic to penicillins, macrolides are recommended.

B. Botulism

1. General characteristics

a. *Clostridium botulinum,* a strictly anaerobic, spore-forming bacillus found in the soil, may inadvertently be packed in food (home-canned, smoked, or commercial), where toxin is produced and stored until ingested. Botulinum toxin inhibits the release of acetylcholine at the neuromuscular junctions.

b. Infant and wound botulism result from exposure to the bacteria or spores and elaboration of the toxin in vivo. Injection drug users are at increased risk of wound botulism. Infants should not be fed honey because of the increased risk of botulism.

2. Clinical findings

a. The initial clinical symptom is visual changes, including diplopia and loss of accommodation. Manifestations typically appear 12–36 hours after ingestion.

b. Additional manifestations include ptosis, impaired extraocular muscles, and fixed, dilated pupils. Other manifestations include cranial nerve palsies, dysphonia, dry mouth, dysphagia, nausea, and vomiting.

c. Mental status changes or sensory deficits do not occur.

d. Respiratory paralysis ensues and, unless mechanic assistance is provided, death.

3. Laboratory findings. The toxin can be identified using specific antiserum after mouse inoculation with the patient's serum.

4. Treatment

a. Botulinus antitoxin is available through the Centers for Disease Control and Prevention (CDC); the CDC also will assist with obtaining assays of serum, stool, or suspect food.

b. Respiratory failure necessitates intubation and mechanical ventilation. If dysphagia persists, IV support and hyperalimentation are required.

C. Anthrax

1. General characteristics

a. *Bacillus anthracis* is a spore-forming, Gram-positive aerobic rod found in sheep, cattle, horses, goats, and swine.

b. It is transmitted to humans via inoculation of broken skin or mucous membranes or via inhalation. Farmers, veterinarians, and tannery and wool workers are at high risk.

c. The organism is a likely candidate for biologic warfare.

2. Clinical findings
   a. Dermatologic
      (1) Approximately 2 weeks after exposure to spores, anthrax causes an erythematous papule at the site of inoculation that becomes vesicular with a purple to black center, which in turn ulcerates, becomes necrotic (eschar), and eventually sloughs. Surrounding skin is edematous and vesicular. The lesion is painless unless secondarily infected with staphylococci or streptococci.
      (2) Regional adenopathy, fever, malaise, headache, and nausea and vomiting may occur. This usually is self-limited.
      (3) Hematogenous spread results in sepsis and hemorrhagic meningitis. This can occur anywhere between 10 days and 6 weeks after exposure.
   b. Pulmonary
      (1) Initially, fever, malaise, headache, dyspnea, cough, and congestion of the nose, throat, and larynx are seen.
      (2) Hours to days later, a fulminating pneumonia or mediastinitis may occur.
   c. GI
      (1) Ingestion of contaminated meat may lead to fever, diffuse abdominal pain, rebound tenderness, vomiting, and change in bowel habits, which may range from bloody diarrhea to constipation. Ulcerations may lead to bowel perforation, dysphagia, or obstruction.
      (2) Although less common, an overwhelming sepsis may develop, causing delirium, obtundation, meningeal irritation, and hemorrhagic meningitis.
      (3) GI anthrax and its complications have not been reported in the United States.
3. Laboratory studies
   a. Skin lesions yield Gram-positive, encapsulated, box-shaped rods in chains; sputum, blood, cerebrospinal fluid (CSF), or skin lesion cultures are positive for *Bacillus anthracis.*
   b. Chest radiography in cases of inhalation anthrax will reveal mediastinal widening secondary to hemorrhagic lymphadenitis.
   c. Any suspected case of anthrax should be reported to the CDC, which can perform immunohistologic testing or polymerase chain reaction (PCR) to confirm.
4. Treatment
   a. Combination therapy is recommended for inhalation anthrax or disseminated disease or cutaneous infection that involves the head or neck.
   b. Ciprofloxacin or another fluoroquinolone is the treatment of choice; doxycycline is the alternative.
   c. An attenuated vaccine is available for persons with a high likelihood of exposure (e.g., laboratory workers).
   d. Prognosis is excellent in cutaneous anthrax. Prognosis for inhalation or GI anthrax is poor (85% mortality) despite treatment; results are best if treatment is begun early.

D. Cholera
   1. General characteristics
      a. *Vibrio cholerae* produces a toxin that activates adenylyl cyclase in intestinal epithelial cells of the small intestine. This results in hypersecretion of water and chloride ion and a massive diarrhea. Death results from hypovolemia.
      b. Epidemics of cholera occur in times of war, overcrowding, and famine and where sanitation is inadequate. Infection results from ingestion of contaminated food or water.
   2. Clinical findings. A sudden onset of severe, frequent, "rice water" diarrhea (gray, turbid, and without odor, blood, or pus); dehydration, hypotension, and electrolyte imbalance develop rapidly.
   3. Laboratory studies. Stool cultures are positive for *Vibrio cholerae*; serum agglutination tests are available.
   4. Treatment
      a. Replacement of fluids and electrolytes is essential. Oral rehydration with water containing salt and sugar is adequate for mild or moderate cases (1 tsp salt, 4 tsp sugar, 1 cup water). Severe cases require IV replacement.
      b. Tetracycline, ampicillin, chloramphenicol, trimethoprim/sulfamethoxazole (TMP/SMX), and fluoroquinolones are effective. Resistance exists, so susceptibility testing is encouraged.
      c. The key to prevention is clean water and food sources as well as proper waste disposal. A vaccine is available, but protection is temporary, with boosters needed every 6 months.

E. Tetanus

   1. General characteristics

   a. *Clostridium tetani* spores are ubiquitous in soil. The spores germinate in wounds where the bacteria produce a neurotoxin (tetanospasmin), which interferes with neurotransmission at spinal synapses of inhibitory neurons. The result is uncontrolled spasm and exaggerated reflexes.

   b. Puncture wounds are most susceptible. The elderly, migrant workers, newborns, and injection drug users are at particular risk. The incubation period is from 5 days to 15 weeks.

   2. Clinical findings

   a. Pain and tingling at the site of inoculation is followed by spasticity of the muscles nearby.

   b. Jaw and neck stiffness, dysphagia, and irritability are common. Hyperreflexia and muscle spasms develop, especially in the jaw (trismus) and face.

   c. Painful tonic convulsions, spasm of the glottis and respiratory muscles, and asphyxia develop if the patient is untreated.

   d. The patient typically is alert throughout the course.

   3. Treatment

   a. Tetanus immune globulin should be given IM. A full course of tetanus toxoid should be administered once the patient recovers. Bed rest, sedation, and mechanical ventilation often are necessary to control tetanic spasms. Penicillin is given to all patients to eradicate toxin-producing organisms. Mortality is high.

   b. Active immunization is recommended starting in childhood. Three to four initial doses are followed by boosters every 10 years. An additional booster is recommended if a major injury occurs after 5 years from last booster. Passive immunization with tetanus toxoid in addition to vaccine is recommended for patients with major wounds and uncertain tetanus status.

F. Salmonellosis

   1. General characteristics. There are more than 2,000 serotypes of salmonellae, all of which are members of the species *Salmonella enterica* and are transmitted by ingestion of contaminated food or water.

   2. Clinical features

   a. Three patterns are recognized.

   b. Enteric fever (typhoid fever)

   (1) The incubation period is 5–14 days. Organisms enter the mucosal epithelium of the intestines and invade and replicate within macrophages in Peyer's patches, mesenteric lymph nodes, and the spleen; bacteremia accompanies infection.

   (2) Onset is insidious, with a prodrome of malaise, headache, cough, and sore throat. Abdominal pain, distention, and constipation and/or diarrhea ("pea soup") develop as the fever increases. Fever reaches a peak on days 7–10, and the patient appears toxic and then generally improves over the next 7–10 days. Relapses are common (15% of cases). Children commonly have an abrupt onset.

   (3) Physical findings include splenomegaly, abdominal distention and tenderness, and bradycardia. A rash develops during the second week; it appears as pink papules, primarily on the trunk, that fade on pressure.

   (4) The organism can be isolated from blood during the first week of the illness; later, the blood cultures will likely be negative. Stool culture is not reliable.

   (5) Complications occur in 30% of untreated cases. Intestinal hemorrhage can be fatal. Other complications include urinary retention, pneumonia, thrombophlebitis, myocarditis, psychosis, cholecystitis, nephritis, osteomyelitis, and meningitis.

   (6) Treatment. Resistance to ampicillin, chloramphenicol, and TMP/SMX is increasing. Resistant strains may be susceptible to ceftriaxone or fluoroquinolones (contraindicated in children and pregnancy). Treat for 2 weeks.

   (7) Prevention. Treatment of carriers often is not effective. Immunization may be provided for household contacts of carriers, travelers to endemic areas, or during epidemics, but it is not always effective. Protection of the food and water supplies as well as proper waste disposal are key to control of the disease.

   c. Gastroenteritis

   (1) This is the most common form of *Salmonella* infection. The incubation period is 8–48 hours after ingestion of contaminated food or drink. Fever, nausea and vomiting, crampy abdominal pain, and bloody diarrhea last 3–5 days. Diagnosis is made through stool culture.

(2) Illness is self-limited, and treatment is symptomatic. Specific treatment with TMP/SMX, ampicillin, or ciprofloxacin is required for severely ill or malnourished patients, sickle-cell disease, or patients who develop bacteremia.

d. Bacteremia

(1) This is characterized by prolonged or recurrent fevers, with bacteremia and local infection in bone, joints, pleura, pericardium, lungs, or other sites.

(2) It is most common in immunosuppressed persons.

(3) Treatment is the same as that for typhoid fever; any abscesses should be drained.

(4) Immunosuppressed patients may benefit from therapy with ciprofloxacin.

G. Shigellosis

1. General characteristics. *Shigella sonnei, S. flexneri,* and *S. dysenteriae* are the most common species that cause dysentery.

2. Clinical findings

a. Illness starts abruptly with diarrhea, lower abdominal cramps, and tenesmus accompanied by fever, chills, anorexia, headache, and malaise.

b. Stools are loose and mixed with blood and mucus. Abdomen is tender; dehydration is common.

c. HLA-B27 individuals may mount a reactive arthritis because of temporary disaccharidase deficiency.

3. Laboratory studies

a. Stool is positive for leukocytes and red blood cells; culture yields *Shigella* spp.

b. Sigmoidoscopy will reveal inflamed engorged mucosa, punctuate lesions, or ulcers.

4. Treatment

a. Replacement of fluid volume is essential.

b. Antibiotics. TMP/SMX is the antibiotic of choice, although ciprofloxacin or a fluoroquinolone may be substituted; amoxicillin is not effective.

H. Diphtheria

1. General characteristics

a. *Corynebacterium diphtheriae* is transmitted via respiratory secretions. The organism has a propensity for mucous membranes, especially the respiratory tract.

b. It produces an exotoxin that causes myocarditis and neuropathy.

2. Clinical findings

a. Nasal infection produces few symptoms other than nasal discharge.

b. Laryngeal infection causes upper airway and bronchial obstruction.

c. Pharyngeal infection is the most common form. A tenacious gray membrane covers the tonsils and pharynx, and patients complain of mild sore throat, fever, and malaise.

d. Myocarditis and neuropathy involving the cranial nerves may develop; untreated cases exhibit toxemia and prostration.

3. Diagnosis is clinical; culture will confirm.

4. Treatment

a. A horse serum antitoxin must be given in all cases of diphtheria. It is obtained from the CDC.

b. Airway obstruction may necessitate removal of the membrane via laryngoscopy.

c. Penicillin or erythromycin is effective. Azithromycin or clarithromycin are effective alternatives.

d. Patients should be isolated until three negative pharyngeal cultures are documented.

e. Contacts should be treated with erythromycin to eradicate carrier states.

5. Diphtheria toxoid is available as a vaccine (DTaP, Td). Unimmunized persons who are exposed to diphtheria should receive active immunization and antibiotic therapy.

III. VIRAL INFECTIONS

A. Epstein-Barr virus (EBV)

1. General characteristics

a. EBV is human herpes virus 4, a universal virus transmitted via saliva.

    b. The most characteristic disease is mononucleosis (the "kissing disease"); it has also been implicated in Burkitt's lymphoma, nasopharyngeal carcinoma, pediatric leiomyomas, collagen vascular diseases, and other disorders.

  2. Clinical findings

    a. After an incubation period of several weeks, patients develop fever and sore throat. Oral lesions include exudative pharyngitis, tonsillitis, gingivitis, and soft palate petechiae. Severe infections also exhibit malaise, anorexia, and myalgias.

    b. Lymph nodes, typically the posterior cervical nodes, are enlarged, discrete, and nonsuppurative, with minimal pain.

    c. Splenomegaly is present in 50% of cases.

    d. A maculopapular and, occasionally, petechial rash develops in 15% of cases; administration of amoxicillin raises the incidence of rash to 90%.

    e. Less common manifestations are hepatitis, mononeuropathy, aseptic meningitis, myositis, gallbladder disease, renal failure because of interstitial nephritis, and dyspnea and cough ("pseudocroup").

    f. Complications include secondary bacterial pharyngitis (most commonly Strep), splenic rupture, pericarditis, myocarditis, aseptic meningitis, transverse myelitis, and encephalitis.

  3. Laboratory studies

    a. An early granulocytopenia is followed by a lymphocytic leukocytosis. Atypical lymphocytes appear as larger cells that stain darker and are frequently vacuolated.

    b. Hemolytic anemia and thrombocytopenia may develop.

    c. Heterophil antibodies and screening mononucleosis tests usually are positive within 4 weeks. A false-positive syphilis test (Venereal Disease Research Laboratory [VDRL] or rapid plasma reagent [RPR]) occurs in 10% of infected patients.

    d. Increased hepatic aminotransferases, increased bilirubin, and decreased cryoglobulins also may be found.

  4. Treatment

    a. Treatment is symptomatic, with nonaspirin antipyretics and anti-inflammatories. Antivirals will decrease viral shedding but do not affect the course of the illness.

    b. Patients with splenomegaly should avoid contact sports.

    c. Steroids are indicated for thrombocytopenia, hemolytic anemia, or airway obstruction secondary to enlarged lymph nodes.

    d. Prognosis is good. Although full recovery may take months, 95% recover without specific treatment.

B. Human papillomavirus (HPV)

  1. General characteristics

    a. HPV is a group of nonenveloped icosahedral virions. There are 77 known types based on DNA sequence.

    b. They invade the cutaneous and mucosal epithelium, proliferate, and cause warts. The local growths commonly regress, but the virus persists and lesions frequently recur.

  2. Clinical findings

    a. Common skin warts are ubiquitous and most commonly occur in children and young adults.

      (1) Most are caused by HPV types 1–4 and typically are asymptomatic.

      (2) Hands and feet most commonly are affected. Plantar warts may cause pain with pressure.

      (3) Warts vary in size, shape, and appearance; they may be flat and superficial or plantar and deep.

    b. Laryngeal warts are caused by serotype 11.

      (1) They are the most common benign epithelial tumor of the larynx.

      (2) In children, they may be life-threatening if they obstruct the airway and must be removed surgically.

    c. Anogenital warts (condyloma acuminata) occur in the squamous epithelium of the external genitalia and perianal area.

      (1) They most commonly are caused by HPV types 6 and 11 and are sexually transmitted. Condoms reduce transmission of the virus.

      (2) They rarely turn cancerous, unless the patient is immunosuppressed.

    d. Cervical warts are found in 5% of females and may be visible only by colposcopy.

(1) Between 40 and 70% will regress.

(2) HPV types 16, 18, and others have been implicated in intraepithelial cervical dysplasia, neoplasia, and invasive carcinoma.

(3) A vaccine against HPV types 6, 11, 16 and 18 is available.

3. Laboratory findings

a. The diagnosis is established by histologic sampling. Hyperplastic prickle cells with excess keratin are found in skin warts. Koilocytotic or vacuolated squamous epithelial cells in clumps on a Pap smear are typical of cervical warts.

b. Molecular probes have been developed to detect HPV DNA in cervical swabs.

4. Treatment

a. Spontaneous remission in months to years is typical of skin warts.

b. The goal of treatment is to reduce the number and frequency of lesions, especially in immunocompromised hosts.

c. Persistent lesions or cosmetically bothersome lesions may be treated medically or surgically.

(1) Medical options include liquid nitrogen, salicylic acid, podophyllum, or topical interferon (Imiquimod [Aldara]).

(2) Surgical options include blunt dissection, electrocautery, or carbon dioxide laser.

d. Recurrence is common.

C. Herpes simplex virus (HSV)

1. General characteristics

a. Humans are the only reservoir of HSV. Transmission is via close contact and inoculation of virus into the mucosal surface or through cracks in the skin. The virus is inactivated at room temperature or by drying.

b. HSV type 1

(1) More than 85% of the U.S. population has evidence of infection with HSV type 1. Transmission is via infected saliva.

(2) Primary infection can be asymptomatic or produce severe disease.

(3) Recurrent, self-limited attacks are common. Precipitating factors include sun exposure, surgery, stress, fever, and viral infection.

c. HSV type 2

(1) About 25% of the U.S. population is infected with HSV type 2. Transmission is via sexual contact or from the mother's genital tract during delivery.

(2) This virus typically causes genital lesions (vulva, vagina, cervix, glans, prepuce, and penile shaft).

(3) Asymptomatic shedding and painful eruptions can be frequent.

d. HSV remains latent within the dorsal root ganglia (HSV-1 has a predilection for the trigeminal nerve and HSV-2 for the sacral root ganglia). Reactivation may be precipitated by fever, stress, menses, trauma, ultraviolet light, weight gain or loss, immunosuppression, or other factors. Reactivation is more frequent and more severe in those who are immunocompromised.

2. Clinical findings

a. Initial infection has a higher rate of systemic signs, longer duration of herpetic symptoms, and a higher rate of complications.

(1) Acute herpetic gingivostomatitis (HSV-1)

(a) Typically occurs in those from 6 months to 5 years of age.

(b) The incubation period is 3–6 days; acute symptoms last 5–7 days. Lesions heal in about 2 weeks, although shedding may continue.

(c) Patients present with abrupt onset, fever, anorexia, listlessness, and gingivitis. Mucosa is red, swollen, and friable. Vesicles appear on the oral mucosa, tongue, and lips; these vesicles may rupture and coalesce to form ulcers and plaques. Regional lymphadenopathy is common.

(2) Acute herpetic pharyngotonsillitis

(a) Common in adults manifesting initial HSV-1 disease, and less common in adults manifesting HSV-2 disease.

(b) Patients present with fever, malaise, headache, and sore throat. Vesicles form on the posterior pharynx and tonsils; these vesicles rupture and form shallow ulcers. A grayish exudate may be present over the posterior mucosa.

(3) Primary genital herpes (invariably HSV-2)

(a) The initial episode may be asymptomatic or severe, with a prodrome of systemic and local symptoms.

(b) Preexisting antibodies to HSV-1 may have an ameliorating effect on the severity of primary HSV-2 infection.

(c) Fever, headache, malaise, and myalgias are common. Vesicles develop on the external genitalia, labia, vaginal mucosa, glans, penis, prepuce, shaft, or perianal area. Nearby cutaneous lesions also may occur.

(d) Vesicles rupture and form tender ulcers, which crust over. Mucosa may be red and edematous.

(e) Females tend to have more severe disease and higher rates of complications. The cervix is involved in more than 70% of female patients, manifesting as ulcerative or necrotic mucosa.

b. Recurrence of HSV lesions is heralded by burning or stinging. Neuralgia also may occur, but constitutional symptoms are unlikely.

(1) Lesions begin as erythematous papules that rapidly develop into tiny, thin-walled, grouped vesicles, which continue to erupt over 1–2 weeks.

(2) Typical locations are the vermillion border (type 1) and the genital area, including the penile shaft, labia, perianal area, and buttocks (type 2).

(3) On average, HSV-1 infections tend to recur twice per year; maximum shedding is during the first 24 hours. The number of episodes tends to decrease with time.

(4) In 90% of cases, HSV-2 can reactivate within 12 months. More than 30% of patients have six episodes per year, and about 20% have more than 10 episodes per year. Reactivation can be subclinical; however, viral shedding leads to further transmission of the virus.

c. Complications of HSV infection

(1) Complications include pyoderma, eczema herpeticum, herpetic whitlow (grouped vesicles on the fingers, common in health-care workers), herpes gladiatorum (disseminated cutaneous infections, common in wrestlers), esophagitis, keratoconjunctivitis (dendritic corneal ulcers, may cause blindness), and disseminated neonatal infection. Viremia may result in visceral infection with multiple organ involvement, leukopenia, thrombocytopenia, and DIC.

(2) Herpes simplex infection of the central nervous system (CNS) may cause aseptic meningitis, ganglionitis, myelitis, or encephalitis. HSV accounts for 10–20% of all encephalitides in the United States. Patients develop headache, meningeal irritation, change in mental status, seizures, and focal necrosis syndromes (temporal cortex, limbic system). CSF shows a moderate pleocytosis of mixed cells, mildly elevated protein, and normal glucose. HSV DNA by PCR or MRI will confirm infection. The mortality rate is greater than 70% without treatment; neurologic sequelae are typical even with treatment.

(3) Genital herpes in pregnancy is dangerous to both the mother and the infant. First infection during pregnancy has a high risk of disseminated infection and maternal mortality. Infants exposed to herpes in utero or during delivery have a high rate of visceral and CNS infection. Mortality and sequelae rates are high. Cesarean section is recommended for women with active infection.

3. Laboratory studies

a. The diagnosis usually is established clinically.

b. Vesicular fluid may be cultured or stained (Tzanck smear), revealing multinucleated giant cells.

c. Antibodies can be identified in the serum by PCR techniques.

4. Treatment

a. Local wound care and supportive therapy are recommended.

b. Treatment is with antivirals (e.g., acyclovir, valacyclovir).

c. Patients with frequent outbreaks may benefit from suppressive therapy. Foscarnet is beneficial in immunocompromised patients with resistant infections.

d. Keratitis is treated with trifluridine.

D. Influenza

1. General characteristics

a. Influenza is caused by an orthomyxovirus. It is readily transmitted through droplet nuclei and occurs in epidemics and pandemics during the fall or winter.

b. Three strains exist (A, B, and C) and are typed based on the surface antigens hemagglutinin and neuraminidase. Influenza A is more pathogenic. Major mutations cause antigenic shifts; minor mutations cause antigenic drifts. Public health authorities follow changes in strains to predict new virus.

c. An avian influenza A subtype (H5N1) has caused epidemic infection in birds and has been transmitted from birds to humans. If a mutation occurs to allow human-to-human transmission, this highly virulent and lethal subtype could become responsible for widespread disease.

2. Clinical findings

   a. After an incubation period of 18–72 hours, patients exhibit an abrupt fever, chills, malaise, muscle aches, substernal chest pain, headache, nasal stuffiness, and occasionally, nausea. The fever lasts for 1–7 days and is accompanied by coryza, nonproductive cough, photophobia, eye pain, sore throat, pharyngeal injection, and flushed facies. Wheezes and rhonchi may be heard, and children often develop diarrhea.

   b. Primary influenza pneumonia may develop in the elderly or those with chronic cardiovascular disease. Patients exhibit progressive cough, dyspnea, and cyanosis.

   c. Complications are especially common in the elderly and the chronically ill. Necrosis of respiratory epithelium results in secondary bacterial infection (*Staphylococcus*, *Streptococcus*, or *Haemophilus* sp.), acute sinusitis, otitis media, and purulent bronchitis.

   c. Reye's syndrome

   (1) Reye's syndrome is defined as a fatty liver with encephalopathy.

   (2) It is rapidly progressive, has a 30% fatality rate, and may develop 2–3 weeks after onset of influenza A or varicella infection, especially if aspirin is ingested.

   (3) Clinical manifestations include vomiting, lethargy, jaundice, seizures, hypoglycemia, increased liver enzymes and ammonia levels, prolonged prothrombin time, and changes in mental status.

   (4) Treatment is supportive.

   (5) The mortality rate is approximately 10%.

3. Laboratory studies

   a. Leukopenia and proteinuria may be found.

   b. The virus can be isolated from the throat or nasal mucosa. Viral cultures take 3–7 days to return. Direct immunofluorescent tests are labor-intensive and less sensitive, but recently developed rapid serology tests are proving to be helpful. The QuickVue test takes 10 minutes and has a sensitivity of 70–80%.

   c. Chest radiography in primary influenza pneumonia will show bilateral diffuse infiltrates.

4. Treatment

   a. All patients require supportive care with rest, analgesics, and cough suppressants as needed.

   b. Amantadine and rimantadine are no longer recommended because of resistance.

   c. Neuraminidase inhibitors (zanamivir inhalation [Relenza] or oral oseltamivir [Tamiflu]) will significantly reduce severity if given within 48 hours of the onset of symptoms. They are effective against both influenza A and B and have fewer side effects than amantadine and rimantadine. These drugs are contraindicated in patients younger than 12 years. Half-strength dosing also may be effective in preventing influenza during times of high transmission.

   d. Prognosis in uncomplicated cases is very good; patients generally recover in 1–7 days. Pneumonia is the cause of most influenza fatalities.

5. Prevention of influenza is through a trivalent influenza virus vaccine.

   a. Its configuration is based on the strains isolated during the preceding year. The vaccine should be given to all patients yearly in October or November and is especially recommended for all people older than 65 years (some sources suggest all people older than 50 years), children or adolescents on chronic aspirin therapy, nursing home residents, patients with chronic lung or heart disease, and all health care workers.

   b. The vaccine is contraindicated in patients with hypersensitivity to eggs or other components of the vaccine, during acute febrile illness, or in cases of thrombocytopenia.

   c. Tenderness, redness, and induration at the injection site may occur; myalgias and fever are rare. It also is available as a nasal spray (FluMist) for those from 5 to 49 years of age.

   d. Immunity is set within 2 weeks of the vaccination. Antibodies wane quickly in the elderly and the sick, but the vaccine has been proven to decrease mortality and morbidity from the flu.

E. Varicella-zoster

1. General characteristics

a. Varicella virus is highly contagious, especially the day before the rash.

b. The incubation period is 10–20 days. A single attack confers lifelong immunity.

c. Most cases occur in late winter or spring.

d. It typically is a benign illness in childhood, but it can be life-threatening, especially in adults or the immunocompromised.

e. Zoster represents reactivation of varicella virus that has been dormant in ganglionic satellite cells.

f. Outbreaks may be precipitated by illness, stress, or advancing age.

2. Clinical findings

a. Varicella is characterized by a generalized eruption that follows a centripetal pattern.

(1) Lesions begin as erythematous macules and papules, form superficial vesicles, and later, crust over.

(2) Lesions appear in "crops," so at any given time, several morphologies can be identified.

(3) The mucous membranes also may be involved.

b. Systemic symptoms are highly variable and include low-grade fever, malaise, muscles aches, arthralgias, and headache. Severe, progressive infections manifest with deeper lesions of the lung, liver, pancreas, or brain; the mortality rate approaches 10%.

c. Complications are varied, including secondary bacterial infection of excoriated lesions, varicella embryopathy, and Reye's syndrome.

d. Zoster is characterized by a painful eruption, usually following a dermatomal pattern. The thoracic and lumbar areas are the most common sites. Trigeminal eruptions that include the tip of the nose risk corneal involvement.

3. Laboratory findings

a. The diagnosis is established clinically.

b. Confirmatory laboratory studies rarely are done, but if necessary, serology and fluorescent microscopy will confirm the diagnosis.

4. Treatment

a. Treatment generally is supportive.

b. Prevention

(1) Prevention of bacterial superinfection involves good hygiene and trimming of fingernails.

(2) Immunocompromised patients exposed to varicella should receive acyclovir and varicella-zoster immunoglobulin.

(3) Anecdotal evidence suggests that steroids may prevent postherpetic neuralgia in some patients. Postherpetic neuralgia rates are higher in the elderly and in patients with trigeminal lesions and can be quite debilitating. Treatment is difficult; choices include tricyclic antidepressants, capsaicin cream, narcotic analgesics, or corticosteroids.

(4) Prevention is through a live attenuated vaccine given at 1–2 years of age. Older patients without evidence of immunity should receive two doses, given 2 months apart. Avoid giving the vaccine during pregnancy.

F. Rabies

1. General characteristics

a. Rhabdovirus is transmitted via infected saliva from an animal bite or an open wound.

b. Vectors include dogs, bats, skunks, foxes, raccoons, and coyotes; rodents and lagomorphs do not transmit rabies.

c. Incubation period between the bite and the onset of symptoms is from 10 days to years (typically 3–7 weeks). A correlation exists between the length of incubation and the distance of the wound from the brain.

2. Clinical findings

a. A history of an animal bite may not be apparent.

b. There typically is pain and paresthesias at the site; the skin is sensitive to changes in temperature and wind.

c. Patients are restless, with muscle spasms and extreme excitability. They exhibit bizarre behavior, convulsions, and paralysis. Thick, tenacious saliva is produced.

    d. Hydrophobia is defined as painful spasms caused by drinking water.

    e. Less commonly, patients may exhibit an ascending paralysis.

3. Laboratory studies

    a. Suspect animals should be sacrificed so that their brains can be tested for the virus using fluorescent antibody markers.

    b. Domestic animals may be quarantined and observed for bizarre behavior.

    c. PCR tests and genetic probes for use in humans are expensive and often negative early in the disease.

    d. CSF may show rabies reverse transcriptase by PCR. MRI may reveal nonenhancing, ill-defined changes in the brainstem, hypothalamus, or subcortical matter.

4. Treatment

    a. No specific treatment against rabies disease is available. Mechanical ventilation and oxygen therapy should be started. Rabies vaccine immunoglobulin is given along with monoclonal antibodies, ribaviron, interferon-α and ketamine. It is almost universally fatal within 7 days, most likely from respiratory failure.

    b. Prevention is key.

        (1) Control of bat populations is helpful in preventing spread.

        (2) All household pets should be immunized. Persons who are exposed regularly (vets, park rangers) also should receive active immunization.

    c. After an animal bite, local care with cleansing, debridement, and flushing is recommended. Wounds should not be sutured.

    d. Postexposure immunization includes rabies immunoglobulin (in the wound and IM at a distant site) and human diploid cell vaccine (HDCV). Five injections of 1 mL IM are given on days 0, 3, 7, 14, and 28. The vaccine may cause pruritus, erythema, and tenderness in 25% of cases, and 20% also develop myalgias, headache, and nausea.

    e. If the patient has received active immunization in the past, immunoglobulin is not given; HDCV doses are given on days 0 and 3 only.

    f. Preexposure vaccination of persons at high risk (vets, animal handlers, Peace Corps volunteers, travelers) is accomplished with IM HDCV doses on day 0, 7, and either 21 or 28. HDCV also can be administered intradermally on days 0, 7, and 28. Rabies antibody titers should be checked every 2 years; boosters are given to persons who become seronegative.

G. HIV and AIDS

1. General characteristics

    a. HIV was first recognized when a cluster of patients with opportunistic infections was identified in 1981. A human retrovirus that requires reverse transcriptase for replication was identified as the cause.

    b. Currently, more than 40 million people worldwide are infected with the virus. The highest prevalence is in Central and East Africa, where approximately one-third of all adults are infected. An estimated 5 million new cases and 3 million deaths occur per year worldwide.

    c. HIV infects all cells containing the T4 antigen, primarily the CD4 helper inducer lymphocytes.

        (1) The result is a disordered function of the immune system.

        (2) HIV attaches to the T4 antigen, replicates, and causes cell fusion or cell death.

        (3) Macrophages serve as a reservoir of virus and promote its dissemination to other organs.

    d. HIV is transmitted through bodily fluids. Risk includes sexual contact, parenteral exposure (blood or blood products, including injection drug use and occupational exposure), and perinatal exposure.

2. Clinical features

    a. The acute HIV syndrome is infrequently identified. It is a cluster of nonspecific findings similar to EBV infection. Some patients may develop persistent generalized lymphadenopathy without symptomatic HIV disease.

    b. HIV disease is a syndrome of nonspecific and specific diagnoses. It can be progressive and insidious, or it can be rapidly fatal. The time from infection to symptomatic disease averages 10 years but is quite variable.

    c. Systemic manifestations include fever, night sweats, and weight loss. The wasting syndrome is a result of increased metabolic rate and decreased protein synthesis. There is disproportionate loss of muscle mass.

    d. Immunodeficiency causes infections and malignant diseases at any site; common sites include the lungs, upper respiratory system, lymph system, CNS, peripheral nervous system (PNS) mouth, GI tract, eyes, and skin.

TABLE 14-1 AIDS Indicator Diseases

Bacterial infections, multiple or recurrent

Candidiasis
    Bronchi, trachea, or lungs
    Esophageal

Cervical cancer, invasive

Coccidioidomycosis, disseminated or extrapulmonary

Cryptococcosis, extrapulmonary

Cryptosporidiosis, chronic intestinal (>1 month)

Cytomegalovirus disease (other than liver, spleen, or nodes)

Encephalopathy, HIV-related

Herpes simplex
    Chronic ulcer(s) (>1 month)
    Bronchitis, pneumonitis, or esophagitis

Histoplasmosis, disseminated or extrapulmonary

Isosporiasis, chronic intestinal (>1 month)

Kaposi's sarcoma

Lymphoid interstitial pneumonia and/or pulmonary lymphoid hyperplasia

Lymphoma
    Burkitt (or equivalent term)
    Immunoblastic (or equivalent term)
    Primary, of brain

Mycobacterium sp.
    M. avium complex or *M. kansasii,* disseminated or any site
    M. tuberculosis, any site
    Mycobacterium, other species or unidentified species, disseminated or extrapulmonary

Pneumocystis jeroveci (nee *carinii*) pneumonia

Pneumonia, recurrent

Progressive multifocal leukoencephalopathy

Salmonella septicemia, recurrent

Toxoplasmosis of brain

Wasting syndrome, HIV-related

e. AIDS is defined by the CDC as a CD4 count (cells/μl) below 200 or the development of an AIDS indicator disease (Table 14-1). A diagnosis of AIDS can be made with or without laboratory evidence of HIV infection.

f. Opportunistic infections and malignancies develop as the CD4 count (cells/μl) drops (Table 14-2). Few patients in the United States develop opportunistic infections or malignancies because of the successes of highly active antiretroviral therapy.

g. The current World Health Organization HIV/AIDS Classification System is based on symptoms: Stage I, asymptomatic disease; Stage II, minor symptoms; Stage III, moderate symptoms; Stage IV, AIDS. In general, as the CD4 count (cells/μl) decreases, the viral load increases, and symptoms of infections and malignancies become more frequent and severe.

3. Laboratory studies

a. Screening for HIV infection detects antibodies. Two enzyme-linked immunosorbent assay (ELISA) tests followed by a confirmatory Western blot analysis confirm HIV infection with a sensitivity of greater than 95%; most patients develop antibodies within 6 months of exposure.

b. Other laboratory findings may include anemia, leukopenia, thrombocytopenia, polyclonal hypergammaglobulinemia, hypercholesterolemia, and cutaneous anergy.

c. The CD4 count (cells/μl) typically decreases as the illness progresses. For best accuracy, it should be measured at the same time of day and by the same laboratory. Patients with a CD4 count (cells/μl) of greater than 350 can have levels measured every 6 months; otherwise, it should be measured every 3 months or with any

TABLE 14-2	HIV-Related Illnesses by Usual CD4 Count
CD4 Count	**Illness**
Any time; generally >500	*Salmonella*, recurrent or septicemia *Clostridium difficile* colitis Kaposi's sarcoma *Mycobacterium tuberculosis*, pulmonary, extrapulmonary, or disseminated Herpes simplex; herpes zoster
<200	*Candida*, esophagus, bronchi, trachea, lungs HIV encephalopathy; AIDS dementia syndrome *Pneumocystis jeroveci* (nee *carinii*) pneumonia
<100	B-cell lymphoma (non-Hodgkin's) Toxoplasmosis *Isospora; Microsporidia* Histoplasmosis Cryptococcosis Coccidioidiomycosis Cryptosporidia
<50	Progressive multifocal leukoencephalopathy (PML) *Mycobacterium avium* complex (MAC) Cytomegalovirus CNS lymphoma

change in patient status. Risk of disease progression increases with a CD4 count (cells/μl) of less than 200 or CD4 (cells/μl) lymphocyte percentage of less than 20%.

d. The viral load is a measure of actively replicating virus, which correlates with disease progression. Changing viral loads also may support treatment response.

4. Treatment

a. Prevention is essential if the HIV epidemic is to end. Primary prevention efforts include safer sex with barrier methods (latex only), harm reduction programs, drug rehabilitation, screening of all blood products, and universal precautions in health care delivery. Development of a vaccine against HIV has been unsuccessful.

b. Secondary prevention efforts include antiretrovirals (Table 14-3) and chemoprophylaxis. Patients should be screened for diseases such as tuberculosis and other infections, and they must be counseled on ways to maintain health and prevent spread of the virus.

c. Postexposure prophylaxis (PEP) may be offered to individuals with a high probability of exposure, including health care workers who sustain occupational injuries. PEP should be started within 72 hours of exposure.

   (1) The chance of contracting HIV from a needlestick injury involving a patient with known HIV disease is 0.3%.

   (2) Health-care workers who sustain an injury must be counseled. Testing should be done on the health care worker and the patient; retesting is recommended in 6 weeks, 3 months, and 6 months.

   (3) Antiretroviral therapy is an option; the decision to begin therapy should be made by the patient. Combination therapy with drugs from different classes should be continued for at least 4 weeks. Full-course PEP reduces the chance of HIV transmission by up to 70%.

d. Pregnant women with HIV disease should be counseled on the risk to the fetus. Antiretroviral therapy to the mother during pregnancy, labor, and delivery and to the newborn reduces the chance of transmission significantly. HIV also can be transmitted through breast milk.

e. Drug treatment of HIV disease includes antiretroviral therapy and treatment of or prophylaxis against opportunistic infections and malignancies.

   (1) The patient must be counseled and made to understand the complexity of treatment. Combination antiretroviral therapy is based on CD4 count (cells/μl), viral load, and overall patient status (nutrition, compliance, access, and acceptance of therapy). Treatment may be aggressive, complex, and toxic.

   (2) Patients must be monitored closely for adherence, effectiveness, adverse effects, and resistance.

TABLE 14-3 | **Antiretroviral Medications**

Drug Category	Drug	Common Adverse Effects
Nucleoside reverse transcriptase inhibitors	Zidovudine (AZT; Retrovir)	Anemia, neutropenia, nausea, malaise, headache, insomnia, myopathy
	Didanosine (ddI; Videx)	Pancreatitis, peripheral neuropathy, hepatitis
	Zalcitabine (ddC; Hivid)	Pancreatitis, peripheral neuropathy, hepatitis
	Stavudine (d4; Zerit)	Peripheral neuropathy, hepatitis, pancreatitis
	Lamivudine (3TC; Epivir)	Peripheral neuropathy, rash
	Emtricitabine (Emtiva)	Dyspigmentation, especially palms and soles
	Abacavir (Ziagen)	Rash, fever
Nonnucleoside reverse transcriptase inhibitors (NRTIs)	Nevirapine (Viramune)	Rash
	Delavirdine (Rescriptor)	Rash
	Efavirenz (Sustiva)	Neurologic manifestations
Protease inhibitors	Saquinavir (Fortovase, Invirase)	Headache, GI dysfunction
	Ritonavir (Norvir)	Peripheral paresthesias, GI dysfunction
	Indinavir (Crixivan)	Renal calculi
	Nelfinavir (Viracept)	Diarrhea
	Amprenavir (Invirase)	Rash, GI dysfunction
	Lopinavir/ritonavir (Kaletra)	Diarrhea
	Fosamprenavir (Lexiva)	GI symptoms, rash
	Atazavavir (Reyatez)	Hyperbilirubinemia
Nucleotide reverse transcriptase inhibitors	Tenofovir (Viread)	GI distress, renal insufficiency
Entry inhibitors	Enfuvirtide (Fuzeon)	Injection site pain, allergic reactions

(3) The goal is suppression of the viral load. A rising or persistently high viral load, clinical progression, or continued immunologic deterioration signals treatment failure.

(4) Prophylaxis against opportunistic infections and malignancies is based on the likelihood of developing disease as judged by the CD4 count (cells/μl) and viral load. Discontinuation of prophylaxis after a sustained response to highly active antiretroviral therapy may be considered.

H. Cytomegalovirus (CMV; human herpes virus type 5)

1. General characteristics

a. Most infections with CMV are asymptomatic.

b. Illness occurs in the immunocompromised, especially patients with HIV disease or posttransplant.

2. Clinical findings

a. Perinatal infection and CMV inclusion disease occurs in 10% of babies born to mothers with primary CMV infection during pregnancy.

(1) The infant may be asymptomatic until later in life.

(2) Clinical findings include jaundice, hepatosplenomegaly, thrombocytopenia, periventricular CNS calcifications, mental retardation, motor disability, and purpura.

b. Acute acquired CMV can be transmitted through sexual contact, breast milk, blood transfusion, or respiratory droplets. Patients develop fever, malaise, myalgias, arthralgias, splenomegaly, abnormal liver enzymes, leukopenia, and atypical lymphocytes. It is similar to EBV infection but without pharyngitis, respiratory symptoms, or heterophil antibodies.

c. Posttransplant patients and patients who are otherwise immunocompromised are at risk for myriad clinical manifestations.

(1) Retinitis occurs with a CD4 count (cells/μl) of less than 50. Examination reveals neovascularization and proliferative lesions, commonly referred to as "pizza pie." With aggressive treatment of HIV disease, the frequency of retinitis can be reduced.

(2) GI manifestations include esophagitis and odynophagia, small bowel inflammatory ulcers, diarrhea, hematochezia, abdominal pain, weight loss, and cholangiopathy. Diagnosis may require biopsy.

(3) Pulmonary manifestations occur in 15% of bone marrow transplant patients; 80–90% of these are fatal.

(4) Neurologic manifestations include polyradiculopathy, transverse myelitis, and encephalitis.

(5) CMV infection is theorized to play a role in the pathogenesis of inflammatory bowel disease, atherosclerosis, and breast cancer.

3. Laboratory studies

    a. Patients may exhibit lymphocytosis or leukopenia.

    b. Culture is very difficult; antigens can be detected in blood, urine, or CSF via PCR.

    c. Tissue biopsy looks for intracytoplasmic inclusions ("owls' eyes").

4. Treatment

    a. Measures to prevent CMV infection include limiting blood transfusions, filtering to remove leukocytes, and restricting the organ donor pool to seronegative donors. CMV immunoglobulin and IV ganciclovir reduce the risk of pneumonia in bone marrow transplant recipients.

    b. Ganciclovir, valganciclovir, foscarnet, and cidofovir are effective against CMV.

        (1) Initial IV loading therapy is followed by maintenance therapy.

        (2) Sustained-release ganciclovir implants for suppression of retinal infections are effective.

IV. FUNGAL INFECTIONS

A. Candidiasis

    1. General characteristics

        a. *Candida albicans* is the most common form of pathogenic *Candida* sp. It is part of the normal flora of human hosts and is an opportunistic pathogen.

        b. Risk factors for disease include neutropenia, recent surgery, chronic illness, broad-spectrum antibiotic therapy, IV catheterization (especially total parenteral nutrition), chemotherapy or corticosteroids, injection drug use, and cellular immunodeficiency, as in HIV.

    2. Clinical findings and treatment

        a. Cutaneous disease

            (1) Diaper dermatitis commonly is caused by *Candida* sp. and does not indicate immune deficiency in newborns. The diaper area is red, with defined margins. Pustules, vesicles, papules, or scales may be seen, and satellite lesions are characteristics.

            (2) Children and adults may develop candidal dermatitis in dark, moist areas, such as axillae or under the breasts or large pannus, especially if the immune system is stressed. Lesions have distinct borders, and satellite lesions are common.

            (3) Treatment is with topical antifungal creams.

        b. Mucosal disease of the mouth and esophagus

            (1) Oral mucosal candidiasis (thrush) causes white plaques that can be scraped off, revealing reddened mucosa. In denture wearers, infection may manifest as a painful red palate.

            (2) Esophagitis is heralded by odynophagia and pain on swallowing. Symptoms resemble gastroesophageal reflux.

            (3) Treatment is with oral fluconazole, itraconazole, or amphotericin B if recurrent or recalcitrant.

        c. Vulvovaginal disease occurs in 75% of females at least once during their lifetime.

            (1) Risk factors include age extremes, pregnancy, uncontrolled diabetes mellitus, corticosteroids, and HIV disease.

            (2) Symptoms include pruritus, burning, dyspareunia, and a white, cottage cheese or curd–like discharge. Physical examination reveals white plaques on vaginal walls.

            (3) Treatment is with topical azoles or oral fluconazole.

        d. Candidal fungemia can be life-threatening.

            (1) It occurs in very ill patients with indwelling instrumentation. Any suspect catheters should be removed.

            (2) IV amphotericin B is recommended. The mortality rate is greater than 40%.

            (3) If disseminated disease develops (positive blood cultures; retinal lesions; infection of skin, brain, meninges, or myocardium), flucytosine should be added; alternatively, fluconazole can be tried.

    e. Hepatosplenic candidiasis occurs in patients with very low WBC counts, such as patients with leukemia.

      (1) With aggressive chemotherapy, the WBC count begins to rise, and the patient develops fever, (RUQ) right upper quodrant, tenderness, and nausea.

      (2) An increase in alkaline phosphatase and multiple low-density defects in the liver, spleen, and kidneys develop. The diagnosis is confirmed with biopsy.

      (3) Treatment is amphotericin B; once the patient is responding, he or she can be switched to fluconazole.

    f. Endocarditis occurs through direct inoculation at surgery, in injection drug users, or in late-stage HIV disease.

      (1) Approximately 50% of cases involve nonalbicans *Candida* sp. and are resistant to treatment. These organisms cause large vegetations.

      (2) Splenomegaly, petechiae, murmur, and large-vessel embolization are common.

      (3) Treatment is amphotericin B, but infected valves must be surgically replaced. Once the patient has recovered, he or she typically will receive lifelong fluconazole.

B. Histoplasmosis

  1. General characteristics

    a. *Histoplasma capsulatum* is a dimorphic fungus found in soil infested with bird or bat droppings.

    b. It is endemic to many areas and is transmitted by inhalation.

  2. Clinical findings

    a. Most infections are asymptomatic or mild and unrecognized. Patients with cellular immunodeficiency are at risk for symptomatic infections.

    b. Acute histoplasmosis occurs in epidemics when soil is disturbed. Patients are prostrate and febrile, with few pulmonary complaints.

    c. Progressive disseminated histoplasmosis may be fatal within 6 weeks. Patients complain of fever, dyspnea, cough, weight loss, and prostration; ulcers may develop in the mouth, pharynx, liver, spleen, adrenals, and elsewhere.

    d. Chronic progressive pulmonary histoplasmosis occurs in older patients, especially those with chronic obstructive pulmonary disease. It manifests as chronic progressive pulmonary changes with calcified nodes and pericarditis.

    e. Disseminated disease occurs in immunocompromised patients, especially those with late-stage HIV disease. It more likely represents reactivation rather than a new acute infection.

      (1) Highest risk is with a CD4 count (cells/μl) of less than 100. Patients develop fever and multiorgan failure; fulminant disease, septic shock, and death are common.

      (2) Chest radiography shows miliary infiltrates.

  3. Laboratory studies

    a. Anemia of chronic disease and increased alkaline phosphate, lactate dehydrogenase (LDH), and ferritin are seen in the severely ill. A pancytopenia also may develop.

    b. A urine antigen assay can confirm the presence of disseminated disease; bronchoalveolar lavage may be done with chronic pulmonary disease.

  4. Treatment

    a. Itraconazole orally for weeks to months is recommended.

    b. Amphotericin B is recommended for patients who cannot tolerate or fail itraconazole therapy or in patients with meningitis or severe disease.

    c. Lifelong suppressive therapy with itraconazole is recommended for the immunocompromised.

C. *Cryptococcus* sp.

  1. General characteristics

    a. *Cryptococcus neoforms* is an encapsulated, budding yeast found in soil contaminated with dried pigeon dung.

    b. It is transmitted through inhalation and causes illness in patients with cellular immune deficiency, such as HIV, cancer, or long-term corticosteroid therapy.

  2. Clinical findings

    a. Pulmonary disease may develop in patients with chronic obstructive pulmonary disease, chronic steroid use, or posttransplant. Fever, cough, and dyspnea occur; chest radiography reveals nodules or pneumonitis.

b. Cryptococcal CNS disease causes headache and meningeal signs. It occurs with a CD4 count (cells/µl) of less than 50. Patients exhibit mental status changes and cranial nerve or visual abnormalities.

c. Cryptococcoma is a rare, intracerebral mass lesion that causes obstructive hydrocephalus.

d. Disseminated disease, although rare, may affect the skin, prostate, osteoarticular surfaces, eye, lymph tissue, or other sites.

3. Laboratory studies

    a. CSF shows variable pleocytosis (predominantly lymphocytes), increased opening pressure, increased protein, and decreased glucose.

    b. Budding, encapsulated fungus may be isolated on culture,

    c. Cryptococcal antigen can be detected in CSF and serum. India ink stain or latex agglutination assay (CRAG) is helpful.

    d. CT or MRI is indicated if cryptococcoma is suspected.

4. Treatment

    a. In patients with HIV disease, oral fluconazole is continued for 10 weeks. In severe infections, amphotericin B can be given for the first 2 weeks, followed by oral fluconazole. Flucytosine may be added in severe disease. Lifelong fluconazole therapy is recommended.

    b. In non-HIV immunocompromised patients, the mortality rate is much higher. Treatment is amphotericin B.

D. *Pneumocystis carinii* pneumonia (PCP; now known as *Pneumocystis jiroveci*)

  1. General characteristics

    a. PCP is caused by a fungus found in the lungs of humans and many animals. Evidence of infection can be found in almost all persons by a young age. It probably is transmitted through the air and lies latent in alveoli.

    b. Premature or debilitated infants in underdeveloped areas are infected during epidemics. Sporadic cases are found in patients with abnormal cellular immunity, such as cancer, severe malnutrition, immunosuppressive drugs, irradiation, or patients with HIV/AIDS and a CD4 count (cells/µl) of less than 200.

    c. PCP is the most common opportunistic infection in HIV disease.

  2. Clinical findings

    a. Typically, PCP disease presents with fever, shortness of breath, and a nonproductive cough. Physical examination findings are disproportionate to imaging results, which show diffuse interstitial infiltrates that may be heterogeneous, miliary, or patchy. Between 5 and 10% of patients have a normal chest radiograph.

    b. Less commonly, patients may present with spontaneous pneumothorax. Recurrent pneumothorax is related to previous pentamidine use.

    c. Patients also may develop fatigue, weakness, and weight loss. Infection is likely to recur without treatment of the underlying disease or chemoprophylaxis.

  3. Laboratory studies

    a. Blood gas reveals hypoxia, hypocapnia, and reduced carbon dioxide diffusion. Lactase dehydrogenase typically is increased, and the WBC count usually is low.

    b. The organism can be demonstrated with specific stains of induced sputum or via bronchoalveolar lavage.

  4. Treatment

    a. Empiric treatment is recommended for immunocompromised patients presenting with cough or dyspnea. The drug of choice is TMP/SMX.

      (1) Patients often get worse at the start of treatment. Steroids are added if the partial pressure of oxygen in arterial blood (PaO_2) is less than 70 mm Hg to prevent deterioration and promote oxygenation.

      (2) Hypersensitivity reactions to TMP/SMX (likely because of the sulfa component) manifest with fever, rash, malaise, neutropenia, hepatitis, nephritis, thrombocytopenia, and hyperbilirubinemia. Systematic desensitization often is successful.

    b. Dapsone is an alternative treatment and is as effective as TMP/SMX. It is more expensive than TMP/SMX, but it is a good choice for patients who are sensitive to sulfa. Side effects include anemia, rash, and fever. It should not be taken with didanoside.

    c. Alternatively, pentamidine can be used either IV or IM. Nebulized pentamide can be used to prevent PCP. Side effects include rash, neutropenia, abnormal liver function, serum folate deficiency, calcium imbalance, hypoglycemia or hyperglycemia, hyponatremia, and nephrotoxicity. Rarely, fatal pancreatitis occurs.

   d. Atovaquone is reserved for patients who cannot tolerate TMP/SMX or pentamidine. It must be taken with a fatty meal and causes mild to minimal side effects.

   e. Once a patient is successfully treated for PCP, prophylaxis is continued. All patients with a CD4 count (cells/µl) of less than 200 also should receive prophylactic treatment. TMP/SMX is the drug of choice.

V. PARASITIC INFECTIONS

A. Amebiasis

   1. General characteristics

      a. Cysts of *Entamoeba histolytica* are viable in the soil and water for weeks to months. Transmission to humans, the only host, occurs through fecally contaminated food or water, fly droppings, or human-to-human contact.

      b. Once ingested, cysts pass through to the intestines where they hatch. Trophozoites invade the mucosa and induce necrosis. Amebic ulcers typically are flask-shaped and occur anywhere in the large bowel or terminal ileum. They usually are limited to the muscularis, but if they penetrate the serosa, they may cause perforation, abscess, or peritonitis.

   2. Clinical findings

      a. Intestinal disease often is asymptomatic.

      b. Colitis can be mild to moderate (few semiformed stools without blood) or severe dysentery (greater number of liquid stools streaked with blood or bits of necrotic tissue).

         (1) Patients may have cramps, fatigue, weight loss, and increased flatulence. Cycles of remission and recurrence are typical.

         (2) Physical examination may reveal distention, hyperperistalsis, and generalized abdominal tenderness during recurrences.

         (3) Patients with severe disease become prostrate and toxic with fever, colic, tenesmus, and vomiting.

         (4) Complications include appendicitis, bowel perforation, fulminant colitis, massive mucosal sloughing, and hemorrhage.

         (5) Localized ulcerative lesions of the colon and localized granulomatous lesions of the colon (ameboma) result in pain, intestinal obstruction, and hemorrhage.

         (6) Amebomas may be single or multiple and must be differentiated from colon cancer, tuberculosis, or lymphogranuloma venereum. Biopsy reveals granulation tissue.

      c. Extraintestinal disease

         (1) Hepatic amebiasis and amebic liver abscess can be asymptomatic or result in symptoms either suddenly or gradually, over days to months.

         (2) Findings include fever, pain, tender hepatomegaly, malaise, prostration, sweating, chills, anorexia, and weight loss.

         (3) Pulmonary symptoms (coughing, right lower lung findings) may occur if the abscess is in the superior liver.

         (4) Abscesses may rupture and spill into the pleural, peritoneal, or pericardial space; this can be fatal.

         (5) Less commonly, amebiasis may metastasize to the lungs, brain or genitalia.

   3. Laboratory studies

      a. Stool specimens reveal cysts or trophozoites. Sigmoidoscopy, colonoscopy, or rectal biopsy shows ulcers; collection of exudates should be examined for trophozoites.

      b. Serology can detect antibodies up to 10 years after infection and, therefore, cannot be used to differentiate past from present infection. Serology will be positive, but stool examination frequently is negative.

      c. WBC count is moderately elevated but without eosinophilia. There will be minimal changes, if any, to liver enzymes.

      d. Ultrasound, CT, MRI, or radioisotope scanning reveals the size and location of hepatic abscesses.

   4. Treatment

      a. Asymptomatic infection should be treated with a luminal amebicide (diloxanide furoate, iodoquinol, or paromomycin).

      b. Mild to moderate infections should be treated with tinidazole or metronidazole plus a luminal amebicide. Alternatives include tetracycline and a luminal amebicide followed with chloroquine.

c. Severe infection also should be supported with fluids, electrolyte replacement, and opioids to control bowel motility and decrease the risk of toxic megacolon.

d. Hepatic abscess is treated with tinidazole or metronidazole plus a luminal amebicide, followed with chloroquine. If there is no response within 3 days of initial treatment, the abscess should be drained. Complications include bacterial infection, bleeding, and peritoneal spillage.

e. Follow up with at least three stool examinations at 2- to 3-day intervals starting 2–4 weeks after the end of treatment.

    (1) Colonoscopy also may be used to confirm treatment success.

    (2) Postdysenteric colitis after severe infections usually is self-limited but may be a trigger for ulcerative colitis.

f. Prognosis with treatment is very good. Without treatment, mortality can be high.

g. Prevention is through adequate control of the food and water supply, proper sanitation, and personal hygiene.

B. Hookworms

  1. General characteristics

    a. Hookworm is endemic to the moist tropics and subtropics.

      (1) Sporadic cases occur in the southeastern United States; 25% of the world's population is infected.

      (2) Humans are the only host.

    b. Eggs are passed in the stool and hatch in moist soil.

      (1) The larvae last for hours to weeks. They penetrate the skin and migrate in the bloodstream to the pulmonary capillaries, where they destroy alveoli and are carried by cilia to the mouth. Once swallowed, the larvae attach to the small bowel mucosa and suck blood. Once mature, they release eggs to continue the cycle.

      (2) A light infection is defined as 1,000 eggs/g feces and moderate infection as 2,000–8,000 eggs/g feces.

  2. Clinical findings

    a. The site of penetration is pruritic. An erythematous dermatitis with maculopapular or vesicular eruption follows; scratching can cause secondary bacterial infections.

    b. The pulmonary stage may cause cough, wheeze, blood-tinged sputum, and low-grade fever.

    c. With a light infection and adequate iron intake, the patient may remain asymptomatic during the intestinal stage. Heavy infection leads to anorexia, diarrhea, vague pain, and ulcer-like epigastric symptoms. Severe infection causes anemia, protein loss, and malabsorption.

  3. Laboratory studies

    a. The eggs can be demonstrated in feces.

    b. Stool is positive for occult blood. A hypochromic microcytic anemia and eosinophilia may be found.

  4. Treatment

    a. Mebendazole (twice per day for 3 days) or either pyrantel or albendazole (once daily for 2–3 days) is effective.

    b. Pyrantel cannot be used in children younger than 5 years; none of the treatments is recommended in pregnancy.

    c. Supportive treatment includes a high-protein diet, vitamins, and ferrous sulfate.

C. Pinworms (enterobiasis)

  1. General characteristics

    a. Humans are the only host for *Enterobius vermicularis*. There is a worldwide distribution, and children are infected more often than adults.

    b. Adult worms are loosely attached to the mucosa, primarily in the cecum. Gravid females pass through the anus to lay eggs on the perianal skin. Each female is capable of producing a large number of eggs. The eggs are viable for 2–3 weeks outside the host and are infective within a few hours.

    c. Infection is easily passed through hands, food, drink, and fomites. The eggs are swallowed and hatch in the duodenum; larvae pass to the cecum and mature in 3–4 weeks. The lifespan is 30–45 days.

  2. Clinical findings

    a. Many patients are asymptomatic.

    b. Characteristic symptoms include perianal pruritus (crawling sensation that is worse at night), insomnia, weight loss, enuresis, and irritability. Examination at night may reveal worms in the anus or in the stool. Scratching causes excoriations and impetigo.

    c. Migration can cause vulvovaginitis, diverticulitis, appendicitis, cystitis, and granulomatous reactions.

3. Laboratory studies. Eggs can be captured on a piece of cellophane tape over the perianal skin; three tries over three consecutive nights is 90% successful.

4. Treatment

   a. All members of the household should be treated concurrently.

   b. Albendazole, mebendazole, or pyrantel is given in a single dose and then repeated 2–4 weeks later.

   c. Hand washing after defecation and before meals must be stressed. Linens should be washed thoroughly.

D. Malaria

   1. General characteristics

      a. *Plasmodium vivax, P. malariae, P. ovale,* and *P. falciparum* are endemic to the tropics and subtropics.

      b. There are 300–500 million cases per year worldwide, with 1 million deaths. There are 800 cases per year in the United States; almost all are imported.

      c. Transmission is through the bite of the *Anopheles* mosquito.

         (1) The mosquito ingests the parasite, and sporozoites mature and get transferred to humans via saliva. Incubation period ranges between 8 and 60 days.

         (2) The sporozoites invade hepatocytes and mature as tissue schizonts. The schizonts escape the liver and invade red blood cells, where they multiply and cause rupture of the cell within 48 hours.

         (3) The cycle of invasion, multiplication, and red blood cell rupture continues.

   2. Clinical findings

      a. The typical malarial attack starts with shaking chills (the cold stage), followed by fever (the hot stage), and finally, diaphoresis (the sweating stage).

         (1) Patients are fatigued between attacks.

         (2) Release of tissue necrosis factors and cytokines contributes to fatigue, headache, dizziness, GI complaints, myalgias, arthralgias, backache, and dry cough.

         (3) There may be liver and spleen enlargement if symptoms continue more than 4 days.

      b. Infection with *Plasmodium falciparum* can be much more severe and can manifest as cerebral malaria, hyperpyrexia, hemolytic anemia, noncardiogenic pulmonary edema, acute tubular necrosis, adrenal insufficiency, cardiac dysrhythmias, and other complications.

   3. Laboratory studies

      a. Blood films are stained with Giemsa or Wright stain and examined at 8-hour intervals for 3 days during and between attacks. The percentage of infected red blood cells ranges from 5 to 20%.

      b. During attacks, leukocytosis or leukopenia may develop.

      c. Severe infections cause hepatic changes, hemolytic jaundice, thrombocytopenia, marked anemia, and reticulocytosis.

      d. Antibodies appear 8–10 days later, which is too late for diagnostic benefit in most cases. Antibodies also persist for 10 years, making the distinction between old and new infection difficult.

   4. Treatment

      a. Prevention is key to the control of malaria. Evaluation and reduction of risk of exposure, prevention of mosquito bites through proper clothing, mosquito repellant, insect spraying programs, and barriers (mosquito netting and screens) is the first step.

      b. Chemoprophylaxis is recommended for patients traveling to areas of endemicity.

         (1) Chloroquine is the drug of choice for both prophylaxis and treatment. It generally is well tolerated and is safe in pregnancy.

         (2) Transient GI symptoms, headache, pruritus, dizziness, blurred vision, malaise, and urticaria can be reduced if taken with meals or given in divided doses twice per week rather than daily.

      c. Severely ill patients can be treated with parenteral quinine, quinidine, or chloroquine plus either doxycycline, clindamyin, or a tetracycline.

      d. Alternative drugs include malarone, mefloquine, hydroxychloroquine, atovaquone/doxycycline, or other combinations, especially if resistance to chloroquine is suspect.

      e. Prognosis is good if treated except for cases involving *Plasmodium falciparum*, which has a mortality rate of 14–17% despite treatment.

VI. SEXUALLY TRANSMITTED DISEASE

A. Syphilis

1. General characteristics

a. *Treponema pallidum* is a spirochete that can affect almost any organ or tissue. Transmission occurs most frequently during sexual contact. There has been a rising incidence of the disease in urban areas, particularly among adolescents and young adults as well as injection drug users.

b. Congenital syphilis is transmitted via the placenta from the mother to the fetus after the 10th week of pregnancy and can result in severe defects.

2. Clinical findings

a. Early infectious (primary and secondary) and late (tertiary) syphilis are separated by a symptom-free latent phase, during which the infectious stage may recur.

b. Primary syphilis is characterized by the chancre, which is a painless ulcer with a clean base and firm, indurated margins. It develops at the site of inoculation, most commonly the genital area. It is associated with regional lymphadenopathy (rubbery, discrete, nontender).

c. Secondary lesions may involve skin, mucous membrane, eye, bone, kidneys, CNS, or liver. There may be relapsing lesions during early latency.

d. Late (tertiary) syphilis includes gummatous lesions involving skin, bones, and viscera; cardiovascular disease; and nervous system and ophthalmic lesions.

(1) Neurosyphilis can result in asymptomatic disease, meningovascular syphilis (chronic meningitis), generalized paresis, or tabes dorsalis (chronic progressive degeneration of parenchyma).

(2) Tabes dorsalis manifests with impaired proprioception, loss of vibratory sense, Argyll Robertson pupil (reacts to light but does not accommodate), or tabes dorsalis crises.

e. Congenital syphilis leads to abnormalities in the skin or mucous membranes, nasal discharge (snuffles), hepatosplenomegaly, anemia, and osteochondritis. If infants are not treated, they may develop interstitial keratitis, Hutchinson's teeth, saddle nose, deafness, and CNS abnormalities.

3. Laboratory studies

a. *Treponema pallidum* may be identified on dark-field microscopy, but the technique is difficult. Immunofluorescent staining techniques are somewhat more reliable. The organism cannot be cultured. Serologic testing is the recommended method for diagnosis.

b. Nontreponemal antigen tests detect nonspecific antibodies to lipoidal antigens.

(1) The VDRL and RPR become positive 4–6 weeks after infection. These tests are positive in 99% of cases during primary and secondary syphilis but may be negative during late forms of syphilis. False-positive results occur, especially in patients with autoimmune disorders.

(2) The nontreponemal tests also are used to assess effectiveness of treatment.

c. Treponemal antibody tests use live or killed *T. pallidum* as antigen to detect specific antibodies.

(1) The fluorescent treponemal antibody absorption test (FTA-ABS) is the most widely used. It is useful in determining whether a positive nontreponemal antigen test is a true positive.

(2) The test is accurate in most patients with primary syphilis and in virtually all patients with secondary syphilis, but it may be falsely positive in patients with Lyme disease, systemic lupus erythematosus, malaria, or leprosy.

d. Specific testing for tertiary syphilis includes lumbar puncture, joint fluid analysis, and biopsy as indicated.

4. Treatment

a. Benzathine penicillin G, 2.4 million U IM in a single dose, is the treatment of choice. Late latent and tertiary syphilis require three weekly injections.

b. Neurosyphilis is treated with aqueous penicillin every 4 hours for 10–14 days. This may be followed with three weekly doses of benzathine penicillin G as above.

c. The Jarisch-Herxheimer reaction (fever, toxic state) occurs when there is a sudden, massive destruction of spirochetes. To prevent this, patients should be given antipyretics during the first 24 hours of treatment.

d. All cases of syphilis must be reported to the appropriate public health agency for contact tracing. All sexual partners who may have been exposed should be treated.

    e. Careful follow-up is essential to monitor the effectiveness of treatment and to identify treatment failures. HIV testing and screening as well as treatment of concurrent sexually transmitted diseases should be done.

B. Gonorrhea

  1. General characteristics

    a. *Neisseria gonorrhoeae* is a Gram-negative intracellular diplococcus that is transmitted during sexual activity.

    b. The highest incidence is found in 15- to 29-year-olds.

  2. Clinical findings

    a. The incubation period is 2–8 days after exposure.

    b. Men

      (1) Men complain of burning on urination and a serous or milky discharge. Then, 1–3 days later, the urethral pain is more pronounced, and the discharge becomes yellow, creamy, profuse, and occasionally, tinged with blood.

      (2) Without treatment, the infection may regress and become chronic or progress to involve the prostate, epididymis, and periurethral glands with acute, painful inflammation. This may progress to chronic infection, resulting in prostatitis and urethral strictures.

    c. Women

      (1) Women often remain asymptomatic or may develop dysuria, urinary frequency and urgency, and a purulent urethral discharge. Vaginitis and cervicitis are common.

      (2) Asymptomatic gonorrhea is a cause of pelvic inflammatory disease and infertility as well as perpetual transmission of the pathogen.

    d. Gonococcal bacteremia is associated with peripheral skin lesions or septic arthritis of the knee, ankle, or wrist.

    e. Conjunctivitis is caused by direct inoculation. Patients present with copious purulent discharge, which usually is unilateral. Global rupture is a risk if the patient is not treated adequately.

  3. Laboratory studies

    a. Gram stain of urethral discharge typically shows Gram-negative intracellular diplococci. Smears are less often positive in women.

    b. Cultures are essential in all cases.

  4. Treatment

    a. Resistance to penicillin, tetracyclines, and fluoroquinolones is widespread. Currently, the treatment of choice is IM ceftriaxone or oral cefixime.

    b. All partners must be treated. Concurrent treatment against *Chlamydia* sp. is recommended.

    c. Infection is reportable in most states.

C. *Chlamydia* sp.

  1. General characteristics. Chlamydiae are a large group of obligate intracellular parasites, including *Chlamydia psittaci* (psittacosis), *C. pneumoniae* (respiratory infections), and *C. trachomatis* (trachoma, inclusion conjunctivitis, pneumonia, and genital infections).

  2. Clinical findings

    a. Lymphogranuloma venereum starts with a vesicular or ulcerative lesion, which may go unnoticed.

      (1) The infection spreads to the lymph nodes, causing inguinal buboes. These may fuse and break down, resulting in multiple draining sinuses and scarring.

      (2) Anorectal disease causes tenesmus, discharge, and fistulae.

    b. Urethritis and cervicitis

      (1) In males, infection with *Chlamydia* sp. is the most common cause of postgonococcal urethritis. Discharge is less painful than with gonococcal urethritis and usually is watery.

      (2) Females typically are asymptomatic or may develop cervicitis, salpingitis, or pelvic inflammatory disease. Infection with *Chlamydia* sp. is a leading cause of infertility.

  3. Laboratory studies

    a. The diagnosis typically is established clinically and is presumptive. Gram stain is negative.

    b. Complement fixation test or immunofluorescence, ELISA, or DNA probes may help to confirm the presence of the disease.

4. Treatment

    a. Azithromycin, doxycycline, and erythromycin are effective. Erythromycin is the drug of choice in pregnant women.

    b. All partners should be treated.

D. *Trichomonas* sp.

    1. General characteristics

        a. *Trichomonas* is a flagellated protozoan.

        b. It infects the vagina, Skene's gland, and lower urinary tract of females and the genitourinary tract of males.

    2. Clinical findings

        a. There is pruritus and a malodorous, frothy, yellow-green discharge.

        b. Diffuse vaginal erythema and red macular lesions may be visible on the cervix.

    3. Laboratory studies. Wet mount reveals motile flagellates.

    4. Treatment

        a. Metronidazole, in a single 2-g dose; it may need to be repeated if infection does not clear.

        b. Both partners should be treated.

VII. SPIROCHETAL INFECTIONS

A. Lyme disease

    1. General characteristics

        a. *Borrelia burgdorferi* is transmitted to humans by *Ixodides*, a small tick that often goes unnoticed. The tick must feed for more than 24–36 hours to transmit the spirochete.

        b. Lyme is the most common vector-borne disease in the United States.

    2. Clinical findings

        a. Stage 1. Early localized infection (7–10 days after bite)

            (1) Erythema migrans, a flat or slightly raised red lesion that expands over several days, typically with central clearing ("bull's eye"). Most common sites are the groin, thigh, or axilla, and it typically resolves in 3–4 weeks without treatment.

            (2) Flu-like illness occurs in 50% of patients.

        b. Stage 2. Early disseminated infection (days to weeks later)

            (1) Manifestations typically involve the skin, CNS, and musculoskeletal system.

            (2) Headache, stiff neck, fatigue, malaise, and intermittent musculoskeletal symptoms are common.

            (3) Cardiac (pericarditis, arrhythmias, heart block) or neurologic (aseptic meningitis, Bell's palsy, encephalitis) manifestations occur in up to 20% of cases.

        c. Stage 3. Late persistent infection (months to years later)

            (1) Musculoskeletal disease includes joint pain without objective findings, frank arthritis (typically large joints), and chronic synovitis. This most likely is an immunologic rather than an infectious phenomenon.

            (2) Central and peripheral nervous system manifestations include subacute encephalopathy (memory loss, mood changes), axonal polyneuropathy (paresthesias, encephalopathy), and leukoencephalitis (cognitive change, paraparesis, ataxia, bladder dysfunction).

            (3) Acrodermatitis chronicum atrophicans, a bluish-red discoloration of distal extremities with atrophy, is seen in Europe but not in the United States.

    3. Laboratory findings

        a. Antibodies can be detected by immunofluorescent assay or ELISA techniques. A Western blot assay is used as a confirmatory test. Immunoglobulin M wanes after 6–8 weeks; immunoglobulin G may persist indefinitely.

        b. Up to 50% of patients with early disease can be antibody-negative during the first few weeks. Acute and convalescent titers can be compared for support of the suspected diagnosis.

        c. The tests lack sensitivity; the probability of a false-positive test may be greater than that of a true positive test. False positive tests are common in patients with rheumatoid arthritis, systemic lupus erythematosus, mononucleosis, endocarditis, and other infections. Therefore, diagnosis of early Lyme disease should be based on clinical findings. Late disease is diagnosed by objective evidence of clinical manifestations and laboratory evidence of disease.

 d. Other laboratory tests, such as CSF, synovial fluid analysis, aspirations, or biopsy, may be helpful in patients with discrete manifestations.

4. Treatment

 a. Doxycycline is the drug of choice in patients with erythema migrans or a suspicion of Lyme disease based on clinical findings (neurologic, cardiac, musculoskeletal) and a history of tick bite. Alternatives include amoxicillin, cefuroxime, ceftriaxone, or cefotaxime.

 b. Symptomatic treatment with analgesics, such as nonsteroidal anti-inflammatory drugs, may be beneficial in patients with musculoskeletal complaints.

 c. Prevention is important. Proper clothing, tick repellent, and a thorough search for ticks after outdoor exposure are essential. Prophylactic antibiotic therapy after tick bite is not recommended.

 d. The LYMErix vaccine is no longer being manufactured. The vaccine was associated with painful and debilitating side effects in some patients.

B. Rocky Mountain Spotted Fever

 1. General characteristics

  a. *Rickettsia rickettsii* is transmitted by the wood tick. Transmission is highest during the late spring and summer.

  b. It most commonly occurs in the eastern United States.

 2. Clinical findings

  a. Fever, chills, headache, nausea, vomiting, myalgias, restlessness, insomnia, and irritability develop 2–14 days after exposure. Less common manifestations include cough, pneumonitis, delirium, seizures, stupor, and coma.

  b. The face typically is flushed and the conjunctiva injected. Faint macules to maculopapules to petechiae develop first on the wrists and ankles and then spread to the extremities and trunk. About 10% of patients do not exhibit a rash.

  c. Less common findings include splenomegaly, hepatomegaly, jaundice, myocarditis, uremia, acute respiratory distress syndrome, and necrotizing vasculitis.

 3. Laboratory studies

  a. Leukocytosis, thrombocytopenia, hyponatremia, proteinuria, and hematuria are common. A transient rise in aminotransferases or bilirubin is possible.

  b. CSF reveals pleocytosis and hypoglycorrhachia.

  c. A rise in antibody titers appears during the 2nd week of illness.

 4. Treatment

  a. Mild, untreated cases wane during the 2nd week.

  b. Prompt treatment with doxycycline or chloramphenicol hastens recovery.

  c. Poor outcomes occur in advanced age and in patients with atypical features. Death is caused by pneumonitis or by respiratory or cardiac failure.

  d. Sequelae of disease may include seizures, encephalopathy, peripheral neuropathy, paraparesis, bowel or bladder incontinence, cerebellar dysfunction, vestibular dysfunction, hearing loss, or motor deficits.

  e. Prevention is key. Protective clothing, tick repellant, and prompt tick removal reduce the incidence of disease.

Surgery

Frank Acevedo

15

I. PATIENT HISTORY

A. A comprehensive patient history should be performed where possible. In emergent situations, the mnemonic **AMPLE** should be followed.

Allergies

Medications

Past medical history

Last meal

Events preceding the emergency

When time and the patient's condition permit, every effort should be made to complete the history.

B. Allergy history should include not only food and medications but also problems with anesthesia and anesthetic agents, including difficult intubation history, malignant hyperthermia, or previous reaction to an anesthetic agent.

C. Medications should be reviewed for any that cause increased bleeding tendencies: aspirin, warfarin, alcohol, non-steroidal anti-inflammatory drugs, chemotherapeutic agents, and antibiotics are the most likely culprits. At particular risk are patients undergoing procedures on the central nervous system or spinal anesthesia. Risk must be reevaluated in the presence of these medications.

D. Conditions in the medical history that significantly alter the surgical risk should be explored. These include significant cardiopulmonary disease, endocrine disorders, cirrhosis, renal disease, immunosuppression, and previous surgical procedures. Assessment of preoperative surgical risk in elective patient populations may require ancillary diagnostic tests, such as stress testing, coronary angiography, carotid artery duplex B-mode scanning, and pulmonary function tests.

E. Events leading up to presentation should be documented. Focus on the seven cardinal signs of the symptom: location of the complaint, quality of the symptom, quantity or severity, timing, setting, alleviating or aggravating factors, and any associated complaints. Determine if the complaint is acute, subacute, or chronic.

II. PREOPERATIVE EVALUATION

A. Routine laboratory assessment

    1. No documentation exists linking a reduction in mortality and morbidity to routine laboratory testing in otherwise healthy patients undergoing elective surgical procedures.

    2. The history and physical examination is the MOST important preoperative evaluation that can be performed by the surgical team.

B. Selective diagnostic tests

    1. CBC. Consider performing if patient has signs and symptoms compatible with anemia or if the loss of blood during the procedure is anticipated to be significant.

    2. Serum electrolytes

        a. Not indicated for patients without medical problems.

        b. Should be considered in patients taking certain medications, such as warfarin, because of the association with potassium abnormalities and toxicity.

        c. More useful as a postoperative laboratory evaluation.

    3. Serum creatinine

        a. Convenient and inexpensive marker for renal function; creatinine levels decrease with age and decreased muscle mass.

        b. Consider following creatinine levels if the patient is going to receive nephrotoxic medications or agents as part of the preoperative workup (i.e., radiologic dyes), if intraoperative hypotension is anticipated, or if cross-clamping of the aorta will be performed.

        c. Preoperative creatinine levels should be obtained in all patients older than 40 years.

4. Blood glucose. Obtain in patients with a personal or family history of diabetes or who will undergo bypass grafting for peripheral vascular disease, abdominal aortic aneurysm repair, or coronary artery bypass grafting.

5. Hepatic enzymes
   a. Not indicated routinely in healthy patients.
   b. Order if clinical signs and symptoms indicate hepatic dysfunction.

6. Coagulation studies
   a. The best determinant of bleeding tendencies during surgery is an accurate history detailing coagulation response to minor traumas.
   b. Bleeding time, activated partial thromboplastin time, and prothrombin time do not reveal a risk of perioperative bleeding in healthy patients.
   c. Results of coagulation studies should be documented in patients taking anticoagulants.

7. Urinalysis
   a. The incidence of asymptomatic urinary tract infections is 2–7%. Asymptomatic urinary tract infections are a concern to the surgical team whenever a prosthetic device is to be used.
   b. Transient bacteremia during vascular procedures can infect the pseudointimal layer of the bladder and may seed to orthopaedic prosthetic devices.
   c. There is no consensus on the routine use of urinalysis in healthy patients.

8. Electrocardiography
   a. Recommended in all patients older than 40 years. The rationale is that preoperative myocardial infarction and arrhythmias are associated with higher morbidity and mortality.
   b. Silent myocardial infarctions are more common in elderly patients and in those with diabetes.

9. Chest radiography
   a. Little evidence supports or refutes routine chest radiography in patients without significant risk.
   b. Chest radiography is indicated in all patients older than 60 years, and it should be performed in all patients, regardless of age, who have any history of significant pulmonary or cardiac disease.

10. Spirometry
    a. The American College of Physicians recommends preoperative spirometry for patients being evaluated for thoracic and upper abdominal surgery and who have a history of smoking or Hyspnea.
    b. It is indicated in abdominal surgery if pulmonary disease is poorly controlled or if the extent of the disease is not clear.

11. Arterial blood gas
    a. Not routinely indicated for preoperative evaluation. Perform if there is any indication of severe underlying cardiopulmonary disease or to confirm acid-base disturbance.
    b. Pulse oximetry should be used before considering an arterial blood gas; often, the oxygen saturation information is enough in the preoperative patient.
    c. Arterial puncture carries the risk of bleeding from the site during the postoperative period.

12. Pregnancy test. Indicated in all women of childbearing age who are undergoing surgery.

C. Risk assessment for postoperative complications. This crucial assessment will look for factors that increase morbidity and mortality.

1. General history and physical examination
   a. Determine previous myocardial infarction, heart failure, chronic pulmonary disease, diabetes mellitus, peripheral vascular disorders, hepatic or renal impairment.
   b. Look for jugular venous distention, cardiac murmurs, irregular pulses, pulmonary rales, abnormal aortic pulsations, and peripheral edema.
   c. Many rating systems have been developed to stratify patients into risk categories, particularly with regard to cardiac disease (Table 15-1).

2. Cardiac complications
   a. Cardiac complications, particularly perioperative myocardial infarction, occur with alarming frequency in certain surgical patients. More than 50,000 perioperative myocardial infarctions occur yearly, with an associated mortality rate of 40%.

TABLE 15-1 **Detsky's Modified Cardiac Risk Index**

	Risk
Age older than 70 years	5
Myocardial infarction	
within six months	10
after six months	5
Canadian Cardiovascular Society Angina Classification*	
Class III	10
Class IV	20
Unstable angina within six months	10
Alveolar pulmonary edema	
Within one week	10
Ever	5
Suspected critical aortic stenosis	20
Arrhythmia	
Rhythm other than sinus or sinus plus atrial premature beats	5
More than five premature ventricular beats	5
Emergency operation	10
Poor general medical status†	5

Class	Points	Cardiac Risk
I	0 to 15	Low
II	20 to 30	
III	31+	High

*Canadian Cardiovascular Society Classification of Angina: 0 = asymptomatic; I = angina with strenuous exercise; II = angina with moderate exertion; III = angina with walking one to two level blocks or climbing one flight of stairs or less at a normal pace; IV = inability to perform any physical activity without development of angina.
†As defined by Goldman risk index.[7]
Adapted with permission from Detsky AS, Abrams HB, McLaughlin JR, Drucker DJ, Sasson Z, Johnston N, et al. Predicting cardiac complications in patients undergoing non-cardiac surgery. J Gen Intern Med 1986;1:213.
Karnath BM: Preoperative cardiac risk assessment. Am Fam Physician 2002;10:1889–1896.

  b. Clinical predictors of significant cardiac risk include recent MI (within 30 days), unstable or severe angina, active heart failure, high-grade atrioventricular block, symptomatic ventricular arrhythmias with underlying cardiac disease, supraventricular arrhythmias with an uncontrolled rate, and severe valvular disease.

3. American Society of Anesthesiologists (ASA) classification (Table 15-2). Although performed by anesthesiologists since 1941, the ASA classification does NOT predict operative risk; instead, it was developed as an aid to assess the physical status of the patient before a surgical procedure and to the choice of anesthetic.

4. Detecting cardiac complications in patients undergoing noncardiac surgery remains a challenge. A commonly used cardiac risk index identifies independent predictors of risk for patients undergoing noncardiac surgery. These predictors include:

  • High-risk surgery
  • History of ischemic heart disease
  • History of congestive heart failure

TABLE 15-2 **Classification by the American Society of Anesthesiologists[a]**

Class 1	Healthy patient, no medical problems
Class 2	Mild systemic disease
Class 3	Severe systemic disease, but not incapacitating
Class 4	Severe systemic disease that is a constant threat to life
Class 5	Moribund, not expected to live 24 hours regardless of operation

[a]The letter e is sometimes added to the class designation to designate an emergency operation.

TABLE 15-3	Classification of Risk for Deep Vein Thrombosis
Low risk	Minor surgery, no risk factor other than age
	Minor surgery, age <40 years, no other risk factor
	Minor trauma or medial illness
Moderate risk	Major general, urological, gynecological, cardiothoracic, vascular, or neurological surgery; age ≥40 years; or other risk factor
	Major medical illness, heart or lung disease, malignancy
	Major trauma or thermal injury
	Minor surgery, trauma in patients with thromboembolism history
High risk	Fracture of orthopaedic procedure of pelvis, hip, or lower extremity
	Pelvic or abdominal surgery for malignancy
	Major surgery or trauma in patients with thromboembolism history
	Lower limb paralysis
	Major lower limb amputation

- History of cerebrovascular accident
- Diabetes requiring insulin
- Serum creatinine >2.0 mg/dL

D. Deep vein thrombosis (DVT) prophylaxis

   1. General characteristics

      a. Classically, the triad described by Rudolph Virchow of stasis, intimal damage, and hypercoagulability has been used to identify patients at risk.

      b. DVT is thought to start at the induction of anesthesia in elective surgical cases, so any attempts at prophylaxis MUST be started preoperatively.

      c. Specific surgical populations are at varying risk (Table 15-3).

         (1) Those patients identified as being at high risk should have preoperative prophylaxis against DVT.

         (2) High-risk populations include patients older than 70 years, those undergoing a surgical procedure anticipated to last longer than 2 hours, those with a history of DVT or pulmonary embolism, patients malignancy, paralysis, polytrauma, or those scheduled to have pelvic procedure (gynecologic or urologic) or lower extremity joint replacement.

      d. Prophylaxis using agents that alter blood coagulability should NOT be considered for procedures within the central nervous system.

   2. Prophylaxis options

      a. Unfractionated heparin, 5000 U subcutaneously either every 8 or every 12 hours, should be started preoperatively and continued until patient is fully ambulatory.

         (1) The every-8-hour dose is associated with a higher incidence of wound complications, such as hematoma formation.

         (2) Heparin therapy is a cost-effective and efficacious method of prophylaxis.

      b. Enoxaprin, 40 mg subcutaneously q.i.d., to be started 12 hours before the procedure and continued until the patient is fully ambulatory or up to 14 days postoperatively.

         (1) Enoxaprin is more expensive per dose than unfractionated heparin, but it may be cost-effective when factoring in other requirements of dosing with low-molecular-weight heparin.

         (2) The dosage may need to be adjusted in cases of renal impairment.

      c. Warfarin has been used primarily in orthopaedic patient populations.

         (1) The dosing regimen typically is 1 mg/day, started 14 days before surgery.

         (2) Dosing is complicated and associated with a higher incidence of bleeding complications.

      d. Fondaparinux is associated with a lower incidence of DVT in hip surgery.

         (1) It works by blocking activated factor X. The dose is 2.5 mg subcutaneously q.i.d., starting 6 hours postoperatively.

         (2) Adjustment is necessary in patients with renal insufficiency.

      e. Nonfitted thromboembolic stockings are not recommended.

(1) The elastic band at the top of the stocking can actually promote a tourniquet effect and stimulate the development of DVT.

(2) Only fitted stockings should be used, if at all; their benefit for preventing thromboembolism in surgical patients is questionable.

f. Sequential compression devices are beneficial in all patient populations.

(1) Application usually is on both lower extremities on call to the operating room, and they are continued until the patient is fully ambulatory. In lieu of bilateral lower extremity application, they may be used on one lower and one upper extremity.

(2) They are the prophylactic measure of choice for patients in whom anticoagulation is contraindicated.

g. Greenfield filter insertion

(1) This is an invasive procedure that allows prophylaxis only from clots that form in the lower extremities.

(2) A filter is indicated in some trauma patients, those who have bled while on anticoagulation, those in whom anticoagulation is contraindicated because of procedure or adverse reaction, those in whom a thromboembolic event has developed while on prophylaxis or full anticoagulation, and those undergoing central nervous system procedures.

h. Dextran

(1) Dextran has been used by some as a prophylactic measure against DVT.

(2) Its use is not associated with significant decreases in the incidence of DVT but is associated with the development of heart failure, renal failure, and difficulties in cross-matching blood.

E. Surgical nutrition

1. General characteristics

a. A malnourished patient is defined as someone who has lost more than 10% of his or her lean body mass and/or has not had adequate nutritional intake for more than 7 days.

b. Expected risks of malnutrition include greater incidence of infection, immune dysfunction, wound complications, and operative morbidity and mortality.

c. Increased nutritional requirements will be present because of the hypermetabolic hypercatabolic response seen in the systemic inflammatory response syndrome. Tumor necrosis factor-α has been shown to enhance muscle catabolism and to promote patient cachexia in metabolic stress.

2. Clinical features

a. Weight loss, reduction of subcutaneous fat stores, and wasting may be apparent.

b. Decreased cognitive function may be associated with severe malnourishment.

c. Subtle changes in skin and hair occur, especially with essential fatty acid deficiency syndromes.

3. Physiologic impact

a. Cardiovascular system will develop decreased myocardial mass, stroke volume, and cardiac output.

b. Respiratory system will undergo catabolism of major muscles of respiration, with decreased vital capacity and difficulty in extubation of patients.

c. GI tract will develop atrophy of villi, with overgrowth of bacteria. Overgrowth of bacteria plus mucosal dysfunction may result in bacterial translocation and subsequent multisystem organ dysfunction.

d. Immune system will develop both impaired cell-mediated and humoral immunity.

e. Ultimately, poor wound healing will develop, with an increased incidence of wound infection, dehiscence, and evisceration.

f. In severe malnutrition, marasmus or kwashiorkor may develop.

4. Diagnostic studies

a. Serum creatinine, creatinine height index, total lymphocyte count, albumin, prealbumin, transferrin may be abnormal.

b. Body mass index, arm circumference, and nitrogen balance are useful parameters to measure overall status.

5. Treatment

a. Treatment aims at replacement of caloric and nitrogen requirements necessary to maintain nutritional homeostasis or at prevention of catabolism and promotion of anabolism.

b. Basal energy expenditure is calculated using the Harris-Benedict equation (Table 15-4). Stress factors can then be used to increase the K/cal calculations dependent upon the severity of the underlying condition.

TABLE 15-4 Calculation of Basal Energy Expenditure (kcal/day)*a*
Men = 66.5 + 13.6(weight) + 5.0(height) − 6.8(age)
Women = 655.1 + 9.6(weight) + 1.9(height) − 4.7(age)
*a*Height and weight measurements are in centimeters and kilograms, respectively. Age is measured in years.

    c. Preferred nutritional replacement is always via the enteral route to maintain GI viability and to aid in the prevention of multisystem organ dysfunction. Another option includes the use of peripheral or central catheters and the infusion of IV hyperalimentation.

  6. Complications

    a. Aspiration

      (1) Enteral feedings should be used in alert patients to avoid the major complication of aspiration pneumonitis.

      (2) Gastrostomy tube feedings are better than nasoenteric tube feedings but are still associated with aspiration.

      (3) Jejunostomy tube feedings are a preferred nonenteral alternative to prevent this complication.

    b. Diarrhea

      (1) Diarrhea caused by osmotic loading is a common complication and can be controlled by limiting the concentration or rate of infusion.

      (2) Never assume that diarrhea is solely from enteral feedings, and always consider *Clostridium difficile* pseudomembranous enterocolitis.

    c. Hyperalimentation complications can be broken down into those related to catheter insertion and those related to the infusion of the solution.

      (1) Catheter-related problems include air embolus, sepsis, pneumothorax, hemothorax, hydrothorax, and cardiac rupture.

      (2) Infusion complications include severe hyperglycemia (including nonketotic hyperosmolar coma), hepatic steatosis, electrolyte abnormalities, and trace element and vitamin deficiencies.

III. TRAUMA

A. General characteristics

  1. Traumatic injuries are the leading cause of death between the ages of 1 and 44 years.

  2. Motor-vehicle accidents are the leading cause of accidental deaths in the United States. Drinking is linked to at least half of all fatal motor-vehicle incidents.

  3. In-field emergency medical services, rapid transport to trauma centers and application of Advanced Trauma Life Support guidelines generate the best results.

B. Primary Survey: ABC (Airway, Breathing, Circulation)

  1. Assuring a patent and functioning airway is the first priority.

    a. Cervical spine stabilization should be provided by a hard (Philadelphia) collar.

    b. Altered mental status is the most common indication for intubation.

    c. Orotracheal intubation is the preferred modality.

    d. Nasotracheal intubation requires that the patient be awake.

    e. Cricothyroidotomy can be performed in emergent situations but only by experienced operators and not in patients under the age of 12 because of the risk of developing subglottic stenosis.

  2. Breathing is the next priority in the trauma patient.

    a. Caregivers should look for the presence of tension pneumothorax, open chest wounds, or flail chest.

    b. Tension pneumothorax is associated with hypotension, tracheal deviation away from the side of injury, jugular venous distention, lack of or decreased breath sounds on the affected side, hyperresonance on the affected side, and subcutaneous emphysema.

  3. Open chest wounds should never be completely occluded with dressings, because this may convert the wound into a tension pneumothorax.

  4. Flail chest is characterized by paradoxical breathing.

    a. Segmental rib fractures cause free-floating segments that move opposite to normal respiratory patterns.

    b. The major problem is not the fractures but, rather, the underlying pulmonary contusion.

  5. Circulatory status should be assessed after the above have been secured.

    a. Cardiopulmonary resuscitation may be necessary.

    b. IV access with at least two angiocatheters (≥16 gauge) should be established.

    c. Initial infusion of balanced solutions, such as Ringer's lactate or normal saline, should be started (fluids should be warmed if large quantities are to be infused).

    d. Persistent hypotension requires the exclusion of tension pneumothorax, myocardial contusion or infarction, or cardiac tamponade. Beck's triad (jugular venous distention, hypotension, and muffled heart sounds) characterizes cardiac tamponade.

C. Secondary survey

  1. After completion of the primary survey and assurance of ABC, a secondary survey should be performed. The focus during this survey is to identify any occult injuries the patient may have sustained.

  2. Thoracic or abdominal injuries, neurologic deficits, lacerations or hematomas, or musculoskeletal injuries must be identified.

  3. Progressive changes or additional clinical manifestations are important indicators of ongoing pathology.

    a. Some major injuries may not be apparent at first inspection.

    b. Continued monitoring of the trauma patient is essential.

  4. Digital rectal examination may detect a high riding prostate and, in association with blood in the urinary meatus, may imply a pelvic fracture.

D. Penetrating chest trauma

  1. Most cases of penetrating chest trauma (95%) can be managed by tube thoracostomy alone.

  2. The remaining cases (5%) must be evaluated regarding clinical indications for operative intervention (Table 15-5).

E. Blunt abdominal trauma

  1. At most major trauma centers, the **F**ocused **A**ssessment with **S**onography for **T**rauma (FAST) has replaced diagnostic peritoneal lavage as the diagnostic test of choice for detecting intra-abdominal injury.

  2. FAST examination evaluates the abdominal cavity for air or fluid collection in the perihepatic, perisplenic, pericardial, and pelvic regions.

    a. A specific diagnosis of an injured organ does NOT have to be made.

    b. CT may be added as needed to clarify the FAST results.

F. Penetrating abdominal trauma

  1. Immediate laparotomy is indicated if a patient exhibits any signs of shock, peritoneal irritation, or evisceration.

  2. Selective laparotomy can be done in the hemodynamically stable patient without any of the above signs after performance of a FAST examination. If the FAST examination reveals intraperitoneal air, laparotomy is indicated.

G. Penetrating flank trauma

  1. Workup in the stable patient includes CT with oral and IV contrast. Penetrating flank trauma is difficult to assess, because many injuries in this region may be retroperitoneal.

TABLE 15-5 Indications for Thoracostomy in Penetrating Trauma
Caked hemothorax unable to drain via thoracostomy tube
Evacuation of 1,500 mL of blood in an injury <3 hours old
Evacuation via tube thoracostomy of 200 mL of blood for three consecutive hours
Signs of cardiac tamponade
Signs of esophageal perforation
Bowel sounds in the chest, indicating diaphragmatic injury
Persistent leakage of air
Development of a bronchopleural fistula

2. Wherever sequential clinical examinations are required, do NOT prescribe analgesics, because they may mask the clinical picture significantly.

H. Vascular trauma

1. Look for signs of arterial injury, such as a pulsatile mass or hemorrhage, expanding hematoma, significant hemorrhage, presence of a thrill or bruit, or acute ischemia to the involved extremity.

2. The presence of a pulse distal to the injury does NOT rule out significant vascular injury.

3. Arteriography and the ankle-brachial index are useful diagnostic tests for determining arterial injury.

I. Head trauma

1. Glasgow Coma Scale (Table 15-6)

a. The Glasgow Coma Scale score should be calculated in all trauma patients.

b. It is useful for triage and prognosis.

2. Basilar skull fractures

a. Basilar skull fractures may be associated with rhinorrhea, otorrhea, ecchymosis of lids (raccoon eyes), and ecchymosis behind the ear (Battle's sign).

b. Be careful with nasogastric tube insertion in this patient population, because a fractured cribriform plate can lead to inadvertent brain cannulation.

3. Epidural hematomas

a. Epidural hematomas usually are caused by injuries to the middle meningeal artery.

b. A brief period of unconsciousness is followed by a lucid interval.

c. Herniation may develop and is heralded by a triad of coma, fixed and dilated pupils, and decerebrate posturing.

d. Diagnosis is established by CT and requires emergent craniotomy.

4. Subdural hematomas

a. Subdural hematomas usually result from injuries to bridging veins.

b. They are associated with severe head injuries and can result in significant axonal injury even after evacuation.

c. Chronic subdural hematoma is more common in alcoholics and elderly patients.

d. It can occur after apparently minor trauma and is associated with mental status changes or focal neurological signs.

e. CT is diagnostic, and once the diagnosis has been established, burr holes over the hematoma are indicated to evacuate the clot.

TABLE 15-6	Glasgow Coma Scale[a]	
Points	**Adults**
Eye Opening	
4	Spontaneous
3	To voice
2	To pain
1	None
Verbal	
5	Oriented
4	Confused
3	Inappropriate words
2	Incomprehensible words
1	None
Motor	
6	Obeys commands
5	Localizes pain
4	Withdraws
3	Abnormal flexion
2	Abnormal extension
1	None

[a]A score of 15 is normal. A score of 13–15 indicates mild head injury, 9–12 indicates moderate head injury, and less than 9 indicates severe head injury.

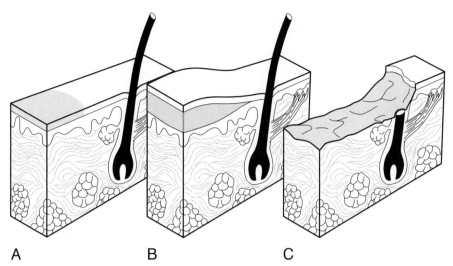

FIGURE 15-1 Types of burns. **A,** First-degree burn. **B,** Partial-thickness burn (second degree). **C,** Full-thickness burn (third degree).

IV. BURNS

A. General characteristics. Burns generally are classified as first, second, third, or fourth degree (Fig 15-1).

   1. First-degree burns involve minor damage to the epidermis.

   2. Second-degree burns are subdivided into superficial partial-thickness burns that extend to the papillary dermis and deep superficial burns that extend into the reticular dermis.

   3. Third-degree, or full-thickness, burns involve and destroy the epidermis and the dermis.

   4. Fourth-degree burns destroy the skin and subcutaneous tissue, with further involvement of fascia, muscle, bone, or other structures.

B. Incidence

   1. More than 1,000,000 burn injuries are seen in emergency departments per year.

   2. Approximately 5,000 deaths per year occur among the approximately 50,000 patients who are hospitalized for burn injuries.

   3. Scald burns are the most common type of burn.

C. Clinical features

   1. First-degree burns are characterized by erythema, tenderness, and the absence of blisters.

   2. Second-degree burns (partial thickness)

   a. Superficial second-degree burns have thin-walled, fluid-filled blisters; are moist; blanche with pressure; and are painful.

   b. Deep second-degree burns have thicker-walled blisters, many of which are ruptured, a mixture of erythema and pallor, and are painful with application of pressure.

   3. Third-degree burns (full thickness)

   a. Third-degree burns give the skin a white, leathery, or charred appearance.

   b. The skin is characteristically dry and without the presence of sensation.

   4. Fourth-degree burns

   a. Fourth-degree burns are characterized by significant charring and exposure of muscle or bone.

   b. The extensive damage to nerves results in little to no sensation of pain.

   5. Any burn that occurs on the face, on the upper torso, or in an unconscious patient should raise the suspicion of associated upper airway involvement.

D. Laboratory Studies

   1. In patients with moderate to severe or extensive burns, required laboratory studies include hematocrit, electrolytes, blood urea nitrogen (BUN) and creatinine, urinalysis, and chest radiography. Depending on extent of the injuries and patient status, also consider obtaining an arterial blood gas, electrocardiography, carboxyhemoglobin, or glucose levels, depending on the history obtained.

2. Direct further laboratory and diagnostic studies once the secondary survey has been performed. Remember that burn patients may have significant associated trauma from falls or blunt injuries.

E. Treatment

1. Maintain ABCs (see above).

2. Estimate the percentage of burn.

   a. Many formulas are available: Rule of 9's, Lund and Broder, and Berkow. (Tidbit: The palm of the victim is roughly equal to a 1% burn.)

   b. Rule of 9's

      (1) The major body areas are divided so that each area is a multiple of nine.

         (a) The head represents 9% of the body surface, and each arm is 9%.

         (b) The front of each leg (extending to the groin) is 9%, and the back is 9%.

         (c) The front of the torso is 18%, and the back of the torso is 18%.

      (2) This formula is accurate for adults only because of the larger head size and smaller thighs in children.

3. Stop the burning process.

   a. Sterile water usually is sufficient.

   b. If dealing with a chemical substance, first identify the substance in question, because specific neutralization measures may be required.

   c. Burns that are caused by white phosphorus may require neutralization with 1% copper sulfate solution and administration of calcium gluconate to address concomitant hypocalcemia.

   d. Hydrofluoric acid burns will require copious lavage for at least 30 minutes, with concomitant application of calcium gluconate gel to the affected area.

4. Manage shock by aggressive fluid resuscitation.

   a. Many formulas exist; choose one and become familiar with it.

   b. Parkland formula: Percentage of burn area × body weight (kg) × 4 mL/hr.

      (1) Half the calculated fluid is given during the first 8 hours, with the rest over the remaining 16 hours.

      (2) Ringer's lactate solution is recommended.

      (3) Colloids can be introduced during the second 24 hours. However, their use remains controversial, because thermal injury of capillaries may make them particularly prone to leak. Administration of colloids with leaky capillaries may cause fluid loss from, rather than retention within, the intravascular space.

      (4) Monitor urine output as a measure of adequate circulation and hemodynamic stability.

5. Insert a nasogastric tube because gastric distention can be problematic and, in severe cases, cause non–fluid respondent hypotension because of mediastinal shift.

6. A Foley catheter should be inserted early and used for monitoring urine output.

   a. Maintain a urine output of at least 0.5 mL/kg/hr in an adult.

   b. Maintain a urine output of at least 1 mL/kg/hr in a child.

7. Address the need for escharotomy in circumferential burns of extremities or the anterior trunk.

8. Silvadene (sulfadiazine) is the MOST commonly used topical burn ointment.

   a. Other preparations, such as Sulfamylon (mafenide) may be used.

   b. Care must be taken when using Sulfamylon, because in large amounts, it can block the action of carbonic anhydrase and lead to severe metabolic alkalosis.

9. Deep dermal burns and full-thickness burns typically are excised on or about day 3.

   a. Coverage is attained by numerous methods.

   b. Autograph is the BEST method, but allographing of skin is acceptable.

   c. Other alternatives include epidermal cell culture, artificial skin, and porcine xenograph.

10. Complications

   a. Common complications of severe burns include inhalation injury, hypovolemic shock, neurogenic shock secondary to pain, renal failure, multiorgan system dysfunction, and gastric ulcerations (termed Curling's ulcers).

b. The most common complication associated with all burns is infection of the burn wound, which has the potential for hematogenous spread.

c. Chronic healing burn wounds can undergo malignant transformation into a squamous cell carcinoma (Marjolin's ulcer).

V. ORTHOPAEDIC INJURIES (SEE CHAPTER 9)

VI. POSTOPERATIVE COMPLICATIONS

A. Postoperative fever

    1. General characteristics. Mnemonic of the five W's is applied (Table 15-7):

        a. Wind

        b. Water

        c. Wound

        d. Walking

        e. Wonder Drugs/Whopper

    2. Clinical Features

        a. Wind (atelectasis)

            (1) Wind usually is the cause of fever in the first 24–48 hours postoperatively.

            (2) Examination may reveal bronchial breathing, and in cases of significant atelectasis, the trachea may be deviated toward the affected side.

        b. Water (urinary tract infections)

            (1) Water usually develops 48–72 hours after surgery.

            (2) Many cases are caused by indwelling urinary catheters or genitourinary instrumentation.

            (3) Patients may complain of dysuria, frequency, or urgency.

        c. Wound infections

            (1) Wound infections are the most common cause of postoperative fever after 72 hours.

            (2) *Staphylococcus aureus* is the most common pathogen.

            (3) Mild elevation in the vital signs is seen early, and pain may or may not be present at the site of infection.

            (4) Superficial infections involve the skin and subcutaneous tissue; deep infections involve areas below the fascia.

TABLE 15-7	Mnemonic of the Five W's	
	Timing	**Findings**
Wind (atelectasis)	First 24–48 hr postoperatively	Bronchial breathing Shift of trachea toward affected side
Water (urinary tract infection)	72 hr postoperatively	Indwelling Foley catheter Genitourinary instrumentation Cloudy urine Positive urine cultures
Wound (wound infection)	After 72 hr postoperatively Most common cause of fever during this time period is wound infection.	Early on, possibly just mild elevation in vitals Undue pain at wound site with erythema and/or drainage
Walking (thrombophlebitis)	After 72 hr postoperatively	Indwelling catheters Cellulitic streaking indicates streptococcal infections; local abscess formation indicates staphylococcal infections
Wonder drugs/**W**hopper (drug fever/abscess)	Fever after 1 week is a serious complication unless caused by drug allergies.	Persistent fever with negative cultures should raise index of suspicion for drug fever Intra-abdominal abscesses may present with blood cultures that are polymicrobial

   d. Walking (thrombophlebitis)

     (1) Superficial thrombophlebitis most commonly is associated with intravascular catheters. Purulent drainage around an indwelling catheter with induration of the vein may be detected on physical examination.

     (2) Deep thrombophlebitis can be associated with indwelling central lines or deep vein thrombosis.

     (3) Thrombophlebitis of the lower extremity may be associated with Homans' sign; this is nonspecific. Unilateral edema of an extremity is a more specific indicator of deep vein thrombophlebitis.

   e. Wonder drugs

     (1) Wonder drugs, such as anesthetics, sulfa-containing antibiotics, and others, often are implicated in drug fever that develops 1 week postoperatively.

     (2) This is a diagnosis of exclusion and should be considered when faced with a negative sepsis workup in a postoperative patient with fever.

   f. Whopper

     (1) Whopper refers to the presence of a postoperative abscess.

     (2) In the case of intra-abdominal fluid collections, an ileus may develop as a sequelae of an occult abscess.

     (3) Blood cultures may be polymicrobial, indicating anastomotic leakage.

3. Imaging studies

   a. A directed workup may include CBC, wound cultures, sputum cultures, blood cultures, chest radiography, and abdominal CT. Intra-abdominal abscesses, if intraloop (i.e., situated between two loops of small bowel), can be associated with a 25–33% false-positive rate when performing CT.

   b. Chest radiography in patients with atelectasis may reveal shifting of the mediastinum toward the affected side, with evidence of loss of lung volume.

   c. When deep vein thrombophlebitis is suspected, B-mode real-time ultrasonography can be used to reveal clots. Venography is still the gold standard for DVT but is invasive and, in some patients, can cause inflammation because of intimal injury.

4. Treatment

   a. Atelectasis

     (1) Atelectasis is best treated by prevention.

       (a) Patients should be instructed to stop smoking at least 2 weeks before any thoracic or abdominal procedure.

       (b) Instruction in using an incentive spirometer should be given and its use encouraged as a preventive measure.

     (2) When atelectasis develops postoperatively, incentive spirometry, mucolytics, expectorants, and β-agonists are beneficial.

   b. Urinary tract infections

     (1) Urinary tract infections should be treated based on culture and sensitivity reports.

     (2) Empirical antibiotics should be chosen to cover organisms that are common in hospitalized patients, including *Proteus mirabilis, Pseudomonas* sp., and *Klebsiella* sp.

     (3) Complicated urinary tract infections warrant an initial choice of an aminoglycoside and cephalosporin. This combination will provide broad-enough coverage until the causative organism is identified.

     (4) In critically ill patients already on multiple antibiotics, a urinary tract infection with *Candida* sp. may be suspected.

   c. Superficial thrombophlebitis

     (1) Superficial thrombophlebitis requires termination of the IV line at the site of infection and use of warm compresses.

     (2) If systemic signs and symptoms are present or if the patient is immunocompromised or diabetic, antibiotics that cover both *Staphylococcus* sp. and *Streptococcus* sp. should be started.

   d. Septic thrombophlebitis requires a vein stripping of the affected site, because it will behave like an abscess and make antibiotic penetration difficult.

   e. DVT

     (1) DVT should be treated with anticoagulation using either heparin or low-molecular-weight heparin.

(2) For patients in whom anticoagulation is contraindicated, vena caval interruption with a Greenfield filter should be considered.

f. Intra-abdominal abscesses

(1) Intra-abdominal abscesses require either surgical debridement or percutaneous drainage, both in combination with appropriate antibiotics.

(2) Percutaneous drainage can be performed as either a CT- or an ultrasound-guided procedure.

(3) Abscesses must be uniloculated to be amenable to percutaneous drainage.

B. Keloids and hypertrophic scars

1. General characteristics

a. Both keloids and hypertrophic scars represent abnormal healing and an imbalance between collagen deposition and degradation.

b. Keloids are more common in African Americans and Asians.

2. Clinical features

a. Keloids tend to extend beyond the original wound or trauma, whereas hypertrophic scars usually are limited to their original boundaries.

b. Hypertrophic tissue usually regresses without intervention, whereas keloid tissue will require intervention.

c. Diagnosis is established based on clinical findings.

3. Treatment

a. No single treatment modality has been shown to be effective across the board in all patients.

b. Topical triamcinolone (Kenalog), 40 mg/ml in a dosage of 2 ml every 6–8 weeks, has been shown to be effective. It can cause dermal atrophy, telangiectasia, and hypopigmentation.

c. Excisional surgery also can be used but is associated with a very high recurrence rate unless combined with other treatment modalities.

C. Decubitus ulcers (pressure ulcers)

1. General characteristics

a. Decubitus ulcers are linked to pressure and shear forces over bony prominences.

b. Most patients who develop this complication have an inability to change position and, thus, sustain long periods of uninterrupted pressure, with subsequent tissue ischemia.

c. Patients with spinal cord injury are at the greatest risk of developing these types of ulcerations.

2. Clinical characteristics. Follow the National Pressure Ulcer Advisory Panel (Table 15-8).

3. Diagnostic procedures. Quantitative wound culture is essential to differentiate between colonization and true infection.

4. Treatment

a. Treatment should encompass a multimodal approach that includes removal of the pressure source, nutritional support, and surgical intervention.

b. Reconstructive procedures are performed only after tissue cultures show that there is no evidence of infection.

c. Treatment can include skin grafts or rotational flaps.

d. Antibiotics should be reserved for those patients who manifest clinical signs of septicemia.

TABLE 15-8	**Classification of Pressure Ulcers**
Stage I	Intact skin with erythema that blanches
Stage II	Partial-thickness skin loss; may present as abrasion, blister, or shallow crater
Stage III	Full-thickness skin loss extending to the subcutaneous tissue but not beyond the fascia; crater with or without undermining of adjacent tissue
Stage IV	Full-thickness skin and subcutaneous tissue loss with extension into muscle, tendons, bone, or joint capsule

D. Necrotizing fasciitis

   1. General characteristics

      a. Although necrotizing fasciitis is a rare complication, it is more common in patients with diabetes, alcoholics, and IV drug abusers. Some case series have identified those with diabetes as accounting for 20–30% of identified cases.

      b. It is associated with mortality rates ranging from 25% to 70% in some studies.

      c. It can be polymicrobial or caused by group A streptococci or clostridial infections. Saltwater necrotizing fasciitis is caused by *Vibrio* sp.

   2. Clinical characteristics. Can present with a multitude of symptoms, including rapidly progressing erythema, tissue crepitus, marked tissue tenderness, high temperatures, tachycardia, hypotension, and an altered mental status.

   3. Diagnostic procedures

      a. Look for the triad: elevated WBC (>14,000 cells/μl), elevated BUN (>15 mg/ml), and hyponatremia (<135 mmol/L).

         (1) This triad is not present in all patients.

         (2) If this triad is present, it should prompt a heightened index of suspicion.

      b. Ultrasonography, CT, and MRI have been used to demarcate the affected regions before surgical intervention.

      c. Plain-film radiographs are of use only if gas is present within the affected tissues.

   4. Treatment

      a. Aggressive surgical debridement is the mainstay of therapy.

      b. Antibiotic therapy should cover all possible pathogens.

         (1) An initial therapeutic choice of triple antibiotics (ampicillin, gentamicin, and clindamycin) is acceptable.

         (2) It is important to monitor renal function and adjust dosages accordingly, because renal impairment is a major hallmark of this disease.

Geriatrics

16

Kathy Kemle

I. BACKGROUND

A. Life expectancy

1. The number of years that an individual can be expected to live at birth is increasing in all industrialized and many developing countries; it is approaching 80 years for both sexes.

2. Life tables predict that persons living until age 65 can expect to live 18 additional years; those living until age 75 can expect to live 12 additional years.

B. Coupled with a declining birth rate, the result is an overall aging of the population; the number of persons older than 65 years is estimated to grow to 70 million by the year 2030.

C. This aging phenomenon brings with it higher burdens of chronic disease and greater use of health care resources.

II. PATIENT CARE

A. Normal changes of aging

1. Individuals and their organ systems age at varying rates, making the elderly the most heterogeneous group in the population.

2. Significant aging changes by system are listed in Table 16-1.

B. Comprehensive geriatric assessment

1. Assessment has been shown to improve patient placement and functional status, and it provides a baseline for comparison for future status changes. Despite the greater number of diagnoses in the elderly, fewer medications are used in patients who are followed by a comprehensive geriatric team.

2. Assessment encompasses cognitive status, physical evaluation, functional status, psychological status, nutritional status, and socioeconomic status. Table 16-2 lists some commonly used assessment instruments.

3. Functional status includes activities of daily living and instrumental activities of daily living (Table 16-3).

4. Assessment of driving skills is difficult because of the multidimensional nature of the tasks involved and the lack of standardized assessment tools.

C. Prevention

1. The efficacy of many preventive services in the elderly is uncertain.

2. Recommendations should be tailored to the individual.

3. Table 16-4 lists routine tests for the elderly and those that generally are not appropriate.

4. Tetanus boosters, the pneumococcal vaccine, and yearly influenza vaccines should be strongly encouraged in the elderly, because these patients are at greater risk for poor outcomes of these diseases.

D. Pharmacology

1. The elderly are particularly vulnerable to the ill effects of medication.

2. Pharmacokinetics (absorption, distribution, metabolism, and excretion) is altered during the aging process, which results in higher frequency of drug-related adverse events.

  a. Altered absorption from the GI tract is not a certainty of aging; however, a decline in gastric acid may affect absorption of some drugs. Drugs that require a low pH may be less readily absorbed.

  b. Interstitial and skin perfusion declines, resulting in slower absorption of topical preparations.

  c. Metabolism of drugs (biomedical modification and degradation mostly as a result of enzymatic processes) is not changed significantly by aging.

  d. Moderate reductions in free water and serum proteins occur with aging, resulting in higher active drug concentrations. Malnutrition adds to the decline in serum proteins.

  e. Decline in liver mass and hepatic blood flow as well as declines in renal clearance affect drug clearance. Dosages of many agents should be reduced.

TABLE 16-1 Common Changes in Aging

Dermatologic	Loss of rete pegs; thinning skin; loss of subcutaneous fat; fragile skin; decrease in collagen and elastin; increased photo-aging
Pulmonary	Decline in forced vital capacity; less effective cough; decline in forced expiratory volume; increased fibrosis; less elastin; decreased chest wall compliance
Immune system	Decline in B- and T-cell function (most changes result from decreased nutrition rather than from aging alone)
Cardiovascular	Decline in compliance; increased wall thickness; decreased maximal heart rate; decreased cardiac output; increased systemic vascular resistance; increased reliance on atrial contraction for ventricular filing; baroreceptor dysfunction
Endocrine	Impaired glucose tolerance; decreased testosterone and estrogen
Gastrointestinal	Impaired swallowing; slower transit time; decreased gastric acid; slight gallbladder duct dilation
Renal	Slow decline, but effect is variable; prostatic hypertrophy
Musculoskeletal	Loss of fluid in collagen; decreased elasticity; decrease in myocytes
Neurologic	Slower response times; decline in vibratory and proprioceptive senses; decline in righting reflexes
Vision	Increased lens opacity; decreased peripheral vision; decreased accommodation
Hearing	Loss of cochlear cells; increased and stickier cerumen

TABLE 16-2 Instruments for Geriatric Assessments

Cognition	Mini-Mental Status Exam Clock Drawing Test Geriatric Depression Scale Yesavage Geriatric Depression Scale Blessed Dementia Rating Categorical Word Fluency Short Portable Mental Status Questionnaire
Function	Physical Self-Maintenance Rating Scale Lawton and Brody function scales Performance of Activities of Daily Living
Nutrition	Mini-Nutritional Assessment Tool and short form
Mobility	Tinetti get-up-and-go test

TABLE 16-3 Activities of Daily Living and Instrumental Activities of Daily Living

Activities of daily living	Bathing Grooming Dressing Mobility Toileting Eating Transferring
Instrumental activities of daily living	Telephoning Meal preparation Shopping Finances Stairs Reading Laundry Housework Transportation Medications Employment

TABLE 16-4	Recommended and Inappropriate Screening Procedures for Older Adults
Recommended Screening Procedures	
Height/weight	At least annually
Blood pressure	At least annually
Vision	Annually
Hearing	Annually
Depression	Uncertain
Alcohol questionnaire	Uncertain; base frequency on patient history
Lipids	Annually
Bone density	Uncertain
Glucose	Uncertain
Mammography	Every 2–3 years
Pap smear	Every 3 years; may cease if all Pap smears have been normal until age 65; if never tested, stop after 2 negative annual smears
Stool Hemoccult	Every 3–5 years
Colonoscopy	At least once
Smoking cessation	Every visit
Dental care	At least annually
Calcium intake	At least annually
Exercise	Each visit
Safety counseling	At least annually
Immunizations	Pneumococcal—at least once Tetanus booster—every 10 years Influenza—annually
Aspirin	81 mg by mouth daily
Inappropriate Screening Procedures	
Annual complete history and physical examination	
Screens for pancreatic cancer, lung cancer, ovarian cancer, and bladder cancer	
Annual blood chemistry panel	
Annual complete blood count	
Annual electrocardiography	
Annual chest radiography	

3. Pharmacodynamics (the effect of medication on targeted tissue) is difficult to measure in the elderly because of altered pharmacokinetics. The elderly are likely more sensitive to the effects of some drugs, such as warfarin and centrally acting drugs.

4. Adverse drug events are the most common medical errors, with rates as high as 74% during long-term care.

   a. Drugs and drug combinations with high risk of adverse consequences should be used with caution and very rarely in the elderly (Tables 16-5 and 16-6).

   b. Any drug with anticholinergic properties is likely to cause confusion in the elderly, and their effects are cumulative. Many commonly prescribed agents not usually suspected of this have anticholinergic effects (Table 16-7).

   c. Side effects and drug interactions may be readily apparent (rash, vomiting) or more subtle (change in personality, somnolence).

5. About 30% of the elderly in the community use some form of alternative therapy, such as saw palmetto for prostatism, glucosamine/chondroitin for osteoarthritis, and melatonin for insomnia.

E. Assessment and management of the hospitalized older adult

   1. Old age itself is not a contraindication to surgical procedures, but mortality/morbidity rates are higher for those with comorbidities.

TABLE 16-5	Drugs Commonly Implicated in Adverse Drug Events
α-Methyldopa	Ciproheptadine
Reserpine	Cyclobenzaprine (and other relaxants)
Propoxyphene ~ *Darvon*	Flurazepam ~ *Dalmane*
Diphenhydramine	Indomethacin (and all NSAIDs)
Ticlodipine	Pentazocine ~ *Talwin*
Doxepin ~ *Sinequan*	Dicyclomine ~ *Bentyl*
Diazepam ~ *Valium*	Chlorpropamide ~ *Diabenese*
Amitriptyline	Chlorpheneramine ~ *Chlor-Trimeton*
Meperidine	Meprobomate ~~~~
Minoxidil	Belladonna
Trazadone	Metoclopropamide ~ *Reglan*

NSAIDs, nonsteroidal anti-inflammatory drugs.

TABLE 16-6	Drug Combinations Commonly Involved in Adverse Interactions
Medication	**Risk**
ACE inhibitor + potassium	Hyperkalemia
ACE inhibitor + potassium-sparing diuretics	Hyperkalemia
ACE inhibitor + salt substitute	Hyperkalemia
Antiarrhythmic + diuretic	Arrhythmias
Benzodiazepine + other sedative	Sedation, confusion, falls
Calcium channel blocker + nitrate	Hypotension, falls
Digoxin + verapamil	Elevated digoxin levels
Digoxin + quinidine	Elevated digoxin levels
Nitrate + vasodilator	Hypotension
Theophylline + other xanthines	Tachyarrhythmias, anxiety
Warfarin + sulfa, quinolones, macrolides, NSAIDs	Increased effect

ACE, angiotensin-converting enzyme; *NSAIDs*, nonsteroidal anti-inflammatory drugs.

TABLE 16-7	Medications with Anticholinergic Effects
Furosemide (all loop diuretics)	Digitalis
H$_2$-blockers	NSAIDs
Clonidine	Amantadine
Opioids	Some antiarrhythmics
SSRIs	β-blockers, especially propranolol
Benzodiazepines	Some antipsychotics
Tricyclic antidepressants	Fluoroquinolones
Antituberculin drugs, especially isoniazid and rifampin	

NSAIDs, nonsteroidal anti-inflammatory drugs; *SSRIs*, selective serotonin reuptake inhibitors.

2. Iatrogenic problems, especially delirium, are more common in older adults.

    a. Delirium is characterized by alteration of consciousness, waxing and waning of symptoms, psychomotor retardation or agitation, and decreased attention span.

    b. Delirium is a medical emergency and should be evaluated promptly. Delirium is associated with poorer outcomes and higher mortality.

    c. Delirium is most common with surgical admissions, especially orthopaedic and urologic procedures.

    d. Evaluation and management of delirium includes the need to:

        (1) Maintain a high index of suspicion.

        (2) Complete physical examination including neurological and rectal exam.

        (3) Identify and treat reversible factors (unnecessary medications, infection, dehydration, congestive heart failure, electrolyte imbalance, central nervous system oxygenation, sensory deprivation, impaction, urinary retention).

        (4) Encourage family visitation, remove/avoid restraints, mobilize the patient, assist with feeding, reduce noise, and provide familiar surroundings.

        (5) Recommend lorazepam or haloperidol if medication is necessary. *[handwritten: Ativan]*

F. Rehabilitation

    1. Sites of care include rehabilitation hospitals, subacute placements in long-term care facilities, outpatient facilities, and the home.

    2. Premorbid function is the best predictor of outcome after stroke or serious fracture.

    3. Mobility aids, such as canes and walkers, as well as functional assistive devices are helpful, especially if used in conjunction with education on their use by a physical or occupational therapist.

G. Palliative care

    1. As it becomes clear that a disease process is not amenable to further treatment or cure, focus shifts to more intense concern with symptom amelioration.

    2. Older adults and demented persons experience pain just as younger individuals do but may have more difficulty in expressing their sensations.

    a. Nocioceptive pain arises in somatic or visceral tissues and usually is described as aching, stabbing, or intense pressure and pain.

    b. Neuropathic pain originates in disordered central or peripheral nerves and is described as electrical, burning, shooting, or stinging.

    c. Pain management involves pharmacologic and nonpharmacologic modalities.

        (1) Pharmacologic

            (a) Dosing of pain medication must be titrated in the elderly, because these patients often are very susceptible to side effects and interactions.

            (b) Nociceptive pain.

                (i) Mild pain should be managed with acetaminophen or tramadol (avoid nonsteroidal anti-inflammatory drugs because of the risk for GI bleed).

                (ii) Moderate to severe pain should be managed with hydrocodone/acetaminophen, oxycodone, morphine, transdermal fentanyl, or methadone.

            (c) Neuropathic pain

                (i) Neuropathic pain should be managed with anticonvulsant medication (especially the pentin agents, such as gabapentin), duloxetine, or lidocaine patch.

                (ii) Avoid tricyclic antidepressants because of their potential for dehydration.

        (2) Nonpharmacologic control of pain can be achieved through distraction (music, relaxation techniques, aromatherapy, massage), cold/warm applications, positioning, splinting, electrical stimulation, hypnosis, or biofeedback.

    3. Nonpain symptoms of chronic disease may be just as distressing as pain.

    a. Nausea, dyspnea, fatigue, and anxiety are common.

    b. Treatment of underlying cause and supportive measures are key to management.

H. Geriatric syndromes

TABLE 16-8	Consequences of Immobility
Deconditioning	Depression
Cardiac deconditioning	Mislabeling (dementia)
Renal lithiasis	Delirium
Pressure wounds	Hyperglycemia
Deep venous thrombosis	Worsened chronic disease
Pulmonary embolism	Constipation
Urinary retention, urinary tract infection	Fecal impaction
Atelectasis	Pneumonia
Reflux disease	Osteoporosis

1. Syndromes are multifactorial and require aggressive, multifaceted investigation.

2. Immobility is the great disabler.

   a. Encouraging the elderly to be active in even a limited exercise program is imperative.

   b. Table 16-8 lists the most common consequences of immobility.

3. Accidents are the sixth-leading cause of death in the elderly, and two thirds of these are falls.

   a. Falls are the result of disordered interaction between the individual and their environment.

   b. Falls may be a sign of acute illness, most often urinary tract infection, exacerbation of congestive heart failure, or pneumonia.

   c. Changes in gait, balance, vision, and hearing as well as disease predispose older adults to falling.

   d. Evaluation of a fall should include a full history, physical examination, assessment and management of any injuries, and a search for the factors that resulted in it.

   e. Many medications are associated with falls (Table 16-9).

4. Urinary incontinence (see Chapter 6)

   a. Incontinence is NOT a normal part of aging

   b. Falls often are the result of an overactive bladder.

   c. Medications used for urge pattern incontinence are anticholinergic and, therefore, of limited utility in the elderly population.

5. Cognitive impairment

   a. Impairment of cognition is NOT a normal part of aging.

   b. Mild cognitive impairment

     (1) Recently recognized, mild cognitive impairment is characterized by deficits in cognition, without deficiencies in activities of daily living.

     (2) It may progress to dementia in susceptible individuals.

     (3) Treatment with acetylcholinesterase inhibitors has not been shown to retard progression to dementia. *Aricept, Namenda*

TABLE 16-9	Common Drug Classes Frequently Associated with Falls
Anticonvulsants	
Antihypertensives (especially central-acting)	
Benzodiazepines (especially long-acting)	
Tricyclic and other antidepressants	
Hypnotics	
Diuretics	
Vasodilators	
Opioids (if oversedating)	

c. Dementia (see Chapter 11)

(1) Dementia is a progressive decline in cognitive function. Unlike delirium, dementia generally is irreversible.

(2) Many causes of dementia are recognized, but all result in loss of intellectual capacity, eventually involving all activities of daily living.

(3) Chronic dementia progresses to a terminal phase that is characterized by immobility, eating difficulties, and frequent infections.

d. Behavioral complications of dementia

(1) Troubling behaviors are common in dementia and cause a great burden for caregivers and safety issues for patients.

(2) Medications do not remove target behaviors and are associated with undesirable side effects.

(3) Behaviors are managed best by environmental manipulation.

(4) Antipsychotic medications are NOT approved by the U.S. Food and Drug Administration for this purpose.

(5) No drug therapy works well.

    (a) Acetylcholinesterase inhibitors and memantine as well as anticonvulsants and β-blockers may be helpful.

    (b) Benzodiazepines, especially lorazepam in small doses, are the recommended agent for sedation if drugs must be used.

(6) Table 6-10 describes common behaviors seen in dementia and their management.

e. Dizziness

(1) One of the three most common complaints in primary care, dizziness is a sensation of light-headedness, spinning, or impending syncope.

(2) It is classified as vertigo (the sensation of rotational movement of self or surroundings) or as nonvertigo (presyncope, disequilibrium, unsteadiness, floating, or light-headedness).

(3) Historical accuracy is the key to successfully establishing the diagnosis.

(4) Examination should include orthostatics, observation of gait, a check for nystagmus, as well as cardiac and neurologic examinations.

(5) Treatment varies with the cause.

(6) Prognosis for recovery is good in three-fourths of patients.

(7) Nonvertiginous

    (a) Disequilibrium is a sensation of unsteadiness and is caused by vestibulopathies, visual and musculoskeletal disorders, and neuropathies or anxiety/depression disorders. Canes or walkers often are useful.

    (b) Presyncope is the sensation that a faint is imminent and is caused by decreased cerebral perfusion, usually because of orthostatic hypotension or vagally mediated cardiac events. Advise the patient to arise slowly, and correct reversible causes.

    (c) Light-headedness is a more vague sensation and often is psychiatric in origin. A trial of antidepressants may be warranted.

TABLE 16-10	Behaviors Seen in Chronic Dementia and Their Management	
Behavior	**Management**
Wandering	Provide safe place to wander Patient identification system (bracelets, MedAlert) Identify and avoid precipitants Sedatives (last resort)
Screaming	Search for source and treat (pain?) Distraction
Aggression	Identify and avoid precipitants Sedatives
Restlessness/agitation	Consider depression
Hallucinations	If bothersome, use atypical antipsychotics If Parkinson's or Lewy body disease, use quetiapine or benzodiazepine

6. Syncope

   a. A sudden, transient loss of consciousness not resulting from trauma, syncope increases in occurrence with age.

   b. Common causes include arrhythmias, aortic stenosis, carotid sinus hypersensitivity, myocardial infarction, hypoglycemia, orthostatic hypotension, postprandial hypotension, psychogenic disorders, pulmonary embolus, and vagal faint.

   c. History and physical examination are key to diagnosis.

   d. Diagnostic tests should be chosen based on the history and physical examination.

   e. Tests include electrocardiography, ambulatory monitoring (Holter), echocardiography, tilt-table test, electrophysiologic studies, and possibly, CT or MRI of the brain.

   f. Treatment varies with the cause.

7. Sensory impairment

   a. Vision

   (1) Declines in accommodation and peripheral vision occur with aging.

   (2) Clouding of the lens occurs even without disease.

   (3) See Chapter 1 for specific conditions.

   b. Hearing

   (1) Cerumen impaction and presbycusis are common causes of hearing loss in the elderly.

   (2) See Chapter 1 for specific conditions.

8. Malnutrition

   a. Undernutrition is the most common disorder but overweight and obesity also are problematic.

   b. Undernutrition (macronutrients)

   (1) The cause is most often "pre-mouth" (i.e., problems with inability to shop for or prepare meals or inadequate assistance with feeding).

   (2) Other causes include mouth disorders, dysgeusia (loss of or abnormal taste), dysphagia, mesenteric ischemia, gastritis, generalized fatigue, endocarditis, malignancy, and pain.

   (3) Water deficit is common, because the elderly lack a thirst response and often are on diuretics, increasing water loss.

   (4) Evaluation should include a complete history, especially regarding medications, food availability and preferences, and pain referable to the GI tract, as well as a search for other medical causes.

   (5) Laboratory studies that may be useful include CBC, electrolytes, renal and liver function, thyroid-stimulating hormone, erythrocyte sedimentation rate, and urinalysis; chest radiography may be useful as well. Other studies may be needed as suggested by the evaluation.

   (6) Treatment is geared toward the cause.

   c. Undernutrition (micronutrients)

   (1) Vitamins C, D, B_{12}, and the other B vitamins are the most common deficiencies in older adults.

   (2) For most, undernutrition results from reduced intake, but declines in gastric acid and intrinsic factor render the elderly especially vulnerable to vitamin B_{12} deficiency.

9. Pressure wounds (see Chapter 13)

   a. Predisposing factors in elderly skin consist of loss of subcutaneous fat, loss of the rete pegs (projections of dermis into the epidermis that help to prevent shearing off of the epidermis), and a decline in elasticity.

   b. Predisposing factors in general include diseases that reduce perfusion or delivery of nutrients to tissue, increased shearing force, moisture (such as fecal or urinary incontinenc), dehydration, and immobility.

   c. Treatment primarily consists of paying attention to systemic factors, including hydration, nutrition, adequate oxygenation and carrying capacity, frequent turning, pressure-relieving devices, optimal management of related diseases, and pain relief.

10. Vertebral compression fractures

   a. Associated with osteoporosis, fractures usually are in the thoracic or lumbar spine and present as deep pain over the site of the fracture, sometimes radiating in the appropriate nerve root distribution.

   b. Trauma may be minimal or absent.

   c. Diagnosis is established by radiography or, occasionally, by MRI.

d. Treatment is symptomatic, with analgesics and vertebroplasty or kyphoplasty.

e. Complications include kyphosis, with possible restrictive lung disease as a result; immobility; chronic pain; and even death.

l. Psychiatric disorders

    1. General characteristics

        a. Older adults tend to be self-reliant and satisfied.

        b. Stoicism and present focus are typical.

        c. They often deny mental illness.

    2. Common disorders

        a. Depression is characterized by sadness, withdrawal from enjoyed activities, and anhedonia, but the elderly concentrate on somatic complaints more than on mood. Typical presentations also include memory impairment, agitation, or anxiety.

            (1) Diagnosis is established by clinical suspicion and completion of a screen, such as the Yesavage Geriatric Depression Scale. One also must rule out depression induced by medical disease, such as an indolent cancer, or by medication.

            (2) Because older adults do not respond as well to psychotherapy, pharmaceuticals are the usual therapy.

                (a) Lower side effects make selective serotonin reuptake inhibitors and agents like mirtazipine the drugs of choice. *Remeron*

                (b) Occasionally, stimulants in low doses, such as methylphenidate, are useful, especially in patients with psychomotor retardation. *Ritalin*

                (c) Avoid tricyclic antidepressants.

            (3) Some patients are resistant to medications. Electroconvulsant therapy has been shown to be very effective and safe even in frail elderly patients.

        b. Anxiety

            (1) Avoid benzodiazepines if possible; if they must be used, shorter-acting agents are preferable.

            (2) Avoid antihistamines, and use buspirone and antidepressants. *BuSpar*

        c. Psychosis

            (1) Senile psychosis is characterized by hallucinations and delusions.

            (2) It is associated with isolation, sensory impairment, and dementia.

            (3) It should not be treated unless it is bothersome to the patient or prohibits the caregivers from providing care.

            (4) Newer antipsychotics in low doses are the agents of choice.

        d. Substance abuse

            (1) Tobacco use is common and should be discouraged even in the very old, because cessation may be beneficial even at the extremes of age.

            (2) Ethanol produces intoxication with ingestion of lesser amounts.

                (a) Hidden sources, such as household cleaners, tonics, and personal hygiene products, are common.

                (b) Withdrawal is more lethal in the elderly.

            (3) Other agents, including prescription drugs, often are misused unintentionally but rarely are directly abused in the elderly population.

III. SELECTED COMMON DISEASES AND DISORDERS WITH UNIQUE FEATURES IN THE ELDERLY

  A. Xerosis (dry skin)

    1. Xerosis is characterized by dry skin, pruritus, and cracking skin.

    2. Treatment consists of decreasing the frequency of bathing and using tepid or cool water followed by emollients.

  B. Oral disorders

    1. Oral disorders frequently result in weight loss.

    2. Dysgeusia may be related to dental disease or sinusitis, but it often is secondary to drugs. Common drugs that cause taste disturbances include any anticholinergic agent, digitalis, and angiotensin-converting enzyme inhibitors.

3. Toothlessness commonly reduces mastication. Dentures may contribute to decreased taste and lead to denture ulcers.

4. Oral candidiasis is common and should be considered in any elderly patient who decreases oral intake, especially if dentures are used, the patient is on steroids or antibiotics, or has diabetes or another immunodeficiency disorder.

    a. White patches are common, but red mucosa may be the only sign.

    b. Treatment is with antifungal agents.

C. Infectious diseases

    1. Decline in B- and T-cell immunity related to aging increases vulnerability to infection.

    2. Fever almost always indicates bacterial infection but sometimes is the result of malignancy or medication intake. Elderly often do not mount a fever.

    3. Pneumonia

        a. Predisposing factors include decreased ciliary activity, less effective cough, and decreased vital capacity.

        b. Presentation often is atypical, with less cough, absent fever, and absent or unimpressive leukocytosis. Often, only confusion and tachypnea are seen.

        c. Aspiration pneumonia is more common in the elderly but usually is not successfully treated by antibiotics. It is not reduced by use of a percutaneous endoscopic gastrostomy (PEG) tube; in fact, it is increased.

    4. Urinary tract infection (UTI)

        a. Urinary tract infection often presents with vague symptoms or confusion.

        b. It is difficult to distinguish from asymptomatic bacteriuria, which is common and should not be treated, because inappropriate antibiotic use leads to resistance and exposes patients to unnecessary risk.

        c. Diagnosis of a UTI requires urinalysis and culture and correlation with signs and symptoms.

        d. Treatment consists of appropriate antibiotics, increased fluids, and attention to hygiene.

D. Respiratory diseases

    1. Pulmonary fibrosis

        a. Increased incidence with aging; limited fibrosis is a part of normal aging.

        b. Fibrosis is characterized by shortness of breath and bibasilar rales.

        c. Treatment is largely symptomatic, including supplemental oxygen.

    2. Chronic obstructive pulmonary disease (see Chapter 2). Avoid theophylline because of the high risk of side effects and interactions.

    3. Pulmonary embolus (see Chapter 2).

        a. Presentation often is less specific, with confusion or arrhythmia or fever.

        b. Diagnosis and treatment are the same as those in younger adults. Spiral CT may be less accessible, however, because many elderly suffer from chronic renal insufficiency, limiting the use of contrast material.

E. Cardiovascular disease

    1. Ischemic heart disease

        a. Ischemic heart disease is very common in the elderly but frequently presents atypically, often with shortness of breath or fatigue, weakness, or confusion rather than with chest pain or tightness.

        b. Elderly patients are more likely to have severe or three-vessel coronary disease.

        c. Cardiac enzymes may not rise as much or may be difficult to interpret secondary to renal disease.

        d. Elderly patients who present with myocardial infarction are more likely to die than younger individuals.

        e. Treatment is the same as in younger adults; be mindful of comorbidities that may affect treatment options.

        f. Age alone is not a contraindication to invasive or surgical therapies.

    2. Hypertension

        a. Hypertension is very common in older adults.

        b. It should be treated aggressively unless side effects (e.g., falls secondary to orthostatic hypotension) preclude lowering the systolic pressure to recommended levels.

        c. Diagnosis and treatment are the same as in younger individuals.

        d. Renal artery stenosis, contributing to secondary hypertension, is more common in the elderly.

    e. Systolic hypertension should be treated, because it is more highly associated with stroke than diastolic hypertension. Thiazide diuretics are first choice for systolic hypertension.

    f. Avoid centrally acting agents because of the high risk of sedation, dry mouth, and depression.

3. Valvular disease

    a. Aortic sclerosis

        (1) Results from thickening of the aortic leaflets.

        (2) Causes a systolic murmur similar to that of aortic stenosis, from which it cannot be distinguished on physical examination.

    b. Aortic stenosis. Elderly patients may not exhibit the classic pulsus parvus et tardus (slow, late pulse indicative of carotid disease) or the typical radiation pattern to the carotids and axillae.

    c. Mitral regurgitation

        (1) May cause heart failure and death.

        (2) Treatment is surgical.

4. Congestive heart failure (see Chapter 3)

    a. Diastolic dysfunction is more common and results in poor compliance and poor filling, leading to heart failure.

    b. Presentation often is sudden shortness of breath and pulmonary edema.

    c. Diagnosis is established clinically and is supported with echocardiography.

    d. Treatment is with angiotensin-converting enzyme inhibitors, β-blockers, and calcium channel blockers.

    e. Diuretics should be used judiciously because of the high probability of renal insufficiency and risk of dehydration.

F. Endocrine disorders

1. Hypothyroidism

    a. Hypothyroidism is a very common problem, especially in elderly women, and may present in typical fashion or quite atypically.

    b. Thyroid dysfunction often mimics changes associated with aging itself. These symptoms include a general slowing of mental and physical function, tendency to low body temperatures and cold intolerance, weight gain, constipation, hardening of the arteries, elevation of serum lipids (cholesterol), elevation of blood pressure, and anemia.

    c. Evaluation is via thyroid function testing (thyroid-stimulating hormone typically is elevated).

    d. Treatment

        (1) Treatment is with levothyroxine, with a goal of restoring the thyroid-stimulating hormone to high normal or just above normal.

        (2) Dosage should be very low, 1.25–2.5 μg/day and increased at 4- to 6-week intervals, because the half life of levothyroxine in the elderly is variable.

2. Hyperthyroidism

    a. Hyperthyroidism may present as hypothyroidism (apathetic hyperthyroidism), as atrial fibrillation with a rapid ventricular response, or dementia.

    b. Evaluation is via thyroid function testing.

    c. Treatment is the same as in younger patients.

G. GI disorders

1. Reflux disease is evaluated and treated as in younger adults; however, prokinetic agents should be avoided, if possible.

2. Peptic ulcer disease is more likely to present with failure to thrive or nausea than with dyspepsia or pain.

3. Constipation

    a. Aged individuals are predisposed to bowel dysfunction due to changes of aging, immobility, inadequate hydration, and medications.

    b. Diagnosis is established by history and physical examination and, occasionally, by abdominal flat plate.

    c. Treatment is increasing fluids and activity, improving mastication, increasing dietary fiber, and use of stool softeners and laxatives/enemas if necessary.

    d. If unrelieved, complications may ensue: impaction, stercoral ulcers (ulcerations of the colon because of pressure and irritation from retained feces), obstruction, and death.

TABLE 16-11	Medicare Coverage	
Plan	**Eligibility**	**Coverage**
Traditional Medicare		
Part A	Social security eligible	Hospitalization Subacute nursing home Hospice Home care Durable medical equipment
Part B	Social security eligible PLUS premium	Physician, PA/NP visits Laboratory tests OT/PT outpatient care Emergency care Ambulance Outpatient mental health Does not cover eyeglasses or hearing aids
Part D	Social Security PLUS premium PLUS co-pay	Prescription drugs Beneficiary chooses plan Formularies vary
Nontraditional Medicare		
Medicare Advantage	Health maintenance organization	Usually 100% coverage, but varies

OT/PT, Occupational therapy/physical therapy; *PA/NP*, physician assistant/nurse practitioner.

H. Neurologic disorders

1. Subdural hematoma

   a. Subdural hematomas may be chronic or acute.

   b. Chronic subdural hematomas are common and may arise with little or no trauma.

   c. Presentation usually is confusion, decreased level of consciousness, and perhaps, focal findings, but may appear to be dementia.

   d. Diagnosis is established via CT.

   e. Treatment may be surgical (burr holes) or, if the hematoma is small and is not progressing, watchful waiting.

   f. Chronic subdural hematomas frequently recur even after surgery.

IV. LEGAL AND ETHICAL ISSUES

A. Competence is a legal term and is determined by a judge.

B. Decisional capacity is determined by a physician and may change depending on circumstances and cognitive ability.

C. Elder mistreatment

   1. Suspicion of abuse requires a report to legal authorities.

   2. Abuse may take many forms, including neglect, exploitation, and verbal, psychological, or physical mistreatment.

   3. Abuse often is associated with caregiver stress, especially if the caregiver is financially dependent on the elder and has psychological or substance abuse problems.

   4. Patterns of injury that are not consistent with the history should raise suspicion.

D. Financing and costs

   1. Elderly patients account for about one-third of U.S. health care dollars. Medicare pays for most of these expenditures.

   2. Eligibility for Medicare depends on Social Security status, which is determined by enrollment in the system, aging and/or disease (end stage renal disease [ESRD] confers automatic status), or disability. (Table 16-11 describes Medicare coverage.)

   3. Hospice is covered under Medicare Part A and is accessed when the enrollee chooses comfort care and a physician certifies a life expectancy of 6 months or less.

   4. Nursing home care for subacute rehabilitation is covered for up to 100 days after a 3-day qualifying hospital stay (20 days fully and 80 days with a co-pay).

   5. Informal caregivers, usually family members, provide the majority of daily care for those in the community who require assistance.

Pediatrics

Patti Pagels

17

I. EXAMINATION OF THE NEWBORN

A. Examination at birth

1. Begin with observation, auscultation of the heart and lungs, and inspection for birth trauma/deformities.

2. Apgar score is assessed at 1, 5, and 10 minutes (see Table 8-9). Apgar scoring is completed in the delivery room; low serial scores alert the clinician to the need for resuscitation efforts.

3. The New Ballard Score is a more complex assessment of activity, position, and tone, which is used to evaluate for neuromuscular and physical maturity. This rubric estimates gestational age. Growth charts plot the number of weeks to birth weight to help determine if the newborn is small for gestational age, large for gestational age, or of normal weight.

  a. Small for gestational age may be caused by maternal drug use, chromosomal abnormalities, exposure to intrauterine viral infection, multiple gestation, advanced maternal age (>35 years), placental insufficiency, or lack of maternal weight gain.

  b. Large for gestational age most often results from maternal diabetes.

B. Nursery examination

1. A complete newborn examination should be completed within 24 hours of birth.

2. Skin. Check for color, temperature, rashes or lesions, edema, and hair distribution.

  a. Erythema toxicum

   (1) Common; first appears 3–5 days after birth as small pustules on erythematous bases.

   (2) Spontaneous resolution within 1–2 weeks is the norm.

  b. Milia

   (1) Very small, white papules concentrated on nose, cheeks, forehead and chin.

   (2) Resolves without intervention in 1–2 months.

  c. Miliaria

   (1) Caused by blockage of eccrine sweat glands, resulting in a flushed macular appearance frequently involving neck, face, scalp, and diaper area.

   (2) Light clothing and decreased humidity speed resolution of the "heat rash."

  d. Mongolian spots

   (1) Common in dark-skinned infants and involves small to large, blue-black macules concentrated on the back and buttocks; these macules frequently are misdiagnosed as bruising.

   (2) Most will resolve spontaneously within 4 years, although they may persist for life.

  e. Hemangiomas

   (1) Occur secondary to areas of surface capillary restriction and frequently on the eyelids, nape of the neck, and forehead.

   (2) Almost always resolve spontaneously in 3–12 months.

  f. Vernix caseosa (greasy covering) and lanugo (fine hairs)

   (1) More abundant in preterm infants.

   (2) Dry, cracking skin and peeling is more likely in postterm infants.

3. Head/face

  a. Craniosynostosis

   (1) Premature fusion of sutures.

   (2) Referral to neurology and genetics is necessary.

    b. Fontanelles

        (1) Anterior: 1–4 cm in size in either direction; closes around 6–12 months of age.

        (2) Posterior: 1 cm in size on average size; closes around 1–3 months.

        (3) A third fontanelle along the sagittal suture may be present and may be associated with trisomy 21.

    c. Hematomas and hemorrhages

        (1) Hematomas frequently appear contained within suture lines (cephalhematoma) or may cross suture lines (caput succedaneum).

        (2) Subgaleal hemorrhages occur beneath the scalp; they are uncommon but may result in enough blood loss to cause hemorrhagic shock.

    d. Odd facies beyond the edema and bruising secondary to delivery may represent an underlying syndrome.

4. Ears

    a. Oddly rotated or low-set ears should prompt suspicion of other congenital anomalies.

    b. Preauricular pits and tags are common and most frequently benign.

    c. Tympanic membrane should be intact and visualized via otoscopy.

    d. Hearing is now best assessed during the newborn period by auditory brainstem response or evoked otoacoustic emission testing. All infants should be screened regularly during development.

5. Eyes

    a. Abnormalities or asymmetry of red reflex warrants immediate referral to a pediatric ophthalmologist. Congenital cataracts, glaucoma, or retinoblastomas present as absent red reflex in the infant.

    b. Brushfield spots (gray or pale-yellow spots at periphery of the iris) are associated with Down syndrome.

    c. Subconjunctival hemorrhages are common benign findings associated with the trauma of delivery. They generally resolve with time.

    d. Strabismus or crossing of the eyes almost always is present during the newborn period and does not represent pathology unless it persists or is fixed.

6. Nose/mouth

    a. Nose

        (1) Nasal patency is best assessed by simply placing a cold metal object below the nose to check for fogging.

        (2) Choanal atresia or stenosis presents with unilateral or bilateral obstruction. Bilateral obstruction results in respiratory distress, because infants are obligate nasal breathers.

    b. Mouth

        (1) Esophageal atresia presents as excessive drooling.

        (2) Epstein pearls appear as small, pearly nodules along the gumline and are benign retention cysts.

        (3) Cleft lip/palate deformities are easily identified via inspection.

        (4) Pierre-Robin syndrome may first be recognized by observation of a small mandible and tongue as well as a clefted soft palate. Prone positioning often will control respiratory difficulties caused by the tongue occluding the airway.

        (5) Infants with trisomy 21 frequently have large tongues that often seem to be larger than the mouth.

        (6) Natal teeth may need to be extracted to eliminate the possibility of aspiration.

        (7) Excessive frenuli should be left alone unless they severely impair sucking. A pediatric otolaryngology referral should be arranged emergently.

7. Neck

    a. Webbed or redundant skin of neck may suggest Turner's syndrome.

    b. Masses

        (1) Midline: thyroid.

        (2) Anterior to sternocleidomastoid: brachial cleft (also may see sinus tract remnants).

        (3) Posterior to sternocleidomastoid: cystic hygroma.

        (4) Within sternocleidomastoid: torticollis, hematoma.

8. Lungs/chest

    a. Fractures resulting from birth trauma may be palpated in the clavicles; examine for tenderness, crepitus or bruising. Treatment usually is not necessary.

b. Decreased or abnormal breath sounds

(1) Grunting is a sign of respiratory distress, and its cause should be aggressively sought. It may be associated with anything from hyaline membrane disease to sepsis.

(2) Decreased breath sounds may indicate pneumothorax or diaphragmatic hernia. A mediastinal shift supports pneumothorax.

9. Heart

a. Heart rate is rapid (average, 140 bpm).

b. Murmurs are common and not always associated with pathology.

c. Cyanosis, congestive heart failure, and diminished peripheral pulses are the most common serious presentations of heart disease in the infant.

10. Abdomen

a. Prune belly or absence of abdominal musculature may be associated with renal anomalies.

b. Severely scaphoid belly plus respiratory distress suggest diaphragmatic hernia.

c. Prominent kidneys are suggestive of hydronephrosis or cystic kidney disease.

11. Genitalia/anus

a. Inspect and palpate for anal patency.

b. Male genitalia

(1) Hypospadius

(a) Abnormal placement of urethra on dorsum of glans or shaft.

(b) Do not circumcise; bilateral renal ultrasonography is warranted to rule out pathology.

(c) Refer to a pediatric urologist.

(2) Empty scrotal sac

(a) Testes usually descend by the third month of life; more than 80% descent by 1 year of age. If not descended by age 1, refer to a pediatric urologist for surgical intervention.

(b) Testicular cancer and infertility are real concerns for these children. Bilateral absence of testes should raise suspicion of an infant not fully virilized. A referral to a pediatric endocrinologist is warranted.

(3) Inguinal hernias

(a) More common in premature male infants.

(b) Observe and palpate for an extrafull scrotal sac after an episode of crying.

c. Female genitalia

(1) Vaginal leucorrhea or bloody discharge along with edematous labia is the result of maternal estrogens. These features usually resolve in 7–10 days, but they resolve more slowly in the breast-fed infant.

(2) Vaginal adhesions (fused introitus). Application of estrogen vaginal cream for 5–10 days usually will resolve the problem; if not, refer to a pediatric urologist.

d. Ambiguous genitalia most often is associated with rare conditions, such as chromosomal anomalies and adrenal hyperplasia affecting the action of testosterone.

12. Skeletal

a. Congenital hip dislocation

(1) Occurs as frequently as 1 in 500 infants and at higher rates for infants delivered from the breech presentation.

(2) Examination techniques

(a) The Barlow maneuver is performed with the infant fully relaxed; it attempts to dislocate the hip via posterior pressure. With the knees fully adducted and flexed at 90°, the examiner's thumb and index finger grasp the knees while the middle finger is placed on the outside of the femur, extending to the greater trochanter. If during this maneuver the femoral head is felt to dislocate or leave the acetabulum, it is considered a positive Barlow maneuver.

(b) The Ortolani maneuver attempts to identify the hip that is dislocated or subluxed. Grasp the medial aspect of the flexed knee with the thumb, and fully abduct the hips. Feel for spasm or a clunk (not a click sound) as the hips are brought to full abduction.

(c) Positive Barlow and/or Ortolani maneuvers require bilateral ultrasonography of both hips and referral to a pediatric orthopaedic surgeon to prevent a lifelong disability.

  b. Extremities

  (1) Inspect for skin tags at the lateral borders of hands and feet, which represent rudimentary digits (polydactyly). Suspect other malformations when these are present.

  (2) Club foot or talipes equinovarus is a fixed, severe eversion of the plantar surface and warrants immediate orthopaedic referral.

  c. Spinal deformities, such as tufts of hair or hemangiomas that cross the midline as well as deep sinus tracts in the gluteal cleft, may represent spina bifida occulta or a tethered spinal cord.

13. Neurologic (reflexes)

  a. Sucking and rooting

  (1) The two earliest reflexes.

  (2) Stroking the face elicits turning of the head toward the stimulus; when offered a nipple or the examiner's finger, the infant will instinctively suckle.

  b. Moro or startle reflex

  (1) Allow the infant's head to suddenly drop 1–2 cm, and observe for abduction at the shoulders and elbows along with spreading and extending of the fingers, followed by adduction and flexion of the same.

  (2) This reflex disappears by 3–4 months of age.

  c. Palmar grasp. Placement of the examiner's finger in the infant's palm should elicit the grasping reflex, which disappears by 4 months of age.

  d. Traction response. Pull the infant by the arms to the sitting position, and observe the head lag initially, finally coming briefly to midline before falling forward.

  e. Placing reflex

  (1) Noted when the infant is dangled above the bed, allowing the toe to have minimal contact with the surface.

  (2) The extremity will respond with flexion or a stepping response.

  f. Deep tendon reflexes

  (1) These reflexes are brisk. Clonus may be noted, and an upward-going Babinski are all normal findings.

  (2) A Babinski may be noted as late as 2 years of age.

II. PROBLEMS COMMON TO THE TERM NEWBORN

A. Hypoglycemia

  1. General characteristics

  a. Defined as blood glucose level of less than 40 to 45 mg/dL.

  b. Most commonly found in infants born to diabetic mothers and intrauterine growth restricted infants.

  2. Physical examination

  a. Infant may be asymptomatic or present with poor feeding, lethargy, jitteriness, tremulousness, irritability, apnea, or seizures.

  b. In cases associated with hyperinsulinemia, cardiac failure may develop.

  3. Laboratory testing

  a. Heel blood and bedside glucometer readings are adequate for screening.

  b. Abnormal results should be confirmed with whole-blood testing.

  c. Normal glucose level is 50–80 mg/dL at 3 hours of age; an abnormal level is anything less than 40 to 45 mg/dL.

  4. Treatment

  a. Bolus of dextrose and water ($D_{10}W$) and IV glucose as needed.

  b. Continue to monitor; resolution usually occurs by the fifth day of life.

  c. Failure to resolve should prompt investigation for less likely causes.

TABLE 17-1 **Characteristics and Management of Neonatal Jaundice**

Type	Onset	Laboratory Tests	Treatment
ABO incompatibility	First 24 hours after birth	Coombs (+) Reticulocytes ↑ Hct/Hgb ↓	Transfusion Phototherapy
Rh isoimmunization	First 24 hours after birth	Coombs (+) Reticulocytes Hct/Hgb ↓	Transfusion Phototherapy
Hereditary spherocytosis	First 24 hours after birth	Coombs (−) Reticulocytes ↑ Spherocytes on peripheral smear	Transfusion if severe Phototherapy
G6PD deficiency	First 24 hours after birth	Coombs (−) Specific test for G6PD	Phototherapy
Physiologic jaundice	Appears after 24 hours Peaks at 3–5 days	Bilirubin increases by <5 mg/dL per day	Phototherapy when bilirubin is >15 mg/dL or not descending
Breast-feeding jaundice	Second to third day of life	Bilirubin ↑ and may persist for 6–8 weeks	Supplement breast milk with formula; feed or pump breast milk every 2 hours until an adequate supply is established Phototherapy when bilirubin is >15 mg/dL

G6PD, glucose-6-phosphate dehydrogenase; *Hct/Hgb*, Hematocrit/hemoglobin.

B. Neonatal jaundice

1. General considerations (Table 17-1)

a. More than 65% of infants experience a bilirubin level of greater than 5 mg/dL in the first week of life.

b. Most common causes are physiologic, prematurity, and breast feeding.

c. Common etiologies are divided into two categories, overproduction of bilirubin and decreased rate of conjugation.

(1) Excess production of bilirubin may result from hemolysis secondary to blood group sensitizations (Coombs' test–positive incompatibilities such as Rh and ABO) or hereditary spherocytosis or glucose-6-phosphate dehydrogenase deficiency (Coombs' test negative). Sepsis and nonhemolytic anemia (extravascular hemorrhage) are other possible causes. Reticulocyte counts are elevated.

(2) Decreased rate of conjugation with normal reticulocyte counts commonly results from physiologic jaundice and uncommonly from Gilbert's or Crigler-Najjar syndrome.

d. Kernicterus results from toxic bilirubin levels of greater than 20 to 25 mg/dL and is associated with encephalopathy.

2. Physical examination

a. Jaundice begins at the head and extends to the chest and extremities as bilirubin levels rise.

b. Scleral icterus and jaundiced oral mucosa help distinguish this in the darkly pigmented infant.

c. Splenomegaly may be present in hereditary spherocytosis.

3. Laboratory tests

a. Helpful laboratory tests include CBC; peripheral smear; total, direct, and indirect bilirubin; reticulocyte count; Coombs test, and glucose-6-phosphate dehydrogenase test if the infant is a male of African, Asian, or Mediterranean descent.

b. Monitor hematocrit and hemoglobin in cases of hemolysis or hemorrhage.

c. Septic workup as indicated.

4. Management and treatment

    a. Transfusion is necessary if the cause is ABO incompatibility, Rh isoimmunization, or nonimmune hemolysis (Coombs' test negative).

    b. Phototherapy benefits all types of jaundice.

        (1) Phototherapy may be started as early as 12 hours of age.

        (2) It is recommended when the bilirubin level reaches 10 mg/dL in ABO incompatibility and 15 mg/dL for most other causes.

C. Respiratory distress in the newborn

  1. General considerations

    a. Common pulmonary causes

        (1) Unilateral or bilateral choanal atresia

        (2) Transient tachypnea of the newborn (resolves in 24 hours)

        (3) Fluid aspiration (blood or meconium)

        (4) Hyaline membrane disease (especially in premature infants)

        (5) Congenital pneumonia (rectal flora pathogens)

    b. Common cardiovascular causes

        (1) Cyanotic lesions

            (a) Valvular pulmonary stenosis (only when severe)

            (b) Pulmonary atresia with ventricular septal defect (the most extreme form of tetralogy of Fallot)

            (c) Tricuspid atresia

            (d) Transposition of the great arteries

            (e) Total anomalous pulmonary venous return

        (2) Mild cyanosis resulting from left-sided outflow tract obstruction

            (a) Hypoplastic left heart syndrome (usually involving atresia of mitral valve, aortic valve, or both)

            (b) Aortic stenosis

            (c) Coarctation of the aorta

    c. Other common causes

        (1) Hyperthermia or hypothermia (hypothermia can be particularly troublesome for the preterm infant)

        (2) Intrauterine exposure to cocaine

        (3) Metabolic acidosis

        (4) Hemorrhage or asphyxia resulting in damage to the central nervous system (can occur as a result of traumatic delivery)

  2. Physical examination

    a. The infant typically appears cyanotic on room air.

    b. Respiratory rate is greater than 60 breaths per minute.

    c. Grunting as well as intercostal and sternal retractions are common.

    d. Cyanosis resolving with supplemental oxygen supports either a pulmonary or noncardiovascular cause.

  3. Laboratory studies

    a. Chest radiography, pulse oximetry, and arterial blood gases provide the basic information.

    b. CBC and blood cultures should be monitored if appropriate.

    c. A complete metabolic profile typically is done on all cyanotic infants.

    d. Echocardiography or CT of the head and chest may be warranted by the suspected cause.

  4. Management

    a. Provide immediate supplemental oxygen with close monitoring.

    b. Begin IV fluids (glucose or saline, as the situation warrants).

    c. Provide intubation if true respiratory failure is present.

    d. Determine the underlying cause, and manage appropriately.

III. DEVELOPMENTAL MILESTONES AND DISORDERS

A. Developmental milestones

    1. General considerations

        a. Typically, developmental surveys are done at each well-child examination; these examinations usually correspond to the typical vaccination schedule.

        b. Developmental screenings are done frequently between birth to 3 years of age and then each year thereafter.

        c. Parents and caregivers are important sources of information regarding the child's abilities.

        d. It is important to distinguish between a child whose pattern of development has slowed or regressed versus a child who has always been developmentally slow, because the causes generally are quite different.

    2. From birth to 5 years of age, the areas that typically are surveyed are gross and fine motor skills, personal and social behaviors, and language; assessment of older children shifts to higher cognitive functions and sexual maturation.

        a. Table 17-2 highlights milestones for children from birth to 5 years of age.

        b. Table 17-3 highlights milestones in the child 6–10 years of age.

        c. Between 10 and 19 years of age, the focus shifts from developmental milestones to physical maturation. The classical and most efficient way to gauge sexual maturation in males and females is by using Tanner Stages (Table 17-4).

TABLE 17-2	Typical Developmental Milestones from Birth to 5 Years of Age			
Age/Skill	**Gross Motor**	**Fine Motor**	**Personal/Social**	**Language**
0–2 months	Turns head side to side	Clenched fist Eye contact	Recognizes human face	Cries Startles at loud noise
2–3 months	Lifts head	Tracks object past midline Hands open	Smiles responsively	Vocalizes in play
4–5 months	Head steady in supported position	Hands together	Shows displeasure through vocalization	Looks for source of sound
6–8 months	Rolls over Sits leaning forward on arms	Reaches for objects Raking grasp	Responds to own name Holds own bottle	Imitates speech sounds Vocal imitation
9–11 months	Stands while holding on	Passes object from hand to hand	Feeds self Imitates waving	Understands *no* May use *mama*
12–14 months	Stands alone for 2 seconds	Bangs two objects together Places pellet in bottle	Hugs dolls or stuffed animals Routinely gestures to meet needs	Uses one or two words with meaning
15–17 months	Stoops and recovers Walks well	Builds tower of two or three cubes	Attempts use of spoon	Waves bye-bye Four or five words
18–21 months	Runs well Kicks large ball Walks backward	Scribbles Turns pages of book	Drinks well from a cup Feeds self Uses a spoon well	Follows simple commands (e.g., *give me*) 20–50 words
24 months	Throws ball overhead Jumps	Turns doorknobs Builds towers of six to seven blocks	Washes and dries hands Little spilling during self feeding	Two or three words combined Points to body parts
36 months	Stands on one foot at least 2 seconds	Copies circle	Takes turns Toilet trained	Uses pronouns (*I, me, you*) Gives name
48 months	Hops on one foot	Wiggles thumb Copies cross	Dresses self	Knows colors Asks questions
5 years	Skips using alternate feet	Holds a pencil correctly	Brushes teeth without help	Easily carries on a conversation May count or recite part of the alphabet

TABLE 17-3	Typical Developmental Milestones from 6 to 10 Years of Age				
	Age 6 (Grade 1)	**Age 7 (Grade 2)**	**Age 8 (Grade 3)**	**Age 9 (Grade 4)**	**Age 10 (Grade 5)**
Language	Speaks using correct sentence structure	Defines words Compares and contrasts Speech reaches adult proficiency	Defines more words Recites days of week	Comprehends absurdities in sentences	Understands abstract words
Hand–eye coordination	Draws more precisely	Legible printing Ties own shoes	Begins to learn cursive writing	Draws person with detail	Draws people with great detail
Calculation and reading	Reads one-syllable words Counts to 20 Later reads simple sentence, adds and subtracts primary numbers	Reads two-syllable words Counts to 100 Adds and subtracts two-digit numbers	Reads many more two-syllable words Performs simple multiplication	Reads three- and four-syllable words Alphabetizes Does simple division Comprehends fractions	Able to read more complex words Easily uses adding, subtracting, fractions, division, multiplication, and estimation

B. Development disorders

  1. General considerations

   a. Disorders of development often are first noted by parents or caregivers when a child fails to meet one or more milestones in development. Areas of concern include motor, visual–spatial, verbal, attention, behavioral, and social abilities.

   b. The most common neurodevelopmental disorder is attention-deficit hyperactivity disorder; the most severe (in terms of affecting all areas of development) is mental retardation.

  2. Evaluation of developmental disorders

   a. A comprehensive history should include a detailed prenatal history, labor and delivery, complications during pregnancy as well as the immediate postnatal period, major illness/hospitalizations, history of metabolic disease, and family history.

   b. A complete physical examination is essential, especially the neurological examination and careful inspection for dysmorphic features.

   c. Referral to appropriate specialists, including speech and occupational therapists, psychologists, and educational specialists, should be made as dictated by the child's needs.

  3. Speech/language delay

   a. Causes are many (e.g., prematurity, severe neglect, congenital syndromes, conductive hearing loss secondary to chronic serous otitis media).

   b. Language delay may be characterized by omitted sounds, difficulty pronouncing certain letters, dysfluency, or failure to have language skill by 2 or 3 years of age.

TABLE 17-4	Typical Tanner Stages for Males and Females from 11 to 17 Years of Age			
Tanner Stage	**2 Age 11–12**	**3 Age 13**	**4 Age 14–15**	**5 Age 16–17**
Males	Straight hair at base of penis	Coarse, dark, and curly pubic hair	Hair is almost completely full	Pubic hair achieves adult appearance
	Age 11	**Age 12**	**Age 13**	**Age 14–15**
Females	Minimal, straight pubic hair	Increased pubic hair that is dark and coarse	Hair approaches normal adult appearance	Pubic hair reaches adult appearance and forms inverted triangle

    c. Hearing should be carefully assessed, especially when speech delay appears to be the only impairment.

    d. Management includes referral to speech and language specialists for specific diagnosis, development of a treatment plan, and monitoring during development.

4. Attention-deficit hyperactivity disorder (see Chapter 12)

5. Pervasive developmental disorders (see Chapter 12)

6. Mental retardation

    a. Mental retardation is defined as an IQ of less than 70 with disturbances in adaptive behavior

    b. Physical examination

        (1) Abnormal muscle tone is seen at 6 months.

        (2) Motor delay is apparent by 1 year.

        (3) All spheres of development are affected to some degree by 2 years.

    c. Laboratory testing is carried out to uncover possible causes and includes CBC to rule out anemia; lead screen; chromosomal studies, especially if the child is dysmorphic; metabolic testing; thyroid studies; electroencephalography; and MRI as appropriate.

    d. Treatment includes referral to special programs for social, occupational, and cognitive support.

7. Spina bifida (myelomeningocele)

    a. Two forms exist.

        (1) Aperta is when the neural tube defect involves the overlying skin.

        (2) Occulta appears as hairy tufts, dimples, or dermal sinus noted in the lumbosacral region.

    b. Risks factors include insufficient intake of folic acid during pregnancy and maternal use of valproate.

    c. Characteristic findings

        (1) Neurologic. Hypotonia, sensory deficits, paralysis, hydrocephalus, or macrocephaly.

        (2). Extremities. Contractures, tethered cord which may cause back pain, club feet, scoliosis, or hip dislocations.

        (3) Urinary. Frequent urosepsis, incontinence.

    d. Treatment includes prompt intervention for hydrocephalus through shunting and referral for supportive services.

8. Cerebral palsy (see Chapter 11)

IV. INBORN ERRORS OF METABOLISM, CHROMOSOMAL ABNORMALITIES, AND COMMON DYSMORPHIC SYNDROMES

A. Inborn errors of metabolism

1. General considerations

    a. All states screen infants for phenylketonuria, congenital adrenal hyperplasia, galactosemia, and hypothyroidism. These disorders are treatable, and testing generally is inexpensive.

    b. In general, more expansive and/or selective screening should be considered under the following conditions.

        (1) Acutely ill infant or neonate

        (2) Developmental delay (index of suspicion should be higher with regression of development)

        (3) Failure to thrive

        (4) Mental retardation

        (5) Organomegaly

2. Management and treatment

    a. Management and treatment of infants with inborn errors of metabolism have the best success when the inborn error is identified early and families both understand and can adhere to treatment regimens.

    b. Table 17-5 describes the specific characteristics, special tests, and management principles for phenylketonuria, congenital adrenal hyperplasia, galactosemia, and hypothyroidism.

B. Chromosomal abnormalities

1. General considerations

    a. Chromosomal abnormalities are found in 1 in 200 live births and approximately 7% of aborted concepti.

TABLE 17-5 **Common Inborn Errors of Metabolism: Epidemiology, Signs, Symptoms, Testing, and Management**

Condition	Signs and Symptoms	Specific Evaluations	Treatments
Hypothyroidism (1:4,500 live births)	Lethargy, mental retardation, eczema, failure to thrive; rarely goiter, thick tongue; up to 75% of newborns are asymptomatic during the first 2 months of life	Serial TSH, free T_4	Replacement therapy with L-thyroxine
Congenital adrenal hyperplasia (1:5,000 live births)	Virilized female; males may have ambiguous genitalia; infants may present early in life with salt-wasting, adrenal crisis	17-Hydroxyprogesterone	Corticosteroid replacement
Phenylketonuria (1:12,000 live births)	Moderate to severe mental retardation, hyperactivity, seizures, autism, and hypopigmentation	Test after 24 hours of protein intake, then quantitative serum phenylalanine determination	Lifetime of low-protein diet; avoid products with phenylalanine
Galactosemia (1:60,000 live births)	Neonatal nausea and vomiting, jaundice, hepatic dysfunction and liver enlargement, mental retardation, cataracts, and death	Galactose-1-phosphate uridyltransferase electrophoresis after galactose intake	Lactose- and galactose-free diet

TSH, thyroid-stimulating hormone; T_4, thyroxine.

b. Occurrence of one or more of the following should prompt further evaluation: certain phenotypes (trisomy 21, 13, and 18), ambiguous genitalia, multiple congenital anomalies, retinoblastoma, Wilms' tumor, mental retardation, abnormal stature, and primary amenorrhea.

c. Types of chromosomal anomalies

    (1) Structural. Deletions, duplications, translocations, inversions

    (2). Numeric. Triploidy and tetraploidy (both lethal), trisomy, monosomy, aneuploidy of sex chromosomes, and mosaicism

d. Initial evaluation when chromosomal abnormalities are suspected should include DNA methylation and fluorescence in situ hybridization.

e. Management is specific to the disorder and may include supportive care, environmental and educational supports, physical therapy, and other modalities.

2. Common chromosomal abnormalities

    a. Trisomy 21

        (1) Incidence is 1 in 750 live births.

        (2) Also known as Down syndrome.

        (3) Frequently associated with advanced maternal age.

        (4) Common characteristics

            (a) Flattened facies and occiput, low-set ears, upward-slanting eyes, large tongue, Brushfield spots in eyes, small ears, and thin hair.

            (b) Palms have prominent simian creases, short fingers, and medial or laterally placed digits.

            (c) Congenital heart disease is present in up to 50% of cases; atrioventricular septal defects are most common.

            (d) Umbilical hernias and diastasis recti.

            (e) Hypotonia and delayed motor skills

    b. Klinefelter's syndrome (XXY)

        (1) Incidence is 1 in 800 live births.

        (2) Common characteristics

          (a) Initially tall, thin, and long-limbed; become obese in the adult years. Scoliosis is frequent.

          (b) Ataxia, expressive language disorders, and usually mild developmental delay.

          (c) Males. Small penis, hypogonadism, scant pubic and facial hair, and gynecomastia.

          (d) Females. Eunochoid habitus.

c. Turner's syndrome (monosomy X)

    (1) Incidence is 1 in 2,000 female live births.

    (2) Common characteristics

          (a) Short stature, webbed neck, prominent ears and low posterior hairline, broad chest with widely spaced nipples, and increased carrying angle.

          (b) Hearing impairment as well as visual and spatial perceptive disabilities.

          (c) Primary amenorrhea, ovarian dysgenesis, and absence of secondary sex characteristics.

          (d) Coarctation of the aorta, horseshoe kidney, and aortic stenosis.

d. Fragile X syndrome

    (1) Incidence is 1 in 1,250 male live births.

    (2) Common characteristics

          (a) Pale blue irides, long narrowed facies, large protruding ears, large protruding jaw, flat feet, and hyperextendible fingers.

          (b) Prepubertal large gonads.

          (c) Autism and/or moderate to severe mental retardation with disorganized speech patterns.

          (d) Mitral valve prolapse.

          (e) Female carriers exhibit mild learning disabilities.

e. Beckwith-Wiedemann syndrome (chromosome 11p15)

    (1) Incidence is 1 in 15,000 live births.

    (2) Common characteristics

          (a) Large-for-gestational-age infants, hypoglycemia during infancy, creases and pits in earlobes, asymmetric limbs, organomegaly, and large tongue.

          (b) At risk for Wilms' tumor and hepatoblastoma.

f. Prader-Willi syndrome (chromosome 15q11)

    (1) Incidence is 1 in 25,000 live births.

    (2) Common characteristics

          (a) Often small for gestational age, hypogonadism, small hands and feet, almond-shaped eyes, and hypotonia.

          (b) Mental retardation, short stature, polyphagia and eventually, obesity.

          (c) Diabetes and Pickwickian syndrome are common complications.

g. Angelman's syndrome (chromosome 15)

    (1) Incidence is unknown but estimated at between 1 in 15,000 and 1 in 30,000 live births.

    (2) Common characteristics

          (a) Severe mental retardation, marked developmental delay, poor language skills, paroxysmal laughter, and tongue thrusting.

          (b) Prognathism, seizures, and abnormal gait and posturing.

C. Common dysmorphic syndromes

  1. General considerations

    a. Dysmorphic syndromes may result from a chromosomal anomaly or single gene defects. Some are multifactorial; others may result from a combination of genetics and environment.

    b. Signs and symptoms that often accompany these chromosomal or genetic anomalies include:

      (1) Multiple anomalies.

      (2) Abnormal growth patterns, both pre- and postnatally.

      (3) Child typically exhibits characteristics not seen in parents or siblings.

      (4) Infant may present with mental retardation, abnormal muscle tone, seizures, sensory deficits, as well as motor and speech delay.

    c. Testing is specific for the syndrome under consideration.

    d. Treatment involves detailed genetic counseling and, in some cases, surgical intervention.

  2. Common dysmorphic syndromes

    a. Ehlers-Danlos syndrome is primarily an autosomal dominant condition (10 syndromes or clinical types are known).

      (1) The primary defect involves collagen, resulting in joint laxity, hyperelastic skin, pectus deformity, and excessive bruising.

      (2) Death often results from ruptured aneurysm.

    b. Marfan's syndrome is an autosomal dominant mutation.

      (1) The primary defect involves a connective tissue protein, resulting in tall, lanky stature, joint laxity, high arched palate, long digits, and myopia.

      (2) Complications result from mitral valve prolapse, aortic root dilation, aortic insufficiency, aneurysms. and spontaneous pneumothorax.

    c. Fetal alcohol syndrome is related to maternal alcohol use.

      (1) These children are born small and may remain small. Characteristics involving the head and facies include microcephaly, long and smooth philtrum, thin upper lip, small palpebral fissures, and small distal phalanges.

      (2) This syndrome is complicated by developmental delay, hyperactivity, moderate retardation, and involvement of internal organs (congenital heart disease, cleft lip/palate, and renal anomalies).

    d. Neural tube defects

      (1) Causes may include genetics and environment.

      (2) Defects may be as severe as anencephaly or as mild as a small spina bifida.

      (3) Folic acid supplementation throughout pregnancy may be protective.

    e. Cleft lip and palate

      (1) Typically, the cause is multifactorial, but cleft lip and palate may result from autosomal dominant, autosomal recessive, or X-linked disorders.

      (2) Various degrees of severity are seen, involving specific deformities of the lip and palate.

      (3) Look for other malformations because, in many cases, this will not be an isolated defect.

      (4) Many cases are amenable to surgery.

    f. Osteogenesis imperfecti is an autosomal dominant condition.

      (1) The defect involves type 1 collagen, resulting in bone fragility and pathological fractures.

      (2) Some cases result in blue-tinted sclera and varying degree of deafness.

      (3) In its severest form, fetal demise may occur.

V. FAILURE TO THRIVE, GROWTH DELAY, AND SELECTED NUTRITIONAL DISORDERS OF CHILDHOOD

A. Failure to thrive

  1. General characteristics

    a. Failure to thrive is defined as a child 2 or less years of age with weight plotting below the fifth percentile for age on more than one occasion or whose weight crosses two major percentiles downward on a standardized growth grid.

    b. Exceptions to this definition are genetic short stature, small-for-gestational-age infants, preterm infants, and overweight infants with decreased rate of weight gain and increased rate of height gain.

    c. Failure to thrive is a syndrome that most commonly is associated with environmental and/or behavioral factors, followed by an organic cause.

  2. Specific causes to be considered include:

    a. Lack of appetite (caused by anemia, psychosocial problems, CNS pathology, chronic infection, or GI disorder).

    b. Difficulty with ingestion (caused by psychosocial problems, cerebral palsy or other CNS disorders, dyspnea, craniofacial abnormalities, myopathies, or congenital syndromes).

   c. Unavailability of food (consider inappropriate feeding techniques, inadequate volume of food, inappropriate food for age, abuse, or neglect).

   d. Vomiting (caused by reflux, obstruction of the intestinal tract, or increased intracranial pressure).

   e. Malabsorption (cystic fibrosis, biliary disease, disorders of metabolism, immune deficiency, inflammatory bowel disease, and celiac disease are the primary causes).

   f. Diarrhea (caused by bacterial gastroenteritis, parasitic infection, or starvation).

   g. Inadequate absorption of calories (caused by hepatitis or Hirschsprung's disease).

   h. Increased metabolism/increased use of calories (caused by chronic or recurrent infection, chronic pulmonary insufficiency, congenital or acquired heart disease, neoplasm, lead poisoning, chronic anemia, or endocrinopathies).

   i. Defective use of calories (e.g., inborn errors of metabolism, renal tubular acidosis, cyanotic heart disease).

3. Laboratory tests

   a. Investigation centers on uncovering any known cause.

   b. Observation by team or in a hospital setting is desired if a behavioral or psychosocial cause is suspected.

   c. Specific laboratory testing is as needed per history and physical examination and may include:

     (1) CBC.

     (2) Urinalysis with culture and sensitivity.

     (3) Serum electrolytes, blood urea nitrogen (BUN), and creatinine.

     (4) Tuberculin skin test.

     (5) Radiography of wrists for bone age.

4. Treatment

   a. Treat the underlying cause.

   b. Remove the child from the home if necessary.

   c. Increase feedings for infants from 100 to 150 kcal/kg/day.

B. Selected causes of growth delay

1. Familial short stature

   a. General characteristics

     (1) Familial short stature is apparent before the second year of life and manifests as a deceleration in height.

     (2) Height is heredity and closely matches parental height.

   b. Physical examination. The child has normal development without other signs or symptoms of disease.

   c. Special testing

     (1) Further testing that may be done to rule out other causes includes CBC; erythrocyte sedimentation rate; urinalysis; BUN and creatinine; serum electrolytes, including calcium and phosphorus; examination of stool for fat content; karyotype (females); and intrinsic growth factor (IGF)-1 and IGF-binding protein 3.

     (2) Radiography of the distal radius will reveal bone age equal to chronological age.

   d. Treatment. Reassure parents that deceleration is normal and expected, especially if both parents are short.

2. Constitutional growth delay

   a. General characteristics

     (1) Often called a "late bloomer" and may have a family history of delayed growth.

     (2) Family members may be of normal height.

     (3) Skeletal bone age will lag behind chronological age.

     (4) Puberty may be delayed.

   b. Physical examination. Except for height, development is normal for age.

   c. Selected testing

     (1) Further testing is driven by the history and physical examination findings; testing is done to rule out other causes as above.

     (2) Radiography of the distal radius reveals chronological age greater than bone age.

   d. Treatment. Growth is delayed, but eventually, the child will reach his or her expected height.

3. Growth hormone (GH) deficiency

    a. General characteristics

        (1) The anterior pituitary produces GH under stimulation from GH-releasing hormone (GHRH) and suppression of somatostatin.

        (2) GH deficiency may be an isolated disorder or may occur as a result of other pituitary hormone deficiencies. The most likely cause is idiopathic; other diagnoses to consider include congenital (empty sella syndrome) and acquired (craniopharyngioma).

        (3) Growth failure caused by GH deficiency may occur during infancy or appear later in childhood and is largely dependent on the underlying cause.

        (4) Laron dwarfism results from a mutation in the GH receptor.

    b. Physical examination

        (1) Decline in growth velocity or subnormal growth is characteristic.

        (2) Children with dwarfism have distinctive facial features.

        (3) Truncal obesity may be present, because GH also promotes lipolysis.

        (4) Impaired peripheral vision with optic chiasm tumors is frequent.

        (5) Delayed puberty and webbed neck are seen in cases of Turner's syndrome.

        (6) Disproportionately short limbs compared to trunk suggest a skeletal dysplasia.

    c. Testing

        (1) As suggested by the history and physical examination and to rule out other causes, as above.

        (2) Radiography of the distal radius for bone age.

        (3) When other causes are ruled out and GH status is equivocal, more provocative studies are warranted.

        (4) In some cases, a trial of human GH may be warranted and may confirm the diagnosis.

    d. Treatment

        (1) Human GH has been approved for specific causes, such as Prader-Willi syndrome, Turner's syndrome, children born small for gestational age who fail to grow, and chronic renal failure.

        (2) Referral to a pediatric endocrinologist is recommended, because tests for GH deficiency often are difficult to interpret and treatment for other causes is controversial.

C. Selected nutritional disorders

    1. General considerations

        a. Nutritional deficiencies may result from internal causes (e.g., blood loss, malabsorption, chronic disease) or external causes (e.g., inappropriate feeding, psychosocial distress, inability to take in sufficient nutrition).

        b. The ideal source of infant nutrition is breast milk because: it contains a perfect mix of nutrients as well as protein, lipids, and carbohydrates; promotes bonding; and strengthens the infant's immune system. Infant formulas today come very close to matching breast milk in terms of providing energy and nutrition.

        c. The typical infant diet should consist of breast milk or formula until 4 months of age. Cereal may be introduced at 4 months, fruit at 5 months, vegetables at 6 months, and complex proteins and whole cow's milk at 1 year.

    2. Calcium, fluoride, vitamin K, protein, and carbohydrate deficiencies (Table 17-6).

VI. IMMUNIZATION OF INFANTS AND CHILDREN

A. General considerations

    1. Combination products (one syringe containing multiple vaccines) are preferred and have not been found to diminish immune response or to increase the rate of adverse events.

    2. Premature infants are immunized just as term newborns in regard to amount and timing. An exception is hepatitis B vaccine, which is recommended for premature infants weighing 2 kg or more.

    3. There are few contraindications to vaccines.

        a. Anaphylactic reaction to previous vaccine or component of a vaccine.

        (1) Neomycin/streptomycin are common preservatives in MMR (measles, mumps, rubella) and IPV (inactivated polio vaccine) and have caused allergic reactions and anaphylaxis.

        (2) Baker's yeast allergy: avoid hepatitis B vaccine.

TABLE 17-6	Selected Nutritional Disorders			
Nutrient	**Risk Factors for Development**	**Signs and Symptoms**	**Laboratory Examinations**	**Treatment**
Protein	Body cannot store protein, so a daily supply is needed Severe skin disease and burns Cystic fibrosis	Impaired growth velocity Severest form is kwashiorkor, resulting in lethargy, irritability, impaired growth velocity, edema, and hepatomegaly	Chemistry panel (may suggest decreased albumin) CBC (may reveal other deficiencies)	Adjust diet; increase daily intake of protein
Carbohydrate	Daily supply is required because of the body's limited ability to store excess Galactosemia (inborn error of metabolism) Diarrhea Malabsorption Improper diet Excess intake results in obesity and increased risk of type 2 diabetes mellitus	Impaired growth velocity Obesity Marasmus is a severe form of malnutrition resulting from multiple dietary deficiencies, including lack of carbohydrates	Chemistry panel (electrolyte imbalances likely) CBC	Dietary adjustment
Vitamin K	Aids in formulation of coagulation proteins Newborns Breast-fed newborns who do not receive Vitamin K prophylactically at birth	Hemorrhagic purpura involving skin, internal organs, and CNS, which may be fatal	Vitamin K levels Prolonged prothrombin time	IM Vitamin K injection
Fluoride	Fluoride is incorporated into the tooth matrix, increasing resistance to dental caries This element is contained in most public water sources	Increased number of dental caries In case of fluoridosis, look for undermineralization and discolored teeth	Dental examinations	Consider supplementation after 6 months of age when the water source does not contain fluoride
Iron	Breast-fed infants Untreated maternal anemia Prematurity Blood loss during the neonatal period	Asymptomatic when mild Pallor Fatigue Impaired cognitive and motor development Pica	CBC with differential Serum ferritin Serum iron Total iron-binding capacity Reticulocyte count	Food with high iron content Supplementation For breast-fed infants, introduce iron-fortified cereals at 4–6 months

CBC, complete blood count; *CNS,* central nervous system.

(3) Allergy to eggs: avoid influenza vaccine.

(4) Gelatin allergy: avoid varicella vaccine.

b. History of encephalopathy within 7 days of giving DTaP or DTP (diphtheria, tetanus, pertussis).

c. Pregnancy. Avoid live vaccines, such as MMR and varicella, and live attenuated influenza vaccine.

d. Avoid MMR and varicella vaccine if immunocompromised.

4. Precautions should be taken with the following vaccines under certain circumstances:

a. Consider rescheduling any vaccine in the presence of moderate to severe illness and/or fever (≥102.5°F).

b. Postpone MMR and varicella vaccine until 3–6 months after administration of immunoglobulin.

c. Carefully consider readministration of DTaP or DTP when side effects, such as high fever (40.5°C/104.5°F), shock-like state, seizure, prolonged and inconsolable crying, or Guillain-Barre syndrome, have occurred with any dose.

    d. Pregnant females should avoid exposure to IPV.

    e. Consider postponing MMR with current or recent history of thrombocytopenic purpura.

    f. Patients immunized with varicella vaccine should avoid family members with immunodeficiency.

  5. Personal or family history of seizures, mild illness with or without fever (≤102.5°F), breast feeding, recent positive PPD or testing, and use of antibiotics are not reasons to postpone vaccines.

B. Thimerosal

  1. Routine childhood vaccines are now manufactured without the use of thimerosal.

  2. Multidose vials of injectable influenza vaccine contain thimerosal, whereas single-dose preparations are free of the mercury-based preservative.

  3. Numerous large studies have failed to link thimerosal to autism, as was initially reported in one study.

VII. COMMON PEDIATRIC POISONINGS

A. General considerations

  1. Each year, 85% of all poisonings occur in children under the age of 5; they generally are accidental and unwitnessed.

  2. Mortality rates are low and likely to involve analgesics, household cleaning products, iron, hydrocarbons, and illicit drugs.

  3. Adolescent ingestions likely are intentional and result from suicide attempts or use of illicit drugs and are 15-fold more fatal than accidental ingestions in small children.

  4. Commonly ingested substances include cosmetic/hygiene products, cleaning products, analgesics, plants, cough/cold preparations, pesticides, vitamins, and hydrocarbons.

B. History and physical examination

  1. Obtain a detailed history of what, when, and how of the ingestion.

  2. The offending substance should be brought to the emergency department if available.

  3. Inventories of household products as well as over-the-counter and prescription medicines should be conducted.

  4. History may reveal the substance in 90% of cases.

  5. Physical examination (Table 17-7)

    a. Note any unusual breath odors (arsenic and organophosphates produce garlic breath).

    b. Check skin for excessive dryness, sweating, discoloration, and fever (anticholinergics cause warm, dry, skin, whereas organic phosphates produces salivation and urination).

    c. Pupillary size as well as lacrimation should be noted.

    d. Vomiting or excessive salivation should be noted.

    e. Neurological changes, such as agitation, ataxia, tremors, convulsion, and coma, often are encountered.

    f. Tachycardia, tachypnea, dysrhythmias (tricyclic antidepressants are notorious for causing prolonged QRS complexes) may occur in some settings.

C. Laboratory testing (Table 17-7)

  1. Calculate the anion and osmolar gaps (alcohol causes an anion gap; methanol causes an osmolar gap).

  2. Perform initial and ongoing electrocardiography.

  3. When substance is unknown, standard emergency department (ED) toxin panels may provide the diagnosis.

  4. Order specific toxicology screens, such as diuretics, ethylene glycol, lithium, aromatic hydrocarbons, and cyanide, as warranted.

  5. Abdominal radiographs, as a rule, are not helpful, because very few agents are radiodense (e.g., heavy metals, iodine, enteric-coated tablets).

D. Management (Table 17-7)

  1. Airway, breathing, and circulation should be the first concern.

  2. Additional management is predicated on the type of ingestion.

TABLE 17-7 Common Toxidromes

Toxin	Physical Findings	Special Tests	Antidotes/Management
Hydrocarbons (benzene, gasoline, petroleum distillates)	Mucosal irritation Vomiting, bloody diarrhea Cyanosis, respiratory distress Tachycardia Fever CNS depression	CXR Urinalysis ECG	Avoid emetics and lavage Oxygen with mist Antibiotics if pneumonia develops
Caustics (toilet bowel cleaners)	Skin, mucosal burns Hematemesis Abdominal pain Respiratory distress Convulsions, coma	EGD to determine degree of esophageal injury ECG	Small amounts of water or milk Avoid vomiting Supportive care
Bases (Clorox, Drano)	Irritated mucous membranes Respiratory distress secondary to edematous epiglottis Perforation of stomach or esophagus	EGD to determine degree of damage to larynx, esophagus, and stomach	Small amounts of water as dilutant Avoid vomiting Supportive care
Acetaminophen	Hepatotoxic	Monitor APAP plasma concentration (use specific nomogram)	Acetylcysteine is the specific antidote
Aspirin (salicylates)	Vomiting Hyperapnea Fever Encephalopathy, convulsions, coma Renal failure Pulmonary edema	Check serum salicylate level Look for metabolic acidosis and decreased K^+ Elevated or reduced serum glucose	Induce emesis Charcoal to bind drug Correct dehydration Hemodialysis
Antihistamines	Agitation and hallucinations Miosis Red eye, dry skin Fever Respiratory failure CV collapse	EC6 ligase chains Pulse oximetry	Activated charcoal Whole-bowel irrigation Physostigmine
Organophosphates (chlorthion, diazinon)	Salivation, lacrimation Diaphoresis Urination, diarrhea Miosis Pulmonary congestion Twitching, convulsions, coma	Measure red cell cholinesterase levels Blood glucose levels	ABCs Decontamination of skin Atropine plus pralidoxime
Iron (vitamins, prenatal vitamins)	Intestinal bleeding Impaired coagulation Acidosis Shock Coma Red urine	Blood indices Metabolic panel Monitor urine output for renal damage Blood type and cross-match LFTs	Evoke emesis Gastric lavage Whole-bowel irrigation Desferoxamine Dialysis

ABCs, airway, breathing, circulation; APAP, N-acetyl-P-aminophenol; CNS, central nervous system; CXR; chest radiography; ECG, electrocardiography; EGD, esophagogastroduodensoscopy; LFTs, liver function tests.

3. General principles of management
   a. Induced vomiting and/or gastric lavage are no longer recommended.
   b. Activated charcoal is used to promote GI decontamination. It is the current first line treatment for most ingested poisons.
   c. Use of sorbitol or other cathartics may accelerate elimination.
   d. Whole-bowel irrigation, dialysis, and hemoperfusion rarely are necessary.
   e. Antidotes exist for specific ingestions.

VIII. COMMON PEDIATRIC DISORDERS (FOR FURTHER INFORMATION AND OTHER DISORDERS, PLEASE SEE APPROPRIATE CHAPTERS)

A. Foreign bodies

    1. Infants and children often place objects in orifices. Common objects include beads, buttons, nuts, foodstuff, and toy parts.

    2. Ear, nose, and throat (ENT)

        a. Unilateral purulent rhinitis, persistent sinusitis, or a blocked nasal passage should prompt consideration of a foreign body in the nose.

        b. Ear pain, drainage, and hearing loss accompany foreign bodies in the ear.

        c. If the object is visible, remove it using a curette, forceps, or catheter. Be sure the child is restrained, and do not blindly probe.

    3. Respiratory tract

        a. Upper airway. Abrupt onset of cough, stridor, choking, cyanosis; complete obstruction leads to inability to cough or choke.

        b. Lower airway. Acute to subacute cough, unilateral persistent wheezing, recurrent pneumonia; complete obstruction may cause a ball-valve effect, resulting in distal hyperinflation and mediastinal shift, which is most apparent on expiratory films.

        c. Attempt the Heimlich maneuver if respiratory distress is apparent and rigid bronchoscopy if the object is lodged in the lower airway.

    4. GI tract

        a. Most objects will pass through the GI tract. Large or irregularly shaped objects may become lodged; sharp objects, such as pins, may cause mucosal tearing.

        b. Removal by esophagogastroscopy is recommended for caustic (batteries), sharp, or lodged objects.

B. Functional (innocent) murmurs

    1. Approximately 40–45% of children have an innocent murmur at some point in their childhood.

    2. Still's murmur is the most common innocent murmur of childhood.

        a. It usually is apparent from 2 years of age through preadolescence.

        b. It is loudest in the apex and left sternal border. It typically is a grade I–III musical or vibratory, high-pitched, early systolic murmur that diminishes with sitting, standing, or Valsalva maneuvers, and it will accentuate with fever.

    3. Venous hum

        a. Grade I or II musical hum that is heard best in the left and right infraclavicular areas and usually is louder on the right.

        b. It typically appears after 2 years of age.

        c. Best heard with the child sitting; diminishes with turning of the head, jugular compression, or supine position.

    4. Innominate or carotid bruits

        a. Typically found in older children and adolescents.

        b. Grade II or III, harsh, systolic ejection murmur.

    5. Pulmonary ejection murmur is a common innocent murmur of older children.

        a. Typically first appears around 3 years of age and continues through adolescence.

        b. Grade I or II, soft, systolic ejection murmur well localized to the upper left sternal border.

        c. It typically becomes louder with the patient supine and diminishes with Valsalva maneuver.

    6. Echocardiography is recommended to rule out pathologic murmurs; other testing should be selected based on patient history, physical examination, and echocardiography results.

    7. The most important components of management are establishing the correct diagnosis and reassuring the parents.

C. Infectious diseases

    1. Coxsackievirus

        a. Herpangina

            (1) Acute onset of fever and posterior pharyngeal vesicles.

            (2) Vesicles are grayish white and quickly form ulcers with erythematous halos. Lesions may be linearly arranged on the palate, uvula, and tonsillar pillars.

TABLE 17-8	**Common Viral Exanthems**				
	Varicella (Chicken Pox)	**Erythema Infectiosum (Fifth Disease, Slapped cheek)**	**Roseola (Roseola Infantum, Exanthem Subitum)**	**Measles (Rubeola)**	**Rubella (German Measles)**
Etiology	A human herpes virus	Human parvovirus B19	Human herpes virus 6 or 7	Measles virus	Rubella virus
Incubation period	10–21 days	4–14 days	10–14 days	8–14 days	14–21 days
Prodrome	Fever, respiratory symptoms (1–3 days)	None	Fever (4 days)	Fever, cough, anorexia, coryza (1–3 days)	None
Rash	Vesicular erythematous, torso and face to extremities (dew drop on rose petal)	Red face ("slapped cheek"); lacy, pink, macular rash on torso	Pink, macular rash	Maculopapular, face to extremities; Koplik spots in mouth	Maculopapular, from head to toe
Comments	Pruritic		Fever resolves before rash		Teratogenic

(3) Dysphagia, fever, vomiting, and anorexia occur. The child will be irritable secondary to pain.

(4) Treatment is supportive (e.g., fluids, antipyretics, topical lidocaine).

b. Hand-foot-mouth disease

(1) Red papules or vesicles occur on the tongue, oral mucosa, hands, and feet.

(2) Fever, sore throat, and malaise usually are mild.

(3) Treatment is supportive.

2. Kawasaki disease (mucocutaneous lymph node syndrome)

a. Etiology is unknown, but a viral cause is suggested.

b. Most patients are younger than 5 years.

c. Fever (>5 days) plus at least four of the following symptoms are needed to make a diagnosis: conjunctivitis; lip cracking and fissuring, strawberry tongue, or inflammation of the oral mucosa; cervical lymphadenopathy, usually unilateral; polymorphous exanthema; or redness and swelling of the hands and feet with subsequent desquamation.

d. Cardiovascular manifestations are worrisome; myocarditis, pericarditis, valvular heart disease, and coronary arteritis and aneurysms are possible. Two-dimensional echocardiography or angiography is recommended in all patients suspected of having Kawasaki disease.

e. Treatment is with IV immunoglobulin and high-dose aspirin; early treatment will reduce the chance of cardiac events. Patients with cardiac disease should receive long-term aspirin therapy and annual follow-up.

f. Patients should be monitored through serial electrocardiography, chest radiography, and echocardiography until they have recovered.

3. Viral exanthems. Table 17-8 depicts the characteristics of some common viral exanthems.

Index

Page numbers followed by t indicate table and f indicate figure.